Essentials of
Community Medicine

Essentials of Community Medicine

(Previously known as Short Textbook of Preventive and Social Medicine)

As per the Competency-based Medical Education Curriculum (NMC)

Third Edition

GN Prabhakara MD MAPHA MIPHA
Former Principal and Professor, Department of Community Medicine
SDM College of Medical Sciences and Hospital
Manjushree Nagar, Sattur, Dharwad
Karnataka, India

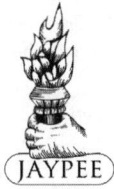

JAYPEE BROTHERS MEDICAL PUBLISHERS
The Health Sciences Publisher
New Delhi | London

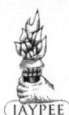 **Jaypee Brothers Medical Publishers (P) Ltd.**

Headquarters
Jaypee Brothers Medical Publishers (P) Ltd.
EMCA House
23/23-B, Ansari Road, Daryaganj
New Delhi 110 002, India
Landline: +91-11-23272143, +91-11-23272703
+91-11-23282021, +91-11-23245672
Email: jaypee@jaypeebrothers.com

Corporate Office
Jaypee Brothers Medical Publishers (P) Ltd.
4838/24, Ansari Road, Daryaganj
New Delhi 110 002, India
Phone: +91-11-43574357
Fax: +91-11-43574314
Email: jaypee@jaypeebrothers.com

Overseas Office
J.P. Medical Ltd.
83 Victoria Street, London
SW1H 0HW (UK)
Phone: +44 20 3170 8910
Fax: +44 (0)20 3008 6180
Email: info@jpmedpub.com

Website: www.jaypeebrothers.com
Website: www.jaypeedigital.com

© 2023, Jaypee Brothers Medical Publishers

The views and opinions expressed in this book are solely those of the original contributor(s)/author(s) and do not necessarily represent those of editor(s) and publisher of the book.

All rights reserved. No part of this publication may be reproduced, stored or transmitted in any form or by any means, electronic, mechanical, photocopying, recording or otherwise, without the prior permission in writing of the publishers.

All brand names and product names used in this book are trade names, service marks, trademarks or registered trademarks of their respective owners. The publisher is not associated with any product or vendor mentioned in this book.

Medical knowledge and practice change constantly. This book is designed to provide accurate, authoritative information about the subject matter in question. However, readers are advised to check the most current information available on procedures included and check information from the manufacturer of each product to be administered, to verify the recommended dose, formula, method and duration of administration, adverse effects and contraindications. It is the responsibility of the practitioner to take all appropriate safety precautions. Neither the publisher nor the author(s)/editor(s) assume any liability for any injury and/or damage to persons or property arising from or related to use of material in this book.

This book is sold on the understanding that the publisher is not engaged in providing professional medical services. If such advice or services are required, the services of a competent medical professional should be sought.

Every effort has been made where necessary to contact holders of copyright to obtain permission to reproduce copyright material. If any have been inadvertently overlooked, the publisher will be pleased to make the necessary arrangements at the first opportunity.

Inquiries for bulk sales may be solicited at: jaypee@jaypeebrothers.com

Essentials of Community Medicine

First Edition : 2002
Reprint : 2003
Second Edition : 2010
Third Edition : **2023**

ISBN: 978-93-5465-124-3

Printed at Rajkmala Electric Press, Kundli, Haryana.

PREFACE TO THE THIRD EDITION

In Indian context of Medical Education, since 1947 till 2022, we saw many changes to fulfil the objectives of medical education.

Medical Council of India gave a new guideline recently which Hallmark the content of medical education and also phase-wise integration of medical subjects.

Third edition has made a venture to incorporate these changes in the syllabus of community medicine, which is taught from 1st year MBBS to final MBSS and also during Internship.

Author has made an effort include two new chapters:
1. Hospital Waste Management
2. Essential Medicine

Effort is made to edit earlier chapters to update the public health information to Medical Professionals, to Heath Science Professionals and Teachers in Medical and Health Science Institutions.

An effort is made to include 13 New Units under recent area of interest in community medicine which is eagerly looked for, both by teachers and students.
1. Ayushman Bharat Programme
2. Dengue Burden
3. Janani Suraksha Yojana
4. Millennium Developmental Goals
5. Nipah Viral Infection
6. Niti Aayog 2017-20
7. National Health Policy 2017
8. National Urban Health Mission (NUHM)
9. Recent Global TB Strategy
10. Rights of Persons with Disability Bill 2016
11. Trends in Recent Immunization
12. Tribal Health
13. Zika Viral Infection

Areas of ethical interest in present day practice is included under medical ethics.

Omission or inclusion of points in the text is solely based on author's personal experience as a teacher over a period of 47 years (1972 to till date), at Central Government Colleges, State Government Colleges and SDM College of Medical Sciences and Hospital Dharwad, Karnataka

It shall serve the present requirement of professionals, teachers and students.

GN Prabhakara

PREFACE TO THE FIRST EDITION

The purpose of this book is to provide a simple and systematic guide to the trainers and trainees in medical science, health science and paramedical science fields, who are involved in community health care in their day-to-day professional activity and research.

The short text is not a compendium on community health (PSM) but a synopsis of essentials of PSM for:
- Medical professionals
- Health science professionals
- Teachers in medical and health sciences students.

Recommendations by universities of health sciences are followed in the syllabus, which is also as per concerned councils of India stipulation.

An effort is made for inclusion of 34 items in a Chapter on Recent Area of Interest, which is eagerly looked for, both by teachers and students.

Omission or inclusion of points in the text is solely based on author's personal experience as a teacher over a period of 32 years, both at Central and State Government Medical Colleges.

I hope that this book will serve the present requirement of professionals, teachers and students.

GN Prabhakara

ACKNOWLEDGMENTS

Students in Medical, Dental, Physiotherapy, Nursing, Public Health Engineering, Home Science and Paramedicals in my walk of life to whom I taught are responsible for bringing out my experience in the form of Short Textbook of PSM.

I am happy to acknowledge that in the span of 18 years, it has seen Third Edition.

Initiation, motivation, guidance, Proofreading and specific appropriations are from:

My wife Mrs Malathi Prabhakara, Former scientist CFTRI, CSIR, Mysuru, Karnataka, India

My son Dr Bharat MP, Director and Consultant Radiologist, Nava Sanjeevini Diagnostics, Shimoga, Karnataka, India

My daughter-in-law Dr Mrs Pooja Bharat, Consultant Anaesthesiologist, Maax Subbaiah Super Speciality Hospital and Subbiah Institute of Medical Sciences, Shimoga

I am very grateful to the whole team of M/s Jaypee Brothers Medical Publishers (P) Ltd, New Delhi, India, who helped and guided me, Shri Jitendar P Vij (Group Chairman), Mr Ankit Vij (Managing Director), Mr MS Mani (Group President), Dr Madhu Choudhary (Director-Educational Publishing), Ms Pooja Bhandari (Production Head), Ms Sunita Katla (Executive Assistant to Group Chairman and Publishing Manager), Ms Samina Khan (Executive Assistant to Director-Educational Publishing), Mr Rajesh Sharma (Production Coordinator), Ms Seema Dogra (Cover Visualizer), Mr Vakil Khan (Proofreader), Mr Kapil Dev Sharma (Typesetter), Mr Sharvan Kumar (Graphic Designer) and their team members, for all their support to work in this project and make it a success. Without their cooperation, I could not have completed this project.

GN Prabhakara

CONTENTS

SECTION 1

1. Concept of Health and Disease — 3
- Holistic Approach of Health (Multifactorial Causation, Web of Causation) 4
- Disease 5
- Triad of Epidemiology (Agent–Host–Environment) 8
- Effective Communication 10
- Health Indicators 11
- Estimates of Demographic Values of India 2019 11
- Role of Health Education in Health Programs 11
- Doctor–Patient Relationship 11
- International Classification of Diseases 12

2. Relationship of Social and Behavioral to Health and Disease — 13
- Terminology Used 14
- Special Terms in Social Medicine 14
- Behavioral Change Communication 14
- Social Problems 15
- Social Area of Interest 15
- Group Behavior 15
- Social Factors in Health and Disease 16
- Clinico-Sociocultural and Demographic Assessment of Individual, Family and Community (Medicosocial Cases) 16
- Sociocultural Factors in Health and Disease 16
- Barrier to Good Health and Health-seeking Behavior 16
- Social and Behavior to Health and Disease (Family in Health and Disease) 16
- Socioeconomic Programs 20
- Present Grouping of the Community 20
- Social Agencies 21
- Interviewing Technique 21
- Medical Economics 21
- Geographic Pathology 21
- Hospital Sociology 21
- Knowledge, Attitude, and Practice 22
- Social Security and Health Care 22

3. Environmental Health Problems — 25
- Evolution 25
- Major Components of Physical Environment 25
- Water and Other Components 25
- WHO Standard for Drinking Water (Bacteriological) 33
- Surveillance of Drinking Water Quality 33
- Swimming Pool Sanitation 33
- National Water Supply and Sanitation Program 34
- Water Pollution Law 34
- Air 34
- Ventilation 35
- Lighting 36
- Noise 36
- Radiation 36
- Meteorology 38
- Housing and Town Planning 39
- Waste Disposal 41
- Human Dead Body Disposal and Environmental Sanitation 48

4. Medical Entomology — 49
- Classification 49
- Mode of Transmission 49
- Vector-borne Diseases 49
- Identifying Features 49
- Insecticides 62
- Zoonoses 64
- Integrated Vector Control 64

SECTION 2

5. Principles of Health Promotion and Education — 67
- Information 67
- Education 68
- Communication 70
- Role of Health Education in Health Programs 70
- Population Education 71
- Cancer Education 71
- AIDS Education 71
- Nutrition Education 71
- Planning and Management of Health Education 71

6. Nutrition and Health — 73
- Main Areas of Study 73
- Terminology 73
- Source of Nutrition 73
- Basal Metabolism 74
- Proximate Principles 74
- Important Nutritional Profile of Foodstuff 75
- Nutritive Value of Common Foods 76
- Nutritional Assessment 76
- Balanced Diet 77
- Nutritional Diseases 79
- Food Poisoning 83
- Food Toxins 83
- Food-borne Diseases 85
- Commercial and Processed Foods 85
- Therapeutic Diets 85
- Indications for Parenteral Nutrition (IV Feeding) 87
- Nutritional Surveillance 87
- Food Surveillance 87
- Food Additives, Food Adulteration, and Food Fortification 88
- Nutritional Program 88
- Nutrition Education 89
- Nutrition Rehabilitation 89
- Calorific Value of Cooked Preparations 90
- Population Nutrient Intake Goals 90
- Integrated Child Development Services Scheme or Integrated Mother and Child Development Services 90

7. Basic Statistics and its Application — 91
- Common Terms 91
- Types 92
- Formulation of Research Question for a Study 92
- Sources of Statistics 101
- Scope of Statistics 101
- Data Collection, Classification, Analysis, Interpretation, and Presentation 101
- Measures of Central Tendency, Measures of Variability and Significance Tests 103
- Measures of Variability 104
- Normal Distribution 104
- Significance Tests 104
- Sampling 107
- Standard Error 107
- Sample Size 107

SECTION 3

8. Epidemiology — 111
- Milestones in Epidemiology 111
- Terms Used in Epidemiology 112
- Types of Epidemiology 114
- Investigation of An Epidemic 117
- Quarantine 118
- Emporiatrics 118
- Desmotology 118
- Disinfection 118
- Dynamics of Disease Transmission 120
- Immunity (Host Defense) 121
- Adverse Event Following Immunization 122
- Prevention and Control of Disease in Man 123
- Epidemiometric Analysis 123
- Screening Tests 124

9. Epidemiology of Communicable Diseases — 128
- Intestinal Infections 128
- Respiratory Infections 143
- Vector-borne Infections 160
- Surface Infections 173
- Zoonotic Infections 191
- Emerging and Re-Emerging Infections 200
- Hospital Acquired Infections (Nosocomial Infection) (Hospital Cross Infection) 202

10. Epidemiology of Noncommunicable Diseases — 204
- Common Noncommunicable Diseases 204
- Epidemiological Findings in Noncommunicable Disease 204
- General Measures in Prevention of Noncommunicable Disease 205
- Selected Noncommunicable Diseases 205

SECTION 4

11. Demography and Vital Statistics — 221
- Demography 221
- Terminology 221
- Process in Demography 221
- Estimates of Demographic Values of India 2019 223

- Demography and Genetics 223
- Demographic Cycle 224
- Major Sources of Demographic Data 224
- Population Estimation/Dynamics 224
- Improvident Maternity 224
- Family Planning (Family Welfare Planning) 224
- Population Education 227
- National Family Welfare Program 229
- National Population Policy—2000 229

12. Reproductive Maternal and Child Health 231

- Basic Elements of Reproductive and Child Health 232
- Child Survival and Safe Motherhood 232
- Delivery Service at Primary Health Care 233
- Emergency Care 234
- Eag (Empowered Action Group) of Health and Family Welfare Service, Government of India 234
- Safe Motherhood 235
- Maternal and Child Health Indicators (RCH Indicators) 238
- Handicapped Children 242
- The Growth 242
- Infant Feeding Practices 244
- Weaning and Supplementation (Addition of Semisolids) 246
- Social Welfare Schemes for Better RCH 247
- Integrated Child Development Services 247
- Key Indicators in Reproductive and Child Health 248

13. School Health 250

- Objectives 250
- Milestones 250
- Health Problems in School Children 250
- Activities 251
- Healthy School Environment 253

SECTION 5

14. Occupational Health Including Social Security 257

- Ergonomics 257
- Occupational Hazards 258
- Pneumoconiosis 260
- Occupational Hazards in Agriculture 260
- Occupational Cancer 260
- Sickness Absenteeism 261
- Industrialization 261
- Occupational Risks of Health Professionals and their Prevention 261
- Prevention of Occupational Diseases 262
- Employees State Insurance Scheme (1948) Amended (1975, 1984, 1989, 2010) 263

15. Geriatrics and Health 265

- Geriatric Health Problems 266
- Nutritional Requirement 266
- Social Welfare Measures 267
- Elderly Citizen Facility Concept 267

16. Genetics and Health 269

- Common Terms 269
- Genetic Basis 270
- Genetic Disorders 270
- Prevention of Genetic Disorders 271
- Population Genetics 272
- Gene Therapy 272
- Heritability 273

17. Mental Health 274

- Current Picture 274
- Common Defense Mechanisms 274
- Mentally Ill 275
- Mentally Well 275
- Mental Illness 275
- Psychophysiological Disorders (Psychosomatic) 275
- Alcohol and Substance Dependence 276
- Childhood Disorders 276
- Modern Therapy 276
- Prevention of Mental Illness 276
- Community Psychiatry 277
- National Mental Health Programme 277

SECTION 6

18. Disaster Management 281

- Terminology 281
- Classification of Disasters 282
- Public Health Tools Available in Disasters 282
- Challenges in Disaster Management 282
- Documentation and Tagging in Disaster Areas 282
- Effects of Inappropriate Humanitarian Assistance 282
- Vulnerability Reduction in Disaster Management 282
- Emergency Preparedness in Disaster 283

- Phases of Disasters 283
- Common Natural Disasters in India 284
- What to Do in An Earthquake 285
- Action Plans on Earthquake by Government of India 285
- Steps in Management of Natural Disasters 286
- Management of Cyclonic Storm Affecting PHC Area 286
- Hazard Description Scales 286

19. Hospital Waste Management 287
- Classification 288
- Hazards 288
- Waste Disposal Container Code at Hospital Waste Management 288
- Treatment Option for Hospital Waste Management 288
- Important Aspects of Hospital Waste Management 288
- Major and Important Instructions in Hospital Waste Management Through Pictures 290

SECTION 7

20. National Health Programs 293
- National Health Problems 293
- National Health Programs 293
- Major National Health Programs 296

21. Health Planning 309
- Elements of Health Planning 310
- Planning Cycle 310
- Health Committee Reports 311
- Goals of National Health Policy By 2005, 2007, 2010 and 2015 312

22. Health Management 313
- Gulick's POSDCORB in Health Management 313
- Inventory Management 314
- Financial Management 315
- Basic Activity of Health Management 316
- Span of Management 316
- Management Methods 316
- Health Policy 318
- Health System in India 320
- Rural Development 322
- Evaluation of Health Services 322
- Milestones in Public Health in India 322

23. Community Healthcare 324
- Concepts of Healthcare 324
- Primary Healthcare 325
- Community Development Program 327
- Essential Healthcare 327
- Health for All 328
- Millennium Development Goals Set By United Nations in 2000 329
- Health Programs 329
- Levels of Healthcare 330
- Healthcare Delivery Systems 330

SECTION 8

24. International Health Organizations 335
- History in Development of International Health 335
- Organizations 335

25. Voluntary Health Organizations 339
- Role of Voluntary Health Organization 339
- Functions of Voluntary Health Organizations 340
- Organizations 340

26. Nongovernmental Health Organizations 343
- Organizations 343

SECTION 9

27. Urban Health 347
- India: Trend in Growth of Urban Population 347
- Urban Health Problems 348
- History of Urban Health 348
- Process of Urban Life 348
- Suggested Education Activity 349
- Service on Urban Slum Areas and Services on Urban Area 349
- Agenda for Sustainable Ecological Balance 350
- Krishnan Committee Report (1982) on Urban Health 350

28. Medical Ethics 351
- Indian Legislations Related to Medical Ethics 352
- Heteronomous and Autonomous Ethics 352
- Major Principles of Medical/Bioethics 352

- Perspectives of Medical Ethics 352
- Ethics of the Individuals 352
- Organ Donation 353
- The Ethics of Human Life 354
- Cloning 354
- Recent Approaches in Gene Therapy 355
- Prolongation of Life 355
- Advanced Life Directives 355
- Death and Dying 356
- Professional Ethics 356
- Research Ethics 357
- Areas of Ethical Interest in Present Day Practice 358

29. Public Health Law 362

- Troubling Problems in Medical Ethics 363
- Legal Rights and Responsibilities in Modern Medicine 363
- Health Law in India 363
- Major Acts 363

SECTION 10

30. Essential Medicine 369

- Criteria for Inclusion of A Medicine in National List of Essential Medicine 369
- Criteria for Deletion of A Medicine From NLEM 370
- History 370
- Uses of Essential Medicine 370
- National List of Essential Medicines 2015 370

31. Rational Drug Management 372

- Types of Irrational Drug Use 373
- Drugs 373
- Prescription 374
- Compliance 374
- Self-Medication 374
- Irrational Use of Drugs 375
- National Drug Policy 375
- Drug Economics 376

32. Health Information System 377

- Qualities of Good Health Information System 377
- Components of Health Information System 377
- Uses of His 378
- Sources of Health Information System 378
- Recent Approach in Medical Informatics and Public Health Informatics 378

SECTION 11

33. Recent Area of Interest in Community Medicine 381

- Acute Flaccid Paralysis Surveillance 382
- Adverse Events Following Immunization 382
- Acquired Immunodeficiency Syndrome Day 384
- Aids Surveillance 389
- Anthrax—Bioterrorism 390
- Avian Influenza (Birds Flu, Avian Flu, or Fowl Plague) 391
- Ayushman Bharat Program 394
- Baby-Friendly Hospital Initiative 395
- Chikungunya Fever Epidemic 395
- Community Dentistry 397
- Community Ophthalmology 397
- Community Psychiatry 398
- Consumer Protection Act 399
- Dengue Burden in India: Recent Trends and Importance of Climatic Parameters 400
- Coronavirus Epidemic 2019–2020 401
- Vaccine Development Cycle 402
- Drastic Preventive Measures 402
- Desmotology 402
- Early Childhood Development 403
- Emporiatrics 403
- Essential Drugs 403
- Family Medicine 404
- Genetic Engineering 405
- Global Warming 405
- Guinea Worm Eradication: Indian Scenario 405
- Handigodu Syndrome (Endemic Familial Arthritis) 407
- Hospital Waste Management 407
- Hypothermia 407
- Intensive Pulse Polio Immunization (IPPI) 408
- Janani Suraksha Yojana 410
- Kangaroo Mother Care 410
- Leptospirosis: An Emerging Public Health Problem 410
- Medical Informatics 412
- Meta-Analysis 413
- The Millennium Development Goals 413
- National Days 413
- National Health Goals By 2015 415
- National Rural Health Mission 415
- National Sociodemographic Goals By 2010 417
- National Urban Health Mission 417

- National Health Policy 2017 418
- Nipah Viral Infection 418
- National Institution for Transforming India Aayog 2015 418
- Poison Control Information 418
- Partogram 419
- Postpartum Program 419
- Recent Global Tuberculosis Strategies 420
- Red Cross Day 420
- The Rights of Persons with Disability Bill 2016 420
- Re-Orientation of Medical Education 421
- Sanitation at Fair, Festival, Pilgrimage 422
- Severe Malaria 422
- Social Accountability of Hospitals and Medical Colleges 423
- Social Marketing 424
- Sociometric Analysis 425
- Substance Abuse 425
- Sulabh Shauchalaya 425
- The Prenatal Diagnostic Techniques and Preconception 426
- Trends in Recent Immunization 428
- Tribal Health 433
- Universal Declaration of Human Rights 433
- World Health Organization Day 436
- Women's Hygiene Kit 443
- Zika Viral Infection 444

Appendix 445

Index 449

COMPETENCY TABLE

Number	COMPETENCY: The student should be able to	Chapter No.	Page No.
	**Topic: Concept of Health and Disease**		
CM1.1	Define and describe the concept of public health	1	3
CM1.2	Define health; describe the concept of holistic health including concept of spiritual health and the relativeness and determinants of health	1	4, 5
CM1.3	Describe the characteristics of agent, host and environmental factors in health and disease and the multi factorial etiology of disease	1	7 8
CM1.4	Describe and discuss the natural history of disease	1	5-8
CM1.5	Describe the application of interventions at various levels of prevention	1	9
CM1.6	Describe and discuss the concepts, the principles of health promotion and education, IEC and behavioral change communication (BCC)	1 2	9,10 14,15
CM1.7	Enumerate and describe health indicators	1	11
CM1.8	Describe the demographic profile of India and discuss its impact on health	1	11
CM1.9	Demonstrate the role of effective communication skills in health in a simulated environment	1 2	10,11 14,15
CM1.10	Demonstrate the important aspects of the doctor patient relationship in a simulated environment	1	11,12
	**Topic: Relationship of Social and Behavioral to Health and Disease**		
CM2.1	Describe the steps and perform clinico-socio-cultural and demographic assessment of the individual, family and community	2	16
CM2.2	Describe the socio-cultural factors, family (types), its role in health and disease and demonstrate in a simulated environment the correct assessment of socio-economic status	2	16-20
CM2.3	Describe and demonstrate in a simulated environment the assessment of barriers to good health and health-seeking behavior	2	16
CM2.4	Describe social psychology, community behavior and community relationship and their impact on health and disease	2	20
CM2.5	Describe poverty and social security measures and its relationship to health and disease	2	22-24
	**Topic: Environmental Health Problems**		
CM3.1	Describe the health hazards of air, water, noise, radiation and pollution	3	28, 34, 37
CM3.2	Describe concepts of safe and wholesome water, sanitary sources of water, water purification processes, water quality standards, concepts of water conservation and rainwater harvesting	3	26-34
CM3.3	Describe the etiology and basis of water-borne diseases/jaundice/hepatitis/diarrheal diseases	3	28-29

Competency Table

Topic: Environmental Health Problems

CM3.4	Describe the concept of solid waste, human excreta and sewage disposal	3	41-47
CM3.5	Describe the standards of housing and the effect of housing on health	3	39, 40
CM3.6	Describe the role of vectors in the causation of diseases. Also discuss National Vector Borne disease Control Programme	4	49-64
CM3.7	Identify and describe the identifying features and life cycles of vectors of public health importance and their control measures	4	50-61
CM3.8	Describe the mode of action, application cycle of commonly used insecticides and rodenticides	4	62-64

Topic: Principles of Health Promotion and Education

CM4.1	Describe various methods of health education with their advantages and limitations	5	68-70
CM4.2	Describe the methods of organizing health promotion and education and counseling activities at individual family and community settings	5	70-72

Topic: Nutrition

CM5.1	Describe the common sources of various nutrients and special nutritional requirements according to age, sex, activity, physiological conditions	6	73-75
CM5.2	Describe and demonstrate the correct method of performing a nutritional assessment of individuals, families and the community by using the appropriate method	6	76-77
CM5.3	Define and describe common nutrition-related health disorders (including macro-PEM, Micro-iron, Zn, iodine, vitamin A), their control and management	6	79-83
CM5.4	Plan and recommend a suitable diet for the individuals and families based on local availability of foods and economic status, etc., in a simulated environment	6	77-79
CM5.5	Describe the methods of nutritional surveillance, principles of nutritional education and rehabilitation in the context of socio-cultural factors	6	87-89
CM5.6	Enumerate and discuss the National Nutrition Policy, important national nutritional programs including the Integrated Child Development Services Scheme (ICDS), etc.	12	247
CM5.7	Describe food hygiene	6	87, 88
CM5.8	Describe and discuss the importance and methods of food fortification and effects of additives and adulteration	6	88

Topic: Basic Statistics and its Applications

CM6.1	Formulate a research question for a study	7	92-100
CM6.2	Describe and discuss the principles and demonstrate the methods of collection, classification, analysis, interpretation and presentation of statistical data	7	101-103
CM6.3	Describe, discuss and demonstrate the application of elementary statistical methods including test of significance in various study designs	7	104-107
CM6.4	Enumerate, discuss and demonstrate common sampling techniques, simple statistical methods, frequency distribution, measures of central tendency and dispersion	7	103-104 107

Competency Table

	Topic: Epidemiology		
CM7.1	Define epidemiology and describe and enumerate the principles, concepts and uses	8	112-113
CM7.2	Enumerate, describe and discuss the modes of transmission and measures for prevention and control of communicable and noncommunicable diseases	8	120-123
CM7.3	Enumerate, describe and discuss the sources of epidemiological data	9	128-129
CM7.5	Enumerate, define, describe and discuss epidemiological study designs	8	114-117 124
CM7.6	Enumerate and evaluate the need of screening tests	8	124-127
CM7.7	Describe and demonstrate the steps in the investigation of an epidemic of communicable disease and describe the principles of control measures	8	117-118
	Topic: Epidemiology of Communicable and Noncommunicable Diseases		
CM8.1	Describe and discuss the epidemiological and control measures including the use of essential laboratory tests at the primary care level for communicable diseases	9	128-203
CM8.2	Describe and discuss the epidemiological and control measures including the use of essential laboratory tests at the primary care level for noncommunicable diseases (diabetes, hypertension, stroke, obesity and cancer, etc.)	10	204-220
CM8.3	Enumerate and describe disease specific national health programs including their prevention and treatment of a case	20	293-307
CM8.5	Describe and discuss the principles of planning, implementing and evaluating control measures for disease at community level bearing in mind the public health importance of the disease	23	327
	Topic: Demography and Vital Statistics		
CM9.1	Define and describe the principles of demography, demographic cycle, vital statistics	11	221-224
CM9.2	Define, calculate and interpret demographic indices including birth rate, death rate, fertility rates	11	222
CM9.3	Enumerate and describe the causes of declining sex ratio and its social and health implications	11	222-223
CM9.5	Describe the methods of population control	11	224-229
CM9.6	Describe the National Population Policy	11	229-230
	Topic: Reproductive Maternal and Child Health		
CM10.1	Describe the current status of reproductive, maternal, newborn and child health	12	231
CM10.2	Enumerate and describe the methods of screening high-risk groups and common health problems	12	232-235
CM10.3	Describe local customs and practices during pregnancy, childbirth, lactation and child feeding practices	12	244-246
CM10.4	Describe the reproductive, maternal, newborn and child health (RMCH); child survival and safe motherhood interventions	12	233-234 238-242

Competency Table

		Topic: Reproductive Maternal and Child Health		
CM10.5	Describe Universal Immunization Programme ; Integrated Management of Neonatal and Childhood Illness (IMNCI) and other existing programs.	12 20	234-238 299
CM10.6	Enumerate and describe various family planning methods, their advantages and shortcomings	11	224-229
CM10.7	Enumerate and describe the basis and principles of the Family Welfare Programme including the organization, technical and operational aspects	12	247
CM10.8	Describe the physiology, clinical management and principles of adolescent health including ARSH	13	251-253
CM10.9	Describe and discuss gender issues and women empowerment	12	247-248
	Topic: Occupational Health		
CM11.1	Enumerate and describe the presenting features of patients with occupational illness including agriculture	14	260
CM11.2	Describe the role, benefits and functioning of the Employees' State Insurance Scheme	14	263-264
CM11.3	Enumerate and describe specific occupational health hazards, their risk factors and preventive measures	14	258-260
CM11.4	Describe the principles of ergonomics in health preservation	14	257
CM11.5	Describe occupational disorders of health professionals and their prevention and management	14	261-263
	Topic: Geriatric Services		
CM12.1	Define and describe the concept of geriatric services	15	265
CM12.2	Describe health problems of aged population	15	266
CM12.3	Describe the prevention of health problems of aged population	15	267-268
CM12.4	Describe national program for elderly	15	267
	Topic: Disaster Management		
CM13.1	Define and describe the concept of disaster management	18	281
CM13.2	Describe disaster management cycle	18	282-284
CM13.3	Describe man-made disasters in the world and in India	18	284
CM13.4	Describe the details of the National Disaster Management Authority	18	285-286
	Topic: Hospital Waste Management		
CM14.1	Define and classify hospital waste	19	287-288
CM14.2	Describe various methods of treatment of hospital waste	19	288-290
CM14.3	Describe laws related to hospital waste management		
	Topic: Mental Health		
CM15.1	Define and describe the concept of mental Health	17	274-275
CM15.2	Describe warning signals of mental health disorder	17	275-276
CM15.3	Describe National Mental Health Programme	17	297

Competency Table

	Topic: Health Planning and Management		
CM16.1	Define and describe the concept of health planning	21	310
CM16.2	Describe planning cycle	21	310
CM16.3	Describe health management techniques	22	313-323
CM16.4	Describe health planning in India and national policies related to health and health planning	21 22	310-312 318-320
	Topic: Health Care of the Communtiy		
CM17.1	Define and describe the concept of health care to community	23	324
CM17.2	Describe community diagnosis	23	327
CM17.3	Describe primary health care, its components and principles	23	325-327
CM17.4	Describe national policies related to health and health planning and millennium development goals	21 22	310-312 318-320
CM17.5	Describe healthcare delivery in India	22 23	320-323 330-331
	Topic: International Health		
CM18.1	Define and describe the concept of international health	24	335
CM18.2	Describe roles of various international health agencies	24	335-338
	Topic: Essential Medicine		
CM19.1	Define and describe the concept of Essential Medicines List (EML)	30	369-370
	Topic: Recent Advances in Community Medicine		
CM20.1	List important public health events of last five years	33	413-415
CM20.4	Demonstrate awareness about laws pertaining to practice of medicine, such as Clinical Establishment Act and Human Organ Transplantation Act and its implications	28	353-354

ABBREVIATIONS

aA	Heterozygous	BHW	Basic Health Worker
AA	Homozygous	BIRD	Bidar Integrated Rural Development Project
ABER	Annual Blood Examination Rate	BIS	Bureau of Indian Standards
AD	After Christ (Anno Domini)	BOAA	Beta Oxalyl Amino Alanine
ADS	Antidiphtheric Serum	BOD	Biological Oxidation Demand
AEFI	Adverse events following immunization	BP	Blood Pressure
AFB	Acid Fast Bacilli	BPL	Betapropriolactone
AFP	Acute Flaccid Paralysis	BR	Birth Rate
AID	Artificial Insemination Donor	BSAM	Bachelor in Ayurvedic Medicine and Surgery
AIDS	Autoimmune Deficiency Syndrome	C	Columb
AIH	Artificial Insemination Husband	Ca	Carcinoma
AIR	All India Radio	CARE	Cooperative for Assistance and Relief Everywhere
ALRI	Acute Lower Respiratory Infection	CCD	Control of Communicable Disease
AM	Arithmetic Mean	CCF	Congestive Cardiac Failure
AN	Antenatal	CD	Communicable Disease
ANC	Antenatal Care	CD	Count Cell Count in AIDS for Immune Response
ANTU	Alpha Naphthyl Thiourea	CDC	Code for Disease Control
APH	Antepartum Hemorrhage	CDPO	Child Development Project Officer
API	Annual Parasitic Index	CET	Corrected Effective Temperature
APT	Alum Precipitated Toxoid	CFR	Case-Fatality Ratio
ARI	Acute Respiratory Infection	CFTRI	Central Food Technological Research Institute
ARS	Antirabies Serum	CGHS	Central Government Health Scheme
ARV	Antirabies Vaccine	CHC	Community Health Centre
ARWSP	Accelerated Rural Water Supply Programme	CHD	Coronary Heart Disease
ASFR	Age Specific Fertility Rate	CHEB	Central Health Education Bureau
ASO	Anti-Streptolysin O	CHO	Carbohydrate
ATS	Antitetanus Serum	CMV	Cytomegalovirus
AURI	Acute Upper Respiratory Infection	CNS	Central Nervous System
AW	Anganwadi	COD	Chemical Oxidation Demand
AWW	Anganwadi Worker	COPRA	Consumer Protection Act
AZT	Zidovudine	CPM	Critical Path Method
BAL	British anti-Lewisite	CSIR	Council of Scientific and Industrial Research
BC	Before Christ	CSSM	Child Survival Safe Motherhood
BCG	Bacilli Calmette Guérin (TB vaccine)	CV	Coefficient of Variation
BD	(Bis in die) twice a day		
BFHI	Baby Friendly Hospital Initiative		
BHC	Benzene Hexachloride		

CVS	Cardiovascular System	EDTA	Ethylene Diamine Tetraacetic Acid
CWR	Child Women Ratio	EFA	Essential Fatty Acid
DALY	Disability Adjusted Life Years	EIUS	Environmental Improvement of Urban Slums
DANIDA	The Danish International Development Agency	ELISA	Enzyme Linked Serum Assay (Immuno)
dB	decibel (loudness)	EPA	Code for Epidemiology
DBT	Dry Bulb Thermometer	EPID	An Epidemiological Number given for a Stool Sample in AFP Surveillance
DD	Diarrheal Disease		
DDC	Diarrhea Disease Control		
DDC	Drug Distribution Centre		
DDK	Disposable Delivery Kit	ESI	Employees State Insurance
DDP	Desert Development Program	ESIS	Employee State Insurance Scheme
DDT	Dichloro Diphenyl Trichloroethane	FAO	Food and Agriculture Organization
DEC	Diethyl Carbamazine		
DF	Day Light Factor	FCU	Filaria Control Unit
DF	Deep Freezer	FNV	French Neurotropic Virus
DG	Director General	FP	Family Planning
DGO	Diploma in Gynecology and Obstetrics	FPAI	Family Planning Association of India
DHEB	District Health Education Bureau	FPO	Fruit Product Order
DHF	Dengue Hemorrhagic Fever	FRU	First Referral Unit
DHFWO	District Health and FW Officer	FS	Ferrous Sulphate
DHO	District Health Officer	FT	Formal Toxoid
DIO	District Immunization Officer	FTD	Fever Treatment Depot
DMAP	Disaster Management Action Plan	FW	Family Welfare
DMPA	Depo Medroxy Progesterone Acetate	GA	General Anesthesia
		GDM	Gestational Diabetic Mellitus
DNA	Deoxy Ribonucleic Acid	GE	Gastroenteritis
DOTS	Directly Observed Treatment Short course	GFI	General Flea Index
		GFR	General Fertility Rate
DPAP	Draught Prone Areas Program	GHG	Greenhouse Gases
DPH	Diploma in Public Health	GI	Gastrointestinal
DPT	Diphtheria Pertussis Tetanus	GMFR	General Marital Fertility Rate
DR	Death Rate	GOI	Government of India
DT	Diphtheria Tetanus	GR	Growth Rate
DTC	District TB Center	GRR	Gross Reproduction Rate
DWACRA	Development of Women and Children in Rural Areas	GU	Genitourinary
		Gy	Gray
E	Ethambutol	H	INH
EAS	Employment Assurance Scheme	HA	Health Assistant
EBV	The Epstein-Barr Virus	HAV	Hepatitis A Virus
ECD	Early Childhood Development	Hb%	Hemoglobin percentage
ECHS	Educational Council for Health Science	HBIG	Hepatitis B Immunoglobulin
		HBS Ag	Hepatitis B Somatic Antigen

HBV	Hepatitis B Virus	ILR	Ice Lined Refrigerator
HCG	Human Chorionic Gonadotrophin	IM	Intramuscular
		IMA	Indian Medical Association
HCH	Hexachlorocyclohexane	IMC	Indian Medical Council
HDCV	Human Diploid Cell Vaccine	IMCD	Integrated Mother Child Development
HDL	High Density Lipoprotein		
HE	Health Education	IMNCI	Integrated Management of Neonatal and Childhood Illness
HFA	Health for All		
HIG	Human Immunoglobulin	IMR	Infant Mortality Rate
HIS	Health Information System	IMS	Indian Medical Service
HIV	Human Immunodeficiency Virus	INC	Intranatal Care
HKNS	Hind Kusht Nivaran Sangh	INH	Isoniazid Hydrazide
HTLV	Human T-lymphotropic Virus	IP	Incubation Period
HTST	High Temperature Short Time	IPD	In-patient Department
HUDCO	Housing and Urban Development corporation	IPP	India Population Project
		IPPI	Intensive Pulse Polio Program
HW	Health Worker	IPV	Injectable Polio Vaccine
HWM	Health Waste Management	IQ	Intelligence Quotient
		IRDP	Integrated Rural Development Programme
IAEA	Indian Atomic Energy Agency		
IARC	Indian Agricultural Research Council	ISWA	International Solid Waste Public Cleansing Association
IAS	Indian Administrative Service	IT	Income Tax
IAY	Indira Awas Yojana	IU	International Units
ICCU	Intensive Coronary Care Unit	IUD	Intrauterine Device
ICD	International Classification of diseases	IV	Intravenous
		J	Joule
ICDS	Integrated Child Development Service	JALMA	Japanese Leprosy Mission for Asia
ICMR	Indian Council of Medical Research	JE	Japanese Encephalitis
		JRY	Jawahar Rozgar Yojana
ICRP	International Commission for radiological protection		
		KAP	Knowledge Attitude Practice
ICSSR	Indian Council for Social and Scientific Research	KFD	Kyasanur Forest Disease
		LAN	Local Area Network
ICU	Intensive Coronary Unit	LB	Live Births
IDD	Iodine Deficiency Disorder	LBW	Low Birth Weight
IDDCP	Iodine Deficiency Disorder Control Programme	LCU	Leprosy Control Unit
		LDC	Lower Division Clerk
IDDM	Insulin Dependent Diabetes Mellitus	LDL	Low Density Lipoprotein
		LEC	Leprosy Elimination Campaign
IEC	Information Education Communication	LGI	Lymphogranuloma Inguinale
		LGV	Lymphogranuloma Venereum
IFA	Iron Folic Acid	LIC	Life Insurance Corporation of India
Ig	Immunoglobulin		
IGT	Impaired Glucose Tolerance		
IH	Infective Hepatitis	LIH	Leptospira Icterohaemorrhagiae
IHD	Ischemic Heart Disease		
ILO	International Labor Organization	LRI	Lower Respiratory Infection

MB	Multibacillary	NET-EN	Norethindrone Enanthate
MBO	Management by Objective	NGO	Non-Governmental Organization
MCH	Maternal and Child Health	NHD	Natural History of Diseases
MCI	Medical Council of India	NHP	National Health Policy
MD	Doctor of Medicine	NIDDM	Non-insulin Dependent Diabetes Mellitus
MD	Mean Deviation		
MDG	Millennium Developmental Goal	NIN	National Institute of Nutrition
MDT	Multi-Drug Regimen	NIS	National Immunization Schedule
MI	Myocardial Infarction	NITI	National Institution for Transforming India
MLEC	Modified Leprosy Elimination Campaign	NIUA	National Institute of Urban Association
MLTU	Mobile Leprosy Treatment Unit		
MMR	Mass Miniature Radiography	NLEP	National Leprosy Eradication Programme
MMR	Maternal Mortality Rate		
MO	Medical Officer	NMCP	National Malaria Control Programme
MOH	Medical Officer of Health		
MP	Malaria Parasite	NMEP	National Malaria Eradication Programme
MPF	Multipurpose Food		
MPW	Multipurpose Worker	NNRTIS	Non-nucleoside Analogue Reverse Transcriptase Inhibitor (a group of AIDS drug)
MRDM	Malnutrition Related Diabetes Mellitus		
MS	Mukhya Sevika	NPP	National Population Policy
MSW	Medical Social Worker	NRHM	National Rural Health Mission
MTM	Multiple Tube Method	NRR	Net Reproduction Rate
MTP	Medical Termination of Pregnancy	NSAP	National Social Assistance Programme
MUAC	Mid Upper Arm Circumference	NTP	National TB Programme
MWS	Million Wells Scheme	NUHM	National Urban Health Mission
MYP	Mid Year Population	NWSSP	National Water Supply and Sanitation Programme
NAB	National Association for the Blind		
NACP	National AIDS Control Program	OBG	Obstetrics and Gynecology
NANB	Non-A Non-B	OC	Oral Contraceptive
NBIN	An emulsion containing 68% Benzocaine and 14% Tween 80 Benzyl benzoate, 6% DDT, 12% diluted 1 in 5 parts water (Scabicidal from National Institute)	ODA	Overseas Development Agency
		OPD	Out Patient Department
		OPV	Oral Polio Vaccine
		ORS	Oral Rehydration Solution
		OT	Operation Theatre
NBO	National Building Organization	P	Probability
NCCF	National Calamity Contingency Fund	P and SM	Preventive and Social Medicine
		P4 SR	Predicted Four Hour Sweat Rate
NCCP	National Cancer Control Programme	PAH	Polynuclear Aromatic Hydrocarbon
NCD	Noncommunicable Disease	PaP	Papanicolaou's stain Test (Cancer Screening Test)
NCDM	National Committee on Disaster Management		
		PASB	Pan American Sanitary Bureau
NEERI	National Environmental Engineering Research Institute	PB	Paucibacillary
		PCT	Presumptive Coliform Test

PEFR	Peak Expiratory Flow Rate	RNA	Ribonucleic Acid
PEM	Protein Energy Malnutrition	RNTCP	Revised National TB Control Programme
PERT	Program Evaluation Review Technique	ROM	Rifampicin Ofloxacin Minocycline
PET	Preeclampsia Toxemia	ROME	Reorientation of Medical Education
PF	Provident Fund		
PFA	Prevention of Food Adulteration Act	RSDI	Retirement Survival Disability Insurance
PG	Postgraduate	RSF	Rapid Sand Filter
PGL Ag	Phenolic Glycolipid Antigen	RT	Radical Treatment
PH	Public Health	RTI	Reproductive Tract Infection
PHC	Primary Health Center	RTO	Regional Transport Officer
PID	Pelvic Inflammatory Disease	RW	Rideal Walker (Coefficient)
PMW	Paramedical Worker		
PN	Postnatal	S	Streptomycin
PNC	Postnatal Care	SAPEL	Special Action Projects for Elimination of Leprosy
POP	Progestin Only Pill		
PPBS	Planning Programming Budgeting System	SAR	Secondary Attach Rate
		SC	Subcutaneous
PPBS	Postprandial Blood Sugar	SD	Standard Deviation
PPC	Postpartum Program Centre	SE	Standard Error
PPD	Purified Protein Derivative	SET	Survey Education Treatment
PPF	Public Provident Fund	SFI	Specific Flea Index
PPI	Pulse Polio Immunization	SHEB	School Health Education Bureau
PPM	Parts Per Million	SHEB	State Health Education Bureau
PQLI	Physical Quality Life Index	SITA	Suppression of Immoral Traffic Act
PRAI	Planning Research Action Institute	SNP	Special Nutrition Program
PT	Presumptive Treatment	SRS	Sample Registration System
PTAP	Purified Toxoid Absorbed in Aluminum Phosphate	SSF	Slow Sand Filter
		STD	Sexually Transmitted Disease
PWD	Public Works Department	STI	Sexually Transmitted Infection
QID	(Quarter in Die) Four Times Daily	TAB	Typhoid Vaccine with A and B Strain
		TAF	Toxoid Antitoxin Floccules
R	Rifampicin	TB	Tuberculosis
RBC	Red Blood Corpuscle	TBA	Traditional Birth Attendant
RBS	Random Blood Sugar	TDS	Three Times a Day (Ter in die)
RCA	Research cum Action	TEPP	Tetraethyl Pyrophosphate
RCH	Reproductive Child Health	TFR	Total Fertility Rate
RDA	Recommended Dietary Allowance	TIA	Transient Ischemic Attack
		TIG	Tetanus Immunoglobulin
RDNA	Recombinant DNA	TRYSEM	Training of Rural Youth for Self Employment
RF	Rheumatic Fever		
RHD	Rheumatic Heart Disease	TT	Tetanus Toxoid
RIG	Rabies Immunoglobulin	TU	Tubercular Unit
RMP	Registered Medical Practitioner	TV	Television

UBSP	Urban Basic Services for Poor
UCD	Urban Coordinated Development
UCI	Universal Child Immunization
UDC	Upper Division Clerk
UGC	University Grant Commission
UHT	Ultrahigh Temperature
UIB	Unemployment Insurance Benefit
UIP	Universal Immunization Program
UK	United Kingdom
UMI	Universal Mother Immunization
UN	United Nations
UNDP	United Nations Development Program
UNFPA	United Nations Fund for Population Activity
UNICEF	United Nations International Children's Fund
UP	Uttar Pradesh
URI	Upper Respiratory Infection
USAID	United States Agency for International Development bacterial culture. (Lab test for *Vibrio Cholera*)
VDRL	Venereal Disease Research Laboratory
VHG	Village Health Guide
VP reaction	Voges-Proskauer reaction—a test for production of acetyl methyl carbinol from glucose in
VR Media	Venkatraman Media
VVM	Vaccine Vial Monitor
VZIG	Varicella-zoster Immunoglobulin
WATSAN	Water Sanitary Program
WBT	Wet Bulb Thermometer
WHK	Women Hygiene Kit
WHO	World Health Organization
WIC	Walk in Cooler
WWW	World Wide Web
XX	Woman
XY	Man
Z	Pyrazinamide
ZP	Zilla Parishad

INTRODUCTION

Hygiene, Public Health, Preventive Medicine, Social Medicine, Community Medicine, Community Health

Long revolutionary history exists in the development of public health. Transformation of individual health care got transformed slowly through the changes in social history of a nation. Preventing illness in epidemics was also rare in those days. Jenner's discovery of vaccination, first pathogenic bacteria demonstration by Robert Koch marks the turning point in public health.

The life in developing countries was one mainly rural and cities with home industries. Transport was insignificant. However there was a stabilized village community.

Mode of farming changed the outlook and later Industrial revolution gave the life a new face with expanding towns. Rapid growth led to development of urban and shanty towns and migration of rural population.

Problem of poverty as a social problem made apparent to adopt in certain welfare schemes to overcome the social problem in the country. Health authorities were after some way to mitigate the obvious social problems of the country. Acts, Amendments and Rules including labor regulations came into existence.

Health institutions in the country started recording events and it became possible to estimate the extent of disease, determinants of disease. This helped in mapping out national level and global level epidemiology of certain diseases.

India had committees in British India and many committees in post independent India that lead to transformation of health care services in the country. This helped in both long-term and short-term planning for the health and welfare of the country. Simultaneously control and eradication programs were planned to reduce morbidity and mortality of Indian population.

Development of District health administration was a turning point. This led to *Panchayat Raj* System viz., rules by the people for the people and of the people. Slowly community participation gave way for the responsibility for the health of the local community. Child health, maternal health, made the contribution of preventive medicine a concrete in the system of health in India. School health, child welfare and home visiting were the basis for preventive and social medicine development in the country.

Social reforms could be seen during 1960 to 1990 which included Education Acts, Industrial Acts, Social insurance and Social assistance. Thus, social security built up in the country made it possible to visualize the development of community health through preventive and social medicine. Simultaneously mental health and environmental health improved that lead to considerable rise in life expectation.

Recent advances like Universal Immunization, screening, survey, surveillance, study of congenital deformities, child education made it possible to consider preventive medicine, social medicine and community health as leading branches of medicine in the country.

There is disparity in distribution of health resources and health services which are coming in the way of sustainable developmental goals. Now all agree that medical knowledge is an essential component of socioeconomic development.

OUR COUNTRY

VILLAGES IN INDIA

About 66.46% of population are rural based and reside in over 6,49,481 villages. Government of India has launched rural health schemes through three-tier system of healthcare delivery. Reach and access of healthcare to rural community through primary health care functionaries viz., village health guide, Anganwadi worker, traditional birth attendant; is the hallmark of our healthcare system. Villages and districts form key unit in all health and welfare activities.

Subcenters at periphery, primary health center a basic unit and upgraded PHC called community health center have been the ladder in healthcare approach.

HEALTH PROFILE

Disease pattern	Mostly infectious
Socioeconomic	Rural
Character	Joint family Agriculture as main occupation Low per capita income Low literacy rate Low standard of living Poor medical care
Demographic	More of young population
Character	More of pediatric problems High birth, death and growth rate High IMR and high MMR Low life expectancy
Health problems	Infection Malnutrition Poor sanitation Shortage of health personnel

INDIAN CULTURAL HERITAGE

Indian culture is based on age old tradition. In spite of the influences of Western culture which has modified this from time to time, yet our culture remains essentially traditional. Indian civilization is mainly social in character and finds expression in art, literature and architecture through the following:

- Tolerance
- Sense of synthesis
- Universal outlook
- Philosophical outlook
- Respect for the individual
- Agreement with source.

Objectives of life

- *Dharma* (duties of an individual)
- *Artha* (gainful occupation and promotion of social life)
- *Kama* (physical and artistic enjoyment)
- *Moksha* (liberation from worldly chain).

Basic ideals of way of life

- *Balya* (childhood)
- *Brahmacharya* (disciplined life)
- *Grihasta* (family life)
- *Vanaprastha* (retired life)

Planning in India derives its objectives and social basis from the directive principles of state policy enshrined in our constitution.

CULTURAL AWAKENING

The movements of religious and social reforms were the part of awakening of the Indian society which affected every aspect of our culture and was further stimulated by development in various aspects of Indian culture. The main areas of cultural awakening have been through the following:

- Literature and art
- Growth of press
- Growth of science.

NATURAL RESOURCES

Agricultural and allied activities still constitute the major source of livelihood for more than 80% of population of India. Hence, Indian society is still agrarian in nature, and natural resources have a major influence on Indian economy.

Renewable resources	Non-renewable resources
Inexhaustible:	Mineral resources:
Sunlight, wind, Water	Metal, oil, coal gas, marble, gold, sand
Exhaustible:	Recyclable:
Soil, groundwater, forest	Metals
	No recyclable:
	Coal, oil, natural gas

INDIAN SYSTEM OF MEDICINE

The History of Indian system of medicine dates back to 5000 BC. Ayurveda and Siddha are still practiced under Indian systems of medicine. According to Ayurveda, God of medicine is *Dhanvantari* and knowledge of *Atharvanaveda* is Ayurveda science.

According to the Indian system of medicine, Atreya of Takshashila is known to have been the first teacher and physician. Descriptions of various diseases, their diagnosis by observation and treatment by herbal medicine have been presented in *Charaka Samhita* by famous ancient Indian Physician Charaka. *Shushsruta* is the father of Indian Surgery. His *Sushruta Samhita* is well known. *Vagbhata* is another known person in Indian medicine.

Vata, *Pitta* and *Kapha* are *Tridosa* theory of illness. Manu has given code of conduct in Indian medicine.

Other systems of traditional medicine which came to India and became indigenous are Unani Tibb and Homoeopathy.

Government of India has stressed the need for primary health care in the National Health Policy with emphasis on prevention, promotion and rehabilitation. Team approach and use of large health manpower from alternative system of medicine, such as Ayurveda, Unani Tibb, Siddha, Homoeopathy, Yoga and Naturopathy are stressed.

COMPLEMENTARY AND ALTERNATIVE MEDICINE (CAM)

Alternative healing through traditional medicine is called CAM. Important complementary and alternative medicines are Ayurveda, Unani, Homoeopathy, Unani Tibb, Acupuncture, Diet Therapy, Herbs, Yoga, Naturopathy and Siddha. This also can include the component of prayer, faith and meditation.

Ayurveda

The Science of Life known to promote spiritual, mental and physical balance. Non-invasive approaches, such as yoga, massage, diet, purification regimen, breathing exercises, meditation and herbs are known to be used in this system.

The ancient *Rishis, such as Shushrutacharya, Charakacharya, Vagbhata, Sarangdhar* discovered truth by means of religious practices, disciplines and through intensive meditations. Balance of *Doshas* which are described as *Tridosha* which contain *Vata*, *Pitta* and *Kapha*.

Vata

Moody, hyperactive, imaginative, impulsive, slender, eats and sleeps frequently, prone to insomnia, muscle cramps, constipation, joint pain and swelling.

Pittha

Efficient, perfectionist, passionate, short tempered, medium build, warm skin, heavy perspiration, thirst present, acne present, ulcers present, piles present, stomach problems present.

Kapha

Relaxed, graceful, sleeps long, pale, oily skin, eats slowly, obese, allergy present and sinus present.

Most of the preparations are from plant extract and herbal preparations. Many are not fit for licensing. Reputed trained practitioner is important in referral and for advice.

Unani

It is of Greek origin. Hippocrates gave the status of science and further development was by Galen, Rhazes, Avicenna found in the history of Egypt, Syria, Iraq, Persia, India and China.

In India, Unani system of medicine was introduced by Arabs. Delhi Sultan, the Khiljis, the Tughlaqs and the Mughal Emperors provided state patronage to the scholars and even enrolled some as state employees and court physicians.

An outstanding physician and scholar of Unani medicine, Hakim Ajmal Khan (1868-1927) championed the cause of the system.

Most of the preparations are animal sources which are processed and given in decided doses.

Homoeopathy

This has the principle of 'like can cure like'

In 1790, Hahnemann built up a symptoms picture of each patient. Then he matched the individual's symptoms picture to the 'drug picture' of various substance. When he established the closest match, he would prescribe a remedy. He found that the closer the match, the more successful the treatment. Thus, a new system of medicine 'Homoeopathy' was discovered.

In 1776, Hahemann published his book *'A new principle for ascertaining the curative powers of drugs and some examination of previous Principles'*, his first work on Homoeopathy. In this book, he explained the key principle that, a drug taken in small amounts will cure the same symptoms it causes in large amounts.

According to Jacobs, there are 10 common conditions for which people use homeopathic medicine. They are:
1. Asthma
2. Allergic rhinitis
3. Headache or migraine
4. Dermatitis
5. Arthritis
6. Hypertension
7. Non-specific allergy
8. Otitis media
9. Depression
10. Neurotic disorders.

In Homoeopathy, law of cure is used to evaluate the effectiveness of a remedy. If there is cure, symptom should go to less vital organ of the body and then should go out to disappear. Worsening of symptoms after remedy is given importance as healing is taking place.

Unani Tibb

Unani Tibb is part of the culture of the Indian subcontinent, and is practiced widely in India, Pakistan, Bangladesh, and other countries. Based upon the concept of the humors and vital forces, which control the functioning of the body, the principles of Unani Tibb are not very different to those of Ayurveda. Besides the curative aspect, Unani medicine is used for the promotion of health and rejuvenation of vigor.

Al-Razi, popularly known by medieval Latinists as Rhazes, was probably the first physician known to have composed a lengthy manuscript *Al-Hawi*.

The detail and accuracy of *Al-Hawi* in recognizing different diseases, differentiating among similar-looking diseases, their classification and the methods adopted to treat them, makes *Al-Hawi* a highly regarded text even today. The treatise on smallpox and measles contains the first definite description of smallpox as a clinical entity.

Delhi, the capital of the Sultans, became an even greater center of culture and glory than Baghdad. The Khilji and Tughluq Sultans nurtured eminent Unani physicians, surgeons, and ophthalmologists. During the reign of Sikander Lodi (1489-1517), Mian Bhowa, an eminent courtier, composed a medical treatise entitled *Madan-ul-Shifa Sikander Shahi* in Persian. The Mughal rulers patronized physicians and surgeons from medical centers in Persia, more particularly from Gilan, Shiraz, and Tabrez.

During the reign of Akbar, there was a mass exodus of learned men from regions where Arabian medicine was taught. These included Hakim Ali Gilani, Hakim Abul Fatah Gilani (who invented the Indian *hookah)*, Ain-ul-Mulk Hakim Sharnsuddin Ali Sherazi, Hakim Hummam, Hakim-ul-Mulk Gilani, and some Hindu physicians, such as Mahadev, Bhim Datt, and Narayan. The English rulers showed no interest in either Unani Tibb or Ayurveda, causing these systems to be further neglected.

Working principles of the body, according to Unani Tibb, can be classified into *amur-e-tabia* or seven main groups:
1. *arkan* or elements, comprising *mitti* (earth), *pani* (water), *hawa* (air), and *aag* (fire) as different states of matter and the materials which make up everything in the universe;

2. *mizaj* (temperament);
3. *akhlat* (humors);
4. *aza* (organs);
5. *arwah* (life, spirits or vital breaths);
6. *quva* (energy); and
7. *afa'al* (action).

Arkan (matter) in its different states, helped by the *amzija*, plural of *mizaj* (temperament), of each of its individual constituents, combines to produce the *aza* or organs and *arwah* or life spirits; the organs with the spirit develop qava or energy which manifests itself in the *afa'al* (actions) of the body.

Each of the elements has its own special qualities: the earth is cold and dry; water is cold and moist; fire is hot and dry; air is hot and moist. When these elements mix with one another qualitatively and quantitatively, there emerges a uniform body possessing an amalgam of these qualities. The resultant quality of the uniform body is called its *mizaj* (temperament).

The temperament of a substance may be a *mizaj-emutadil* (balanced one) or a *mizaj-e-ghairmutadil* (imbalanced one). Different types and shades of imbalanced temperaments are described in the Unani System.

In the human body, there are four humors. These are *balgham* (phlegm), *khoon* (blood), *safra* (yellow bile), and *sauda* (black bile).

A Unani physician does not prescribe the strongest drug at the onset of the treatment.

Since in Unani Tibb, health and disease depend upon the equilibrium or disequilibrium of the four humors, a thorough examination of the *nabz* (pulse) is undertaken to determine which humor is dominant at the time. The detailed examination of the pulse is an art and some hakims are known to depend largely upon it for diagnosis of a disease. The pulse is examined for the frequency of its beats (slow or fast), its force (whether the pulse beats hard or soft against the examining fingers), dilation (how much it dilates), the pause between the two beats of the pulse against the examining fingers, and many other details. Unani Tibb seems to be lagging behind in research and modernization.

The scope of Unani Tibb is similar to that of Ayurvedic medicine. Even though Unani Tibb is based upon ancient Greek medical concepts, over the centuries, it has adapted itself to Indian conditions and made use of the drugs available in India. People understand the basic concepts of the system and believe in it in the same manner as they do in Ayurveda.

Acupuncture

In Latin 'Acus' means needle and 'Punctura' means penetration or prick. Acupuncture is an ancient Chinese art of Healing. Acupuncture also known as needling is the insertion of fine steel, silver or gold needles into selected areas of the skin as a remedy for disease. There are more than 1,000 Acupuncture points in the human body located along 12 main pathways or channels in each half of the body and two channels in the mid-line of the body. To treat a given case, an acupuncturist has to select about 8–12 points out of these 1,000.

The 'Huang Di Nei Jing' is the foundation stone of traditional Chinese medicine. It is said to be the oldest medical text in the world. A special section of it, called Ling Shu is devoted to Acupuncture and moxibustion (a method of Acupuncture without needles). The Chinese traditionally consider it more as a preventive science than a curative science.

Pain relief is most common reason people seek acupuncture.

OTHER METHODS

Diet Therapy

Specific dietary supplement of vitamin E for arthritis and heart disease is known.

Herbs

Garlic as antioxidant, Ginkgo biloba in Dementia, Valerian as sedative, ginger as digestant, Chamomile as intestinal sedative, are known herbs.

Meditation

It is an act of momentary concentration. This can be a relaxation response found useful in stress, anxiety, pain and high blood pressure.

Naturopathy

Patients are guided and treated for unhealthy practices, helped to cultivate healthy lifestyle, natural use of herbs, homeopathic remedies, diet therapy and exercise. Types of Naturopathy are water therapy, air therapy, fire therapy, space therapy, mud therapy, food therapy, massage therapy, acupressure, magnetotherapy, and chromotherapy.

Vincent Priessnitz (1799-1851) who was a farmer by profession has been known as "Father of Naturopathy". The word "Naturopathy" has been coined by Dr John Scheel in the year 1895 and was propagated and popularized in the western world by Dr Benedict Lust.

In short, Nature Cure includes all the available non-invasive treatments and diagnostic modalities which do not interfere with the body's natural functional capacity and healing process and are in affirmative with Nature's constructive Principles.

Siddha

Siddha system is one of the oldest systems of medicine in India. The term Siddha means achievements and Siddhars were saintly persons who achieved results in medicine. Eighteen Siddhars were said to have contributed towards the development of this medical system. Siddha literature is in Tamil and it is practiced largely in Tamil speaking part of India and abroad. The Siddha System is largely therapeutic in nature.

According to tradition, the origin of Siddha system of medicine is attributed to the great Siddha Ayastiyar. Some of his works are still standard books of medicine and surgery in daily use among the Siddha Medical practitioners.

Like Ayurveda, this system believes that all objects in the universe including human body are composed of five basic elements namely, earth, water, fire, air and sky. As in Ayurveda, this system also considers the human body as a conglomeration of three humors, seven basic tissues and the waste products of the body such as feces, urine and sweat. The food is considered to be basic building material of human body which gets processed into humors, body tissues and waste products. The equilibrium of humors is considered as healthy and its disturbance or imbalance leads to disease or sickness.

In general, this system is effective in treating all types of skin problems particularly Psoriasis, STD, urinary tract infections, diseases of liver and gastrointestinal tract, general debility, postpartum anemia, diarrhea and general fevers in addition to arthritis and allergic disorders.

Prayer

Scientific evidence is being searched for prayer and faith healing. This is to be remembered since majority have the faith in faith healing.

Yoga

Siddhartha Gautama, who was skilled in Meditation and also the first Buddhist who studied Yoga, attained enlightenment at the age of 35.

The Gita's message is to oppose evil in the world. The Gita earned its relevance because of its attempt to blend Jnana-Yoga. Bhakati-Yoga and Karma-Yoga together unifying these various Yogic traditions.

After the turn of the millennium, the spread of Yoga in its diffcrent forms gave rise to the need for standardization. Thus in the second century CE, Patanjali composed a seminal text, Yoga-Sutra and defined Classical Yoga. The 195 aphorisms or sutras that comprise the Yoga-Sutra, expound upon Raja-Yoga (the eightfold Yoga path). The Yoga-Sutra is meant to be memorized as a means of internalizing its wisdom. The eight limbs of classical Yoga are:
1. Yama, or restraint,
2. Niyama, or observance of purity, tolerance and study,
3. Asana, or physical exercises,
4. Pranayama or breath control
5. Pratyahara, or preparation for meditation
6. Dharana, or concentration,
7. Dhyana or meditation and
8. Samadhi or absorption in the sublime.

Patanjali advocates studying the sacred scriptures as part of the Yoga practice, which becomes Classical Yoga's distinct feature.

Five principles of Yoga are:
1. Proper relaxation (savasana),
2. Proper exercise (Asanas),
3. Proper breathing (pranayama),
4. Proper diet (vegetarian), and,
5. Positive thinking and meditation (dhyana).

Now that we know how *Yoga* originated let's take a look at the various types of *Yoga*. Medical science has begun to pay attention to the effects of Yoga as a therapy in recent times. Studies have shown, the relaxation in the corpse pose effectively relieves high blood pressure and that regular practice of the poses or postures (Asanas) and breathing exercises (Pranayama) can help such a variety of ailments, such as arthritis, sclerosis, chronic fatigue, asthma, varicose veins, cardiac conditions, and women's health problems. Laboratory tests have also confirmed Yoga's ability to allow one to consciously control autonomic (involuntary) functions of the body such as temperature, heart rate and blood pressure. But before you start the practice of Yoga, it is essential to know which type of Yoga would be best suited to you. You should make this decision keeping your own nature in mind. Decide which form appeals to you the most. Yoga can be broadly classified into 8 main categories.

They are Bhakti Yoga, Karma Yoga, Jnana Yoga, Raja Yoga, Mantra Yoga, Laya Yoga, Tantra Yoga, and Hata Yoga

Yoga which also means union of body, mind, spirit can be adapted at any level and at any capability so that it can be easily used.

Massage

Manipulation of soft tissue by pressing, tapping movements is called massage.

If massage is done with deep tissue manipulation it is called bodywork.

If healing meditation is done it is called touch therapies.

Types of massages have been:
- *Healing touch:* Energy healing technique, a component of massage, where multilevel therapeutic touch is undertaken.
- *Reike:* It is under a massage, where the therapy uses techniques to direct universal life energy to specific site.
- *Rolfing which is called structural integration:* Here manual manipulation and stretching of body's fascial tissues to establish balance and symmetry.
- *Alexander technique:* Balanced posture and coordination by gentle hands on guidance and verbal instruction is followed.
- *Swedish massage:* Uses long strokes, friction and kneading of muscles.
- *Trager approach:* Gentle, rhythmic rocking to promote relaxation and energy flow.
- *Reflexology:* Pressure application to pressure points on the hands and feet that correspond to various parts of the body.
- *Movement re-education:* By using gentle manipulations to heighten awareness of the body as described by Feldenkrais.

Tai Chi

This is an art of stimulating life energy, a Chinese medicine. This is done by slow graceful dance with controlled movements of arm and leg.

It is used for pain relief and wound healing. It is used in Germany and Japan with the help of specified magnets. Variety of forms, variety of strengths and in different prices magnet is available. Magnet mattresses, magnet jewelry are also available. Magnet therapy is not to be used on a Person using pacemakers and on the abdomen of pregnant abdomen.

ENVIRONMENT AND SUSTAINABLE DEVELOPMENT

The constant interaction of all surrounding living and non-living form Mega Environment. They can be physical, chemical, biological, psychological, sociological or spiritual.

Physical environment: Water, air, soil, housing, climate, heat, light, noise, radiation.

Chemical environment: Organic and inorganic chemicals.

Biological environment: Bacteria, virus, rickettsia

Psychological environment: Content, need, anxiety, stress

Social environment: Culture, custom habit, belief, education, lifestyle.

Spiritual environment: Mental stability, broadmindedness.

Environmental resources:
- Energy
- Air
- Water
- Soil
- Minerals
- Plants
- Animals

Impact of environment when used:
- Deforestation
- Air pollution
- Water pollution
- Climate changes
- Depletion of resources

Environmental action for sustained development:
- Environment projection and conservation
- Soil conservation
- Vanamahotsava
- Appiko chaluvali
- Wildlife Protection Act
- UN environmental programs
- Social forestry
- National park, Zoo
- Bird sanctuaries
- Law making

FIELD PRACTICE AREA

Looking into the need of the country Re-Orientation of Medical Education (ROME) is brought to action since 1976 in India. More focus is given on teaching and training to students, House surgeons and postgraduates at family side clinics (rather than bedside clinics) in rural and urban Field Practice Areas.

Primary health center as RHTC and an urban health center as UHTC are adopted or owned as field practice areas for medical college. This also helps specialists and students to understand rural India and understanding of disease in rural background. Further, training is offered on management of cases within available resources at Field Practice Areas.

Main activities in the FPA are:
- UG Training Progrmme
- PG Training Programme
- Interns Training Programme
- School health check up
- Immunization
- MCH and FP work
- Periodic survey
- Subcenter clinics
- Anganwadi visits
- Implementation of National Health Programmes
- Health education talks
- Project works

Specialist/Specialties made available are:
- Pediatrics
- Orthopedics
- Trauma care
- Skin care
- OBG services
- Eye care services
- Dental care
- X-ray service

Lab services made available are:
- Routine blood examinations
- HB percentage
- Blood count
- Blood grouping
- Peripheral smear for malaria

MAN TOWARDS HEALTH FOR ALL

INTRODUCTION
There has been a significant change in the present healthcare system from age old practices of managing illness through magic, herbal drugs, prayers and cosmic effect. But certain time-tested remedies are still prevalent in one form or the other. However, education, science and technology have revolutionized the healthcare systems.
- *Curative medicine:* Treatment of disease by drugs, intervention to neutralize illness.
- *Preventive medicine:* Study covering communicable disease, environmental, social, economic and general preventive actions.
- *Social medicine:* Study of man as a social being in his total environment.
- *Family medicine:* Family-oriented medicine for healthcare delivery.
- *Community medicine:* Management of health and health-related problems, covering total environment in the community. Now it is termed as community health.

EVOLUTION OF COMMUNITY MEDICINE (HISTORY OF MEDICINE)
Stages seen in the history of medicine.
- Stone age
- 5000 BC: Indian medicine in Vedic times
- 2700 BC: Chinese medicine (Principles of Yang and Yin, system of barefoot doctor, system of acupuncture)
- 2000 BC: Egyptian medicine (manuscript of Papyrus)
- 2000 BC: Mesopotamian medicine (Babylonian code of Hammurabi)
- 800 BC: Atreya and Shushruta: Golden age of Indian medicine
- 460 BC: Greek medicine (Hygiea the daughter of Aesculapius, Hippocratic Oath)
- 130 AD: Roman medicine (Galen)
- 200 AD: Charaka
- Up to 800 AD: Dark age of medicine
- 900 AD: Arabic medicine (Rhazes, Avicenna)
- 1500 AD: Revival period (theory of contagion of Fracastorius, blood circulation by Harvey, microscope by Leeuwenhoek, vaccination by Jenner)
- 1800: Sanitary awakening
- 1810: Homoeopathy (Hahnemann)
- 1850: Rise of Public Health (Epidemic of cholera by John Snow, typhoid by William Budd, Sanitary reforms by Chadwick and Sir John Simon)
- 1860: Germ theory (Demonstration of bacteria by Louis Pasteur in 1860, anthrax by Robert Koch in 1877, gonococci in 1847, typhoid and pneumococci in 1880, Mycobacterium in 1882, vibrio in 1883, diphtheria in 1884)
- 1883: Birth of preventive medicine (Anti-rabies vaccine, cholera vaccine, typhoid vaccine, diphtheria antitoxin, antiseptics and disinfectants)
- 1896 to 1900: Disease transmission demonstrated (Sleeping sickness by Dr Bruce, Malaria by Dr Ross, Yellow fever by Walter Reed)
- 1900: Multifactorial causation of disease
- 1911: Social medicine
- 1920: Measures against disease control
- 1923: Development of family medicine
- 1940: Social revolution
- 1951: Birth of concept of community development program
- 1966: Development of community health (community medicine)
- 1978: Concept of primary health care
- 1982: 20 Point Programme and National Health Policy
- 1985: Universal Immunization Programme
- 1989: Blood safety activities
- 1990: ARI Programme
- 1992: Child Survival and Safe Motherhood Programme
- 1993: RNTCP and DOTS activities
- 1994: Panchayat Raj system in the country

- 1995: PPI followed by IPPI
- 1995: RCH Programme
- 2000: National Population Policy and Millennium Development Goals
- 2002: National Health Policy
- 2004: Integrated Disease Surveillance Project
- 2005: National Rural Health Mission Janani Suraksha Yojana Achieved Leprosy Elimination Target
- 2006: RNTCP covers whole country IMNCI launched
- 2007: Senior Citizen Bill passed
- 2008: NCD projects launched
- 2009: New Mother Child Protection Card came to use.: Guidelines for Human Stem Cell Research by NIH
- 2010: Nutrition Standards for Indians set by ICMR
- 2011: 14th Decennial Census of India: Patient Protection and Affordable Care Act enacted
- 2013: National Health Mission launched
- 2014: India declared Polio Free
- 2015: NITI Aayog replace earlier Yojana Aayog: IPV vaccine reintroduced in Schedule Swatch Bharat Abhiyaan launched
- 2016: Malaria Eradication Plan launched (2016 to 2030 plan): Sustainable Development Goals came into force: Public Health adopted bOPV
- 2017: National Health Policy 2017
- 2018: National Health Protection Scheme
- 2019: World Health Summit in Berlin

APPROACHES TO PROVIDING HEALTH CARE

- Comprehensive health care is interpreted as curative and preventive care from womb to tomb; to all.
- Basic health care is a network of coordinated, peripheral and intermediate health units capable of performing effectively with essential healthcare services by basic health workers.
- Primary health care is an essential health care made universally accessible to individuals and community; their full participation and at a cost the community and country can afford.
- Health for all refers to the attainment of a level of health that will enable every individual to lead to socially and economically productive life.
- Millennium development goals on seven areas are:
  1. Provision of peace, security and disarmament
  2. Development and poverty eradication
  3. Protecting our common environment
  4. Protecting human rights, democracy and good governance
  5. Protecting the vulnerable
  6. Meeting the special needs of developing countries
  7. Strengthening the United Nations.

SECTION 1

Section Outline

Chapter 1. Concept of Health and Disease
Chapter 2. Relationship of Social and Behavioral to Health and Disease
Chapter 3. Environmental Health Problems
Chapter 4. Medical Entomology

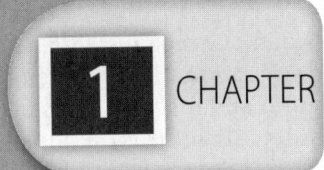

CHAPTER 1: Concept of Health and Disease

CHAPTER OUTLINE

- Definitions
- Holistic Approach of Health
- Triad of Epidemiology
- Natural History of Diseases
- Modes of Intervention
- Effective Communication
- Health Indicators
- Estimates of Demographic Value of India 2019
- Role of Health Education in Health Programs
- Doctor–Patient Relationship

DEFINITIONS

Health

Health is a state of complete physical, mental and social well-being and not merely an absence of disease or infirmity (WHO).

Standard of Living

This refers to the scale of expenditure, goods we consume, and services we enjoy, the level of education, the employment status, and items of modern living, such as food, dress, house, amusements and comforts (WHO).

This consists of health, food consumption, education, occupation, working condition, housing, social security, clothing, recreation, leisure and human rights (United Nations).

Quality of Life

The condition of life resulting from the combination of the effects of the complete range of factors, such as those determining health, happiness, education, social and intellectual attainments, freedom of action, justice and freedom of expression (WHO).

Physical Quality of Life Index

This varies from "0" to "100". Three indicators are consolidated in Physical Quality of Life Index (PQLI). They are:
1. Infant mortality
2. Life expectancy at age one
3. Literacy

Human Development Index

This varies from "0" to "1". This reflects human achievements and his capabilities. Three dimensions are consolidated in Human Development Index (HDI). They are:
1. Life expectancy at birth
2. Literacy/knowledge
3. Per capita gross domestic product (GDP)/income.

Comparative Table for PQLI and HDI:

Physical quality of life index	Human development index
Commonly known as PQLI	Commonly known as HDI
It is a composite index	It is a composite index

Contd...

Contd...

Physical quality of life index	Human development index
Derived from infant mortality rate (IMR), life expectancy at 1 year and literacy status	Derived from expectation of life at birth, mean year of schooling and expected years of schooling
0 = Worst performance 100 = Best performance	0 = No development category 1 = Very high development category
It is a measure for well-being of a community	It is a measure for country's development *Dimension before 2010* • Life expectation at birth • Adult literacy • Standard of living by purchasing power *Dimension after 2010* • Life expectation at birth • Education index • Decent standard of living

Health Team

The health team is a group of skilled persons who share a common goal and common objectives, which are determined by the needs of the community. Each member in a health team has specific and recognized function.

Health for All

This is an attainment of a level of health that will permit them to lead to a socially and economically productive life.

Primary Health Care

Primary health care is "an essential health care based on practical, scientifically sound and socially acceptable methods and technology made universally accessible to individual and families in the community through their full participation and at a cost that the community and the country can afford to maintain atevery stage of their development in the spirit of self-determination."

Health System

Health system is intended to deliver health services for the community. This involves planning, identifying priorities, finding out resources in terms of money manpower and material, periodic evaluation. Health system has concept of health and disease, ideas of coverage and equity, structures, such as hospital or centers, community with service givers and consumers.

Hygiene

Hygiene is the science of health and embraces all factors that contribute to healthful living.

HOLISTIC APPROACH OF HEALTH (MULTIFACTORIAL CAUSATION, WEB OF CAUSATION)

It is a combination of social, economical, political and environmental influence of health. The person is seen in the context of his environment. All factors, viz. food, education, housing, animal husbandry, agriculture, industry, information technologies, etc., which have an impact on health, are considered. Promotion and protection of health is possible by the approach of multifactorial causation.

Health Dimension

Functioning and interaction of many health dimensions are observed in the concept of health. They are:
- Physical
- Emotional
- Environmental
- Mental
- Vocational
- Nutritional
- Social
- Socioeconomic
- Philosophical
- Spiritual
- Cultural

Health Concepts

- Germ theory (Biomedical)
- Environmental (Ecological)
- Social, economic, and cultural (Psycho-somatic)
- Multidimensional (Holistic), and
- Biological average (Relative concept)

Chapter 1: Concept of Health and Disease

Health: A Relative Concept

When we say average height of Australians is 6'3" and of British 6'1", they are local standards based on statistical averages. Culture and social class among Australians and British influence health. Thus, health standards, by average and local condition, form a relative concept of health.

Determinants of Health

There are many interacting factors that influence and decide health. These are called health determinants. They are:
- Heredity
- Environment
- Ways of living
- Personal hygiene
- Economic status, and
- Health service availability

Ecology of Health

It is a science of mutual relationship between man and his environment. Physical, chemical, biological, social and environmental factors determine man's health. These influencing factors are studied with respect to disease under ecology of health.

Spectrum of Health (Table 1.1)

Many possibilities are seen in the dynamic phenomenon of health. At a given point of time, we come across all possible combinations of health status.

Table 1.1: Influencing factors in health status.

↓	Health	↑
↓	Apparently healthy	↑
↓	Acutely ill	↑
↓	Chronically ill	↑
↓	Dying	↑
↓	Dead	↑
Efforts (surrounding factors)	Efforts (medical profession)	

Health or well-being is determined by:
- Quality of life (PQLI)
- Level of living, and
- Standard of living (lifespan, literacy and HDI)

Health and Development

Development from all sectors brings about positive health in man. Socioeconomic development and cultural development bring about health development resulting in a continuous improvement of health status of a population. Physical and mental health is inextricably interwoven with socioeconomic growth.

Health and Service

1. *Level (primary):* Essential primary health care [Subcenter, primary health centers (PHC), clinics]
2. *Level (secondary):* Referral service (Taluka hospital, district hospital)
3. *Level (tertiary):* Hi-tech service (Regional hospital, teaching hospital, railway hospital, specialty service hospital).

Health examinations are by:
- Survey
- Screening, and
- Surveillance

Equality in Health

Attainment of level of health by people which will permit social, economic and productive life. Health for All (HFA) is a new philosophy of health care which has the following characters (primary health care).
- Socially acceptable
- Universally accessible
- Community participation
- Affordable

DISEASE

Disease, as name implies, is departure from state of health, interrupting in normal functioning of the body.

Causes of Disease

Causes of disease are depicted in **Figure 1.1**.

Definitions

Hygiene: Science of health that embraces all factors which contribute to healthful living.

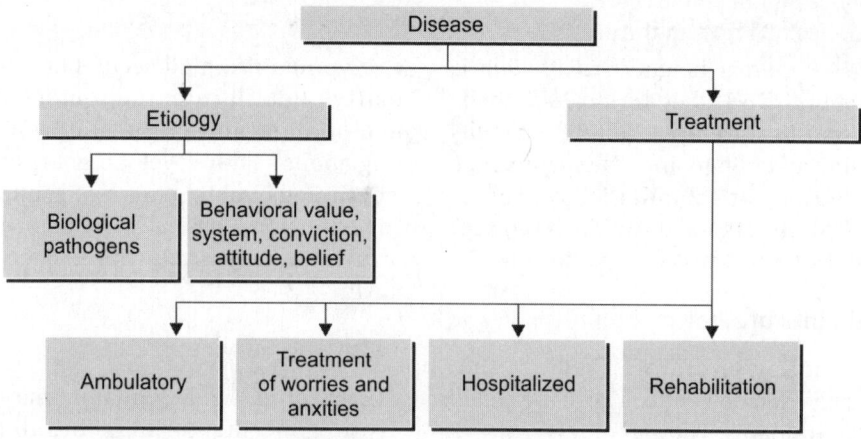

Fig. 1.1: Causes of disease.

Sanitation: Individual and community surrounding which are depicted through personal hygiene and environmental hygiene.

Public health: Science and art of preventing disease, preserving life, promoting health and efficiency through organized community efforts.

Preventive medicine: It is a science that includes specific medical measure and specific community measure in preventing diseases or ill-health status.

Social medicine: The study of man as a social being in his total environment.

Preventive and social medicine: Area of discipline covering individual health measure, community health medicine, special health measures and studying the man in his total environment.

Community medicine: It is the successor of public health. It has concept and scope of public health, preventive medicine and social medicine.

Community health: Latest concept, which includes all personal health and environmental health of human community.

Community diagnosis: Application of medical knowledge to diagnose pathology in the community. Here, pattern of diseases is identified along with factors influencing disease, e.g., protein–energy malnutrition (PEM), iodine deficiency disorder (IDD), and cholera epidemic in the community.

Clinical examination and laboratory examinations are essential for the diagnosis of illness of the patient. Even it will have differential diagnosis (DD) in the beginning followed by final diagnosis.

In a society, occurrence of illness is checked by manifestations, by epidemics, by more morbidity, by more mortality, supplemented with serological investigations. All these arrive at community diagnosis. Community diagnosis also includes social, behavioral, existing customs, existing traditions and existing beliefs.

Thus, examination, investigation, survey, screening, surveillance of group of people or a community in case of group illness constitute *community diagnosis.*

Community diagnosis is influenced by following data:
- Age distribution
- Sex distribution
- Race distribution
- Occupation distribution
- Socioeconomic group distribution
- Culture distribution
- Environment group distribution
- Morbidity rates
- Mortality rates
- Fertility rates
- Vital events in the area

Chapter 1: Concept of Health and Disease

- Incidence of illness in the area
- Prevalence of illness in the area

Community diagnosis is a tool in identifying the uses of epidemiology. Community diagnosis quantifies the problems of health in a group of population.

Community diagnosis gives an idea of health needs of a community and also gives a picture of risks to which a community is exposed.

We can infer disease control measures by systematic community diagnosis.

Surveys and studies done for community diagnosis also help as a basic data in future community diagnosis.

Investigation of an epidemic is a tool in community diagnosis.

Community treatment: Action, in terms of health measures in the community to manage community-illness diagnosed by community diagnosis, e.g., nutrition supplementation and nutrition education in PEM. Iodized salt supply in IDD, protected water supply to the community in cholera epidemic.

Hospital and health centers: An establishment to provide medical care, follow-up and rehabilitation. It takes care of ambulatory patients, nonambulatory patients and the community.

Physicians: A recognized and registered medical practitioner who has acquired prescribed knowledge through course of studies in medicine and who is legally licensed to practice medicine.

A basic doctor: One who is well-conversant with common health problems, providing curative and preventive health services, capable of managing common illness and referral of the needy and who can give life-saving aid.

Surveillance: Continuous scrutiny of the factors that determine the occurrence and distribution of disease.

Monitoring: Routine watching over, aiming at detecting changes in health status.

Sentinel surveillance: Identification of missed cases and further notifying them. Selected institutions do the job of sentinel surveillance.

Population medicine: Medicine as applied to the community through public health, community health and preventive and social medicine.

Triad of epidemiology: Agent, host and environment that can determine disease in an individual or in the community. Case occurrence or epidemics are determined by these determinants.

Web of causation of disease: All precipitating factors, all perpetuating factors and all predisposing factors are considered in the causation of a disease. Understanding of chains of illness can help us to delink to eliminate such disease.

Disease Spectrum

Similar to light spectrum, the disease gives its pattern at a given point of time in the community. Such spectrum contains subclinical cases, mild illness, moderate illness, early severe stage of illness, late severe stage of illness and advanced stage of illness. Dying and dead are also seen in the spectrum.

Germ theory: It is single cause theory. Definite causative agent causing disease is one of the revolutionary concepts.

Multifactorial cause: A modern concept which carries many factors including risk factors in the causation of disease. Social, economic, cultural, genetic and psychological factors are equally important in disease causation.

Agent, host and environment: It is called epidemiological triad commonly used in infectious diseases. Basic factors of causative agent, influencing environment and person who hosts the disease are studied.

Natural history of disease: It is a trademark of disease occurring in nature foreseeing all events from the beginning of illness to death. Recovery and disability are usual course in the history. Before its occurrence and after its occurrence are visualized over a disease **(Fig. 1.2)**.

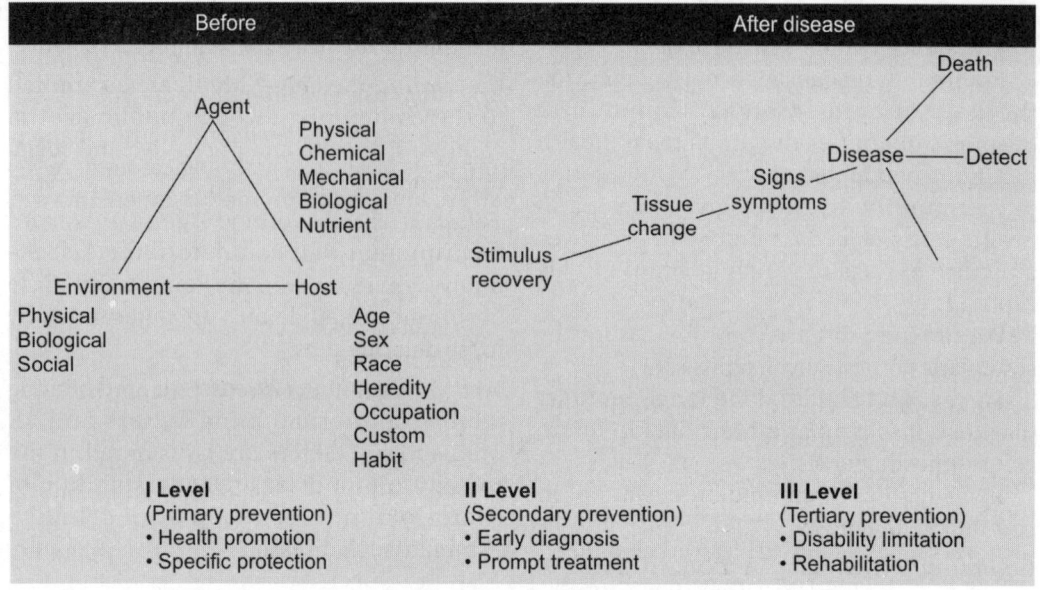

Fig. 1.2: Natural history of disease (NHD).

Risk Factors (Table 1.2)

An exposure that is significantly related with development of disease, e.g., high cholesterol and heart disease.

Group of people exposed to risk are called *risk group*.

Appropriate action to prevent risk is *risk approach*.

Iceberg Phenomenon of Disease

Diseases seen in the community is similar to that of the tip of an iceberg. Most of the illnesses are not seen at the outset. Phenomenon of small portion of symptomatic disease seen and a big portion of a symptomatic disease that is not seen is called iceberg phenomenon.

Table 1.2: Examples of risk factors.

Fatty diet, obesity	Diabetes
Alcohol	Cirrhosis of liver
Smoking, radiation	Cancer
High cholesterol, obesity	
Type of a personality	Heart disease
Smoking, high BP, High cholesterol	Stroke
Alcohol consumption, ignorant about traffic signal	Accident

TRIAD OF EPIDEMIOLOGY (AGENT–HOST–ENVIRONMENT)

Natural History of Disease

The disease spectrum of a disease in a population is constructed with the help of its pattern in the community.

Table 1.3 depicts the differences between control and eradication.

Table 1.3: Differences between control and eradication.

	Control	Eradication
Definition	To reduce incidence to acceptable level, e.g., cholera control	Total extirpation of disease agent, e.g., polio eradication
Objective	To reduce mortality and morbidity (no more a public health problem).	To uproot the disease
Area of operation	In high incidence area	Total coverage
Duration of operation	Indefinite	Time limited

Contd...

Contd...

	Control	Eradication
Economic aspect	Recurring	Cheap
Case finding		
Confirmation		
Epidemiological Investigation	Not important	Very important

Prevention

Promoting, preserving and restoring positive health are basic aspects of prevention of disease in the community.

Levels of Prevention

a. *Primordial:* Attack at emergence or attack on risk factors including lifestyle constitutes primordial prevention, e.g., regular exercise in cardiovascular disease prevention, smoking regulation in cancer prevention.
b. *Primary prevention:* Action taken before the onset of disease, disallowing disease, population strategy and high-risk strategy in the prevention of chronic diseases.
c. *Secondary prevention:* An action to halt the progress of a disease.
d. *Tertiary prevention:* Intervention in the late pathogenic phase to reduce disability and to promote adjustment to disease condition.

Modes of Intervention

Health Promotion

It is a process of enabling people to increase and improve health
- Health education
- Environmental modification
- Nutritional intervention
- Lifestyle changes
- Behavioral changes

Specific Protection

It is a process to totally avoid disease or illness.
- Immunization
- Nutritional supplement
- Chemoprophylaxis
- Immunoprophylaxis
- Protective device in industry
- Protective device in traffic accident
- Protective device against carcinogen
- Protective device against allergen

Early Diagnosis and Prompt Treatment

It is a process of early detection of transformation from physiological to pathological status, e.g., early diagnosis and prompt treatment of:
- Hypertension
  - Ca breast
  - Ca cervix
  - Tuberculosis
  - Leprosy
  - Mass treatment in trachoma and malaria

Disability Limitation (Disability Prevention)

It is a process involving interaction to prevent disability.
- Disability limitation in nerve damage in leprosy
- Physiotherapy in polio lameness

Impairment

Any loss of abnormality of psychological, physiological or emotional stress and functions, e.g., impaired vision, hard of hearing, mental retardation.

Disability

Any restriction or lack of ability to perform an activity in the manner or within the range considered normal for a human being, e.g. loss of both lower limb, loss of hand, blind.

Handicap

It is the disadvantage for the person because of disability or impairment that disallows the role to play, e.g., loss of property, loss of wealth, loss of family, unemployment.

Rehabilitation

It is a combined and coordinated use of medical, social, economical, vocational and psychological measures to make an individual or community function normally.

Medical rehabilitation

Helping medically to restore (physical rehabilitation) organ function, e.g., reconstructive surgery of hand (fitting artificial limb after an accident).

Social rehabilitation
Restoration of family relation and social relation, e.g., widow marriage, employment on compassionate ground.

Economic rehabilitation
Financial assistance to recover from handicap, e.g., loan under self-employment scheme.

Vocational rehabilitation
Restoration of capacity to earn livelihood, e.g., leprosy patients are put to garden work which enables them to have an earning.

Psychological rehabilitation
Restoration of prestige, dignity and confidence, e.g., tuberculosis patient after full course of treatment and becomes noninfectious.

Disease pattern is depicted in **Table 1.4**.

EFFECTIVE COMMUNICATION

Communication deals with transmission of information or ideas. They are done through:
- Expressing our feelings
- Facial expression
- Gesture of face, hand
- Spoken words
- Songs
- Improved language
- Written script

Major components of communication are as following:
- Source (sender)
- Content (message), and
- Audience (receiver)

Main Aim of Communication
- To help acquire the knowledge (cognitive domain)
- To help acquire skill (psychomotor domain)
- To inform, educate, motivate, and persuade for high standard of health

Communication Media
Communication media are:
- Interpersonal media
- Mass media (recent)
- Folk media (tradition)

Table 1.4: Disease pattern in developing and developed countries.

	Developing	Developed	
I. Disease pattern	Infection Malnutrition Helminthic infestation		Metabolic diseases Cancer Autoimmune disease
II. Socioeconomic characters	Rural Joint family Agriculture ↓ Per capita income ↓ Literacy ↓ Standard of living ↓ Medical care		Urban Single family Industry ↑ ↑ ↑ ↑
III. Demography	Young Pediatric ↑ ↑ ↑ ↑ ↑	Population Problem Birth rate Death rate Growth rate Infant mortality rate (IMR) Maternal mortality ratio (MMR) Life expectancy	Older Geriatric ↓ ↓ ↓ ↓ ↓
IV. Health problem	CD	Population explosion Social problem of developing countries Malnutrition Environmental sanitation Medical care	NCD Re-emerging infectious disease Social problem of developed countries Overnutrition

Chapter 1: Concept of Health and Disease

Communication Types

* One way (Didactic method)
* Two way (Socratic method)
* Visual way
* Verbal way
* Soft skills, such as gesture, posture, body movement, facial expressions, smiling, frowning, staring, gazing, etc.
* Nonformal way
* Formal way
* Internet way

Communication Barriers

* Physiological: Difficulty in hearing
* Psychological: Emotional disturbance
* Environmental: Loud noise
* Cultural:
  * Urban—rural
  * Foreign—national
  * Positive and negative attitude

HEALTH INDICATORS

Valid, reliable, sensitive and relevant indicators which determine health development are called health indicators.

* *Mortality indicators:* Death rate, lifespan, IMR, child mortality rate, MMR, case fatality rate, proportion mortality rate
* *Morbidity indicators:* Disease rates (Incidence, prevalence)
* *Disability indicators*: Hospitalization, loss of work, Sullivan's index, (when bed disability is subtracted in lifespan, it is Sullivan's disability free of life), DALY (Disability adjusted life years) which express loss of year of health life
* *Nutritional indicators*: Anthropometric values, low birth weight
* *Healthcare indicators*: Staff population ratio
* *Utilization indicators*: Fully immunized, bed turn out
* *Socioeconomic indicators*: Per capita income, family size.

Millennium developmental goals indicators:
* Provision of peace, security and disarmament
* Development and poverty eradication
* Protecting our common environment
* Protecting human rights, democracy and good governance
* Protecting the vulnerable
* Meeting the special needs of developing countries
* Strengthening the United Nations.

ESTIMATES OF DEMOGRAPHIC VALUES OF INDIA 2019

* Population   1359.8 million (as per 2018)
* Birth rate   20
* Death rate   6
* Growth rate   1.2%

Most densely populated states are UP, Maharashtra and Bihar.

* 0–4 age group   8.5%
* 0–14   27%
* 65+   5.4%
* Sex ratio   1000: 898
* [Societal dependency ratio 32.4% (0–14 age and 65+) age]

Density of:
* Population   876/sq km
* Family size   2.3
* Urbanization   31.8%
* Urban:rural ratio 32 : 68

ROLE OF HEALTH EDUCATION IN HEALTH PROGRAMS

Health education brings about reformation by adaptations which will bring about behavioral changes.

It also can bring about transformation by a social change.

In health programs for an effective health education, following essentials are drafted:
1. Rural community can have traditional folk media for an effective communication. Regional local language usage is a must.
2. Urban community can have recent mass media for an effective communication. National or international language is more effective.

DOCTOR–PATIENT RELATIONSHIP

All social factors are implicated in this relationship. If doctor is authoritative, conflict starts between doctor and patient. Success of a doctor lies in his communication skills, giving sympathetic ear, understanding patient's cultural background, and giving psychological satisfaction to the patient.

Doctor–patient relationship in the practice of modern medicine lies in making patient co-operative from noncooperative.

INTERNATIONAL CLASSIFICATION OF DISEASES

Definition

International Classification of Diseases (ICD) is a system of classification of illness/disease which helps in uniformity of notification and international comparison. ICD-10 (10th revised) has 21 major chapters.

Examples

Chapter 2: Neoplasm (COO-D48), Each chapter contains three character categories to cover its content.
- Z72—problem related to lifestyle.
- For new diseases, unclassified and for research "u" code is used.
- u49 disease of unknown etiology.

ICD-10 has three volumes dealing as under:
Vol. I   Body of ICD with nomenclature
Vol. II Instruction manual
Vol. III Index

Uses
- Uniform classification for accurate comparison
- Decision making in disease prevention
- Health care management
- Research

SUMMARY

Various definitions are given. Highlighted NHD, triad of epidemiology and modes of intervention. Demographic values for 2019 are given. Described holistic approach and doctor–patient relationship.

VIVA VOCE

1. Define health.
2. Mention determinants of health.
3. Define community diagnosis.
4. Define surveillance.
5. What are the risk factors in diabetes?
6. What are the risk factors in accident?
7. Give examples of mortality indictors.
8. What is present birth rate?
9. What is present death rate?
10. What is present growth rate?
11. What are the uses of ICD?

CHAPTER 2: Relationship of Social and Behavioral to Health and Disease

Chapter Outline

- Clinico-Sociocultural and Demographic Assessment of Individual, Family and Community (Medicosocial Case)
- Sociocultural Factors in Health and Diseases
- Barrier to Good Health and Health-Seeking Behavior
- Social and Behavior to Health and Diseases
- Social Security and Health Care

INTRODUCTION

Society, social context and social obligations have highlighted social aspect of health and disease. Social medicine, called medical sociology, deals with social epidemiology, study of cultural factors, study of social relations both in health and disease. It also includes social principles in medical organization.

Social Science

This mainly deals with man in his society. They include history, geography, civics, political science and other discipline which are dealt under behavioral sciences.

Behavioral Science

It deals with sociology, anthropology, psychology, and psychiatry. They do the scientific examination of human behavior.

Medical Sociology

It deals with social anatomy, social physiology, social pathology and social therapy of man acquiring many interactions in his social group.

Examples:
- Social anatomy—age, sex of given population
- Social physiology—good environment of air and water, ideal food for better nutrition
- Social pathology—malnutrition, infant mortality
- Social therapy—personal hygiene to prevent typhoid, wearing *chappal* to prevent hookworm infection.

Tradition, value system, culture, and custom which play a major role in health and disease are studied.

Anthropology

Physical, cultural, social and medical anthropology which determine health status.

Example: Erect posture of man versus varicose vein as physical anthropology.

Psychology

Study of human behavior with response to stimuli in his society.

Psychiatry

Clinical discipline which treats mental illness.

TERMINOLOGY USED

Society: A developed system of interrelationship of man in his group.

Role play: Day-to-day acceptance of placement such as son, father, patient, teacher.

Medicosocial: Study of cultural factors and social relations in connection with illness and social principles in medical organization and in medical treatment.

Problem family: Where members are unable to discharge or prevented from discharging minimum family responsibilities.

Broken family: Where father or mother or both absent on account of disease, deficiency, destitution, dependence, despondency, delinquency or degeneracy.

Belief: Things derived from parents, grandparents and other people which are accepted without trying them to prove they are true.

Poverty line: According to Planning Commission of India report, it is as under:
- Urban area—per capita per month below 264 Rupees or consuming less than 2,100 kcal/capita/day of diet.
- Rural area—per capita per month below 229 Rupees or consuming less than 2,400 kcal/capita/day of diet.

Custom: It is the right way of doing things which is also called folkway.

Mores: Stringent customs are called mores.

Culture: Learned behavior which is socially acquired.

Acculturation: Mix up of two culture and adaptation to new culture.

Case study: Studying and analysing a social unit.

Emotion: Strong feeling of a man/woman.

Motivation: Making a man/woman to accept an action which is installed with reasoning.

Habit: Routine doing of a thing by reflex.

Family: Basic unit of society.

SPECIAL TERMS IN SOCIAL MEDICINE

Social security: Security given to man by social organization for risks to which he/she is exposed such as sickness, death, etc. This aspect includes insurance and assistance. They are categorized as under:
- Life Insurance Corporation of India, Public Provident Fund under public security
- Pension, gratuity under civil service security
- Employees State Insurance Scheme under industry security.

Social defense: For protection against antisocial, criminal behavior of man such as beggary, prostitution, and alcoholism. It is a system developed to defend a society against crime by treating and defending the offended.

Social insurance: Risk of death, risk of accident, risk of fire, risk of disability is covered under insurance schemes. This may be done either by the government, a government organization or by a private organization.

Social diet: Adaptation of eating food, food serving, food catering which are determined by social status, changing custom and civilization.

Social disease: Diseases that have social stigma and human interaction such as tuberculosis, leprosy, etc.

BEHAVIORAL CHANGE COMMUNICATION

It is an interactive process for interventions, be it at individual level or at community level.

Behavioral change communication provides a supportive environment for positive health.

New terminology is *communication for development*.

Use pretested material in communication.

Tools used are:
- Radio
- TV
- Billboard
- Print material
- Internet
- Group presentation
- Community mobilization

Chapter 2: Relationship of Social and Behavioral to Health and Disease

Steps in behavioral change communication:

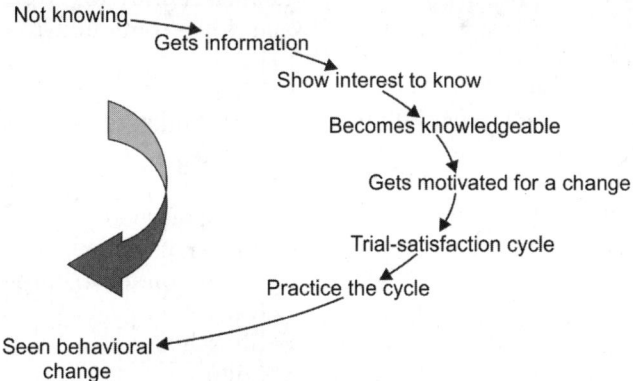

SOCIAL PROBLEMS

We follow social norms. They are the outcome of socialization that means they are conventions that we are used to doing. Social norms are accompanied by sanctions that promote conformity. There are people who refuse to live by the rules that majority of us follow. When people do not show confirmatory to a given set of norms that are accepted by significant number of people in a community, we notice social problems. They are:

- Alcoholism
- Drug abuse or substance abuse
- Sexually transmitted diseases
- Juvenile delinquency
- Prostitution
- Violent criminals
- Unmarried mothers
- Physically challenged

SOCIAL AREA OF INTEREST

Social anatomy: Structure of a society of which it is made of such as age, sex, etc.

Social physiology: Nutrition and ventilation are examples of social physiology.

Social pathology: Social condition causing disease such as Protein-energy malnutrition, diabetes.

Social therapy: Social and political action in disease treatment.

For example: Advice to typhoid patient to avoid relapse (through personal hygiene).

Advice to protect from hookworm infection (wearing chappal when they walk on open defecated area.)

Social obstetrics: Interaction of social and environment on reproductive child health.

Social pediatrics: Application of social medicine in child care for an organized total care.

Socialization: Learning of custom, tradition and belief by man by interaction with his fellow beings. Common types of socialization are:

1. *Primary socialization:* Learning of newborn under mother's care
2. *Secondary socialization:* Late learning of a boy in his school.
3. *Resocialization:* Learning for survival when a person goes to foreign country.

GROUP BEHAVIOR

Social behavior followed by interaction of an individual in a group is called group behavior. Activities of man are regulated by custom, law and social obligations. Always groups are led by a leader. By maintaining solidarity of the group behavior, we have group morale.

Psychosocial events in a society are group activities, group discussions, group opinions and group reactions. Because of group behavior, we come across either progressive reformation or civil unrest. Socialization of an individual and social attitude of society is determined by group behavior.

SOCIAL FACTORS IN HEALTH AND DISEASE

It is known that health and disease are influenced by social factors. Primarily, the level of socioeconomic development of man determines his health status. Common social factors that determine health of an individual as well as a community are:
- Per capita income
- Standard of living
- Family size
- Literacy status
- Poverty
- Malnutrition
- Unemployment

Standard of Living

Standard of living is reflected by ways of living. This is demonstrated by spending capacity and acquiring capacity. Major influencing factors of standard of living are:
- Net national product
- Agricultural product
- Industrial product
- Purchasing capacity
- Population growth
- Educational level
- Per capita income

Standard of living is related to health and disease. High standard of living brings down diarrhea, cholera, tuberculosis, and it improves standard of health status in population. Standard of living determines; (a) Birth, (b) Death, (c) Nutritional level, and (d) Expectation of life.

CLINICO-SOCIOCULTURAL AND DEMOGRAPHIC ASSESSMENT OF INDIVIDUAL, FAMILY AND COMMUNITY (MEDICOSOCIAL CASES)

See **Appendix 1**

SOCIOCULTURAL FACTORS IN HEALTH AND DISEASE (TABLE 2.1)

Cultural factors have stood in the way of health programs. Belief and practice have determined culture, which in turn determine health and disease. Following are common cultural factors in a community:
- Habit
- Belief
- Superstition
- Mores
- Folkway
- Wrath of God
- Breach of taboos
- Sin committed in the past life
- Evil eye
- Ghost action
- Culture
- Tradition
- Food as hot or cold
- Water as holy (even contaminated)
- No "greens" in pregnancy (believed to produce black skin)
- *Purdah* among women
- Circumcision among some religious sects
- Child marriage

BARRIER TO GOOD HEALTH AND HEALTH-SEEKING BEHAVIOR

See **Table 2.1**.

SOCIAL AND BEHAVIOR TO HEALTH AND DISEASE (FAMILY IN HEALTH AND DISEASE)

Biologically related individual live together as family which is the smallest unit of society. There are many family associated functions, which are attached to human behavior. They do have an impact on health and diseases. Family impact is seen in following situations:
- Marriage, pregnancy and lactation
- Infant feeding practices
- Polygamy, polyandry
- Working mother
- Socialization at school
- Son following father in accepting alcoholism, gambling
- Care of the old in a joint family
- Familiar susceptibility for color blindness, schizophrenia, hemophilia
- Broken family
- Family in backward and poor condition

Chapter 2: Relationship of Social and Behavioral to Health and Disease

Table 2.1: Examples of tradition, habit, custom and belief.

Tradition	Habit	Custom	Belief
• Sending pregnant woman for first delivery to her parent's house • Men eat first and later women • Touching the feet of elders • Puncturing ear and nose • Offering pan supari after food in social gathering	• Nail biting • Applying kajal to the cheek of child • Walking barefoot • Application of turmeric powder before bath by women	• No colostrums to the newborn • Onion and garlic not consumed • Apply cow dung to the floor before religious function • Holy dip in river	• Chickenpox is due to wrath of goddess • Leprosy is due to sin of past life • Spirit of ghost cause hysteria • Papaya causes abortion

Problem Family

Where members are unable to discharge or prevented from discharging minimum family responsibilities.

Social Classification (Tables 2.2 To 2.5)

According to Registrar General of England (occupation) oldest.

By Income (Per Capita Income in ₹)

Income alone is not considered for social classification. It gives value of socioeconomic grouping. However, with other variables, many methods are adopted in research methodology.

Table 2.2: Social classification.

Social class	Occupation
I	Professional
II	Managerial
III	Skilled
IV	Semiskilled
V	Unskilled

$$CF = \frac{(\text{Cost inflation index}) \times (\text{Current price index})}{100}$$

1991 inflation index = 206, consumer index = 4.96

$$\text{Correction factor} = \frac{206 \times 4.96}{100} = 10.2176$$

Table 2.3A: Prasad classification (updated).

Social class	Prasad 1961	Updated(1) 1991	Updated(2) 2001	Updated(3) 2019 (Rounded off to hundreds)
I	100 and above	1021 and above	20,503 and above	13,580 and above
II	50–99	510–1020	10,230–20,499	6,800–13,580
III	30–49	306–509	6,130–10,229	4,100–6,800
IV	15–29	154–305	3,076–6,129	2,050–4,100
V	Below 15	Below 153	Below 3,075	Below 2,050

1991 inflation index = 206, 1991 consumer index = 4.96, 1991 correction factor (CF) = 10.2176, 2019 inflation index = 280, 2019 consumer index = 4.85, CF = 13.5800 (correction factor)

2001 inflation index = 406, consumer index = 5.05

$$\text{Correction factor} = \frac{406 \times 5.05}{100} = 20.503$$

2006 inflation index = 480, consumer index = 5.45

$$\text{Correction factor} = \frac{480 \times 5.45}{100} = 26.160$$

2010 inflation index = 635, consumer index = 11.89

$$\text{Correction factor} = \frac{635 \times 11.89}{100} = 75.5015$$

2019 inflation index = 280, consumer index = 4.85

$$\text{Correction factor} = \frac{280 \times 4.85}{100} = 13.5800$$

Note: CF (correction factor) is calculated based on cost inflation index (GOI) and current price index for the year 1991, 2001, 2006, 2010 and 2019 are considered.

$$CF = \frac{(\text{Cost inflation index}) \times (\text{Current price index})}{100}$$

As per calculation:
100 of 1961 is equal to 1,021 at 1991
1,000 of 1991 is equal to 20,503 at 2001
1,000 of 2001 is equal to 26,160 at 2006
1,000 of 2006 is equal to 75,501 at 2010
1,000 of 2010 is equal to 13,580 at 2019

Note: Estimates are done by the author for teaching purpose and the source is from Reserve Bank of India Bulletin December, 2019, The Economic Times, IIM Lucknow and newkerala.com and the indiapost.com.

Table 2.3B: Economic indicators showing cost inflation.

Year	Inflation index	Consumer index	Correction factor	Cost
1961				100.00
1991	206	4.96	10.2176	1021
2001	406	5.05	20.503	20503
2006	480	5.45	26.160	26160
2010	635	11.89	75.5015	75501
2019	280	4.85	13.5800	13580

Note: ₹100/- of 1961 is equal to ₹13,580/- of 2019

Table 2.4: Kuppuswamy classification (modified) for urban areas.

Item			Score
A. Education	Professional, PG		7
	Graduate		6
	Inter		5
	High school		4
	Middle school		3
	Primary		2
	Illiterate		1
B. Occupation	Profession		10
	Semiprofession		6
	Clerk, shop, form		5
	Skilled		4
	Semi-skilled		3
	Unskilled		2
	Unemployed		1
C. Income (per capita)			
	800 and above*	(13,580 and above)@	12
	400–799	(6800–13,580)	10
	300–399	(4,100–6,800)	6
	200–299	(2050–4,100)	4
	120–199	(1,840–2,050)	3
	40–199	(230–1,840)	2
	Below 40	(Below 230)	1

*As per 1988–89 index
@ As per 2019 index

Total score = A + B + C

Social class	Score (total)	Income as per 2019 index
I	26–29	₹ 13,580 and above
II	16–25	₹ 6,800 to 13,580
III	11–15	₹ 4,100 to 6,800
IV	5–10	₹ 2,050 to 4,100
V	Below 5	Rs. Below 2,050

Chapter 2: Relationship of Social and Behavioral to Health and Disease

By Pareek Method
(Pareek Classification for Rural Areas)

For rural areas, Pareek has evolved a method by considering caste, occupation, education, social participation, land holding, housing, farm power, material possession and type of family. It is a form of scoring system for social stratification.

This is based on the following characteristics:
1. Caste
2. Occupation of head of the family
3. Education of head of the family
4. Social participation level
5. Land holding by the head
6. Farm power in terms of bullocks, tractors, ox, sheep, horse
7. Housing
8. Material possession
9. Family type

Socioeconomic Scoring by Grades

Caste
OC	10
BC	8
SC	6

Occupation
Professional	10
Semiprofessional	6
Clerks, shopkeepers	5
Skilled worker	4
Semiskilled worker	3
Unskilled worker	2
Not employed	1

Literacy
PG	7
UG	6
Inter	5
Matric	4
Middle school	3
Primary school	2
Illiterate	1

Literacy of housewife
Degree	8
Inter	7
Matric	6
Primary	6
Illiterate	1

Type of family
Nuclear	6
Joint	4

Housing
Own	6
Rented	2

House type
Pucca	10
Semipucca	6
Kutcha	3

Land holding
Dry land 30 acres/wet land 15 acres	10
20–30 acres/10–15 acres	8
10–20 acres/5–10 acres	6
5–10 acres/2–3 acres	4
Below 5 acres/below 2 acres	3
No land/no land	1

Farm power
Tractor	12
Bullock/ox	2 each
Horse, cow, buffalo	3 each
Donkey	1 each
Sheep or goat	½ each

Material possession
AC	12
Color TV	8
Air cooler	6
Fridge	6
B/W TV	4
Fans	2 each

Social participation
Good	6
Rare	3
Nil	1

Total score
90 and +	Upper class
75–90	Higher middle
60–75	Middle
45–60	Lower middle
30–45	Lower classes
Below 30	Below poverty line (BPL)

Table 2.5: Prabhakara classification (Belonging and achievement), 1982.

	Score			
	0	1	2	3
House	Rented	Lease	Own	-
Room	Nil	1–2	3+	-
Toilet	Shared	Separate	-	-
Kitchen	Not separate	Separate	-	-
Vehicle	Nil	Two wheeler (mechanised)	Two wheeler (auto driven)	-
Radio/Tape recorder	Nil	Own one	Own two	-
Father's education	Illiterate	Primary	Secondary Technical	University
Number of living children	7	3–6	1–2	-

Social class	Score
I	13–15
II	10–12
III	7–9
IV	4–6
V	0–3

SOCIOECONOMIC PROGRAMS

1. *Panchayat Raj* (Power to people)
2. IAY (*Indira Awas Yojana*) shelter to shelterless
3. JRY (*Jawahar Rojgar Yojana*) sustained employment
4. EAS (Employment Assurance Scheme) assured employment
5. MWS (Mission Wells Scheme)
6. IRDP (Integrated Rural Development Program): Provision of asset for production
7. DWACRA (Development of Women and Children in Rural Areas) for economic self-reliance
8. TRYSEM (Training of Rural Youth for Self Employment)
9. Supply of tool kits for rural artisans
10. DPAP (Drought Prone Areas Programme)
11. DDP (Desert Development Programme)
12. Rural Water Supply and Sanitation Programme
13. NSAP (National Social Assistance Program)
14. Old age pension
15. Family benefit
16. Maternity benefit
17. Land reforms
18. Wasteland development

PRESENT GROUPING OF THE COMMUNITY

- *Rural community:* Villages form a specified boundary, specified independent occupation and specified administrative setup.
- *Standard urban area:* A town with a population of 50,000 having encroachment of rural community with mutual socio-economic link.
- *Urban agglomeration:* A few cities with good growth with delineated boundary.
- *Urban community:* Population density is seen of >400 people/sq km and is declared urban area by government.
- *Cosmopolitan community:* Mega cities with above 3-lakh population specified geographic boundary and defined under city municipal corporations.

Chapter 2: Relationship of Social and Behavioral to Health and Disease

SOCIAL AGENCIES

Social agencies carry out social welfare services as an integral part of community development. There are about 60,000 voluntary organizations in India doing yeomen services. They do the job of social activities which can b: (a) general welfare activities, (b) women welfare activities, (c) child welfare activities, (d) specific disease control, and (e) specific welfare activities.

India is becoming welfare state in the sense that it is ensuring a minimum standard of living for all people as a right of citizenship. It is trying to provide economic justice and equalities. Welfare is introduced in factory, for old aged and many more areas. Common welfare services for the old age are—(a) home care of aged sick, (b) meals on wheels (low cost or free), (c) hospital conveyance to the sick, (d) performance of household chores by home help, and (e) companionship to the lonely old.

INTERVIEWING TECHNIQUE

It is part and parcel of survey and investigation. Main aim is to collect correct and proper information required for the survey or investigation.

Types

1. Predetermined question method (structured)
2. On the spot question method (unstructured)
3. Situation method (focused)
4. Re-interview method (impact study)

Characters of good interview are as follow:
- Calm atmosphere maintained
- Good contact is established
- Methodical approach to recall all questions
- Greater care in personal matters
- Guidance and encouragement given frequently
- Recording in short form not wasting much time
- Bringing to close with thanksgiving
- Report prepared on the same day

The personnel who has done special training course in social work (MSW) is appropriate since he is trained in interview techniques.

MEDICAL ECONOMICS

Sickness bringing loss of productivity and costing the exchequer have led to the concept of medical economics. Optimum use of health resources in treatment through cost benefit, cost effectiveness, and budgeting help in maximizing health situation and upbringing socioeconomic development.

Attending to only required investigation and required treatment by an essential drug commands significant enlistment to a common man.

Drug indenting through ABC analysis in a hospital (large quantity of bulk purchase of cheaper drugs to many)—(a) sufficient quantity of average costing drugs to be selected, (b) small quantity of costly to be elective (c) help a good budgeting which can run over a period of few months.

Treating and managing the case suiting to his family's economic background is a typical example of medical economics.

GEOGRAPHIC PATHOLOGY

It is also known as geomedicine or medical ecology. Maladjustment to environment peculiar to a given geographical area determines disease process.

Understanding geographic pathology helps to take up community treatment with community diagnosis.

Examples:
a. Malaria rampant in swampy district
b. Typhus is more in hilly areas among military troops
c. Leprosy is hyperendemic in eastern coastal regions
d. Trachoma is hyperendemic in Rajasthan.

HOSPITAL SOCIOLOGY

Structure:
- Made of different units/departments with category of manpower class IV to class I working force
- Drugs, medicaments, equipment, furniture

Functions:
- Treatment ambulatory
- Treatment inpatient
- Laboratory investigations
- Surgical procedures

Characters:
- Ethics and code on medical, nursing, dental profession
- Doctor–patient relationship

Pathology:
- Interprofessional disagreement
- Medical industry—high fee for service

Therapy:
- National policy of insurance
- Medical social workers to link between patient and hospital
- Consumer Protection Act.

KNOWLEDGE, ATTITUDE, AND PRACTICE (TABLE 2.6)

Knowledge, attitude, and practice (KAP) is the basis of IEC (information, education and communication) (health education) where a person gets information by many modes which becomes his knowledge, then gets motivated to have attitude and adopts to maintain a practice. Current KAP helps to set up health campaign. Uses of KAP are:
1. Can find people's health behavior
2. Impact of a health program is known, such as Universal Immunization Programme (UIP) or Intensified Pulse Polio Immunization (IPPI)
3. Early detection and prevention is easy

Table 2.6: Examples for knowledge, attitude, and practice (KAP).

Knowledge	Attitude	Practice
Heard of leprosy	Penicillin cures pneumonia (positive attitude)	Leprosy child attends school
Seen a case of leprosy	Leprosy is incurable (negative attitude)	HIV-positive person works as typist

4. Need of special health education like AIDS education, cancer education, and population education is established in a community.
5. Health services utilization is maximized.

SOCIAL SECURITY AND HEALTH CARE

Security provided by the society through an organized effort against risks to which members are exposed is called social security. Common risks are sickness, invalidity, maternity, and death.

Society has responsibility to poor, old, disabled and dependants for their welfare and security. Tax supported rehabilitations have come up recently. It attacks on five giants, viz., wants, disease, ignorance, squalor and idleness.

Social security for industrial workers is:
1. Workmen's Compensation Act, 1923
2. Employees' State Insurance Act, 1948
3. Central Maternity Benefit Act, 1961
4. The Family Pension Scheme, 1971.

Definition

Social security comprises of all schemes providing for income security and social service through appropriate organization. In developed countries, social security covers the following areas:
- Retirements, Survival, Disability Insurance (RSDI)
- Unemployment Insurance (UI)
- Old age, blind aid and disabled aid.

Based on above schemes, India has following categories of security to its citizen:
- *Civil services*
  - Pension
  - Gratuity
  - Provident fund
  - Family pension
  - Comprehensive medical care [Central Government Health Scheme (CGHS)]
- *Armed force*
  - Pension
  - Insurance

Chapter 2: Relationship of Social and Behavioral to Health and Disease

- *Industrial workers:* Benefits like maternity, sickness, medical, disability, dependant and funeral
- *Public*
  - Life insurance
  - Accident insurance
  - Fire insurance
  - Crop insurance
  - Insurance on theft
  - Public Provident Fund

Legislative Support for Social Security

- Borstal Schools Act for Adolescent
- Gambling Act, 1867
- The Prison Act, 1894
- Employees State Insurance Act (ESIC) 1948
- IFA, 1948
- Central Probation of Offenders Act, 1951
- Employees Provident Fund Act, 1952
- Central Children Act, 1960
- The Reformatory School Act, 1897
- Suppression of Immoral Traffic Act to protect young girls (SITA)

Social Security

Main approaches to social security:
- Social assistance
- Social defense
- Social insurance

Social Assistance (Noncontributory)

Many areas of needed assistance are catered through social assistance. This forms a wall of security to certain selected category of people in a society.

For example, old age pension, widow pension, assistance to leprosy patients, family planning assistance, geriatric care through old age homes, employment scheme to unemployed graduates.

Social welfare department of Government of India and state governments, women welfare organizations, child welfare organizations have various programs under social assistance. Recent welfare schemes are:
- Maternity assistance to the poor by state government
- Senior citizen facility in state and central government

Social Defense (Protection)

It is mainly protection of society from antisocial, criminal conducts.
For example:
- Criminal punishment
- Deviant counseling under care
- Anti-dowry Act
- Juvenile delinquency control
- Eradication of beggary
- Welfare of prisoners
- Prohibition for regulation of alcohol
- Drug abuse management
- Gambling control
- Prostitution control
- Suicide counseling

Under the Department of Social Welfare, National Institute of Social Defence is regulating above activities in India.

Social Insurance (Contributory)

To protect the interest of each individual in a society, insurance has become part of social security.
For example:
- ESI benefits
- Crop insurance
- Accident insurance
- Workman
- Compensation
- Employee provident fund provision
- Family pension
- Insurance against theft
- Insurance for health

These insurance facilities in society takes care of all risks which are seen in the form of sickness, invalidity, maternity, old age, death, loss of property, etc. Both public and private agencies are involved in this provision.

Comprehensive Social Security

Under the Constitution of India (Article 41 and 42, of part II), a new venture is made to provide comprehensive social security to each and every individual in the society through various Acts passed in the Parliament.

They are:
- Social service like education, employment, medical care through organized institutions.
- Social welfare for the weaker section of society,
- Social insurance to provide income security,
- Social assistance to the needy, and
- Social defense to protect the society.

In all, security of employment, income and power to work form the aim of comprehensive social security. Comprehensive social security includes holistic health care, protection, rehabilitation and motivation for gainful employment, economic growth, specific protection against social evils, health aspect of special groups, legislation and community approaches to protect social structure.

SUMMARY

Social sciences and behavioral sciences are related to health and disease. Sociocultural factors are described. Social security and health are described.

VIVA VOCE

1. Give examples for social therapy.
2. Define problem family.
3. Name common social diseases.
4. Give examples for common cultural factors in community.
5. Expand DWAKRA.
6. What is ABC analysis in hospital drug management?
7. Define KAP and mention its uses.
8. Mention three approaches in social security.

CHAPTER 3: Environmental Health Problems

CHAPTER OUTLINE

- Major components of physical environment
- Water and other components
- Meteorology
- Housing and town planning
- Waste disposal
- Human body disposal and sanitation

EVOLUTION

- Environmental hygiene
- Environmental sanitation
- Environmental health

Definition—Environmental Sanitation

Control of all those factors in man's physical environment which exercise or may exercise a deleterious effect on his physical development, health and survival [World Health Organization (WHO)].

Mega environment includes:
- Physical environment
- Biological environment
- Social environment
- Chemical environment
- Spiritual environment

Relation to Health

Ill-effects of Atmospheric Pollution

- Air pollution
- Water pollution
- Noise pollution
- Soil pollution

Environmental Health Services

- Drinking water
- Solid waste disposal
- Excreta disposal
- Prevention of food adulteration
- Prevention of industrial hazard
- Prevention of vector-borne disease
- Prevention of rodent-borne disease
- Safe housing
- Management of people congregation areas.
- Biomedical waste management
- Greenhouse effect management
- Management for sustained development

Access to safe water is 88% and access to adequate sanitation is 31% in India.

MAJOR COMPONENTS OF PHYSICAL ENVIRONMENT

- Water
- Meteorology
- Air
- Housing
- Ventilation
- Waste disposal
- Lighting
- Noise
- Radiation

WATER AND OTHER COMPONENTS

Water is an essential component of life. It is an integral part of reproductive and child health (RCH), food and nutrition, and health education.

Requirement: 150–200 liters per day per head.

Safe and Wholesome Water

Usable (potable) water with acceptable taste and free from chemicals and pathogens.

Uses

- *Domestic:* Cooking, drinking, bathing, garden, ablution
- *Public:* Swimming pool, fountain, pond, tank, public garden (park)
- Industry
- Agriculture
- Electricity production

Sources (Fig. 3.1)

- *Rain water:* Follows water cycle. It is pure. It has less impurities and is less tasty.
- *Surface water:* Collected water, such as *artificial lake*. This cannot be stored for longer time. There is a likelihood of contamination by animal and human activities.

Running water, such as *river* is comparatively clean since natural purification by aeration, oxidation, and dilution takes place. Chance of contamination by animal and human activities exists.

Tanks and *ponds* do not have elements of self-purification in them. They need periodic cleaning.

Impounding reservoirs are artificial lakes that are good source of water to cities. Water is drained from "catchment area", which are the places for human and animal intrusion.

- *Underground water:* It is a major source of water in India.

Following are the types of well in India:
- Kucha well
- Pucca well
- Step well (connected with eradicated guinea worm infection)
- Artesian well
- Dug well
- Tube well

Difference between Shallow and Deep Well

Shallow well
- Taps water from above impervious layer
- Soft (less mineral)
- Gross contamination
- Dries up

Deep well
- Taps from below impervious layer
- Hard

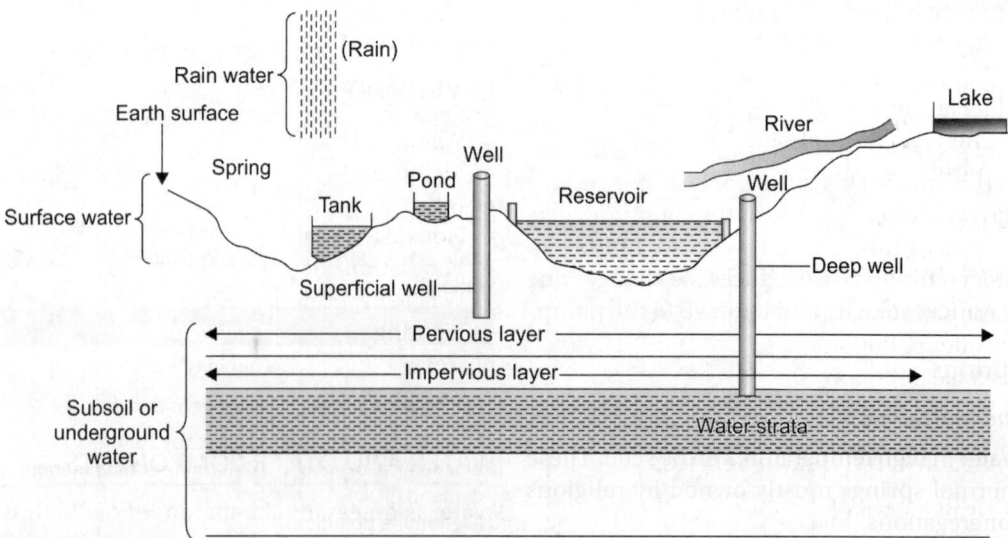

Fig. 3.1: Source of water.

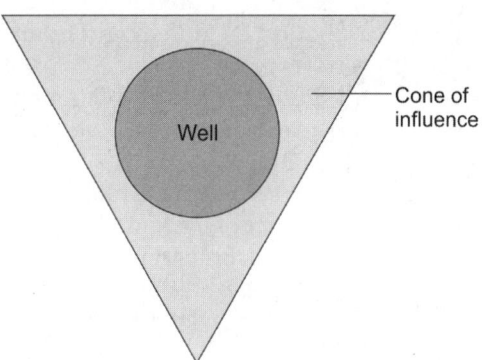

Fig. 3.2: Zone of influence.

- Least contamination
- Continuous supply

Zone of influence (cone of influence) **(Fig. 3.2):** Area under influence for well contamination which is considered for a sanitary well.

Criteria for sanitary well:
- Good location
- Good cement lining
- Good parapet and platform
- Good drain
- Cover and a hand pump.

Tube Well

They are driven wells yielding potable water. Highest number of tube wells is seen in Chandigarh.

Critical Velocity

By continuous use over 12 hours a day by a hand pump, the water in geological strata may go less and, later, sand and water will start coming. This is the point of appearance of *critical velocity, which* is the common cause of spoiled tube wells. Five to six hours gap after continuous use reduces the changes due to critical velocity and damage to the pump.

Springs

Thermal Springs

Water in high temperature can be seen. These thermal springs mostly owned by religious congregations.

Mineral Springs

Water contains sulfur. Sanctity is associated with therapeutic value for skin infection.

Shallow Springs

Easily gets contaminated.

Deep Springs

It is a continuous source.

Hardness of Water

Soap-destroying power of water is hardness.

Temporary hardness: It is by bicarbonate of calcium and magnesium (carbonate hardness). It is removed by boiling, addition of lime, addition of sodium bicarbonate and permutation process.

Permanent hardness: It is by sulfates of calcium and magnesium (noncarbonate hardness). This is removed by the addition of sodium carbonate and by base exchange process.

Degree of Hardness

Soft—below 50 ppm (Below 1 mEq/L)

Hard—50–300 ppm (1–3 mEq/L)

Very hard—above 300 ppm (Above 3 mEq/L) (50 ppm = 1 mEq/L)

Public Health Importance

Continuous soft water consumption is related with arteriosclerosis, atherosclerosis, hypertension, IHD.

Water Pollution (Table 3.1)

Table 3.1: Difference between pollution and contamination.

Pollution	Contamination
Turbidity+	Turbidity + or –
Pathogens doubtful	Pathogens definite
Suspended solids and biochemical oxygen demand (BOD) (Determine pollution)	Microscopy culture (Determine contamination)

Waterborne Disease (Direct Cause)

- Bacterial—cholera, typhoid, GE
- Viral—IH, polio, *Rotavirus*
- Protozoa—amoebiasis, giardiasis

Etiology of Waterborne Diseases—Jaundice, Hepatitis, Diarrhea

Waterborne diseases are by microbes spreading via contaminated water. Using infected water for drinking, food preparation, and washing clothes precipitates the infection. It affects children who have poor personal hygiene and weak immunity. Sometimes, it becomes life threatening. Nearly 900 million people lack basic drinking water. Majority is dependent on surface water. Additionally, fecal contamination of water makes the situation worse causing 6 lacs diarrheal deaths every year.

Water forms part of every walk of life and hence can get contaminated causing waterborne diseases. Further, it is aggravated by the fact that water is associated with culture and spiritual walks of life. Biological agents that cause **waterborne diseases** are:

- *Bacterial:* Typhoid, paratyphoid, dysentery, infantile diarrhea, cholera
- *Viral:* Hepatitis, polio, infantile *Rotavirus*
- *Protozoal:* Amoebiasis, giardiasis
- *Helminthic:* Roundworm, threadworm
- *Leptospiral:* Weil's disease
- *Others:* Schistosomiasis, Guinea worm, fish tapeworm

Jaundice

It is associated with chronic active hepatitis which includes following pathogens:

- Hepatitis A virus (HAV)
- Hepatitis B virus (HBV)
- Hepatitis C virus (HCV)
- Hepatitis D virus (HDV)
- Hepatitis E virus (HEV), and
- Hepatitis G virus (HGV)

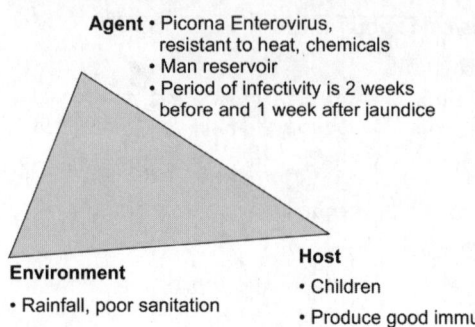

Epidemiology of hepatitis A

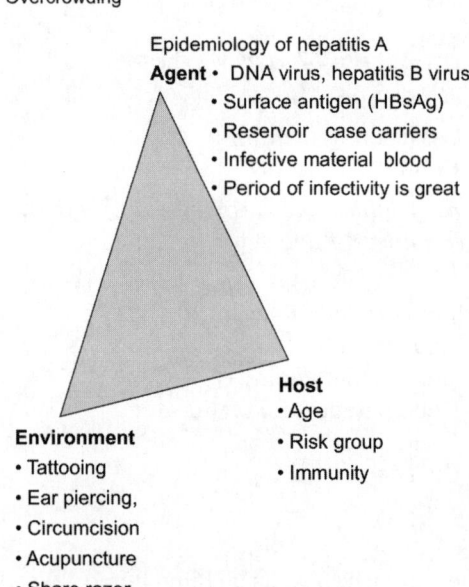

Epidemiology of hepatitis B

Detail of the disease is described under communicable diseases.

Similarly, etiology and epidemiology of diarrhea is detailed under communicable diseases.

Water-related Disease (Indirect Cause)

- Helminthic infestation
- Leptospiral infection
- Schistosomiasis
- Guinea worm infection
- Fish tapeworm

Public Health Chemistry of Water

It considers qualitative analysis of water by physical, chemical, biological, virological, and radiological examinations.

Physical Examination

* Turbidity
* Color
* Taste
* Odor

Chemical Examination

a. *Definitely toxic:*
   * Lead   0.01 ppm
   * Arsenic   0.01 ppm
   * Cyanide   0.07 ppm
   * Cadmium   0.003 ppm
   * Selenium   0.01 ppm
   * Mercury   0.001 ppm

b. *Possibly toxic:*
   * F_2 0.5–0.8 ppm
   * NO_3 45 ppm
   * PAH   0.2 mg

c. *Probably toxic:*
   * Total solid 500 ppm
   * Hardness   100 ppm
   * SO_4 200 ppm
   * Cl_2 200 ppm
   * Calcium   75 ppm
   * Magnesium   30 ppm
   * Zn   5 ppm
   * Fe   0.1 ppm
   * Mn   0.05 ppm
   * Cu   0.05 ppm
   * Phenolic substance   0.1 ppm

Chemical Indicators of Water Pollution

* Chloride   (600 ppm)
* Free ammonia   (0.05 ppm)
* Albuminoid ammonia   (0.1 ppm)
* N_2 as NO_2 (Zero)
* N_2 as NO_3 (1 ppm), and
* O_2 dissolved   (5 ppm)

Tolerable Daily Intake

Estimation of a chemical substance in water in mg per kg body weight or in mg per kg body weight which is ingested every day but do not produce toxicity. This can be found out by:

$$\text{Tolerable daily intake} = \frac{\text{Lowest observed adverse effect level}}{\text{Uncertainty factors}}$$

For the purpose of risk calculation, guideline values are calculated by using available tolerable daily intake by the following formula;

$$\text{Guide line value} = \frac{\text{Tolerable daily intake} \times \text{Body weight} \times \text{Fraction of allocated TDI in Water}}{\text{Quantity of water consumed in a day}}$$

Bacteriological Analysis

Presumptive coliform test (PCT) is done by multiple tube method (MTM). Coliform organisms, such as *Escherichia coli, Clostridium perfringens* and fecal streptococci, which are present in human excreta, even in small quantity, confirm fecal contamination.

PCT = No. of coliform per 100 mL.

PCT guidelines:
* Excellent—Zero/100 mL
* Satisfactory—1–2/100 mL
* Suspicious—3–10/100 mL
* Unfit—10+/100 mL

Virological Examination

Culture for virus should not yield any plaque-forming units (PFU) on culture.

Biological Examination

Microscopic examination should show water free from pathogens of any kind.

Radiological Examination

Water should not contain α and β activity (3 picocuries and 30 picocuries, respectively).

Purification of Water for Domestic Purposes (Small Scale)

* *Boiling:* 10 minutes of boiling kills bacteria, removes temporary hardness, but must be kept in the same container in which the water was boiled.
* *Ozone:* Costly, not applicable.
* *Ultraviolet rays:* Costly, not recommendable.
* *Lime:* Cheap, helpful in only gross contamination. There is usefulness as disinfectant but not in practice.

- *Iodine:* High cost and its thyroid activity do not permit. It is only accepted as emergency water purification.
- *Bleaching powder:* Very common agent, it is a white amorphous powder, contains 33% of available chlorine.
  In case of stabilized bleach,
  = $CaOCl_2$ + Excess lime – 70% available Cl_2
  Requirement
  - 1 ounce per 1,000 gallons of water
  - Should yield residual chlorine of 0.2 ppm after 30 minutes of contact period

  But, turbid and polluted water cannot be disinfected.
- *$KMNO_4$:* An oxidizing agent; it kills *Vibrio cholerae*. Drawback is its color, smell and taste.
- *Chlorine tablet:* Costly and cannot be used for turbid water
  1 tablet (0.5 G) for 20 liters; Double action tablet by National Environmental Engineering Research Institute (NEERI).
  = Alum + $CaOCl_2$ + $NaHCO_3$ + Talc
  In District Health Policy, halazone tablets for solution are supplied in 1,000 packs. Each tablet contains 4 mg and one tablet per one liter and a minimum of contact period of 15 minutes is advocated.
- *Filters:*
  - Chamberland (Porcelain),
  - Berkefeld (Infusorial), and
  - Katadyn (Silver coated).

Filter brings about bacteriological purity. Since they cannot filter viruses, they are not useful in prevention of polio, jaundice, *Rotavirus*, GE of viral origin.

Well Disinfection

Step 1: Volume of water is determined by:
a. British value (foot)
   Circular well $D^2 \times W \times 5$ = gallons
   (D = Diameter in ft., W = Depth of water in ft).
   Square well $L \times B \times H \times 6.25$ = gallons (L = Length (ft), B = Breadth (ft), Height in ft).
b. Metric value (meter)
   $$\frac{3.14 \times d^2 \times h}{4} \times 1000 = \text{Liters}$$
   d = Diameter (meter)
   h = Depth (meter)

Step 2: Chlorine demand is found out by Horrock's test.

Apparatus
- Six white cups
- One black cup
- One scoop (2 g capacity)
- Stirring rods
- Glass pipette
- Reagent—cadmium iodide bottle
- Reagent—starch bottle

Procedure
Six white cups are filled with sample of water up to the mark. They are labeled numerically (1 to 6). Standard solution of bleaching powder is prepared in black cup by mixing one scoop $CaOCl_2$. This is taken in pipette to add one drop to first, two drops to second, till six drops to sixth. By doing with periodic stirring, it is allowed for 30 minutes for reaction to take place.

After 30 minutes, three drops cadmium iodide and 1 mL starch solution is added to all white cups. Blue color appearance is noted. From this, chlorine demand is calculated. (If no blue color, again experiment is repeated with 6–12 drops of stock solution).

For example, if 5th cup onward blue color, then $5 \times 2 = 10$ g/100 gallon is Cl_2 demand.

Step 3: Required quantity of bleaching powder is taken, prepared to paste in the beginning and later to solution.

Step 4: Mixing is done with supernatant clear solution obtained in step 3 (Better done in late evening).

Step 5: Allowed for half an hour (Better overnight).

Step 6: Residual chlorine is found out which should be 0.2 ppm [By orthotolidine (OT) test and orthotolidine-arsenite (OTA) test].

Double Pot Method
It is a NEERI device.
Mixture of $CaOCl_2$ and sand (1:2) in inner pot, which is kept in outer pot.

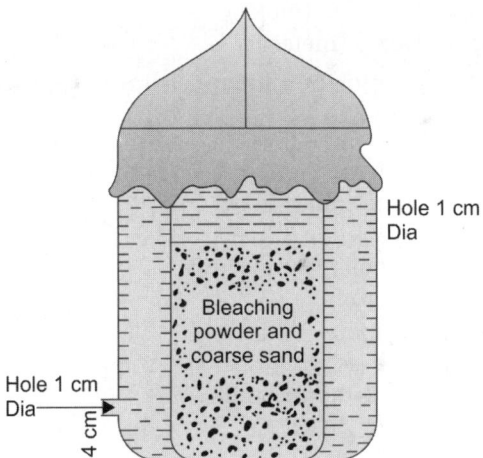

Fig. 3.3: Double pot method.

This double pot, when immersed, is found useful to disinfect a well for a period of over 2 weeks **(Fig. 3.3)**.

Purification in Large Scale

Storage in reservoir
* Suspended impurities will settle down
* Aerobe oxidises organic matter
* Bacterial count drops down, and
* Can be stored for 15 days.

Slow Sand Filters (Table 3.2)

Effective size of sand = 0.15–0.30 mm

First mechanical strain occurs. Later, vital layer is formed by algae, bacteria, plankton, and diatoms (It is also called biological layer or zoogleal layer). The development of vital layer is called ripening of filter, which:
* Removes organic matter
* Holds bacteria
* Oxidizes organic material.

Table 3.2: Difference between slow sand filter (SSF) and rapid sand filter (RSF).

	SSF	RSF
Vital layer	+	–
Alum as coagulant	–	+
Area of operation	Big	Small
Sand size	0.15 mm	0.45 mm
Scraping	Manual	By power
Quality	Very good	Fair

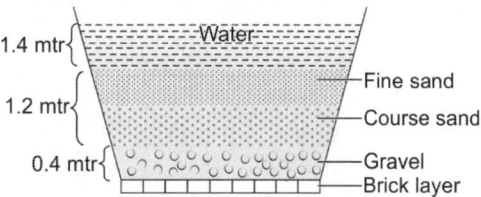

Fig. 3.4: Slow sand filter.

Till biological layer forms, water run to waste. Yield—2–3 million gallons/acre/day **(Fig. 3.4)**.

Loss of Head

When vital layer increases in thickness, *loss of head* occurs. If this is above 4 feet, "scraping the filter" is needed (a manual process) **(Figs. 3.5A and B)**.

Advantages
* Simple
* Economic
* High quality

Rapid Sand Filters (Fig. 3.6)

This was introduced to the world 80 years after the discovery of slow sand filter.

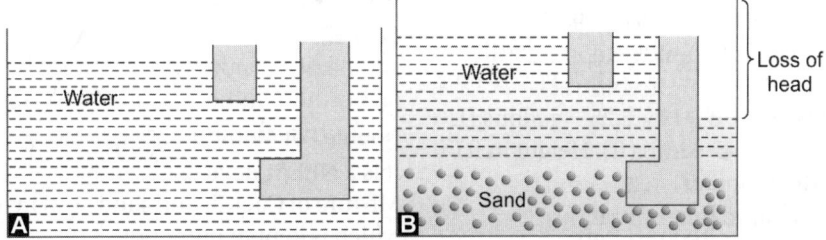

Figs. 3.5A and B: Loss of head.

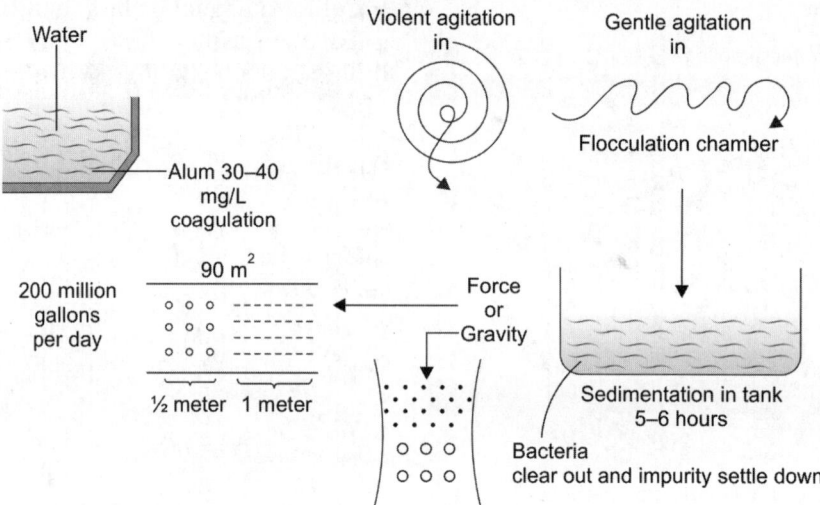

Fig. 3.6: Rapid sand filter.

a. Gravity type, e.g., Paterson filter.
b. Pressure type, e.g., Candy filter.

Here, no vital layer is needed. Alum flock brings about changes in surface tension which help clear out of impurities.

Advantages:
- Directly done
- Less space needed
- Rapid filtration
- Washing easy (back-wash)

Chlorination

By
- Chlorine gas—cheap, quick, efficient and easy
- Chloramine—bad taste, slow action
- Perchloron—65% available Cl_2
- Bleaching powder ($CaOCl_2$)—best
- Liquid chlorine

Principle
- Water must be clean and clear.
- Chlorine demand should be known.
- Contact period 30 minutes (overnight).
- Margin of safety (residual Cl_2 0.2 ppm after 30 minutes contact).

Types
- Prechlorination (before filtration)
- Postchlorination (after filtration)
- Combined (pre and post)
- Super chlorination (excess quantity of $CaOCl_2$ added), and
- Breaking point chlorination (break point).

Breakpoint chlorination (Fig. 3.7)

It refers to a point at which no chlorine, no bacteria, no oxidizable matter are present in the process of chlorination and that point is called breaking point chlorination (break point).

Water sampling (Tables 3.3 to 3.5)

It is a collection of water for public health analysis.

For physical and chemical analysis: Glass stopper, clean natural glass made bottle with two-liter capacity (Winchester quart bottle).

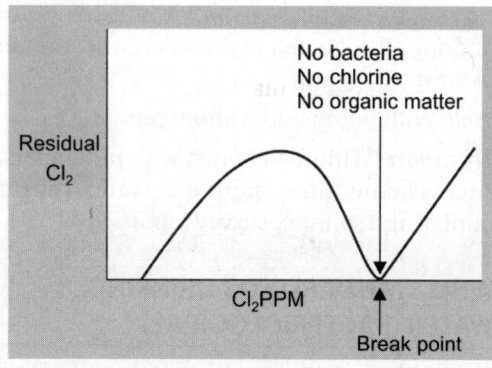

Fig. 3.7: Breakpoint chlorination.

Chapter 3: Environmental Health Problems

Periodicity

Table 3.3: Water sampling.

Population	Sampling
5,000	Once in 30 days
10,000	Once in 15 days
20,000	Once in 7 days
50,000	Once in 3 days
100,000	Everyday

Time Limit of Water Sampling
a. Physical and chemical

Table 3.4: Time limit of water sampling.

Type	Before
Unpolluted	Within 72 hours
Fairly pure	Within 48 hours
Polluted	Within 12 hours
Sullage and sewage +	As soon as reaches

b. For bacteriological

Table 3.5: Time limit of water sampling.

Type	Before
Pure	Within 12 hours
Impure	Within 6 hours

For bacteriological analysis: Neutral glass made of glass stopper bottle with 200–250 mL capacity (If water contains chlorine, sodium thiosulphate is used to wash bottle before sterilization).

Method of Collection

Tap: Regularly used and not in use. After heat sterilization of tip of a tap, midstream is collected.

River: Not too near or too far off from point of draw off collected in direction with stream of flow.

Well: With pump and without pump.

Transport: Within 48 hours, with particulars, such as date, time, source of water, recent rainfall and sanitary survey report.

WHO STANDARD FOR DRINKING WATER (BACTERIOLOGICAL)

1. In 95% sample, no coliform at any time.
2. No *Escherichia coli* in any sample in 100 mL.
3. Coliform should be less than 10/100 mL (MPN).
4. Should not be positive in two consecutive samples.

SURVEILLANCE OF DRINKING WATER QUALITY

It is a public health measure to prevent waterborne diseases.

Elements

- Sanitary survey
- Water sampling
- Bacteriological surveillance by PCT and colony count
- Biological examination, and
- Chemical surveillance

Surveillance Function

- Approval of new water source
- Water store protection
- Water filtration plant maintenance
- Periodic sanitary survey of water source
- Monitoring of public health laboratory services
- Good sanitary contractorship in well construction and in pump installation
- Quality control of bottle water
- Quality control of ice factory

SWIMMING POOL SANITATION

Public health importance
- Athlete foot (fungal infection)
- Infection of eye, ear, nose, throat
- URI
- Intestinal parasitism
- Accidents

Special Note: HIV/AIDS is not transmitted through swimming pools.

Public Health Measure in Swimming Pool

- Personal hygiene by users (not to urinate, etc.)
- About 15% of water supplementation every day.
- Chlorination of 1 ppm.
- Periodic water examinations for pathogens.

NATIONAL WATER SUPPLY AND SANITATION PROGRAM

It was instituted in 1954.

In 1972, Accelerated Rural Water Supply Program (ARWSP) was started as a special program.

In Five-Year Plan, rural water supply is included in Minimum Needs Program.

Problem Village (If anyone is present)
- No source of water is available within a radius of 1.6 km.
- Water is available at a depth of below 15 meters.
- Water source has excess salinity, iron, fluorides or toxic elements.

Current access of water: With one hand pump per 250 population by the program (1981). About 88% are accessible to water supply.

WATER POLLUTION LAW

Passed in 1974 as legal protection to water pollution. Power is vested with Central and State Water Boards.

AIR

Air pollution involves dust, smoke, toxic gases, chemical vapor, and pathogens.

Composition of Air

- Nitrogen 78.1%
- Oxygen 20.9%
- Carbon monoxide 0.03%, and
- Remaining—traces of gases (argon, neon, krypton, xenon, helium).

Overcrowding

Physical Effect
- Temperature increases
- Humidity increases
- Air movement decreases, and
- Dust and bacteria become evident

Chemical Effect
- Oxygen decreases, and
- Carbon monoxide increases

Discomfort and heat retention by physical changes through skin are major effect.

Indicators for Comfort
- Cooling power of the air
  Temperature 70–80°F comfort zone humidity 40–50%
- CET (Globe thermometer is used which records temperature by radiant heat also)
- Predicted 4-hour sweat rate (P_4SR)—three is the upper limit of comfort zone.

Source of Air Pollution

- Industries
- Combustion
- Vehicle

Indicators of Air Pollution

- Carbon monoxide (8-hour average concentration)
  RTO criteria of emission in standard petrol vehicle
  - Four wheeler—3.0%
  - Three wheeler—4.5%
  - Two wheeler—4.5%
  Diesel vehicle—65 units (hartridge)
- Sulfur dioxide
- Lead
- Carbon dioxide
- Cadmium
- Hydrogen sulfide
- Ozone
- Polycyclic aromatic hydrocarbons (PAHs)
- Hydrocarbons
- Particulate matter

Effects of Air Pollution

- Acute bronchitis
- Chronic bronchitis
- Carcinoma lung
- Bronchial asthma
- Respiratory allergy

Inversion in Air Pollution

It is the dangerous state of air pollution. Dissemination of pollutants depends upon air movement and air temperature. Vertical

Chapter 3: Environmental Health Problems

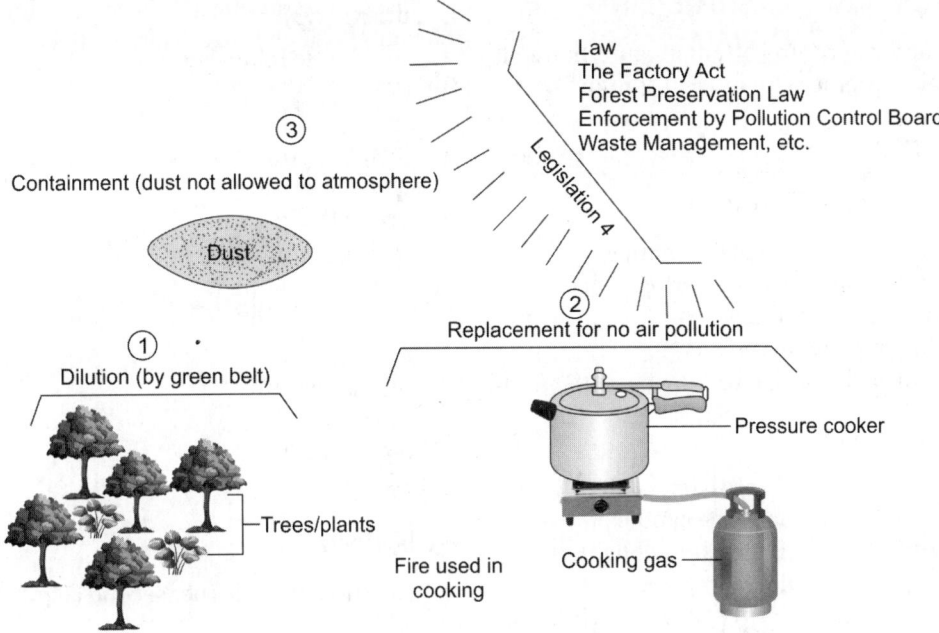

Fig. 3.8: Air pollution control.

temperature gradient determines pollutant dispersion in atmosphere. If hot air layer overlies cold air layer, vertical motion is stopped and pollutants remain trapped in lower level. This process is called *inversion*.

Control of Air Pollution (Fig. 3.8)

Air disinfection done by:
- Mechanical ventilators
- Ultraviolet radiation
- Use of triethylene glycol

VENTILATION

Natural Ventilation

- Perflation, aspiration, diffusion and inequality of temperature
- Inlet
  - Sash window
  - Brick perforated
  - Tobin tube
  - Sherringham value, and
  - McKinnell ventilator
- Outlet
  - Top window (ventilator)
  - Louvered outlet, and
  - McKinnell ventilator

Mechanical Ventilation

- Exhaust ventilation
- Plenum ventilation
- Combined ventilation
- Air conditioning

Cross Ventilation

Quality of air is maintained by easy flow of air, by entry and exit at same level, which helps to obtain required temperature, humidity and purity of air **(Fig. 3.9)**.

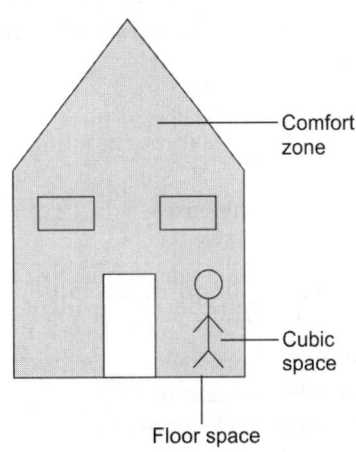

Fig. 3.9: Standards of ventilation.

Air Conditioning

Simultaneous control of temperature, humidity and air movement for human comfort.

LIGHTING

Uses of Proper Lighting

- Body temperature maintenance
- Good physical activity performance
- Skin pigment synthesis
- Vitamin D synthesis
- Good acuity of vision

Measurement

Foot candle: Expression of light at one foot of a candle
Lumen: Expression of light in 1 sq. ft area
Foot Lambert: Expression of light for brightness

Daylight factor (DF)

$$= \frac{\text{Indoor illumination}}{\text{Outdoor illumination}} \times 100$$

(normal requirement of DF = 8–10%).

Types

1. Natural light by sunlight (direct or reflection).
2. Artificial light by filament lamp and fluorescent lamp (direct, indirect, direct-indirect).

Recommended Standard (Illumination)

- 400 lux for general work
- 800 lux for skilled work
  (Sunlight is 100,000 lux, moonlight is 0.1 lux)

NOISE

It is unwanted sound in unwanted place causing nuisance. It is the price paid for civilization.

Loudness (dB)

$$dB = \frac{\text{Sound in question}}{\text{Smallest audible noise}}$$

- Whisper 30 dB
- Usual talk 60 dB
- Street 90 dB
- Road-roller 120 dB

Acceptable Levels

- Residence 25
- Commercial 40
- Industry 40
- Education 30
- Hospital 20

Pitch (Hertz)

It is measured in cycles per second (**Fig. 3.10**).

RADIATION

Importance

- It is a part of environment.
- Radiation hygiene is important in science and technology.
- Role of International Commission on Radiological Protection (ICRP), International Atomic Energy Agency (IAEA), and WHO is stressed.
- Effect on genetic, water, and atomic energy.

Measurement

r = Amount of radiation absorbed in air at a given point [No. of ions produced in 1 mL air (equivalent to C = coulomb)]. SI unit coulomb per kilogram (C/kg) is used. This is the unit for exposure.

Rad = Radioactive energy absorbed per gram of tissue (dissipation of 100 ergs per gram of exposed tissue) (equivalent to Gy = gray). As SI unit gray (Gy) is the unit of absorbed dose.

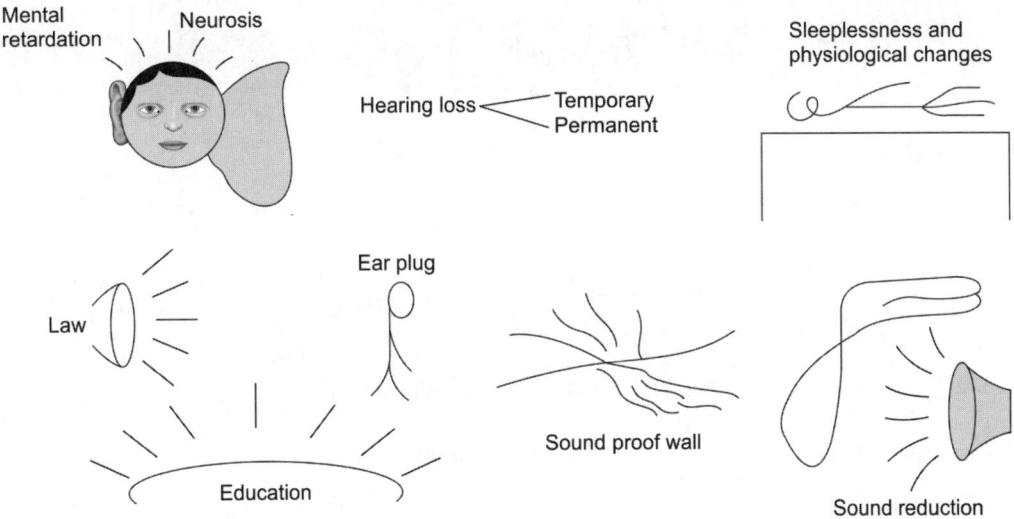

Fig. 3.10: Effect and control of noise pollution.

Rem = The device of potential danger to health. As SI unit Sievert (Sv) is dose equivalent. (Rad + factor of potential danger) [equivalent to J (Joule)].

Dose Equivalent

Present concept is dose equivalent which is obtained by multiplying absorbed dose and quality factor.

Dose equivalent = (Absorbed dose) × (Quality factor)
$$H = (D) \times (Q)$$

Types

1. Natural
   - Cosmic rays
   - Thorium, uranium, radium (radioactive elements)
   - Thoron, radon (radioactive gases)
2. Artificial
   - X-ray
   - Nuclear explosion

Difference between Radiation and Ionizing Radiation

- Radiation is energy particle or electromagnetic waves.
- Ionizing radiation is radiation which has the power to penetrate tissues and infuse the energy into them.

Effect

Acute
- Radiation sickness
- Radiation syndrome

Delayed
- Leukemia
- Malignancy
- Fetal anomaly

Penetrating Ability Protection (Table 3.6)

1. Normal allowable outer space 0.1 rad/year.
2. Permissible in investigation 5 rad/year (e.g., fluoroscopy 4 rad/min).

Table 3.6: Penetrating ability of rays.

	Air	Tissue	Lead
α	4 cm	0.05 mm	Zero
β	300 cm	4.0 mm	0.3 mm
γ	400 m	50 cm	30 mm
X	200 m	30 cm	0.3 mm
Cosmic	Zero	Some	Zero

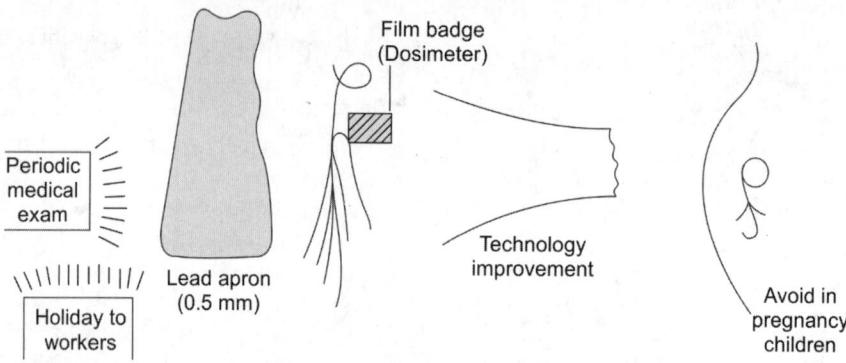

Fig. 3.11: Prevention of radiation hazards.

Prevention

See **Figure 3.11**.

METEOROLOGY

Elements

- Altitude
- Temperature
- Humidity
- Rainfall
- Air movements
- Cloud and weather

Altitude

It is measured in millimeters of mercury by Fortin's barometer and barograph.

- High altitude
  - Air is less dense
  - Low partial pressure of oxygen
  - Breathing equipment needed above 25,000 feet
  - Respiratory rate increases
  - Hb% increases
  - Cardiac output increases
  - Clinical condition—acute mountain sickness and pulmonary edema.
- Low altitude
  - Air is dense.
  - High partial pressure of O_2, CO_2, and N_2 are dissolved in blood
  - Convulsion and death by O_2
  - Narcotic mental dysfunction by N_2
  - CO_2 enhances narcosis of N_2
  - Clinical condition—caisson disease

Temperature

- Mercury and alcohol thermometers are used to measure temperature.
- Mercury has expansible power; records maximum temperature.
- Ether has condensation power; records minimum temperature.

Thermometer

- Dry bulb thermometer (DBT)
- Wet bulb thermometer (WBT)
- Maximum thermometer
- Minimum thermometer
- Six's maximum and minimum thermometer
- Globe thermometer **(Fig. 3.12)**
- Records air temperature
- Radiant heat and temperature
- Kata thermometer is used to measure the cooling power of the air **(Fig. 3.13)**.

Types:

1. *Dry kata:* 6 and more than 6 (comfort)
2. *Wet kata:* 20 and more than 20 (comfort)
3. *Standard kata (red):* 100–95 range
4. *High temperature kata (dark blue):* 130–125 range.
5. *Extra high temperature kata (magenta):* 150–145 range.

Heat stress indices:

- CET (Corrected effective temperature)
- P_4SR (Predicted 4-hour sweat rate)

Heat stress effect:

- *Heat exhaustion*
  - Water and salt loss
  - Circulation failure

- Trench foot
- Numbness

Methods for preventing high temperature heat stroke
- Water and salt replacement
- Regulation of work
- Proper clothing
- Use of protective device, and
- Good working environment

Humidity

Water content in atmosphere is expressed in:
a. Relative humidity (percentage)
b. Absolute humidity (wt./cub. mm)

It is measured by hygrometer (dry and wet bulb thermometer).

Sling psychrometer:

Dry and wet bulb thermometer is kept in such a way that it can be whirled to record atmospheric temperature and inference is drawn with the help of a chart called psychrometric chart or nanogram.

Rainfall

1" rainfall = 2.5 cm rainfall
= 4.7 gallons/sq yard
= 22,000 gallons/acre

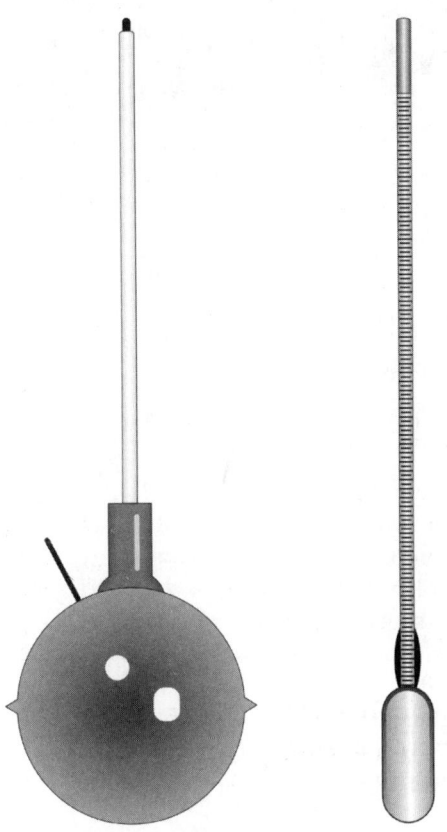

Fig. 3.12: Globe thermometer. **Fig. 3.13:** Kata thermometer.

Air Movement

Anemometer is used to measure air velocity.
- Light air: 1–3 miles/hour
- Light breeze: 4–7 miles/hour
- Strong breeze: 25–30 miles/hour
- Gale: 30–60 miles/hour
- Storm: 60–70 miles/hour
- Hurricane: 70–140 miles/hour

- Collapse
- Management by rest
- Saline
- Cardiac stimulant
- *Heat stroke* (sunstroke)
  - Failure of heat regulating mechanism
  - Body temperature 110°F
  - No sweating
  - Mortality 40%
  - Management by ice bath, ice enema (Make body hypothermic)
- *Heat cramps*: Painful spasmodic contraction of skeletal muscles (chloride loss).
- *Heat syncope*
  - Soldier's parade
  - Rest brings reversible change.
- *Heat hyperpyrexia*: Mild heat stroke at 106°F
- *Heat stress* effect by low temperature
  - Frost bite

Cloud and Weather

They have the bearing on air temperature and environmental pollution.

HOUSING AND TOWN PLANNING

The WHO, National Buildings Organization (NBO) and Environmental Hygiene Committee have defined the need of housing in healthy living. According to NBO (2011), their achievements are 110 million houses in urban area and 220 million houses in rural area. NBO has estimated slum dwellers to 48 million.

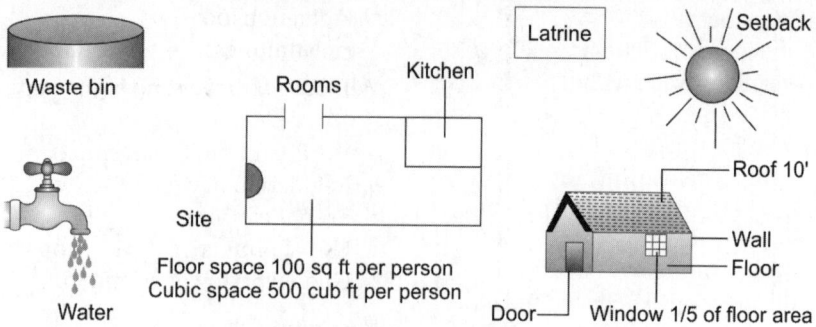

Fig. 3.14: Housing standards.

Need (Fig. 3.14)

Physical Needs

- Temperature, air, humidity
- Noise, lighting, rest, and
- Recreation, exercise.

Physiological Needs

Privacy, family, community

Health Needs

Water, excreta disposal, cooking, protection from insects.

Protective Needs

Accidents, fire, electricity
Site: Good, hard–even surface away from industry.
Setback: For good light and ventilation
Floor: Pucca, minimum 70–90 sq ft per person to avoid overcrowding.
Rooms: According to the size of family
Window and doors: About 40% of the space of the floor.

Indicators of Good Housing

- Physical facility
- Property value
- Social facility

(No illness, good comfort, social well-being).

Overcrowding is Defined by (NBO Standard)

- Person per room
- Sex separation
- Floor space per person.

Public Health Importance

- Respiratory infection
- Skin infection
- Home accidents
- Rodent-borne infections
- Arthropod-borne infections
- Psychological effects

Power of Town Planning under Corporation and Development Authority

- Road
- Electricity
- Minimum space to be left
- Drains
- Park
- Civil amenities
- License issue

Housing Activity Promotion Organization

- NBO
- National Buildings Construction Corporation Limited
- Housing and Urban Development Corporation (HUDCO)
- Hindustan Housing Factory (Ministry of Housing and Works)

According to Environmental Hygiene Committee, rural housing includes the following:

- Two rooms
- Verandah space
- Plinth area to be 1/3rd of total area
- Separate kitchen

- A sanitary latrine
- Window shall be 10% of floor area
- Facility of drinking water within reach (well)
- Separate cattle shed
- Arrangement for waste water flow
- Arrangement for refuse and garbage

Under Rural Landless Employment Guarantee Program, Indira Awas Yojana is introduced for house construction with minimum one room, one kitchen, one sanitary latrine, one bath and one smokeless chullah.

WASTE DISPOSAL

Types

- *Solid waste*—Refuse, garbage, ash, etc.
- *Liquid waste*—Sullage, sewage.

Terminology

Refuse (Litter): Dust, ash, vegetable, putrefiable matter, paper, packing material.

Night Soil: Human excreta

Sewage: Waste water mixed with human excreta.

Sullage: Waste water unmixed with human excreta.

Rubbish: Paper, clothing, bits of wood, waste metal, glass waste, dust and dirt.

Garbage: Waste from kitchen preparations.

Ash: Residue from fire used for cooking, heating, industry and waste disposal.

Organizations which support:
- WHO
- ISWA (International Solid Waste Public Cleansing Association)
- Pollution Control Board.

Solid Waste

Garbage, rubbish, demolition products, dead animal, manure and discarded material constitute solid waste. Normally, 1–2 kg/head/day is the solid waste produce.

Types (Depending on Source)
- House refuse
- Street refuse
- Industry refuse
- Market refuse
- Stable refuse
- Hospital refuse

Health Hazards
- Air pollution by dust, ashes
- Fly breeding
- Rat menace by garbage
- Water pollution by fermented refuse
- Esthetic purpose

Storage
- House—dust bin
- Street—public bin
- Industry—big bin
- Stable—stable bin
- Market—market bin
- Park—use me bin
- Hospital—indicated specific bins.

Collection
- House-to-house collection from bins
- Other by vehicles and closed vans.

Disposal
- *Recommended and sanitary methods*
  - Urban life
    - Controlled tipping/sanitary landfill
    - Incineration
    - Composting
      » Bangalore method
      » Mechanical
  - Rural life
    - Manure pits
    - Gobar gas plant
  - Camp life
    - Burial
    - Burning to ashes
- *Not recommended, not sanitary methods*
  - Dumping
  - Aerobic composting
  - Sea disposal
  - River disposal

Controlled tipping/sanitary landfill
- When land, ground level available (Trench method) **(Fig. 3.15)**
- When land sloppy (Ramp method) **(Fig. 3.16)**
- When land with depressions (Area method).

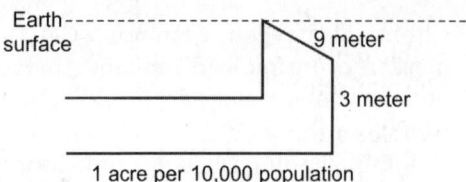

Fig. 3.15: Trench method tipping.

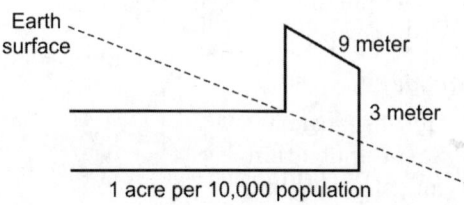

Fig. 3.16: Ramp method tipping.

Filled and sealed temperature at 60°C kill pathogen and make refuse harmless.

Incineration

It is a hygienic and common hospital refuse disposal method. They are burnt in an incinerator. It needs preliminary separation of dust.

Advantages: No fear of pathogen.

Composting

Bangalore method of composting **(Fig. 3.17)** is a method of disposal of refuse and night soil which is also called hot fermentation process.

Mechanical composting is a method where waste is cleared from salvageable material, then pulverized with equipment to reduce size; then mixed with sewage, sludge or night soil in a rotary machine and incubated.

Manure Pit

- To dump refuse to manure pits.
- Two pits are alternated in the backyard.
- Later used as manure **(Fig. 3.18)**.

Liquid Waste

Liquid waste consists of waste water and human excreta termed as sullage and sewage, respectively.

The liquid waste is carried away from dwelling places by systems called water carriage system **(Fig. 3.19)**.

Water carriage system consists of:
- Household fittings and sewers
- Street sewers and sewage pipes, and
- City sewers and big drains. It is tested for no leakage of:
  ◆ Water
  ◆ Air
  ◆ Smoke
  ◆ Chemicals

Collection and transportation of sullage and sewage is a method of disposal of liquid waste by water carriage system.

Trap

- Water close (First)
- House to public road (Second)
- Surface drain to drain (Third) (Gully trap)

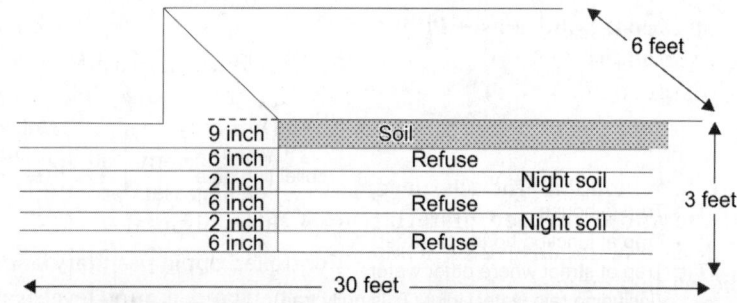

Note: • Ground layer refuse 6 inches
• Alternated with 2 inches night soil, 6 inches refuse
• Top layer 6 inches refuse
• Above top layer refuse soil cover of 9 inches

Fig. 3.17: Bangalore method of composting.

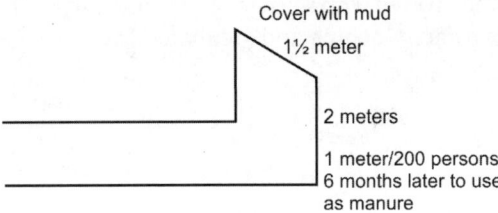

Fig. 3.18: Burial.

Composition of Liquid Waste

Waste water, suspended solids, night soil, pathogens

Measurement of Pollutants

- Biochemical oxygen demand (BOD)—measure of biological load
  Amount of oxygen absorbed by sewage during 5 days at 18°C

Five days 18°C	Dissolved O_2 for aerobic oxidation, etc.	100 ppm = Weak 300 ppm = Strong

- Chemical oxygen demand (COD)—measure of organic load: Amount of oxygen of organic material available for chemical oxidation.
- Suspended solids: It is an indicator of strength of sewage—
  100 ppm = Weak
  500 ppm = Strong

From the water carriage system, drained liquid waste undergoes decomposition by:
- Aerobic process
- Anaerobic process.

Disposal of Night Soil

Only 31% of urban population has amenity of sewerage system.

Public Health Importance

- Fly breeding
- Soil pollution

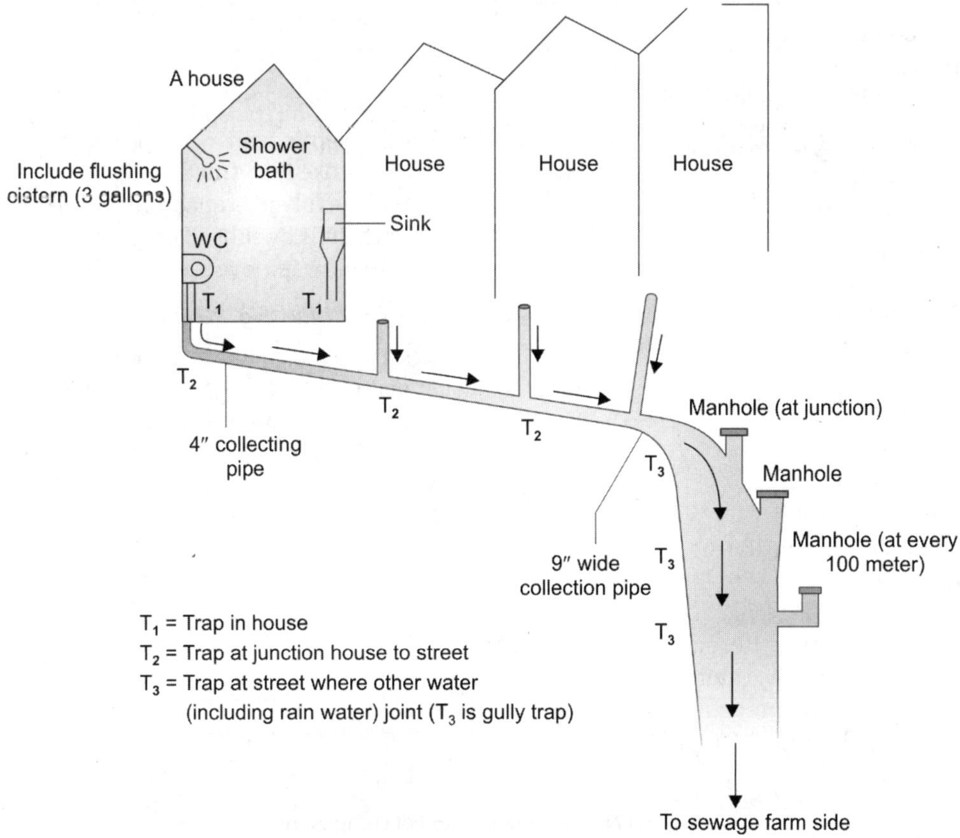

T_1 = Trap in house
T_2 = Trap at junction house to street
T_3 = Trap at street where other water (including rain water) joint (T_3 is gully trap)

Fig. 3.19: Water carriage system.

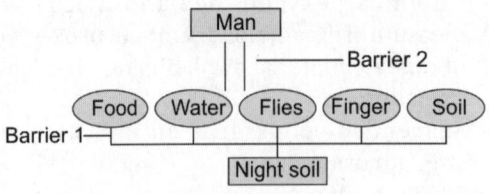

Fig. 3.20: Barriers in fecal-borne diseases.

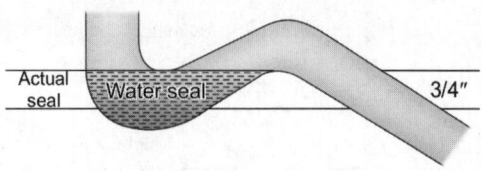

Fig. 3.21: Trap (Water seal).

- Water pollution
- Food contamination

Fecal-borne Diseases (Fig. 3.20)

- Typhoid
- Paratyphoid
- Dysentery
- Cholera
- Hookworm infection (habit of open air defecation)
- Viral hepatitis

Recommendable Methods of Disposal of Night Soil

- Trenching
- Incineration (camp), and
- Composting, Bangalore method

Not Recommendable Methods

- Conservancy
- Dumping
- Sea outfall
- River outfall
- Oxidation pond
- Sewage forming without treatment

Sanitary Latrines (Residential)

- Aqua privy
- Bore-hole latrine
- Chemical closet
- Dug-hole/pit-hole latrine
- Septic tank
- Water seal latrine **(Fig. 3.22)**
- PRAI (Planning, Research and Action Institute, Lucknow, Uttar Pradesh)
- RCA [Research-cum-action, Government of India (GOI)] **(Figs. 3.21 and 3.22)**

Sanitary Latrines (Camp Life)

- Shallow-trench latrine
- Deep-trench latrine

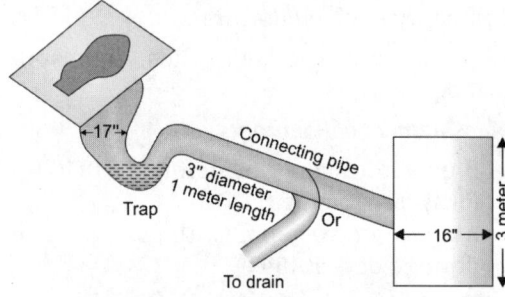

Fig. 3.22: Indirect type water seal latrine.

- Bore-hole latrine
- Dug-hole latrine

Aqua Privy (Fig. 3.23)

- It is like septic tank.
- Six years use for a small family
- Process involved is anaerobic digestion
- Treatment is by subsoil irrigation
- Sludge to be removed at intervals.

Bore-hole Latrine (Fig. 3.24)

- It is a product of Rockefeller Foundation.
- Auger is needed to bore the hole
- Comes for 1 year for a family
- Conversion by anaerobic digestion
- Merits and demerits are listed.
- Not very much in use today.

Fig. 3.23: Aqua privy.

Chapter 3: Environmental Health Problems

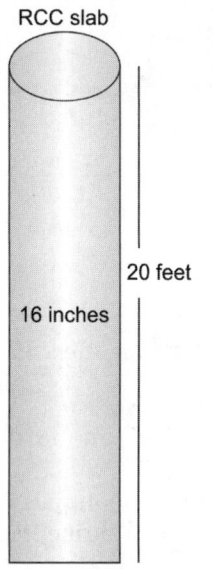

Fig. 3.24: Bore-hole latrine.

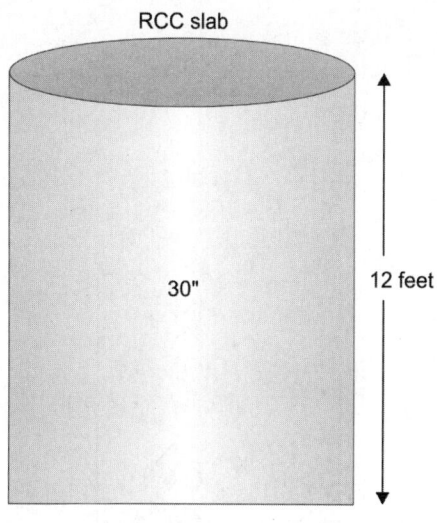

Fig. 3.26: Dug hole latrine.

Chemical Closet (Fig. 3.25)

Functions of chemical closet:
- Caustic soda disintegrates and dissolves excreta
- Phenol kills bacteria.
- Crude oil prevents odor.

Uses—Boats, caravan, aircraft.

Dug Hole Latrine (Fig. 3.26)
- It is a product of Singur study.
- It serves 5 years for a family.
- Easy to construct and longevity is good.
- The action is anaerobic digestion.

Septic Tanks (Fig. 3.27)
- Capacity is 500 gallons
- Retention period is 24 hours
- Sludge undergoes anaerobic digestion (one stage action)
- Scum (effluent) is let to subsoil to undergo aerobic digestion (second-stage action)
- Digested sludge bailed out once a year.

Water Seal Latrines (Fig. 3.28)

Proper maintenance requires good awareness. RCA latrine costs less and 50% is borne by Block Development Office under available scheme.

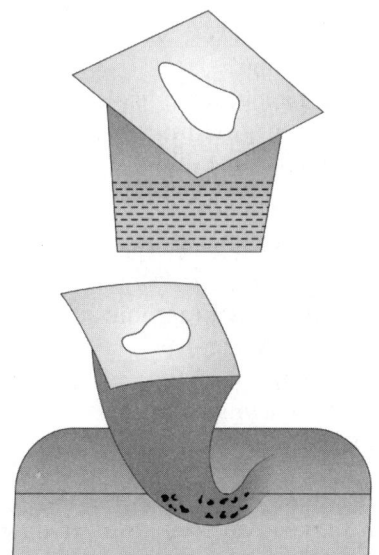

Fig. 3.25: Chemical closet.

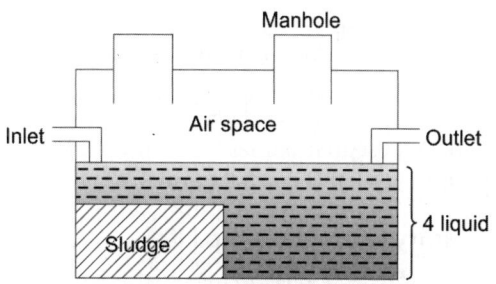

Fig. 3.27: Septic tank.

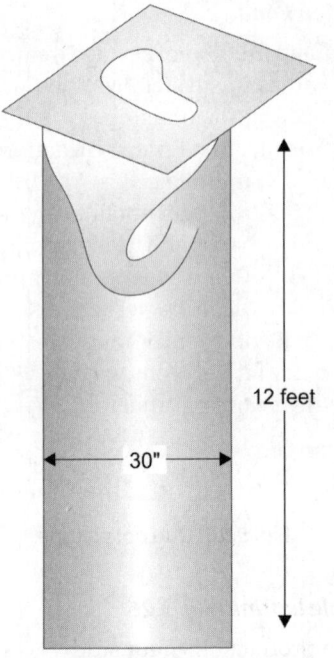

Fig. 3.28: Direct type water seal latrine.

Shallow Trench Latrine

- Separate trench for men and women needed
- Instruct to cover feces with mud each time
- Useful for 1 week (camp) **(Fig. 3.29)**
- When filled, should be covered with earth and compacted.

Deep Trench Latrine

- Useful for camps of longer duration (several months)

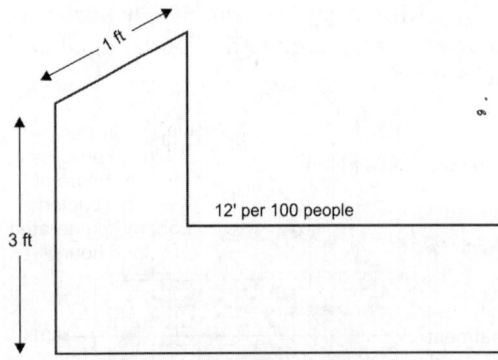

Fig. 3.29: Shallow trench latrine.

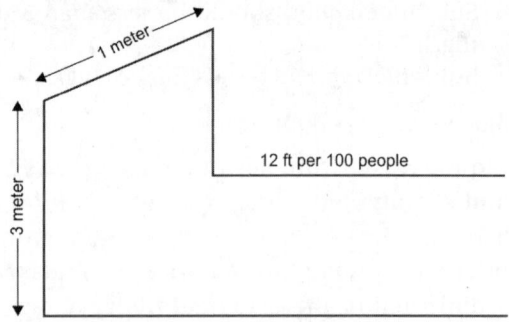

Fig. 3.30: Deep trench latrine.

- Superstructure can be built by local materials
- Other requisite materials are similar to superficial trench latrine **(Fig. 3.30)**.

Modern Sewage Treatment

Sewage contains solid and liquid excreta from residences of a community. Habit of the people and use of water determine quantity of sewage. Usual sewage flow in 24 hours is called "dry weather flow." Sewage strength is expressed by the following:

- BOD—amount of oxygen absorbed by sewage during 5-day period at 20°C which is used by living organisms
- COD—oxygen available which is used in oxidation.
- Suspended solids—available suspended solids in sewage.

Based on biological principles of anaerobic and aerobic digestion, modern sewage treatment plants are built.

Sludge

- One million gallon sewage gives 20 tons of sludge (black mass)
- Sewage treatment (aerobic autodigestion which yields sludge)
- To sea (sludge pumping)
- To land (trenching) farming
- To composting

Effluent

Before leaving to river and stream the permitted dilution is:

Chapter 3: Environmental Health Problems

- Suspended solid should be less than 30 mg/L
- 5-day BOD should be less than 20 mg/L.

Modern Sewage Treatment

Liquid waste from sewerage is screened and sedimented. Later, it is subjected for aerobic oxidation either by trickling filter or by activated sludge process. Later, secondary sedimentation allows to treat sludge and to dispose effluent **(Fig. 3.31)**.

Sewage Farming (Board Irrigation)

Sewage fed to furrow intermittently for growing fodder grass, potatoes, fruit trees (plantation).

If sewage farming is badly managed, it will result in sewage sickness.

Oxidation Pond

It is a cheap method of sewage treatment. It is also called as waste stabilization pond, redox pond or sewage lagoons.

Historically, first known oxidation pond is well recorded in Bhilai.

The organic matter contained in the sewage is oxidized by bacteria. The algae with sunlight utilizes CO_2, water and inorganic minerals for their growth. Algae, bacteria and sunlight are must for oxidation pond. Cloudy weather lowers the efficiency of the process. Here, we see both aerobic digestion and anaerobic digestion.

Oxidation Ditches

It is also a low-cost treatment method for purification of sewage.

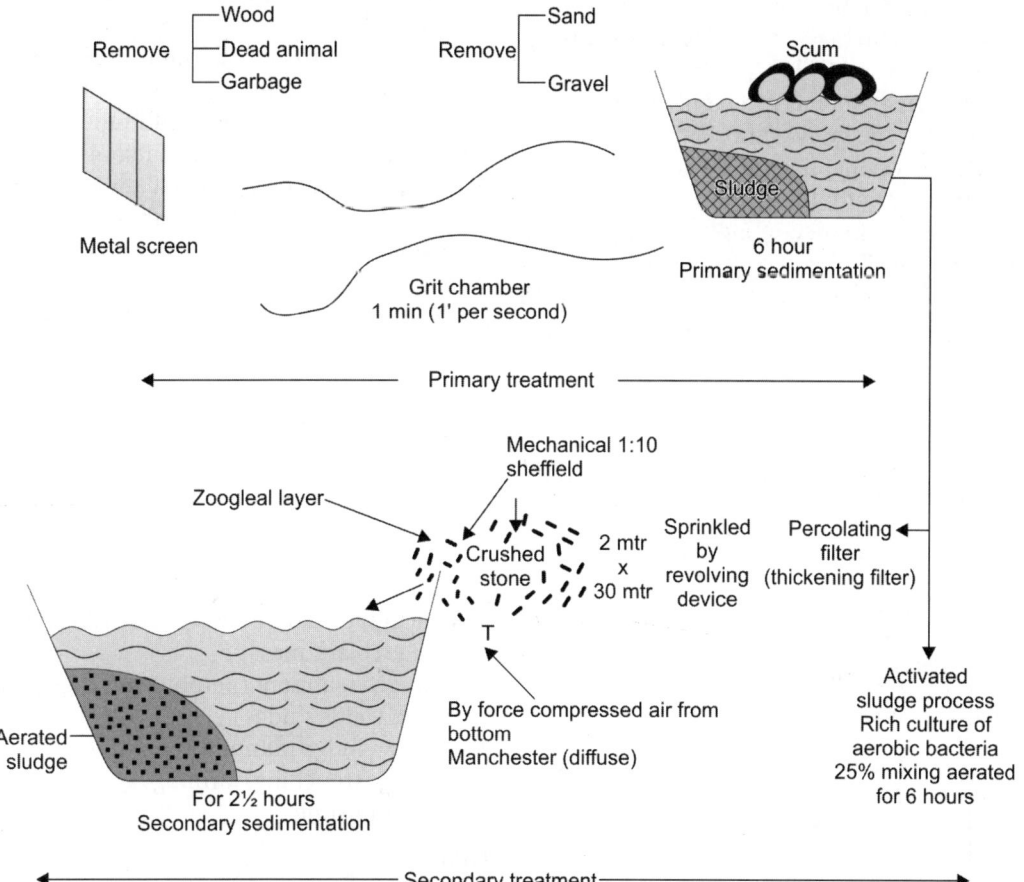

Fig. 3.31: Modern sewage treatment plant.

Sociological Aspect of Excreta Disposal

Open field defecation is an attached cultural behavior in India and is the main content of rural sanitation. Accepting a sanitary latrine in the house and its use needs public awareness and this is possible through health education.

HUMAN DEAD BODY DISPOSAL AND ENVIRONMENTAL SANITATION

This is associated with religious rituals and varies from country to country or from place to place. Practice of throwing dead body to vultures or to river poses health hazards. Sanitary methods of disposal of human dead body have been burning and burial. Burning called cremation is satisfactory method for dead body disposal. Electric crematorium has solved urban problem of dead body disposal. Burial is done in corporation-allocated areas.

Municipal Act has given guidelines for the disposal of the body of those who died due to acute infectious diseases. These guidelines are to be strictly followed. Handling of the dead needs the use of gloves and personal protection. Bed cover dipped in formalin is worn over the body and tied properly. In case of burial, it shall be deep burial, namely more than 3 feet depth and additional of lime crystals with mud covering.

SUMMARY

Major components of physical environment are described. Meteorology, housing, town planning, waste disposal and human body disposal are described in the chapter.

VIVA VOCE

1. Name the components of physical environment.
2. What is safe and wholesome water?
3. What are the differences between shallow well and deep well?
4. What is zone of influences?
5. Mention criteria of a sanitary well.
6. Name waterborne diseases.
7. Mention the steps of disinfection of a well.
8. Mention differences between slow sand filtration and Rapid sand filtration.
9. What is breakpoint chlorination?
10. What are the effects of radiation?
11. Mention uses of kata thermometer.
12. Define overcrowdings in housing.
13. What is BOD?

CHAPTER 4

Medical Entomology

Chapter Outline

- Classification
- Identifying Features
- Insecticides
- Zoonoses
- Integrated Vector Control

DEFINITION

The study of insects of public health (PH) importance.

CLASSIFICATION

1. *Insects:* Winged, have biting instruments, e.g., mosquitoes, flies, lice.
2. *Arachnida*
   - No antennae
   - No wings
   - Terrestrial

   For example, ticks (hard and soft), mite (trombiculid and itch)
3. *Crustacea*
   - No wing
   - Aquatic

   For example, cyclops.

MODE OF TRANSMISSION

- *Direct contact*, e.g., scabies, pediculosis
- *Mechanical*, e.g., flies
- *Biological*:
  - Propagative, e.g., plague
  - Cyclopropagative, e.g., malaria
  - Cyclodevelopment, e.g., filaria

VECTOR-BORNE DISEASES

Mosquitoes: Malaria, filaria, dengue

Flies: Typhoid, dysentery, trachoma, kala-azar, oriental sore, sandfly fever, sleeping sickness

Flea: Plague, endemic typhus

Lice: Epidemic typhus, relapsing fever, trench fever

Ticks and mites: Typhus, encephalitis, relapsing fever, scrub typhus, scabies

Cyclops: Guinea worm, *Diphyllobothrium latum*.

IDENTIFYING FEATURES

Mosquitoes

Anopheles Eggs (Fig. 4.1)

Habitat
Clean water, wells, streams, tanks, etc.

Identification
- Found singly
- Both ends tapering
- Boat-shaped

Float and frill on either side: The floats are seen as bulge on each side of the egg and they show striations called *float ridges* form patterns.

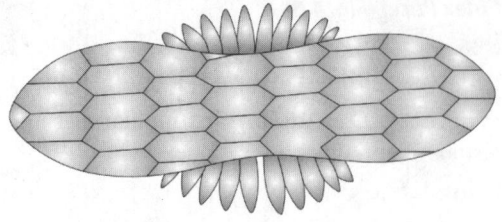
Form patterns

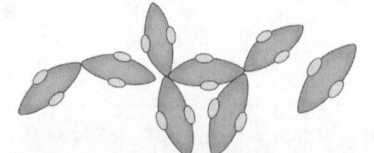

Fig. 4.1: Anopheles eggs.

Anopheles Larva (Fig. 4.2)

- Consists of a head
- It has a segmented body—body covered with hair.
- Lies parallel with and just below the surface of the water.
- Respiratory opening on the dorsum of the 8th segment.
- Siphon tube absent.
- Presence of palmate hair on abdomen.
  PH importance: Adults transmit malaria.

Anopheles Adult Male (Fig. 4.3)

- Palpi are as long as the proboscis and clubbed at its end.
- Antennae long and feathery.
- Proboscis not adapted for piercing and sucking blood.
- Of no PH importance as they do not bite and live on vegetables and fruit juice.
- Wings spotted
- While resting proboscis, head, thorax and abdomen make an angle with the surface.
- Breeds in clear water and slow-running streams.

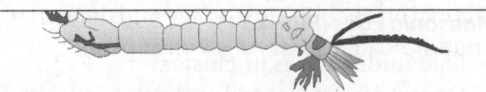

Fig. 4.2: Anopheles larva.

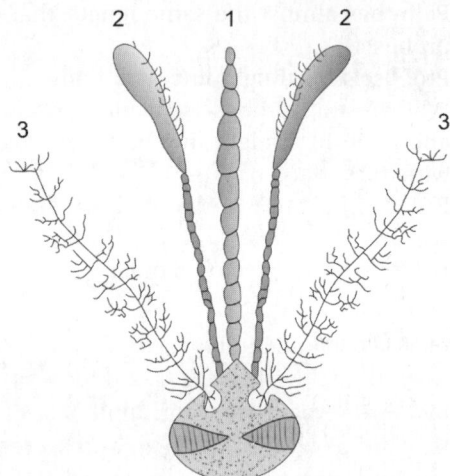

Fig. 4.3: Anopheles adult male—(1) Proboscis, (2) Palpi, (3) Antennae.

Anopheles Adult Female (Fig. 4.4)

Salient Features

- Wings spotted.
- Head has a proboscis and a pair of compound eyes, antennae and palpi.
- Proboscis specially adapted for piercing the skin and sucking the blood.
- Antennae with hairs are short and scanty.

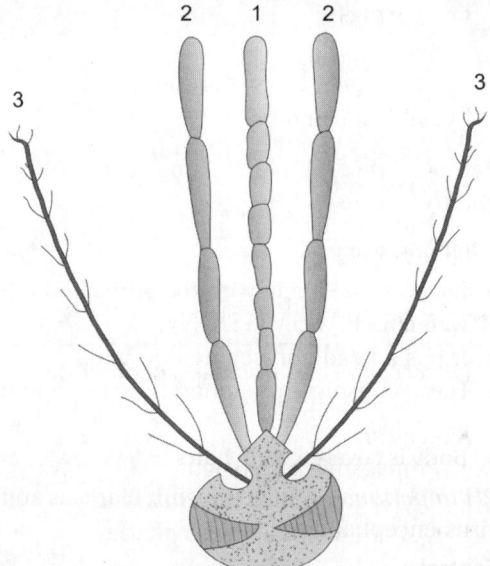

Fig. 4.4: Anopheles adult female—(1) Proboscis, (2) Palpi, (3) Antennae.

Chapter 4: Medical Entomology

- Palpi has almost the same length that of proboscis.
- Proboscis in straight line with body.
- While resting, proboscis, head, thorax and abdomen in straight line make an angle with the surface.
- Breeds in clean water and slow-running streams.

PH importance: Vector of malaria.

Prevention

Antilarval and antiadult measures.
- Insecticide with DDT residual spray, pyrethrum space spray for adult
- Insecticide with Paris green and mineral oils for larvae
- Mosquito net
- Antimosquito cream (repellants).

Culex Eggs (Fig. 4.6)

Habitat

Sullage water collections and sewage contaminated water drains and cesspools.

Identification

Eggs are cemented together in the form of ovate shape in rafts.

Individual eggs are cigar-shaped prominent micropillar process. The upper end being narrower—each raft consists of 200–500 eggs.

PH importance: Female adults—filariasis and encephalitis.

Control

Remove breeding places—drainage—oiling for larval stage.

Culex Larva (Fig. 4.7)

- Lies with an angle with the surface of the water.
- It has a head and segmented body.
- Has a conspicuous siphon tube (long and slender)
- Body is covered with hairs.

PH importance: Adults transmit filariasis and virus encephalitis.

Control

Drainage—oiling—fill up hollows.

Culex Pupa (Fig. 4.8)

- Comma-shaped—large eyes.
- Two breathing trumpets—long and narrow.

PH importance: Adults transmit filariasis and virus encephalitis.

Control

Same as in larva.

Culex Male (Fig. 4.9)

- Antennae feathery
- Palpi long and tapering
- Proboscis bent at an angle with the body.
- Abdomen, head and thorax make an angle with the proboscis which is parallel to the surface.
- Breeds in dirty water like cesspools, stagnant drains containing organic materials and polluted water.

No PH importance.

Culex Female (Fig. 4.10)

- Palpi shorter than proboscis—1/3.
- Antennae—short with some hair.
- Proboscis adapted for piercing the skin and sucking the blood.
- Abdomen, head and thorax make an angle with the proboscis which is parallel to the surface.
- Breeds in dirty water like cesspools, stagnant drains containing organic materials and polluted water.

PH importance: Vector of urban filariasis and virus encephalitis.

Control

- *Adult:* Spraying with pyrethrum extract (space spray).
- Use mosquito curtain—use of antimosquito cream.
- Drainage for larval control.
  Difference between *Anopheles* and *Culex* is depicted in **Figure 4.5 and Table 4.1**.

Mansonia Eggs (Fig. 4.11)

- Laid under leaves in cluster.
- One end is conical and projecting (attached to the undersurface of leaf).

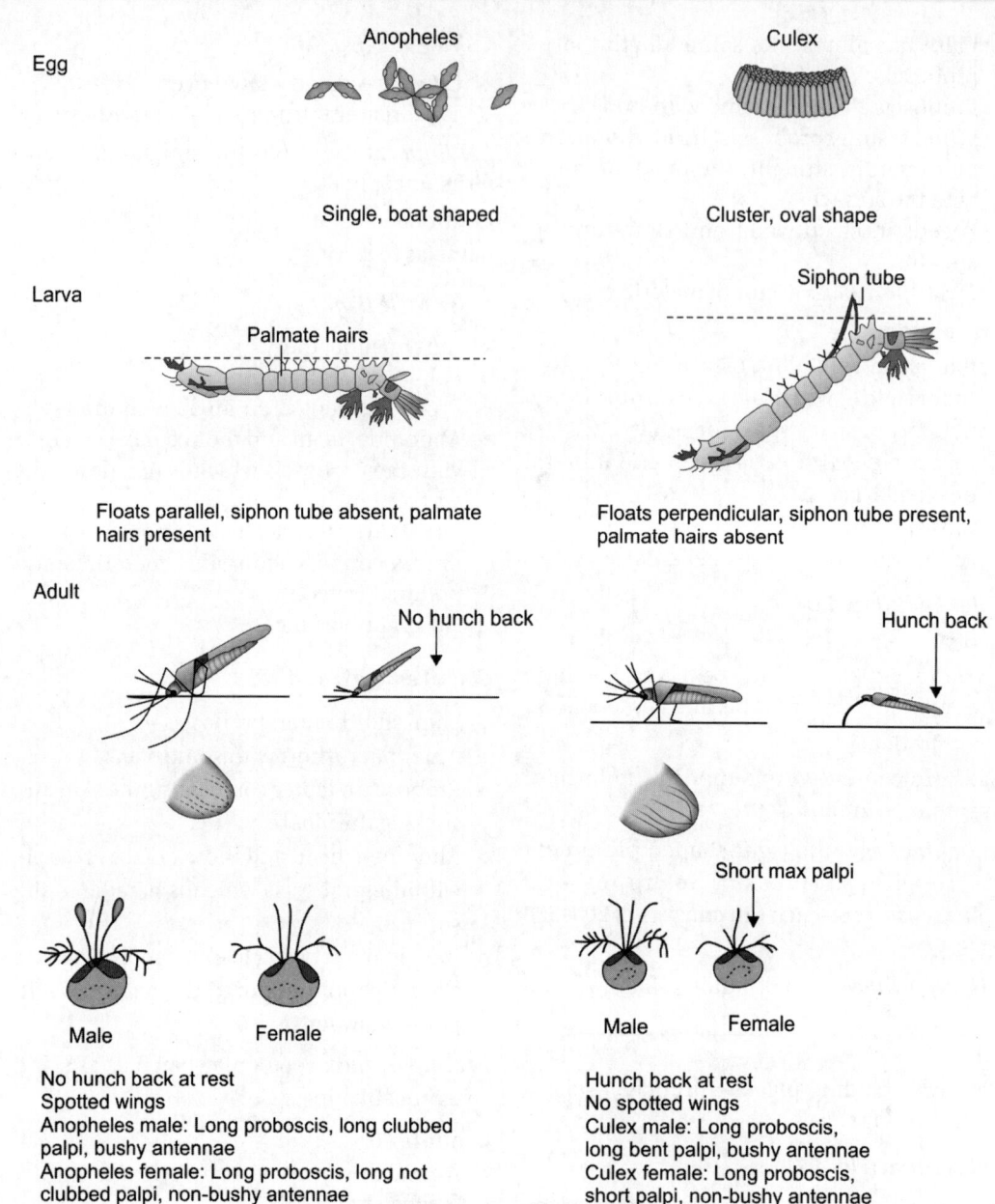

Fig. 4.5: Difference between *Anopheles* and *Culex* mosquitoes.

PH importance: Female adults transmit *Brugia malayi*.

Control
Removal of water plants (*Pistia* plants and water hyacinth).

Species of Mosquitoes
Anopheles
- *Anopheles annularis*
- *Anopheles culicifacies*
- *Anopheles fluviatilis*

Chapter 4: Medical Entomology

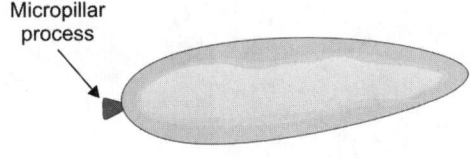

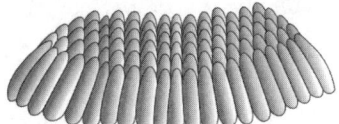

Fig. 4.6: *Culex* eggs.

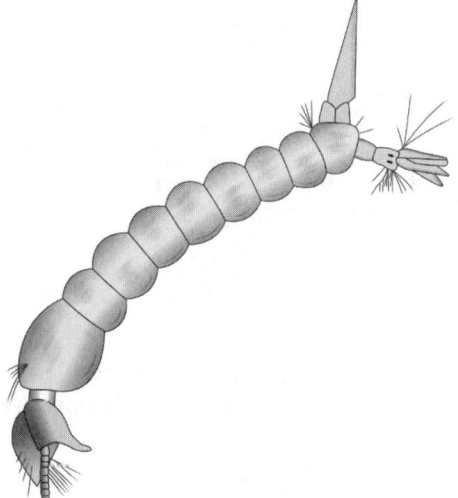

Fig. 4.7: *Culex* larva.

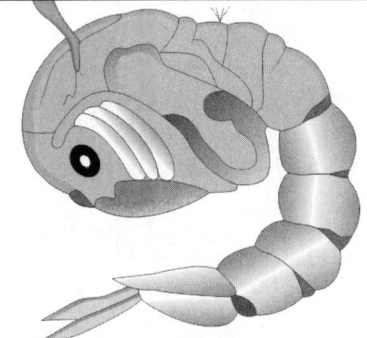

Fig. 4.8: *Culex* pupa.

- *Anopheles minimus*
- *Anopheles philippinensis*
- *Anopheles stephensi*

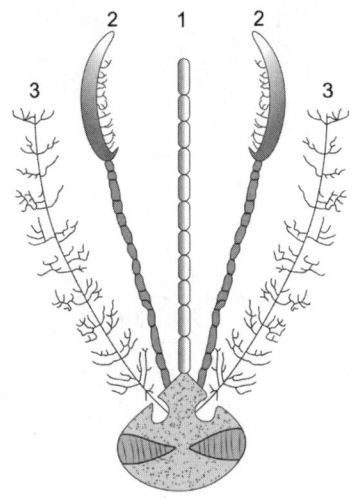

Fig. 4.9: *Culex* male—(1) Proboscis, (2) Palpi, (3) Antennae.

Table 4.1: Distinguishing features of *Anopheles* and *Culex*.

	Anopheles	Culex
Egg	Boat-shaped, single dust-like	• Cigar-shaped in rafts • Easily seen
Larva	• Floats parallel to the surface • Palmate hair present • No siphon tube	• Makes an angle with surface • Palmate hair absent • Siphon tube present
Adult	• Head, thorax, abdomen in a straight line • Spotted wings • Breeds in clean, fresh water	• Not spotted wings • Breeds in cesspool drain, dirty water

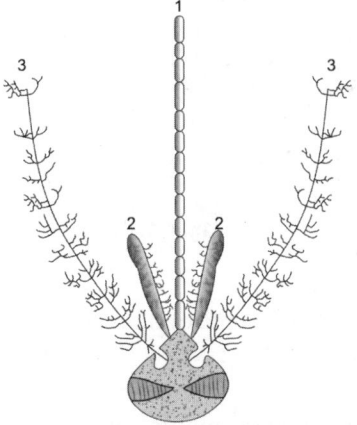

Fig. 4.10: *Culex* female—(1) Proboscis, (2) Palpi, (3) Antennae.

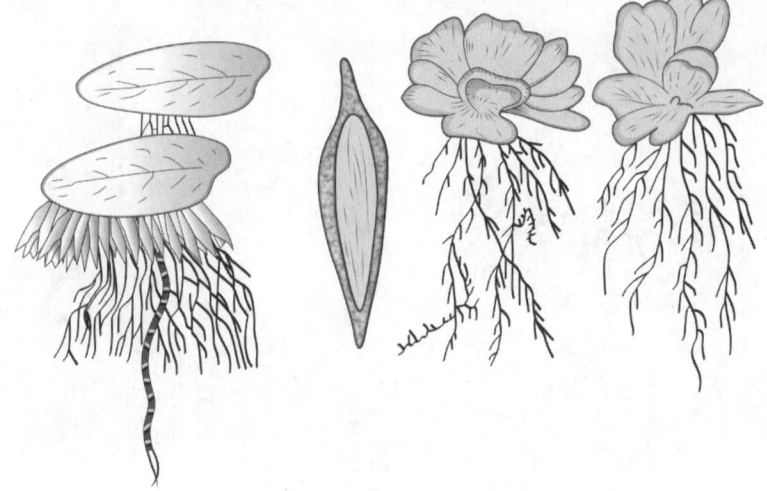

Fig. 4.11: *Mansonia* eggs.

- *Anopheles subpictus*
- *Anopheles sundaicus*
- *Anopheles umbrosus*
- *Anopheles varuna*

Culex
- *Culex fatigans*

Aedes
- *Aedes aegypti*
- *Aedes vittatus*
- *Aedes albopictus*

Mansonia
- *Mansonia annularis*
- *Mansonia uniformis*
- *Mansonia indiana*
- *Mansonia longipalpis*

Diseases Transmitted

- *Anopheles*: Malaria
- *Culex*:
  - Filaria
  - Japanese encephalitis
- *Aedes*
  - Dengue
  - Chikungunya
- *Mansonoides*: Rural filaria

Habit

- Anthropophilic
- Zoophilic

- Others bite at night except Aedes.
- They rest at dark place.
- Breed in:
  - *Anopheles*—clean water.
  - *Culex*—dirty water.
  - *Aedes*—artificial collection of water.
  - *Mansonia*—vegetation (Waterplant).

Control measures are depicted in **Figure 4.12**.

Flies

The Housefly

- Phylum: Arthropoda
- Class: Insecta
- Order: Diptera
- Family: Muscidae
- Genus: *Musca*
- Species: *Musca domestica*

The importance is that it is mechanical transmitter of diseases by its habit.

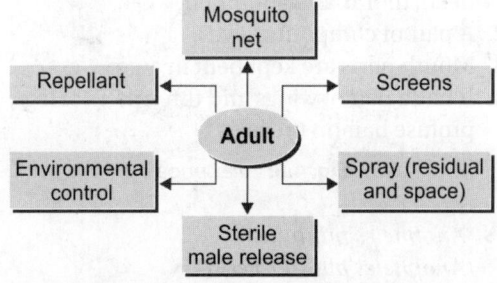

Fig. 4.12: Mosquito control measures.

Chapter 4: Medical Entomology

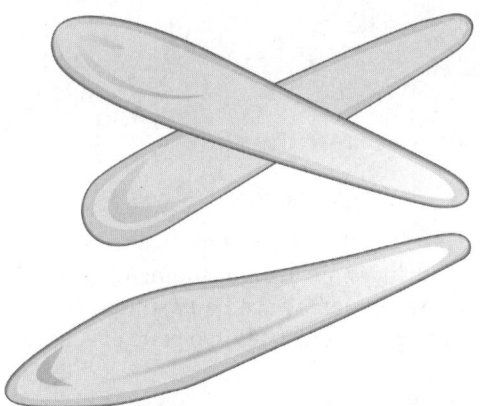

Fig. 4.13: Housefly—eggs.

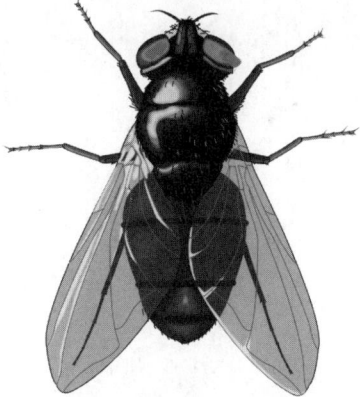

Fig. 4.15: Housefly—adult.

Musca Domestica

Housefly—Egg (Fig. 4.13)
- Measures: 1 mm in length.
- Resembles polished rice grains—found in fresh manure or refuse collections.

PH importance: Adults transmit cholera, dysentery, poliomyelitis, conjunctivitis.

Control Sanitation
Proper disposal of rubbish and excreta fly traps, fly baits, pyrethrum spraying.

Housefly—Larva (Fig. 4.14)
Measures: ½ in length, hairless maggot, very active, found in fresh manure or refuse.

Identification: Cylindrical—anterior end narrow and tapering. Note the single oral hook and dark spot seen through translucent skin at the anterior end.

PH importance and control: Similar to the mentioning in egg.

Housefly—Adult (Fig. 4.15)
1. Large insect, dark in color, body divided into head, thorax and abdomen.
2. A pair of compound eyes.
3. Mouth parts are kept bent in a groove.
4. It has a pair of wings and three pairs of legs, profuse hair on the legs.
5. On the dorsal aspect of thorax are four broad bands.

PH Importance and Control
Similar to the mentioning in housefly—egg.

Morphology
Body is divided into head, thorax and abdomen. Head consists of compound eyes and a hidden retractile proboscis. Abdomen is segmented. Thorax consists of wings and three pairs of legs. Numerous bristles are found over legs and body.

Lifecycle
Passes through egg, maggot, pupa and adult. Eggs are laid on decaying manure, cow-dung, 300 at a time. Hatches to larva in 24 hours which is eyeless, hairless, feetless maggot. Voracious eating for 5 days, it transforms to pupa which is pale yellow, green or brown at a later period. Pupa transforms to adult in 7 days.

Disease Transmitted
Cholera, typhoid, paratyphoid, dysentery (amebic and bacillary), ascariasis, polio and hepatitis.

Control
- Larvicide
  - 5% cresol
  - 5% Borax, Gammexane
- Adult
  - Formalin water
  - Breeding place elimination
  - Baits (cheap is formalin + milk + sugar or water)

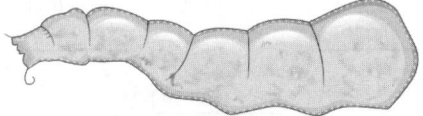

Fig. 4.14: Housefly—larva.

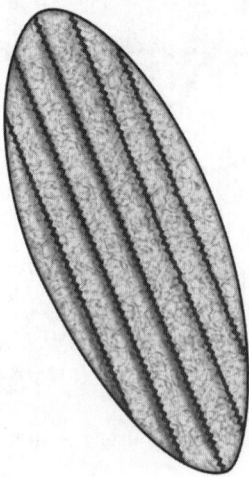

Fig. 4.16: Sandfly—egg.

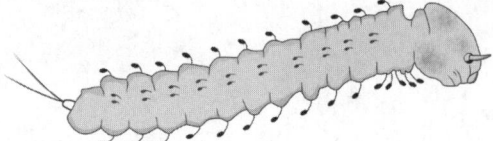

Fig. 4.17: Sandfly—larva.

- Head highly chitinous and conspicuous.
- Four hairs are seen at the head end.
- Body segments have hairy spines.
- Posterior end carries two pairs of very long caudal hairs.
- Inner pair longer.
- Yellow in color and covered with fine hairs.

Sandfly—Male (Fig. 4.18)

- Smaller than mosquito.
- Whole body covered with profuse hairs.
- Abdomen is short and spindle shaped.
- Legs are thin and long. Eyes are very prominent.
- Proboscis starts from a projecting snout.
- Palpi are longer than proboscis and curved downward.
- Wings are kept vertically at rest.
- Posterior end of abdomen resembles the tail of an airplane (because of external genitalia). Sandfly male does not transmit any disease.

Phlebotomus Sandfly—Female (Fig. 4.19)

- Smaller than mosquito.
- Whole body covered with profuse hairs.
- Abdomen is short and spindle-shaped.
- Legs are thin and long. Eyes are very prominent.

- Sprays
- Fly paper (Resin and castor oil) (2 pounds/pint)
- Metal screen to kitchen windows.
- Health education on food sanitation.

Sandfly

Sandfly—Egg (Fig. 4.16)

- Size 0.4 mm × 0.12 mm, torpedo in shape, convex dorsally and concave ventrally.
- Dark yellow in color.
- Laid in moist aerated soil with contaminated organic material.

PH importance: Adult female transmits kala-azar, sandfly fever and oriental sore.

Control

- Removal of poultry and cattle from dwelling houses.
- Cracks and crevices to be plastered.
- Sulfur fumigation or formalin cresol or DDT (Dichlorodiphenyltrichloroethane) spray to kill adult fly.
  - 5% DDT in kerosene oil.
  - Repellants like demethyl-phthalate 1–5%
  - Sandfly nets 45 mesh per inch.
  - Adult male does not transmit any disease.

Sandfly—Larva (Fig. 4.17)

- Consists of a head, neck and 12 body segments—elongated.

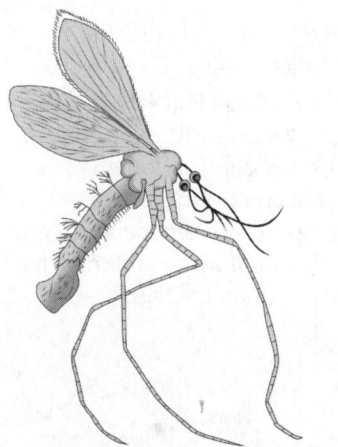

Fig. 4.18: Sandfly—male.

Chapter 4: Medical Entomology

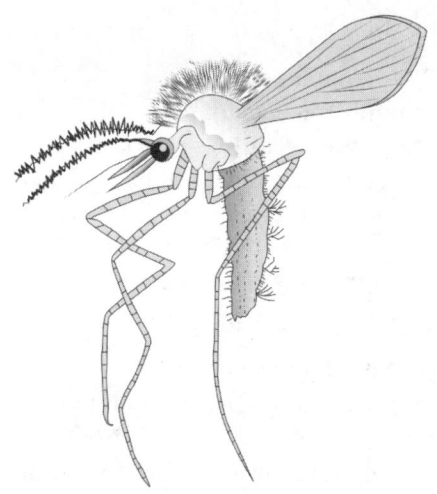

Fig. 4.19: Sandfly—female.

* Proboscis starts from a projecting snout.
* Palpi are longer than proboscis and curved.
* Wings are kept vertically at rest (Downward) (Only the females bite and suck blood).

Diseases: Vector of kala azar; tropical sore and sandfly fever.

Control

* Keep the places clean especially the cow sheds and surroundings.
* DDT sprays of the building, cow sheds, etc.
* Sleep under sandfly net.
* Repellents use.
* Cracks and crevices to be plastered.
* Sulfur fumigation, formalin, cresol or DDT.

Species: Phlebotomus papatasi
Phlebotomus sergenti
Sergentomyia punjabensis.
Adults: Smaller, lanceolate-shaped wings, disproportionate legs, hairs all over.
Diseases: Kala azar, Sand fly fever, and oriental sore.
Control: Control of breeding place
Insecticide
Clear the vegetations and shrubs.

Tsetse Fly

Species: Glossina palpalis
Glossina tachinoides
Glossina morsitans
Glossina pallidipes

No egg stage. It has a lifespan of 100 days with larva, pupa and adult stage.
Disease: Sleeping sickness
Control: Insecticide
Clear the vegetation
Biological sterile male release.

Black Fly

Species: *Simulium indicum*—
It is robust, broad wings, short proboscis.
Vector of *Onchocerca volvulus*
Control: DDT

Flea

They are temporary ectoparasites, bilaterally compressed with chitinized body. They belong to order Siphonaptera. Their host specificity is not rigid. Among them, rat fleas are medically important being the transmitter of plague.

Rat Flea (Fig. 4.20)

Xenopsylla cheopis female

Body

* Flattened laterally and well-segmented
* Body covered with bristles
* No wings
* Both sexes bite

Mesopleuron has a vertical thickening at the center.

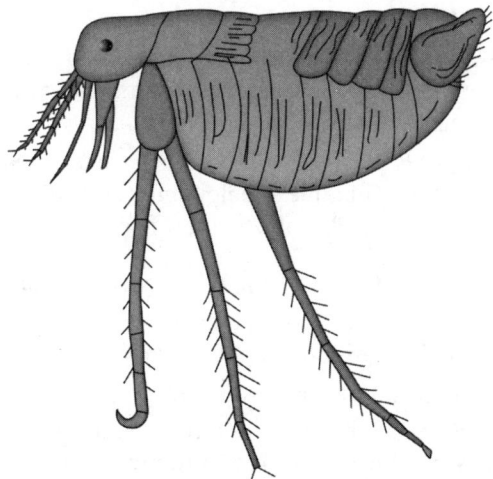

Fig. 4.20: Rat flea—female.

Female: Spermatheca is well marked and semicircular. The head, body and tail of spermatheca are of the same width.

Morphology: Body is divided into head, thorax and abdomen covered by sclerites. Spermatheca in female and aedeagus (coiled penis) in male are distinguishable points. Pygidium and antepygidial bristles are distinguishable to *Xenopsylla* genus.

PH importance: Transmits plague, endemic typhus (Murine typhus).

$$\text{Flea index} = \frac{\text{Number of fleas}}{\text{Number of rats}}$$

Types
1. *Rat flea:*
   - *Xenopsylla astia*
   - *Xenopsylla brasiliensis*
   - *Xenopsylla cheopis*
   - *Nosopsyllus fasciatus*
2. *Human flea: Pulex irritants*
3. *Dog flea: Ctenocephalides canis*
4. *Cat flea: Ctenocephalides felis*
5. *Sand flea: Tunga penetrans*

Diseases transmitted
- Bubonic plague
- Endemic murine typhus
- Sometimes tapeworm (*Hymenolepis diminuta*)
- Partially blocked fleas are dangerous.

Life cycle: Pass through egg, larva, pupa and adult.

Flea index: Ratio obtained by considering number of rats examined and number of fleas found out (Number of flea per rat).

Specific flea index: Number of a particular flea found out. This index if below one, there will be no danger at all. If above one, endemicity can be expected.

If above five, definitely it will be epidemic.

Control of flea: DDT, benzene hexachloride (BHC), malathion, repellents; rodent control.

Control of Rats and Rat Flea
- Fumigation of burrows with cyanogas.
- Insufflation of rat burrows and rat harborages with 10% DDT suspension.

Lice
- *Class:* Anoplura
- *Family:* Pediculicide

They are wingless, dorsoventrally compressed permanent ectoparasite of man. Both male and female are responsible for disease transmission. Entire life cycle takes place on the body of the host.

Pediculus Humanus: Male

Body Louse: Ectoparasite

Entire life history takes place on the human body.
- Wingless insect living on mammalian blood.
- Long and narrow body—well-segmented abdomen.
- Conical head—A proboscis, a pair of jointed antennae and a compound eye.
- Male smaller than female.
- Claws on legs.

PH importance: Vector of typhus, relapsing fever and trench fever.

Prophylaxis: Personal cleanliness and avoidance of contact with verminous person.

Control: Apply DDT powder 10% after washing and drying hair. Dust, DDT in between the skin and clothes, and in between the layers of clothing. Steam the clothes **(Fig. 4.21)**.

Pediculus Humanus: Female
- Larger than male.
- Has a deep notch at the apex of the last abdominal segment. Deposits 300 eggs on hair or cloth.

Phthirus Pubis: Pubic Louse (Fig. 4.22)

Crab Louse

Small size—square body, blunt and truncated head.

Strongly developed legs with claws at the end of the legs.

PH importance: Does not transmit any disease but produces irritation. They are found in the pubic region.

Control: Dust DDT 10%.

Chapter 4: Medical Entomology

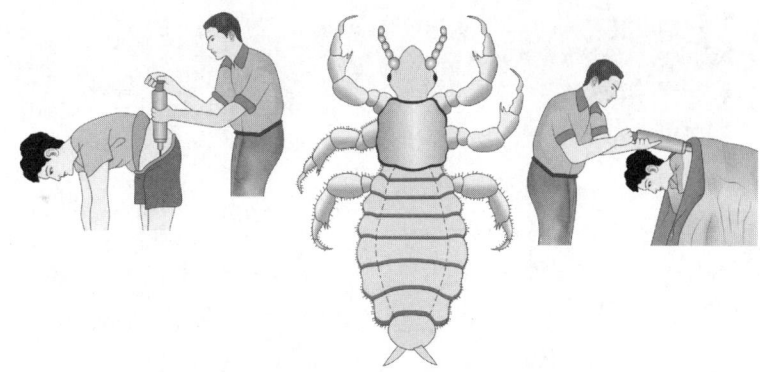

Fig. 4.21: Pediculus humanus: male.

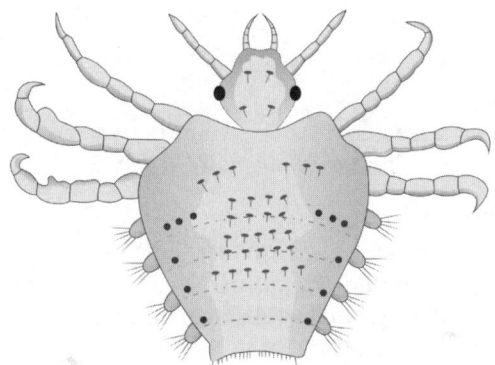

Fig. 4.22: Pthirus pubis—pubic louse.

Morphology

Body is divided into head, thorax and abdomen. The body is dorsoventrally compressed. Body is covered by shiny covering (kitenous plate). Head possesses five jointed antennae, thorax with three pairs of legs.

Life Cycle

Eggs transforms to nit in 8 days. Larva and nymph stages pass on to adult. It takes 14 days for one life cycle.

Species

- *Pediculus humanus capitis* (head louse)
- *Pediculus humanus corporis* (body louse)
- *Phthirus pubis* (pubic louse)

Diseases

Epidemic typhus, relapsing fever, trench fever, Vagabond's disease

Control

- Use of 5% DDT, shaving of hairs, burning the combed hair, 25% benzyl benzoate emulsion
  - NBIN emulsion
  - 68% benzyl benzoate
  - 6% DDT
  - 12% benzocaine
  - 14% TWEEN 80
  - Dilute in water (1:5)

Ticks

Class: Arachnida

They are temporary ectoparasite of warm-blooded animals, including man. Their vector potentiality is greater. The entire body looks like a fused saccular mass. It possesses four pairs of legs.

Hard and Soft Ticks (Fig. 4.23)

- Body compressed dorsoventrally consisting of the thorax and abdomen—body oval and elongated.
- Provided with four pairs of legs.
- Hard ticks provided with a chitinous shield on the dorsal surface.

Hard tick possesses hard structure scutum. It possesses a false head and feeds frequently when compared to soft tick.

PH importance: Hard ticks vector of:

- Tick paralysis
- Tick typhus
- Q fever
- Tularemia

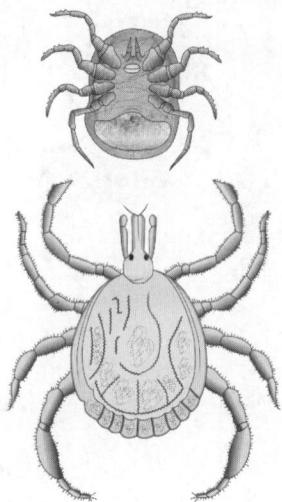

Fig. 4.23: Hard and soft ticks.

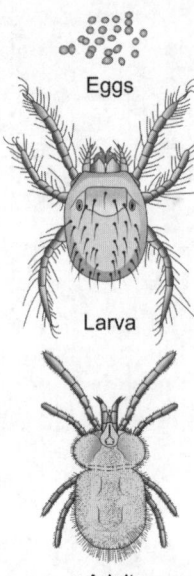

Fig. 4.24: Morphology of mites.

- Encephalitis
- Hemorrhagic fever

Soft ticks—vectors of relapsing fevers.

Species

- *Dermacentor andersoni* (typhus)
- *Haemaphysalis spinigera* (KFD)
- *Ornithodoros moubata* (relapsing fever)

Control in Man

- Avoid sleeping in endemic areas
- Wear long pants and over boots
- Use tick repellants—dimethyl phthalate
- Use of insecticides 5% DDT or 0.5% lindane

Control in Animals

Arsenic dip* to infected animals like cattle, horse, dog.
Use of repellents: 10% of DDT
Arsenic trioxide: 8.0 lb; Pine tar 1 gallon; Water 500 gallon)

Mites

They are very small organisms with the size of pin head. Owing to their appearance, they are called *velvet mites*.

Life Cycle

Passes through stages of egg, larva, nymph and adult. Larva possesses three pairs of legs. Adults have four pairs of legs (**Fig. 4.24**).

Species

- *Trombicula deliensis* (scrub typhus)
- *Trombicula akamushi* (relapsing orientalis)

In mites, except larval stage, other forms are free living forms.

Sarcoptes Scabiei

Morphology (Fig. 4.25)

Itch mites are minute globular parasites; these are visible to naked eyes. They are worldwide in distribution, more in overcrowded areas. Male measures 2.5–3.0 mm and female 3.5–4.0 mm. Adults possess four pairs of legs. They form permanent ectoparasites of man, with their entire life span on the skin of the host. For the disease to spread, contact is essential. The larva after entering the hair follicle grows into adult. Entire cycle completes in 10–14 days.

Public Health Importance

It is not a vector. It directly causes scabies (itch). If secondary infection occurs, they cannot thrive and cannot be seen in scrapings.

Control: Isolation, treatment of all members of the family.

- Hygienic measures (daily bath)

---

*Sodium bicarbonate 24.0 lb.

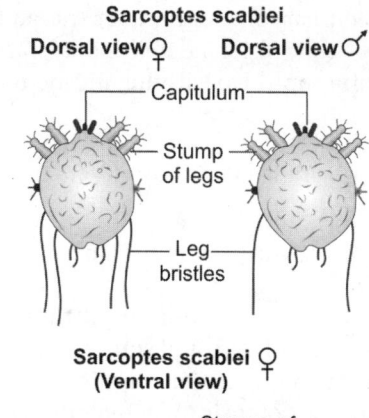

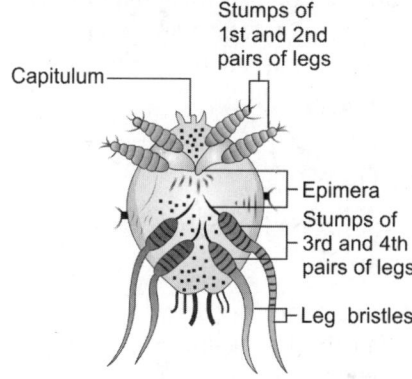

Fig. 4.25: Morphology of itch mite.

- 25% benzyl benzoate (applied to all parts of body below chin and allowed to dry. Later repeated after 12 hours. Further 12 hours later thorough bath is given, all clothing are immersed in boiling water and washed with detergent powder. Application is limited to 2 per week).
- 10% sulfur ointment
- 1% HCH (lindane)
- 5% tetmasol

Cyclops

Morphology (Fig. 4.26)

Salient Features

They are pear-shaped, semi-transparent, and of 1 mm length.
Types: Mesocyclops
Paracyclops
Microcyclops
1. A freshwater crustacean 1/20 inch × 1/8 inch

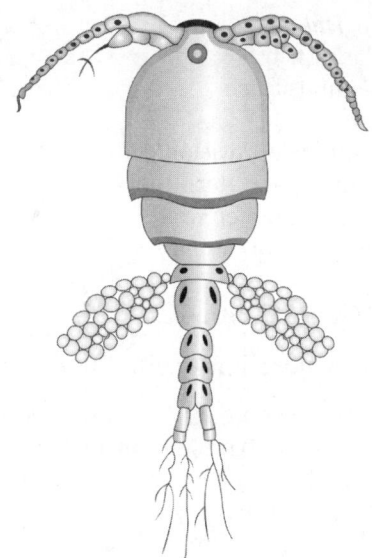

Fig. 4.26: Morphology of cyclops.

2. Has pear-shaped symmetrical body, forked tail, three pairs of antennae, five pairs of swimming legs and one eye
3. Lifespan about 3 months.

PH importance: They are the intermediate hosts for *Dracunculus medinensis* and *D. latum*.

Cyclops Female
- It has a pair of egg sacs.
- *Diseases transmitted:*
  - *D. medinensis*
  - *D. latum*

Prophylaxis

Cyclops can be destroyed by:
- Superchlorination of the water.
- Drinking filtered or boiled water only.
- Cyclopicidal fish—*Barbus puckelli*.
- 50% DDT, once in 6 weeks—in 6 ppm
- Convert step wells into draw wells.

Control
- *Physical:*
  - Straining of water (Muslin cloth)
  - Boiling water
- *Chemical:*
  - 5 ppm chlorine
  - 1 g/gallon lime

- *Biological:*
  - Barbel fish
  - Gambusia fish
- *Others:*
  - Tube well provision
  - Controlled water supply
  - Abolishing step well
  - Provision of sanitary wells.

INSECTICIDES (FIG. 4.27)

DDT—Dichlorodiphenyltrichlorethane

Pure DDT or its solution or emulsions are not used nowadays. Chlorinated hydrocarbon DDT is commonly used now as 10% DDT powder and 50% DDT wettable powder.

Uses

- 10% DDT powder is used on a large scale; has an antiplague measure by insufflating into rat burrows and dusting of runs and rat harborages and also for control of lice infestation.
- 50% DDT wettable powder is used to prepare 2½ or 5% DDT

Suspension: For spraying the floor, wall and roof for plague control, for indoor residual spraying, for malaria control to kill adult mosquitoes.

Action

Acts as a residual contact poison.

Advantages

- DDT is extremely stable and has a prolonged residual action.
- Minute doses are enough to kill the insects.
- It resists wind, rain and sun.
- It needs to be applied only once in 3–6 months.
- Ordinarily not toxic to animals or man.
- Does not spoil water.
- Effective against all insects.

Disadvantages

Some insects like bugs, fleas, flies, etc., become resistant to DDT.

BHC—Benzene Hexachloride (Gammexane)

- It is a residual insecticide.
- Used for the destruction of insects especially houseflies.

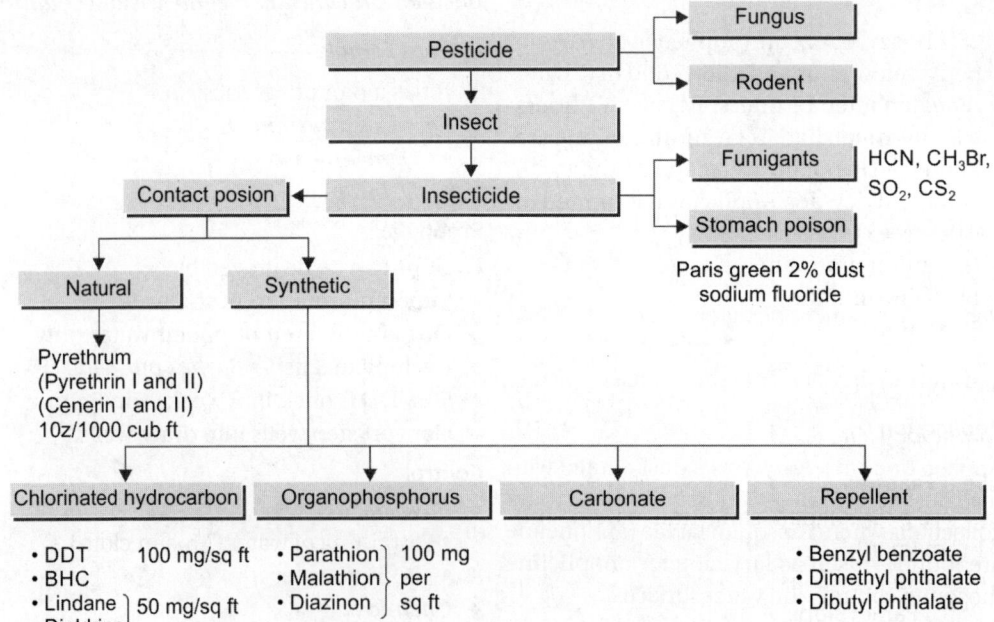

Fig. 4.27: Classification of insecticides.

- It is a white crystalline substance insoluble in water but soluble in inorganic solvents.
- It is a contact poison.

Pyrethrum Extract

- Petroleum extract from pyrethrum flowers.
- Contains alkaloids pyrethrum I and pyrethrum II.
- Used as 1% spray in kerosene 2 ounces per 1,000 cubic feet.
- Immediate knock-down effect.
- It is an insecticide.
- Contact poison.
- Used as space spray.

Malariol

Resembles coal tar disinfectant in color and consistency.

Use

As a larvicide against all mosquitoes except *Mansonia*.

Action

By choking the siphon tubes and suffocating the larvae—also acts as a direct poison. It should form a thin layer over the entire water surface.

Disadvantages

- Weeds should be removed.
- Cannot be used in drinking water or in paddy fields.

Paris Green

Composition

Acetoarsenite of copper, green in color, should be in fine powder so that it may float on water and add through larval mouth (stomach poison).

Application

Applied once in a week—as a dust diluted with road dust, or fine ash—1% dust is used over water collections where mosquito larvae (anopheline are found)—used as larvicide for anopheline mosquito control—on water surface.

Apparatus

- Hand duster: 1%
- Aeroplane spray: 2.5%

Advantages

Weeds removal not necessary.

Disadvantages

- Larvae of *Culex*—are not killed.
- Not useful to destroy pupae.

Commonly used Insecticides

- DDT
- BHC
- Lindane
- Pyrethrum
- Malariol
- Paris green

Rodents (Figs. 4.28A and B)

Disease: Typhoid, leptospirosis, amebiasis, ringworm.

Difference between domestic and norvegicus is depicted in **Table 4.2**.

Anti-rodent Measures

1. *Sanitary*: Houses, food, garbage
2. Trapping

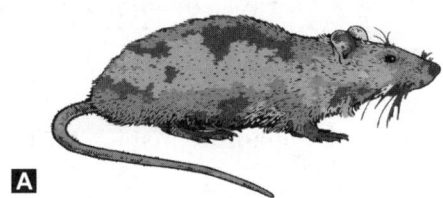

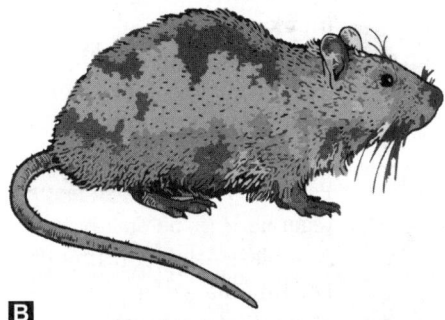

Figs. 4.28A and B: (A) *Rattus rattus* and (B) *Rattus norvegicus*.

Table 4.2: Difference between *Rattus rattus* and *Rattus norvegicus*.

R. rattus		R. norvegicus
Slim, slender	Body	Heavy, large
Sharp	Muzzle	Blunt
Larger	Tail	Shorter
Large	Ear	Small
Big	Eye	Small

3. Poisons:
   $BaCO_3$ (white tasteless)
   Zinc phosphide (black)
   Na Fluoroacetate-alpha-naphthylthiourea (ANTU)
   Arsenous oxide
   Warfarin (anticoagulant)—Multidose
4. Fumigation: $CaCN$, CS_2, CH_3Br, SO_2

ZOONOSES

Diseases of vertebrate animals to man.

Bacterial: Tuberculosis—cattle, goat
Brucellosis—cattle, goat, swine
Plague—rat
Typhoid—mammals, birds
Light induced hypertrichosis (LIH)—rodents
Rat bite fever—rat
Anthrax—sheep, goat, horse
Glanders—horse
Tularemia—sheep, rabbit
Relapsing fever—rodents

Fungal: Dermatophytosis—cat, dog, horse
Ringworm—poultry

Viral: Rabies—dog, wolf
Kyasanur forest disease (KFD)—monkey, cattle

Rickettsial: Endemic typhus—rat
Rickettsial pox—mice
Scrub typhus—rodent
Q fever—cattle, sheep
Psittacosis (ornithosis)—parrot, pigeon

Protozoa: Amebiasis—lower primates
Leishmania—dog
T. gondii—mammal
Trypanosoma—dog

Helminthic: Hydatid—dog
Taenia—swine, cattle
Trichinella—swine
Fasciola—dog, swine
Ankylostoma—dog

Arthopod: Scabies—domestic animals
Tunga—mammals

INTEGRATED VECTOR CONTROL

In case of mosquitoes, "integrated approach" is advocated which allows the combination of one or more methods with a view to obtain maximum results with minimum input. This will disallow excessive use of any one method. Integrated vector control prevents environmental pollution with toxic chemicals.

Integrated Approach to the Environmental Problems

All aspects of a health problem are considered from all angles. This suggests the cooperation between different health care services and many disciplines. For the promotion of health in human environment United Nations, World Health Organization and UNESCO are providing an unprecedented cooperation.

SUMMARY

Effort is made for identifying features of insects of medical importance. Zoonoses and insecticide are described. A note on integrated vector control is given.

VIVA VOCE

1. Mention types of biological transmission.
2. Mention fly borne diseases.
3. Give identifying points of anopheles female mosquito.
4. Differentiate egg of anopheles and culex.
5. Define specific flea index.
6. What is the public health importance of Cyclops?
7. Differentiate domestic rat and Norwegian rat.
8. Give examples of zoonoses.
9. Define integrated vector control.

SECTION 2

Section Outline

Chapter 5. Principles of Health Promotion and Education

Chapter 6. Nutrition and Health

Chapter 7. Basic Statistics and its Application

CHAPTER 5: Principles of Health Promotion and Education

Chapter Outline

- Methods of Health Education
- Health Education Approach
- Planning and Management of Health Education

INFORMATION

Information on health, event, disease, and impact is the requisite of education and communication.

Projects, such as BIRD (Bidar Integrated Rural Development) have given the requisite information for IEC (Information, education and communication) components. They are:

Means

- Health practices
- Health aids
- Health staff
- Health systems
- Walkie-talkie

Materials

- Leaflet
- Posters
- Cinema slide
- Radio
- Folklore
- Publicity

Organization

- Committee
- Government field
- Publicity
- Voluntary organization
- Local leaders

Content

- About diseases
- About life prolongation
- About death prevention
- All free from government

Action

- Film
- Meeting
- Helping immunization
- Exhibition
- Review

Conventional information: They conform and change is brought out (accepting).

Progressive information: They reform and behavior change is brought out (adopting).

Liberating information: They transform and social change is brought out.

Following are the basic areas where information is available to health professionals:
- RCH: Nutrition
- School health: Environmental sanitation
- CD: Geriatrics
- NCD: Mental health
- Demography: Accidents
- Personal hygiene: Family health service available.

Developed area of information for health education.
- Nutrition education
- AIDS education
- Cancer education
- Population education
- Human belief
- Family health

EDUCATION

It is a process of acquiring knowledge and skill through the process of behavior centers through learning by doing which discipline the primitive desires **(Fig. 5.1)**.

Types of Education

- Primary education
- Secondary education
- Collegiate education
- Technical education
- Medical education
- Health education
- Adult education

Health Education

- Sex education
- Nutrition education
- Population education
- Extension education
- Cancer education
- AIDS education

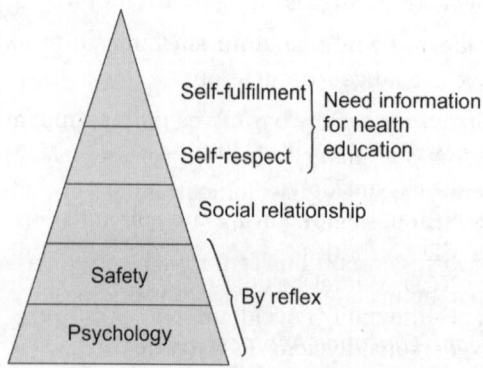

Fig. 5.1: Need, IEC (Information, education and communication) based.

Definition of Health Education

"It is a process that informs, motivates and helps people to adopt and maintain health practices and lifestyle; it emphasizes the need for environmental changes to achieve this goal and conducts professional training and research to the same end".

Human behavior and group behavior decide the acceptance and adaptation. This is facilitated through health education.

Principles of Health Education

- Interest (felt need)
- Trustworthy (credibility)
- Desire to learn (motivation)
- Active learning (participation)
- Knowing the level of understanding (comprehension)
- Repetition at intervals (reinforcement)
- Learning by doing
- Takes from known to unknown
- Preach as you do
- Good human relations
- Get the result (feedback), and
- From respected and regarded people (Zila Panchayat leader, village leader, religious leader)

Methods of Health Education

Auditory Aid
- Tape recorder
- Radio
- Microphone

Visual Aid
- Posters
- Exhibition
- Model
- Specimen
- Chart

Audio-video Aid
- TV
- Cinema

Difference between health education and health propaganda is shown in **Table 5.1**.

Single person approach (individual)
- Interview
- Visits, and
- Postal approach

Chapter 5: Principles of Health Promotion and Education

Table 5.1: Health education and health propaganda differentiated.

	Health education	Health propaganda
Knowledge	Acquired	Instilled
Skill	Acquired	Instilled
Animal instinct	Taken away	Put to action
Action	Think and act	By reflex act
Emotion	No	Yes
Reasoning	Yes	No
Attitude	Positive	Negative

Many persons approach (group)
- Lecture
- Colloquium (interaction between experts and audience with the help of a moderator)
- Dialogue (mutual discussion on a topic by two experts which will benefit audience)
- Step-by-step demonstration (Actual carrying out of an activity)
- Face-to-face interaction of a group
- Group discussion (Large scope for free discussion and exchange of views among teachers and students) **(Figs. 5.2 and 5.3)**.

Examples of mass media
- Newspapers
- Posters
- Flashcards [cards of about 20 inches (40 cm × 50 cm) on a theme in the form of picture]
- Flannel board (card cut outs on khadi cloth displaying pictures)
- Museum
- Radio
- Printed publications

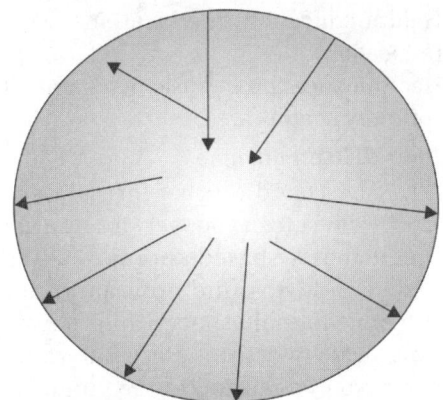

Fig. 5.3: Unequal participation in group discussion.

- TV
- Internet

Examples of folk media
- Dance
- Mono-acting
- Puppet show
- Yakshagana
- Harikatha
- Dramas
- Kirtan
- Gazal
- Qawwali
- Street play

Recent group approach
Panel discussion: Qualified people through the topic and discussion.
Symposium: Series of speeches on a selected subject.
Workshop: Series of meeting emphasizing on a topic.
Role play: It is a social drama dramatizing the topic.
Conference: Broad comprehensive topic at national- or state-level discussion.
Seminar: Single major topic at national or state level discussion.
Buzz session: In small group, allowed to buzz on a theme, later merged for the findings.

Health Education Approach
- Health education in health service (service)
- Health education in health regulation (law)

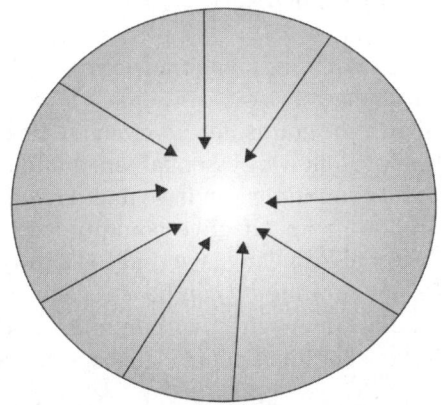

Fig. 5.2: Equal participation in group discussion.

- Health education in educational service (education)
- Health education in basic need approach (primary health care).

Child-to-child programme

In 1977, Dr David Morley formulated an idea of health care of younger sibs by a child. Through activity-based approach, NCERT has tried child-to-child program through health educational aspect. Child power to communicate relevant messages to younger children, to parents and to the community is described in "Manual for teachers from NCERT".

Activities are:
- Care for the young child
- Influence on health practice of parents
- Influence health practice of other members in the community
- Environmental improvement in terms of sanitation, tree planting, etc.

COMMUNICATION

Learning educational communication is of great importance because education implies transfer of knowledge and skill. Information has to be gathered in the process of learning. Skill has to be observed, practiced and developed. Hence, communication forms an important component in the process of education and learning.

Communication deals with transmission of information or ideas. They are done through:
- Expressing our feelings
- Facial expression
- Gesture of face, hand
- Spoken words
- Songs
- Improved language
- Written script

Major components of communication are as following:
- Source (sender)
- Content (message), and
- Audience (receiver)

Main aim of communication:
- To help acquire the knowledge (cognitive domain), and
- To help acquire skill (psychomotor domain)
- To inform, to educate, to motivate, and to persuade for high standard of health

Communication media are:
- Interpersonal media
- Mass media (recent)
- Folk media (tradition)

Communication types are:
- One way (Didactic method)
- Two way (Socratic method)
- Visual way
- Verbal way
- Soft skills, such as gesture, posture, body movement, facial expressions, smiling, frowning, staring, gazing, etc.
- Nonformal way
- Formal way
- Internet way

Communication Barriers

- Physiological: Difficulty in hearing
- Psychological: Emotional disturbance
- Environmental: Loud noise
- Cultural: Urban—rural, foreign—national, positive and negative attitude

ROLE OF HEALTH EDUCATION IN HEALTH PROGRAMS

Health education brings about reformation by adaptations which will bring about behavioral changes.

It also can bring about transformation by a social change.

In health programs, for an effective health education, following essentials are drafted:
- Rural community can have traditional folk media for an effective communication. Regional local language usage is a must.
- Urban community can have recent mass media for an effective communication. National or international language is more effective.

Chapter 5: Principles of Health Promotion and Education

POPULATION EDUCATION

Definition

An educational program is an organized effort which provides the situation for a better development of responsible attitude towards population growth.

Content

- National demographic situation
- National political commitment to population growth
- Educational goal for population growth
- Benefit of small family norms, economics of population growth
- Sociology of population growth
- Statistics of population growth
- Levels of living by population growth.

CANCER EDUCATION

Cancer education program is an organized effort which provides the study of cancer situation for a better development of responsible attitude toward cancer control.

Content

- Warning signs (danger signs of cancer)
- Risk factors in cancer
- National cancer situation
- Political commitment for cancer centers
- Educational goal for cancer centers
- Benefits of simple living
- Economics of smoking
- Economics of alcoholism
- Occupational aspect of cancer
- Carcinogens in atmosphere
- Cancer screening programmes, and
- Available treatment for cancer

AIDS EDUCATION

AIDS Education Programme is an organized effort which provides the study of AIDS situation for a better development of responsible attitude toward AIDS control.

Content

- Making life-saving choices
- Guidelines for prevention of AIDS
- Nature of AIDS
- Transmission of AIDS
- Risk factors in AIDS, and
- National AIDS situation

There should be a high political commitment for AIDS control. Education goals for AIDS control should be to create self-awareness on benefits of living in simple and self-cultured and available treatment for AIDS facilities and clinics to be expanded

NUTRITION EDUCATION

This is aimed at providing a study of nutritional situation for a better development of responsible attitude toward better nutrition and better health.

Contents

- Malnutrition
- National nutritional status
- Political commitment for better nutrition
- Education goal for better nutrition
- Food hygiene
- Special group requirement
- Prevention of Food Adulteration (PFA) Acts
- National programs on nutrition
- Balanced diet
- Nutritional assessment, and
- Nutrition and health

PLANNING AND MANAGEMENT OF HEALTH EDUCATION

It has to be done with specific health programs. Strategies are laid down according to social, economical, cultural and political status of the community. After implementation and monitoring, evaluation is required to be done as a feedback.

Health Education Administration

In 1956, Central Health Education Bureau (CHEB), New Delhi, was established to promote and coordinate health education work in India. We have Central Health Education Bureau in the Ministry of Health, State Governments have State Health Education Bureau and Districts have District Health Education Bureau. Of late, School Health Education Bureau is functioning in health education activities in school health activities.

No department or organization is spared from the health education activity in India.

Other Official Agencies
- Directorate of Advertising and Visual Publicity (DAVP)
- Press Information Bureau
- Doordarshan
- All India Radio
- Indian Red Cross
- International Union for Health Education
- Division of Publication, Information and Public Relation, WHO
- Regional Bureau of Health Education.

SUMMARY

In this chapter, method of health education is described. This is followed by Health Education Approach. Planning and Management of Health Education is described in detail.

VIVA VOCE

1. What are the principles of health education?
2. Describe the methods of health education.
3. What are the differences between health education and health propaganda?
4. Give example for group approach in health education
5. What is child-to-child programme?
6. Mention communication barriers.
7. What is population education?

CHAPTER 6: Nutrition and Health

CHAPTER OUTLINE

- Proximate Principles
- Nutritional Assessment
- Nutritional Diseases
- Therapeutic Diets
- Nutritional Surveillance
- Food Surveillance
- Food Additives, Food Adulteration, Food Fortification
- Nutritional Program

INTRODUCTION

Next to the brilliant achievement of discovery of bacteria, chemistry of body with biochemical lesion and chemical pathology have led to next best discovery of nutrition.

MAIN AREAS OF STUDY

- Not enough food (quantitative)
  - Subnutrition
  - Frank starvation
- Wrong food (qualitative)
  - Malnutrition
- Too much food
  - Obesity

TERMINOLOGY

- *Food:* Item we eat in day-to-day practice.
- *Nutrition:* Science of food in our health.
- *Nutrient:* Food factor identified as body need.
- *Macronutrient:* Proximate principles, viz., carbohydrate, protein, fat.
- *Micronutrient:* Small quantity required nutrient, viz., vitamin, mineral, trace elements.
- *Diet:* Food recipe in servable form (Food and drink regularly confirmed or prescribed allowance of food on health ground).
- *Dietetics:* Practical application of diet.

SOURCE OF NUTRITION

- *Energy yielding:* Cereals, pulses, oilseeds, and fruits, such as orange, malta, mosambi, banana, pineapple, peach, apple, quince, plums, coconut, bitter guard, ears of wheat, *Colocasia*.
- *Body building:* Fish, liver, egg
- *Protective:* Fruits, such as mango, malta, grape, banana, quince, apple, pear, spinach, tomato, *Colocasia*, amla, turnip, carrot, drumstick, egg, meat, liver.
- *Vitamin A:* Liver, egg yolk, butter, ghee, cream milk, whale fish liver oil, carrot, spinach, winter squash, pumpkin, *Amaranthus* leaves, mango, papaya.
- *Vitamin D:* Milk, ghee, butter, egg yolk, cod liver oil, halibut oil, mustard oil.
- *Vitamin E:* Butter, cream, egg yolk, liver, fish liver oil.
- *Vitamin C:* Amla, citrus fruits, strawberries, cantaloupe, tomato, green pepper, cabbage, potato.
- *Vitamin K:* Leafy vegetables, pork, liver, fat, soybean, other vegetable oils.
- *Vitamin B:* Pork, liver, meats of organs, wheat grains, nuts, legumes, potatoes, yeast, wheat germ.
- *Riboflavin:* Liver, milk, meat, egg, enriched bread, green leafy vegetable, yeast.

- *Niacin:* Liver, fowl, meat, fish, wheat grain, legume, mushroom, yeast.
- *Pantothenic acid*: Liver, meat or organs, egg, peanut, legume, mushroom, salmon, wheat grain, yeast, wheat germ.
- *Pyridoxine:* Pork, meat of organs, legumes, grains, potatoes, banana, yeast, wheat germ.
- *Biotin:* Liver, meat of organ, peanut, egg, milk, mushroom, yeast.
- *Calcium*: Egg, milk, cheese, sesame, *Amaranthus* leaves, drumstick, Bengal gram, ragi, crab, fish.
- *Phosphorus:* Banana, nuts, butter, milk, pulses.
- *Iron:* Spinach, *Amaranthus* leaf, gram leaves, drumstick, whole cereal grain, dates, dried yeast.
- *Protein:* Egg, lean fish, lean meat, milk, pulses, nuts.

BASAL METABOLISM

"The energy metabolism of a subject at complete physical and mental rest and having normal body temperature and in the postabsorptive state (i.e., 12 hours after the intake of last meal)."

Basal metabolic rate (BMR) is closely related to body surface area and less directly related to weight or height of an individual.

DuBois and DuBois formula for calculation of body surface is as under:

$A = (W^{0.425}) \times (H^{0.725}) \times (71.84)$

where
A = Body surface (sq. cm)
H = Height (cm)
W = Weight (kg)
Log A = (Log W) × (0.425) + (Log H) × (0.725 + 1.8564)

Examples: When height is 140 cm, weight is 45 kg, body surface is 1.30
When height is 150 cm, weight is 55 kg, body surface is 1.56
When height is 160 cm, weight is 60 kg, body surface is 1.62

PROXIMATE PRINCIPLES

Carbohydrate

It is the main source of energy.
- Four calories per gram
- Starch, sugar, and the cellulose are the components
- Dietary fiber from carbohydrates protects gastrointestinal system.
- *Requirement*—50–60% of total calories must be carbohydrates.

Protein

Functions: Growth, development, repair, antibody, enzyme, hormone.

Source: Animal protein, vegetable proteins.

Essential amino acids: Body cannot synthesize, obtained from diet. They are leucine, isoleucine, lysine, methionine, phenylalanine, threonine, valine, tryptophan, histidine.

Limiting amino acids:
- No methionine in pulses
- No lysine in cereals

Requirement: 1 g per kg body weight.

Reference protein: Milk and egg are animal proteins, have high biological value and are comparable as standard proteins.

$$\text{Net protein utilization} = \frac{\text{Digestibility coefficient} \times \text{Biological value}}{100}$$

Fat

Saturated fatty acids:
- Lauric acid
- Palmitic acid
- Stearic acid

Unsaturated fatty acids:
- Oleic acid
- Linoleic acid [Essential fatty acid (EFA)]

Invisible fat: Milk, egg, meat, nuts.

Public health importance—Obesity, coronary heart disease (CHD), Ca. colon, Ca. breast, skin lesions.

Requirements: About 15–20% of total calories.

Chapter 6: Nutrition and Health

Effects and Requirements of Vitamins and Minerals

See **Tables 6.1** and **6.2**.

Table 6.1: Effects and requirements of vitamins.

Vitamins	Disease	Requirement
Vitamin A	Night blindness	RDA = 600 µg/ (adult)
	Bitot's spot	
	Xerosis of conjunctiva	
	Xerosis of cornea	
	Keratomalacia	
Vitamin D	Rickets	RDA = 100 IU (adult)
	Osteomalacia	
Vitamin E	Nil	0.8 mg/g of EFA
Vitamin K	Bleeding disorder	RDA = 0.03 mg/kg (adult)
Thiamine	Dry beriberi	RDA = 0.5 mg/1,000 cal (adult)
	Wet beriberi	
	Wernicke encephalopathy	
Riboflavin	Angular stomatitis	RDA = 0.6 mg/1000 cal (adult)
	Cheilosis	
	Glossitis	
	Nasolabial dyssebacia	
Niacin	Pellagra	RDA = 6.6 mg/1,000 cal (adult)
Vitamin B_6	Peripheral neuritis	2 mg/day (adult)
Pantothenic acid	Nil	10 µg/day (adult)
Folic acid	Megaloblastic anemia	100 µg/day (adult)
Vitamin B_{12}	Megaloblastic anemia	1 µg/day (adult)
Vitamin C	Scurvy	60 mg/day (adult)

(RDA: recommended dietary allowance)

Table 6.2: Effects and requirements of minerals.

Minerals	Disease	Requirement
Calcium	Bone dysfunction	500 mg/day (adult)
	Teeth problem	
Phosphorus	Bone dysfunction	Not specified
	Teeth problem	
Sodium	Muscular cramp	15 g/day (adult)
Potassium	Nil	Not specified
Magnesium	Tetany	300 mg/day (adult)
Iron	Anemia	28 mg/day (adult)
Iodine	Iodine deficiency disorders	150 µg/day (adult)
Fluorine	Skeletal fluorosis	No specification
	Dental fluorosis	
Zinc	Growth failure	15 mg/day (adult)
	Sex dysfunction	
Copper	Neutropenia	2.2 µg/day (adult)
Cobalt	Nil	Not specified
Chromium	Nil	Not specified
Selenium	Selenium deficiency	Not specified
Molybdenum	Nil	Not specified

Recommended Intake of Nutrients

See **Table 6.3**.

IMPORTANT NUTRITIONAL PROFILE OF FOODSTUFF

Rice: Thiamine, riboflavin and protein are lost by milling. Hot soaking process of parboiling is suggested to retain the nutritive value of rice.

Parboiling: Paddy is soaked in hot water at 70°C for 4 hours. Water is drained, soaked paddy is steamed for 10 minutes, dried and milled.

Jowar: Being a staple diet and containing high leucine content, is found greatly associated with occurrence of pellagra.

Ragi: Richest source of calcium.

Table 6.3: Recommended intake of nutrients.

Item		Requirement
Calorie		Male 2,425 to 3,800 calories Female 1,875 to 2,925 calories (Pregnancy + 300, lactation + 550)
Protein		1 g/kg, children more (Pregnancy +15 g, lactation +25 g)
Carbohydrate		50–60% of total calories
Fat		15–20% of total calories
Vitamin	A	600 µg
	D	100 IU
	E	0.8 mg/g EFA
	K	0.03 mg/kg
	B_1	0.5 mg/1,000 calories
Riboflavin		0.6 mg/1,000 calories
Niacin		6.6 mg/1,000 calories
Folic acid		100 µg
B_{12}		1 µg
C		60 mg
Minerals	Ca	500 mg
	Fe	28 mg
	I_2	150 µg

Soybean: Richest among pulse with 40% protein.

Kesari dal: Associated with lathyrism.

Groundnut: Central Food Technological Research Institute (CFTRI) work—Indian multipurpose food (MPF), Balahar, malt food.

Tender coconuts: 1 liter = 3 mg Na, 74 mg K, 200 calories

Green leaves: Low-calorie bulk food in obesity.

Fruits:
- Rich source of Ca: Dates (120 mg/100 g)
- Rich source of Fe: Dates (7.3 mg/100 g)
- Rich source of vitamin A: Papaya (2740 µg/100 g)
- Rich source of vitamin C: Amla (600 mg/100 g)
- *Skimmed milk:* Fat removed milk
- *Toned milk:* Blend of natural milk and made up milk and reduced fat content.

Vegetable milk: CFTRI work from groundnut, from soybean.

Boiled egg: Nutritionally superior to raw egg.

Testing the egg for freshness is by (a) Fresh egg sinks in water (b) rotten egg floats due to evaporation of water and liberation of gases.

Cook or boil for 7 minutes or pouched for 5 minutes to kill *Salmonella* in egg.

NUTRITIVE VALUE OF COMMON FOODS

See **Table 6.4**.

NUTRITIONAL ASSESSMENT

Objectives of nutritional assessment are:
- To map out the magnitude of malnutrition.
- To find out ecological factors.
- To prevent malnutrition and to develop a health care program.

Methods of Assessment

- *Clinical examination* is undertaken with Indian Council of Medical Research (ICMR)-recommended nutritional assessment schedule.
- *Anthropometric examination* is undertaken with height, weight, head circumference, chest circumference and mid-upper arm circumference (MUAC) among 0–6 age children.
  Height and weight for age among adults are undertaken.
- *Laboratory examination*
  - Hb%, urine and stool examinations are commonly done.
  - Serum level of vitamin A (retinol), folic acid, vitamin B_{12}, and albumin are undertaken in selected cases.
  - Prothrombin time and urinary iodine are considered in selected cases.
- *Functional index test*
  - Capillary fragility (Vitamin C)
  - Prothrombin time (Vitamin K)
  - Sperm count (calorie and zinc)
  - Nerve conduction (Vitamin B12)
  - Heart rate (work capacity).

Chapter 6: Nutrition and Health

Table 6.4: Nutritive value of common foods (per 100 grams).

Foodstuff	Protein (in grams)	Fat (in grams)	Carbohydrates	Calories (in grams)
Cereal	9.9	2.3	71.0	344
Bread	7.8	0.7	51.9	245
Salted biscuit	6.6	32.4	54.6	534
Sweet biscuit	6.4	15.2	71.9	450
Pulses	22.6	2.0	58.4	342
Green leafy vegetables	3.8	0.6	6.0	45
Root, tubers	1.2	0.2	16.0	70
Other vegetables	2.2	0.3	6.3	36
Nuts, oil seeds	15.2	46.6	20.4	578
Condiment, spice	9.8	6.6	40.6	261
Fruits	1.1	0.4	7.6	79
Meat	21.0	4.9	0.8	131
Egg	13.3	13.3	0.0	173
Milk	3.6	5.8	4.7	85
Curd	3.1	4.0	3.0	60
Butter	0.0	81.0	0.0	729
Ghee	0.0	100.0	0.0	900
Oil	0.0	100.0	0.0	900
Sugar	0.1	0.0	99.4	398
Honey	0.3	0.0	79.5	319
Jaggery	0.4	0.1	95.0	383
Sago	0.2	0.2	87.1	351

- *Diet survey*
  - Weighment of raw foods
  - Weighment of cooked foods
  - Stock inventory method
  - Postal questionnaire method
- *Vital statistics*
  - Low birth weight (LBW)
  - Lifespan

Table 6.5: Guideline for balanced diet construction.

Nutrients	Basic requirements
Protein	1 g per kg body weight
Fat	15–20% of total calories
Carbohydrate	50–60% of total calories
Iron	28 mg
Retinol	600 mg (2,400 IU)
Thiamine	1.2 mg
Riboflavin	1.4 mg
Nicotinic acid	16 mg
Pyridoxine	2.0 mg
Vitamin C	40 mg
Folic acid	100 µg
Vitamin B_{12}	1 µg

- *Ecological factors*
  - Per capita consumption of calories
  - Per capita consumption of protein
  - Infant feeding practices
  - Immunization services
  - Intestinal parasitism

BALANCED DIET

It is defined as a diet which contains adequate quantity of proximate principles, vitamins, minerals, trace elements and calories for a given age, sex and nature of work. This should be adequate to meet maintenance of health and well-being. It should also be given an extra allowance for a lean period. It is an accepted means to safeguard population from nutritional deficiencies.

In constructing the balanced diet, following guidelines are used as baseline (**Table 6.5**).

Balanced Diet for Adult Man

Refer **Table 6.6**.

Table 6.6: Balanced diet for adult man.

Items (in grams)	Sedentary	Moderate work	Heavy work
Cereals	460	520	670
Pulses	40	50	60

Items (in grams)	Sedentary	Moderate work	Heavy work
Leafy vegetables	40	40	40
Other vegetables	60	70	80
Roots and tubers	50	60	80
Milk	150	200	250
Oil and fat	40	45	65
Sugar and jaggery	30	35	55

Balanced Diet for Adult Woman (Table 6.7)

Table 6.7: Balanced diet for adult woman.

Items (in grams)	Sedentary	Moderate work	Heavy work
Cereals	410	440	575
Pulses	40	45	50
Leafy vegetable	100	100	50
Other vegetable	40	40	100
Roots, tubers	50	50	60
Milk	100	150	200
Oil, fat	20	25	40
Sugar, jaggery	20	20	40

Balanced Diet for Children (Table 6.8)

Table 6.8: Balanced diet for children (in grams).

Items (in grams)	1–3 years	4–6 years
Cereals	175	270
Pulses	35	35
Leafy vegetables	40	50
Other vegetables	20	30
Roots, tubers	10	20
Milk	300	250
Oil, fat	15	25
Sugar, jaggery	30	40

Recommended Dietary Allowances for Industrial Workers (Table 6.9)

Table 6.9: Dietary allowance for industrial workers.

Items	Moderate work	Heavy work
Calorie (kcal)	2,800	3,900
Protein (g)	55	55
Calcium (g)	0.5	0.5
Iron (mg)	24	24
Retinol (µg)	750	750
Thiamine (mg)	1.4	2.0
Riboflavin (mg)	1.7	2.3
Nicotinic acid (mg)	19	26
Vitamin B6 (mg)	2.0	2.0
Vitamin C (mg)	40	40
Folic acid (µg)	100	100
Vitamin B_{12} (µg)	1	1
Vitamin D (IU)	200	200

Recommended Dietary Allowance for Athletes (Table 6.10)

Table 6.10: Recommended dietary allowance (RDA) for athletes.

Item	RDA
Cal (kcal)	3,000–5,000
Protein (g)	60–90
Fat (g)	80–150
Calcium (g)	0.6–0.8
Iron (mg)	20–30
Vitamin A (µg)	750–1,000
Thiamine (mg)	2.0–3.0
Riboflavin (mg)	2.0–3.2
Nicotinic acid (mg)	26–36
Vitamin C (mg)	50–80
Folic acid (µg)	50–100
Vitamin B12	2–4
Vitamin D (IU)	400

Additional Allowance in Balanced Diet in Special Group (Table 6.11)

Table 6.11: Special group balanced diet allowance.

	Pregnancy*	Lactation**
Cereals	35	60
Pulses	15	30
Milk	100	100
Fat	-	10
Sugar	10	10

*293 calories ** 521 calories

Habitual Diet of Pregnant and Lactating Woman in India (Low Cost Diet–Rural) (Table 6.12)

Balanced diet at low cost (ICMR Nutrition Expert Group) suggests liberal amount of cereals, pulses, nuts, green leafy vegetable and very small amount of milk, egg, meat, fish and fat.

Table 6.12: Habitual diet of pregnant and lactating woman in India (Low cost diet–rural).

Gram per day	Pregnant	Lactating
Cereals	276	333
Pulses	21	15
Leafy vegetable	8	9
Other vegetable	12	23
Roots, tubers	8	3
Fruits	26	4
Milk	41	23
Fat, oil	20	12
Sugar, jaggery	14	15
Supplement to habitual diet		
Ragi	100	100
Other cereals	100	200
Multipurpose food (MPF)	25	50
Leafy vegetable	100	100
Roasted groundnut	-	50

Table 6.13: Special group requirement.

	0–6 months	Preschool (1–5 years)	School age (5–15 years)
Calorie Protein Vitamin C and Fe need	120 cal/kg 2–3 g/kg	1,200–1,500 cal/day 1.6 to 1.9 g/kg	1,700–2,060 cal/day 1.0–1.2 g/day Mid-day meal Menu
Supplement 4th month			Mid-day meal menu Cereal 75 g Pulse 30 g Oil 8 g Leafy vegetables 30 g Nonleafy vegetables 30 g
	Pregnant woman		**Lactating mother**
Calorie	+ 300	(additional)	+ 550
Protein	+ 65 g	(additional)	+ 75 g
Calcium	1,000 mg/day	(regular)	1,000 mg/day
	Fe 38 mg/day		30 mg/day

Requirement of Special Group (Table 6.13)

Prudent Diet

This is the diet developed by National Nutrition and Food Policy to achieve highest level of health. It is called prudent diet if following criteria are adopted in the diet:

- Fat intake below 20–30% of total calories
  - Saturated fat below 10% of total calories
  - Carbohydrate should contain high fiber
  - Fats, alcohol restricted
  - Salt below 5 grams per day
  - Protein below 15–20% of daily intake
  - Junk foods avoided (ketchup, cola, etc.)

Balanced Diet for Elderly People above 65 years

See **Table 6.14**.

NUTRITIONAL DISEASES

Protein–Energy Malnutrition (PEM)

- One of the major nutritional diseases in India
- Common cause for child mortality

Table 6.14: Balanced diet for elderly.

	Woman (>65 years)	Man (>65 years)
Cereals	225	350
Pulses	40	50
Vegetables	150	200
Green leafy vegetable	50	50
Roots and tubers	100	100
Fruits	200	200
Milk, milk products	300	300
Sugar	20	20
Fats and oils	20	25

- Common cause for child morbidity
- Influences physical growth
- Influences mental growth.

Clinical Type
See **Table 6.15**.

Socioeconomic Factors
- Low socioeconomic condition
- Poor environmental hygiene
- Large family size
- Failure of lactation
- Weaning and supplementation practice
- Cultural practice in child rearing
- Poverty and ignorance.

Basic Etiology of Protein–energy Malnutrition (Ecology of Malnutrition)
- Inadequate diet in terms of quantity
- Inadequate diet in terms of quality
- Infections particularly measles and diarrhea
- Parasite infestations, particularly roundworm
- Poverty and ignorance.

Prevention of Protein–energy Malnutrition
- Adequate treatment by energy and protein
- Treatment of infection
- Treatment of worm infestation.

Energy and protein supplements
1. MPF (plain and spiced CFTRI)
   Groundnut flour, Bengal gram, minerals, vitamin
   Yield: 42.9 g protein/100 g 387 calories/100 g.
2. Balahar—70% wheat, 25% defatted groundnut meal and 5% skimmed milk.
3. Hyderabad mix (NIN)—roasted wheat 40 g, Bengal gram 16 g, groundnut 10 g, jaggery 20 g
   Yield: 330 calories/86 g
   11.3 g protein/86 g
4. Protein mixture (CFTRI)
   Mix: I   57 g rice + 57 g MPF
         II 57 g wheat + 57 g MPF
         III 57 g ragi + 57 g MPF
         IV 57 g jowar + 57 g MPF

Classification of Malnutrition (Table 6.16)
Grade III and IV malnutrition need special attention with therapeutic nutrition (double the quantity of supplementary nutrition), i.e., 600 calories and 20 g protein.

Table 6.15: Protein–energy malnutrition (PEM) manifestations.

	Kwashiorkor	Marasmus
Muscle wasting	–	+
Fat wasting	–	+
Edema	+	–
Weight reduction	+	+++
Mental change	Irritable	Quiet
Skin change	+	–
Hair change	+	–
Plasma/amino acid ratio	Elevated	Normal

Incidence of PEM: 2% of preschool age group.

Table 6.16: Grades of malnutrition.

Malnutrition	% of expected weight	Grade	Position in growth chart
–	80–100%	Normal	Above upper line
Mild	70–79%	Grade-I	Between lines one and two
Moderate	60–69%	Grade-II	Between lines two and three
Severe	50–59%	Grade-III	Between lines three and four
Severe	Below 50%	Grade-IV	Below line four

Chapter 6: Nutrition and Health

Mild and moderate malnutrition are given supplementary nutrition with 300 calories and 10 g protein.

Weight recording is done once a month for 0–3 age group, for any illness lasting for 5 days in a month and for all severe malnourished children.

Normal children and children of 3–6 years of age group are weighed once in 3 months (growth monitoring).

Community Action in Protein-energy Malnutrition

Health promotion
- Good antenatal care (ANC)
- Good postnatal care (PNC)
- Promotion of exclusive breastfeeding
- Weaning and supplementation practice
- Nutrition education
- Small family norm
- Home economics

Specific protection
- Nutritional care of special group of children
- Immunization
- Food fortification.

Early diagnosis and prompt treatment
- Nutritional surveillance
- Infection and parasitosis
- Oral rehydration solution (ORS)
- Deworming.

Rehabilitation
- Nutritional rehabilitation

Vitamin A Deficiency

It is a common cause of preventable blindness in India. It is common among the age group of 1–3 years and is related to weaning. **Figure 6.1** depicts the manifestations of vitamin A deficiency.

Socioeconomic causes are as follows:
- Low standard of living
- Low income
- Ignorance
- Faulty feeding practices
- Diarrhea
- Measles

Treatment

It is an emergency treatment to prevent blindness. Oral administration of 200,000 IU vitamin A on 2 successive days is sufficient in early stage. In severe deficiency, parenteral administration is very much needed.

Vitamin A Deficiency Treatment Schedule
- On diagnosis 200,000 IU oral
- Next day 200,000 IU oral
- After 4 weeks 200,000 IU oral

Criteria for determining the public health significance of vitamin A deficiency:

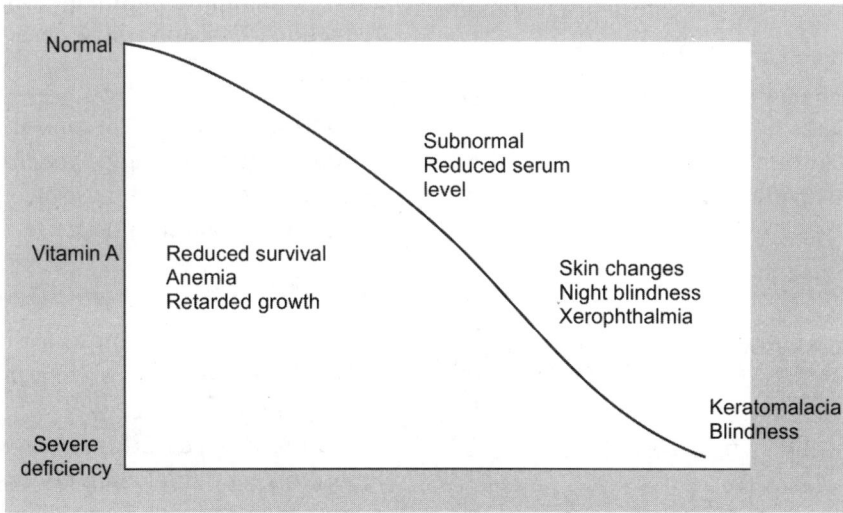

Fig. 6.1: Vitamin A deficiency manifestations.

Criteria	Prevalence (%)
Night blindness	1.0
Bitot's spot	0.5
Keratomalacia	0.01
Corneal ulcer	0.05

Children between the ages of 9 months to 3 years must be given vitamin A at monthly intervals. The first dose of 100,000 IU is to be given at 9 months along with measles vaccine. Subsequent doses are of 200,000 IU at the interval of 6 months.

Community Measures

- Fortification of vitamin A with Dalda
- Generous use of dark green leafy vegetables
- Promotion of breastfeeding
- Safe water supply
- Coverage of children for full immunization
- Nutritional education

Nutritional Anemia

Clinical condition of reduced Hb% as a result of essential nutrients and most common causes being iron deficiency and folic acid deficiency. The criteria for anemias as per WHO is given in **Table 6.17**.

Incidence

Sixty percent of women and children suffer from iron deficiency anemia. 25% of pregnant women suffer from folate deficiency anemia.

Factors

- Pregnancy and associated conditions
- Malaria
- Hookworm infection
- Inadequate intake
- Poor bioavailability

Table 6.17: WHO criteria for anemia.

Criteria for anemia (Hb%)	
Male	13 g%
Female	12 g%
Pregnancy	11 g%
Children (6 months to 6 years)	11 g%
Children aged enough to be in school	12 g%

- Poverty
- Ignorance

Prevention

- Iron and folic acid (IFA) tablets (60 mg) twice a day for 100 days to pregnant women (this is doubled for anemia)
- Hookworm treatment by Mebendazole (100 mg) twice a day for 3 days
- Dietary intake of iron-rich foods
- Birth-spacing by at least 3 years
- Children with anemia treated with IFA (Pediatric) 20 mg. Iron + 0.1 mg folic acid
- Salt fortification with iron [National Institute of Nutrition (NIN)]
- Changing dietary habit
- Control of parasite infection
- Nutritional education

Iodine Deficiency Disorder

India is one of the major endemic iodine deficiency countries in the world. Goiter, cretins and mild neurological disorders are very common in the affected areas.

Figure 6.2 gives an analysis of iodine deficiency disorder (IDD) and **Figure 6.3** depicts the ill effects of IDD.

Cause

It is a geographic pathology where source reduction in soil and food is observed.

Control

- Iodized salt (15 ppm at consumer level).
- Iodine monitoring and surveillance.
- Legal enforcement for use of iodized salt.
- Public education on IDD.

Fluorosis

Excess fluorine in drinking water has been the cause of dental fluorosis, skeletal fluorosis and genu valgum.

Community health survey has shown "mottling" of dental enamels, loss of shiny appearance on teeth, bony changes leading to crippling.

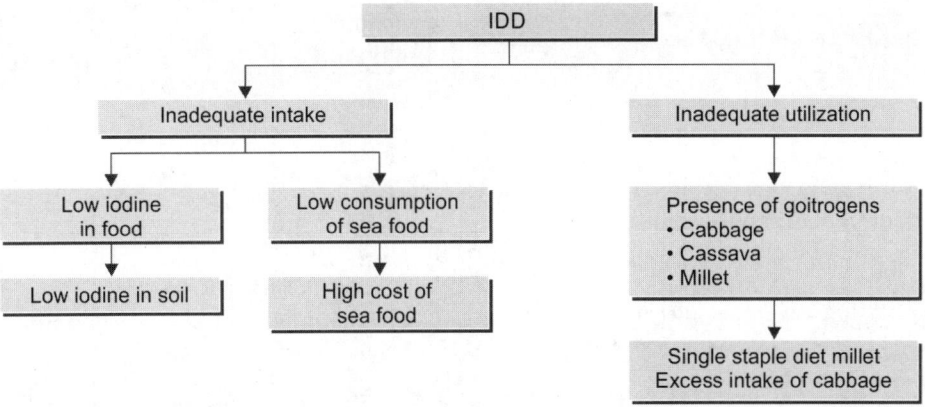

Fig. 6.2: Analysis of iodine deficiency disorder (IDD).

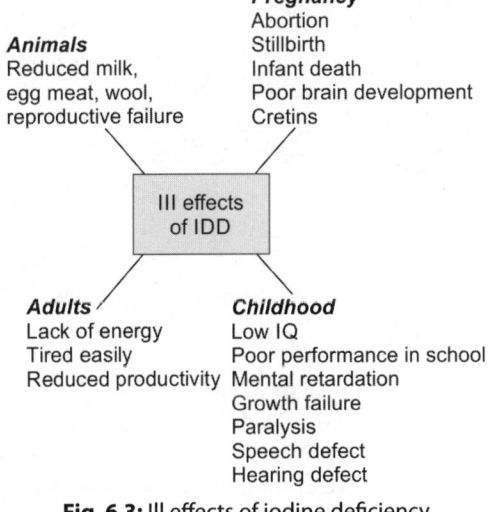

Fig. 6.3: Ill effects of iodine deficiency disorder (IDD).

Preventive Steps

1. Changing to water source which has fluoride level 0.5–0.8 mg/L.
2. Chemical treatment by Nalgonda technique (Defluoridation) **(Fig. 6.4)**.
3. Regulation on fluoride toothpaste, mouthwash in endemic areas.

FOOD POISONING

Types

- Poisonous food, e.g., death cap, mushroom, fish.
- Chemicals

- Bacteria
  a. Toxin type—staphylococcal (enterotoxin), botulism (exotoxin canned bottle), *Clostridium perfringens* (α and β) (exclude cholera, bacillary dysentery, arsenic poison)
  b. Infective type—*Salmonella* food poisoning.

Control

- Food sanitation
  - Meat hygiene
  - Personal hygiene
  - Food handlers
  - Pasteurization of milk
  - Health education
- Protect food
- Refrigeration
- Regulate canned food

FOOD TOXINS

Common food toxins of public health importance are:
- Lathyrism (*Lathyrus* seeds)
- Epidemic dropsy (*Argemone* oil contamination with mustard oil)
- Aflatoxicosis (mycotoxin by fungi).

Lathyrism

Neurological involvement in man (neurolathyrism) is an analog to bone involvement of

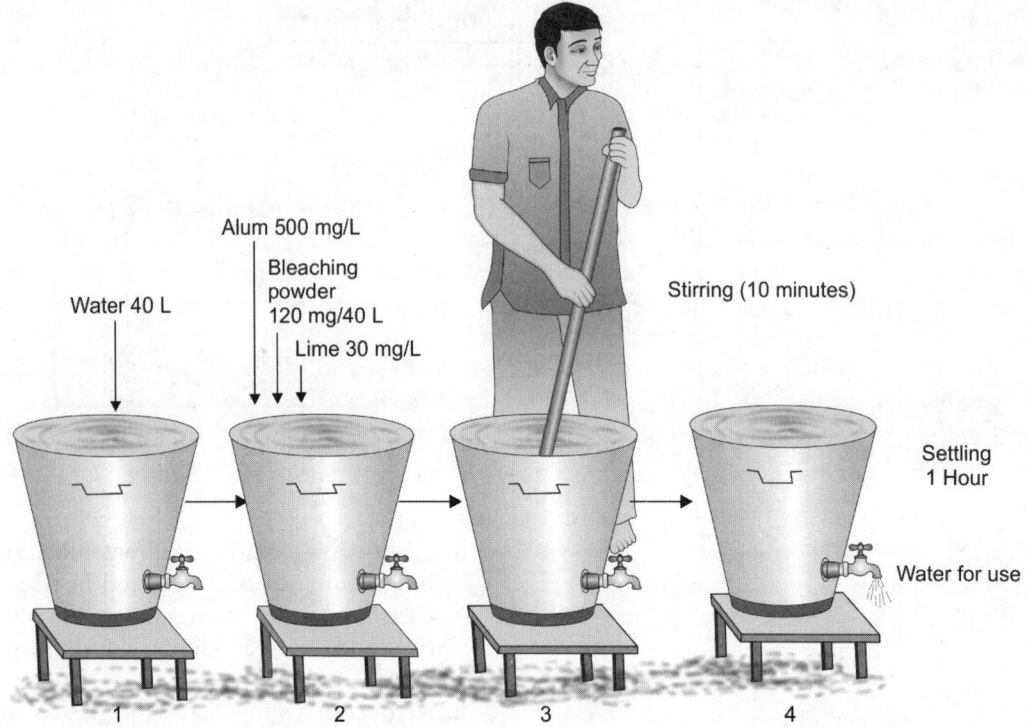

Fig. 6.4: Defluoridation at domestic level (Nalgonda technique).

animals (osteolathyrism). Most of the states in northern and central India have experienced lathyrism which is due to consumption of kesari dal (*Lathyrus sativus*). The toxin identified is beta-N-Oxalylamino-L-alanine (BOAA).

The disease clinically shows five stages in its intensity of development:
1. Latent stage
2. No-stick stage
3. One-stick stage
4. Two-stick stage, and
5. Crawling stage.

Preventive Measures in Lathyrism

- Treatment of case with high dose of vitamin C (1,000 mg per day for 8–10 days)
- Banning the crop
- Steeping method (soaked in hot water for two hours, drained, cleaned, dried)
- Parboiling
- Public awareness
- Growing low-toxin variety plant
- Socioeconomic change

Epidemic Dropsy

Contamination of mustard oil with argemone oil was identified in 1926. Sanguinarine, a toxic alkaloid present in argemone oil, is found to interfere with oxidation of pyruvic acid which accumulates in blood.

Diarrhea, bilateral swelling of legs, dyspnea, cardiac failure, and glaucoma are common clinical manifestations. Tests are available to detect the presence of argemone oil.

Prevention

- Cleaning and removal of *Argemone* weeds
- Enforcement of Prevention of Food Adulteration Act (PFA)
- Public awareness

Aflatoxin

Fungal toxin by *Aspergillus flavus*. Common food grains attacked are groundnut, maize, wheat, and tapioca. It is a hepatotoxin. It is an attributed factor in Indian childhood cirrhosis.

Chapter 6: Nutrition and Health

Prevention
- Proper storage
- Maintaining low moistures (<10%)
- Public awareness

Other Toxins

Ergotism

It is a field fungus found on wheat and bajra called *Claviceps fusiformis*.

Nausea, vomiting, drowsiness, painful cramps in limbs, and peripheral gangrene are usual manifestations.

Prevention
- Floating in 20% salt water, ergot is removed.
- Air flotation removes ergot.

Favism
- Hemolytic anemia by *Vicia faba* glycosides hemagglutinins
- Ricin in castor seeds
- Ackee fruit poisoning by *Blighia sapida* toxin hypoglycin A

Pressor Amines

Endomyocardial fibrosis by high serotonin from plantains.

Endemic Ascites

Millets getting contaminated with weed seeds of *Crotalaria* (*Jhunjhunia*). It contains a hepatotoxin called pyrrolizidine alkaloid. Ascites and jaundice are usual manifestations.

Prevention
- Public awareness
- Deweeding of weed seeds
- Sieving of millets before use.

Fusarium Toxin

Fusarium incamatus, field fungus attacking rice known to cause health hazard.

Other Fungal Toxins

Claviceps, Aspergillus, Penicillium, Mushroom.

FOOD-BORNE DISEASES

Bacterial: Typhoid, staphylococcal toxin, botulism, *Escherichia coli*, diarrhea.

Viral: Viral hepatitis.

Parasites: Tapeworm, roundworm, amebiasis, threadworm.

COMMERCIAL AND PROCESSED FOODS

In certain nutritional disorders, low intake by anorexia and restriction makes it difficult to make up by diet alone. In such occasions, commercial or processed foods come in handy for supplementation.

- Casilon (whole protein food with essential amino acids).
- Complan (milk protein, vegetable fat, minerals and vitamins).
- Farex (reinforced cereal food for growing children).
- Amul milk (infant milk food).
- Proteinex (protein hydrolysate).
- Uniprotein (milk protein with papain).
- Balahar (weaning, preschool children).
- MPF (for PEM).
- Maltodex (assimilated carbohydrate).
- Threptin biscuit (milk protein).
- Cocoa maltine (beverage).

THERAPEUTIC DIETS

Liquid Diet (1,500 calories) (Table 6.18)

See **Table 6.18**.

Table 6.18: Liquid diet.

Milk	1 L
Sugar	100 g
Orange juice	250 g
Vegetable soup	200 g
Skimmed milk	50 g
Salt	5 g
Tea or coffee	7 g/15 g
Provide	
Calories	1,500
Protein	50 g
Fat	40 g
CHO	235 g
Sodium	840 mg

Low Calorie Diet (Table 6.19)

Food to avoid: Whole milk, cream, butter, oil, ghee, fried food, honey, sugar, sweets, cheese, banana, mango, potato, alcohol, dried fruits.

Free foods: All vegetables, pepper water, clear soups.

Low Cholesterol Diet (1,200 calories)

See **Table 6.20**.

Diabetic Diet (1,500 calories)

See **Table 6.21**.

Fruit Portion

Following are equivalents—apple 100 g, grapes 150 g, kharbooja 150 g, watermelon 300 g, orange 100 g, papaya 100 g, pomegranate 100 g, banana 50 g, mango 50 g.

Prohibited Food

Glucose, sugar, honey, all sorts of sweets.

Foods to avoid

Potato, mango, banana, alcohol.

Table 6.19: Low calorie diet.

Skimmed milk	500 mL
Bread	25 g
Cereals	100 g
Curd	200 g
Channa	50 g
Dal	25 g
Greens	500 g
Oil	10 g
Tea/coffee	7/15 g
Salt	10 g
Condiment	15 g
Fruit	Two portions
Provide	
CHO	183 g
Protein	47 g
Fat	30 g
Calorie	1,200

Table 6.20: Low cholesterol diet.

Skimmed milk	600 mL
Bread	25 g
Cereals	100 g
Curd	300 g
Channa	50 g
Dal	25 g
Vegetables	400 g
Seasonal fruit	150 g
Honey	20 g
Sugar	10 g
Oil	10 g
Tea/Coffee	7 g/15 g
Provide	
Carbohydrate	214 g
Protein	54 g
Fat	13 g
Calorie	1,200

Table 6.21: Diabetic diet.

Milk	300 mL
Curds	200 g
Dal	25 g
Atta	100 g
Bread	25 g
Oil	10 g
Channa	10 g
Paneer	100 g
Fruit	1 portion
Vegetables	400 g
Tea/Coffee	7 g/15 g
Salt	10 g
Condiment	15 g

Free food

Leafy vegetables, cucumber, radish, black coffee, pepper water.

Purine Free Foods

White bread, wheat, barley, rice, sago, butter, ghee, cream, egg, milk, rose.

Renal calculi of uric acid and urate, following are eliminated:

Meat, shellfish, dals, peas, beans, spinach.

Chapter 6: Nutrition and Health

Renal calculi of oxalate, following are eliminated:

Green plantain, spinach, sweet potato, beetroot, almond, cashew nut, grapes.

INDICATIONS FOR PARENTERAL NUTRITION (IV FEEDING)

- Cancer
- Inflammatory bowel diseases
- Short bowel syndrome
- Preoperative
- Gastrointestinal fistulae

NUTRITIONAL SURVEILLANCE

It assists in keeping a watch over nutrition of a community to take decision on required improvement for better nutrition. It helps in long-term planning, management, evaluation, and to get over nutrition crisis.

Indicators that are used in nutrition surveillance are:

- Birth weight
- Proportion of breast feed
- Proportion of weaned feed
- Height for age
- Weight for age
- Weight for height
- Clinical signs

Each State has a unit to monitor this surveillance, called State Level National Nutrition Monitoring Bureau.

Table 6.22 depicts the difference between nutritional surveillance and growth monitoring.

Table 6.22: Difference between nutritional surveillance and growth monitoring.

Nutritional surveillance	Growth monitoring
Detect undernutrition by diagnosis	Preserve normal growth by health education
A sample study	All 0–6 years age children
By trained workers	By educating mothers
Precise instrument used	Simple instrument used
Referral to hospital	Referral to primary health care (PHC)

FOOD SURVEILLANCE

All conditions and measures that are necessary during production, processing, storage, distribution and preparation to make food safe for human consumption.

Food Hygiene

Production, handling, distribution and serving of all types of food is included. Prevention of food poisoning and food-borne diseases is the main motto of food hygiene.

Milk Hygiene

- Clean and safe milk supply
- Pasteurization: Heating of milk to a temperature which destroys pathogens.
  - *Holder method* (vat): Milk is kept at 66°C for 30 minutes and cooled to 5°C quickly.
  - *High temperature short time method* (HTST): Rapidly heated to 72°C, held for 15 seconds, rapidly cooled to 4°C.
  - *Ultra-high temperature (UHT) method:* Milk is rapidly heated in two stages to 125°C (II stage is under pressure), kept for few seconds, and then rapidly cooled.

Pasteurized milk is tested by:

- Phosphatase test
- Standard plate count
- Coliform count

Milk-borne diseases:

- Tuberculosis
- Brucellosis
- Streptococcal infection
- Salmonellosis
- Q fever
- Anthrax

Meat Hygiene

This measure is to prevent:

- Tapeworm infestations (*Taenia solium, Taenia saginata, Trichinella spiralis, Fasciola hepatica*)
- Bacterial infections (anthrax, food poisoning)
- Meat inspection by qualified staff
- Slaughterhouse sanitation

Fish Hygiene [*Dibothriocephalus Latus* (Tapeworm), Vibrio Infection]

- Fish inspection
- Inspection of tinned fish

Egg Hygiene

- Proper egg preservation
- Egg inspection

Fruit and Vegetable Hygiene

- Sanitation of eating place
- Examination of food handlers

FOOD ADDITIVES, FOOD ADULTERATION, AND FOOD FORTIFICATION

Food Additives

Addition of non-nutritious substances which are added in small quantity to improve appearance, flavor, texture, storage, e.g.:

- Coloring agent—saffron, turmeric
- Flavoring agent—vanilla
- Sweetening agent—saccharin
- Preservative—sorbic acid

It is regulated by PFA and Fruit Products Order (FPO).

Food fortification: Nutrients are added to improve the quality of a diet of a group or community, e.g.

- Vitamins A and D in vanaspati
- Salt with iodine
- Salt with iron

Food Adulteration

It includes mixing, substitution, and concealing the quality; unsafe food sold; misbranding; and addition of toxicants.

Effect

- Economic loss
- Ill-health

  For example:
  - Dal with *kesari* dal
  - Haldi with lead chromate
  - Pepper with papaya seed
  - Coffee with chicory
  - Mustard seed with argemone seed
  - Ghee with vanaspati, mashed potato, pig's fat
  - Milk with water, starch, paper pulp
  - Edible oil with mineral oil
  - Tea or coffee with dust, husk, tamarind seed powder
  - Cereals with stone, mud
  - Honey with sugar, jaggery

Food Fortification

Reinforcement of nutrients with additional supplies to prevent deficiency.

Examples

- Ghee with vitamin A and vitamin D 2,500 IU and 175 IU, respectively, per 100 grams.
- Salt with potassium iodide
- Sugar with vitamin A
- Milk with vitamin A and D
- Bread with lysine

Food Standards

1. Codex Alimentarius
2. PFA standard
3. The Agmark standard
4. Bureau of Indian Standards (BIS) mark

Prevention of Food Adulteration Act (1954) Amended In 1964, 1976 and 1986

The Act is implemented to certify food adulterated and not confirming to minimum standards through food and public health laboratories. Food inspectors, food analysts and food officers are trained in this aspect.

Provision

- Fine of ₹ 1,000/-
- Six months imprisonment
- For death and grievous hurt, fine of ₹ 5,000/- and life imprisonment
- Consumer can take the sample to submit for testing
- Voluntary organizations can collect sample to submit for testing.

NUTRITIONAL PROGRAM

For Overall Nutritional Status

- Applied Nutrition Programme
- Special Nutrition Programme

Chapter 6: Nutrition and Health

- Balwadi Nutrition Programme
- Mid-day Meal Programme (Central Government)
- Mid-day Meal Programme (State Governments)

Specific Programs

- Vitamin A Prophylaxis Programme
- Prophylaxis against nutritional anemia
- Control of IDDs.

Other Indirect Programmes

- Integrated Child Development Services (ICDS) Scheme
- IPP

NUTRITION EDUCATION

Awareness of the community on habit, custom, preparation, diet, nutrients, and rehabilitative procedure constitute nutrition education as a specific area of health education.

Components

- Infant and child nutrition
- Nutrition in pregnancy, lactation
- Elderly and sick nutrition
- Management in malnutrition.

Food Myths

- Brown egg is not nutritious.
- Papaya leads to abortion.
- Nonvegetarian foods give more strength.
- Indian foods lack in protein.
- Fish eating increases brain power.
- B complex for more strength and more protection
- Bread toast is more nutritious.
- Drinking water leads to increase in body weight.

Contents

- Malnutrition
- Food hygiene
- Special group requirement
- Ongoing nutritional program
- Balanced diet

NUTRITION REHABILITATION

Malnutrition in a community needs nutrition rehabilitation. It is of two specific situations:
1. Family situation
2. Disaster situation

Family Situation

- Home diet improvement
- Changing family diet
- Choosing local foods at reasonable cost
- Cooking and feeding trainings
- Kitchen garden improvement
- Availability of pediatrician
- Establishment of residential rehabilitation centers
- Making local food palatable by different menu
- Making local food acceptable by community
- Possession of cattle, buffalo, sheep, goat for non-dependant yield of milk and also partial scope for earning
- Facility for poultry under rehabilitation for food and also partial scope for earning
- Rehabilitation training through locally available means (three stone kitchen where twigs of wood for fuel is used, etc.) (Village methods of preparing food)
- Making "Best buy" in terms of nourishment
- Facility for cowshed, fodder is co-related factors in nutrition rehabilitation
- Growing fodder in waste bath water is a clue to many other ideas.

Disastrous Situation

After some disaster, there may be substantially decreased food, nutritional deficiency and starvation. Immediate cause of death in disaster is by infectious diseases than by starvation.

Emergency Nutritional Rehabilitation

- Distribution of general food ration.
- Targeting supplement to high risk
- On-site feeding centers' establishment
- Local-cum-culturally acceptable is better than donor provided, since donor provided results in iatrogenic micronutrient deficiency.

- ❖ Accompaniment by environmental sanitation and infectious diseases' control
- ❖ Restoring indigenous food economy rather than emergency feeding should be borne in mind.

Pneumonia and diarrhea are common complications of severe malnutrition. This needs therapeutic nutrition for grade III and grade IV malnutrition. Nutritional rehabilitation centers are established for such causes to save many lives.

CALORIFIC VALUE OF COOKED PREPARATIONS (ICMR) (TABLE 6.23)

Table 6.23: Calorific value of cooked items.

Food preparations	Calorific value
1 cup rice	170
1 puri	100
2 slice bread	170
2 idli	150
1 dosa	125
1 cup sambar	110
1 cup gravy	170
1 boiled egg	90
1 omelette	160
3/4th cup chicken curry	240
2 piece fish fried	220
8 bajji	280
2 vada	140
2 masala vada	150
1 masala dosa	200
1 samosa	200
1 vegetable puff	170
2 tablespoon chutney	120
2 piece barfi	400
½ cup srikhand	380
1 cup tea	75
1 cup coffee	110
1 cup cow milk	180
1 cup buffalo milk	320
1 glass lassi	110
1 bottle cold drinks	150
10 cashew nuts	85
1 apple	65
1 banana	90
1 mango	180
1 sapota	80

POPULATION NUTRIENT INTAKE GOALS (WHO)

Under protein and amino acid requirements in human nutrition, WHO has recommended dietary factor for the goal in % of total energy, total fat, total carbohydrate, total protein, cholesterol, salt, fruits and vegetables, dietary fibers and nonstarch polysaccharides.

INTEGRATED CHILD DEVELOPMENT SERVICES (ICDS) SCHEME OR INTEGRATED MOTHER AND CHILD DEVELOPMENT (IMCD) SERVICES

See Chapter 12 on Reproductive Maternal and Child Health (RCH).

SUMMARY

In this chapter, in the beginning proximate principles are highlighted. Individual nutritional diseases are described. Therapeutic diets are illustrated. Nutritional surveillance and food surveillance are detailed. Food additives, food adulteration and food fortification are discussed. At the end, National Nutritional Programme is highlighted.

VIVA VOCE

1. Mention food source for vitamin D.
2. Define proximate principles.
3. What are the objectives of nutritional assessment?
4. Mention methods of nutrition assessment.
5. Define balance diet.
6. Define prudent diet.
7. What are the differences between kwashiorkor and marasmas.
8. What is Hyderabad mix?
9. What is the criterion to say anaemic among men and women?
10. What are the ill effects of iodine deficiency disorder?
11. Mention common food toxins.
12. Enumerate foodborne diseases.
13. Describe methods of pasteurization.
14. Mention common food adulteration.

CHAPTER 7: Basic Statistics and its Application

Chapter Outline

- Formulation of Research Question for A Study
- Data Collection, Classification, Analysis, Interpretation, Presentation
- Measures of Central Tendency, Measures of Variability and Significance Tests
- Sampling

INTRODUCTION

All health activities of present world and their impact on a country's economy is expressed in numbers. Medical, dental, nursing, pharmacy and the like are indebted to numerical expression which always desire for quantitative expressions. Our knowledge will have a sound scientific base if we can measure and express our knowledge in numbers.

Plural form statistics denote collection of numbers, facts and figures. In singular, it is science of figures.

DEFINITION

"Science of collection, processing, analysis and transformation of data which is required for organizing and implementing health services."

As such, collected figure is data which when analyzed yields information. By experience when information is put to practice, it becomes intelligence.

COMMON TERMS

Data: Attributes or variables without any meaning

Chance: Occurrence of events in nature which are occurring as though they are occurring in nature.

Inference: From sample data, population parameters are estimated in inference.

Null hypothesis (NH): We assume that the difference is zero, i.e., no true difference exists.

Rate: The number of events (cases) in a period of time over the population exposed to the risk of the said event.

Significant test: It is a test of NH. If NH is rejected, it is significant and the specified alternative hypothesis is accepted.

Sample: It is a portion of a universe or population about which information is actually collected.

Attribute: It is a variable that describes a characteristic by classifying it into categories. It has the quality of possessing or not possessing a property.

Variable: Any attribute, any phenomenon or any event that can have different values.

Tabulation: It is a process of data grouping into intervals or groups to which the range of the variable are divided and put.

Percentile: The position of a character or variable when they are arranged in ascending or descending order in an array of one hundred.

Type I error: The error risk is α, an arbitrary level of significance is predetermined. The NH is true but is rejected because the observed result falls in rejection area of NH curve.

Type II error: The error risk is β which cannot be readily determined. The NH is false, but is accepted because the observed results falls in 1-α region of NH curve.

P: Probability that an outcome (unusual) and is sum of probabilities of all chance outcomes.

Contingent table: Qualitative data classification into row and column for application of χ^2 test.

Degree of freedom: Number of independent contributions to a theoretical sampling distributions such as χ^2, student 't' test, F test.

Analysis of variance (ANOVA): A method of partitioning variance into parts (between and within) so as to yield independent estimate of the population variance. This is tested with F distribution. It is a method of testing sample means significance.

Ratio: It is the fraction a/b for two mutually exclusive groups with elements 'a' and 'b'.

TYPES

Biostatistics: Related to biological events.

Medical statistics: Data from clinical profession which usually tells us the proportion of change.

Vital statistics: Data from all vital events.

Population statistics: Data from demography.

Hospital statistics: Morbidity, mortality, hospital service, utilization.

Health statistics: Data of wide health sciences, for most of the occasions quantitative data.

FORMULATION OF RESEARCH QUESTION FOR A STUDY

Research

Science is the development of specialty due to keen observation and experimentation of man by his knowledge. Direct or indirect methods of demonstration are possible to answer our biological questions. Documentation of such observation based on scientific approach constitutes science.

Philosophy of science is to apply the knowledge of science for the welfare of mankind, for resource development and for maintenance of positive health.

Man has shown adventure in finding an answer for unanswered questions since his evolution. For survival of his species "*Homo sapiens,*" he adopted many devices to develop understanding through—(a) observation, (b) natural course of events, (c) interaction in the community, (d) adaptation of education system, and (e) research.

Research is the systematic study of one or more problems, usually posed as questions that need answer. Specific approved methods are adopted to study such problems by developing hypothesis and proving such postulated hypothesis. Question taken will have the potential contribution to existing body of knowledge and it should benefit the nursing profession and the community.

Definition

Research is defined as a systematic study of selected problem through specific methods of scientific basis of specified disciplines. It includes experiment, survey, correlation studies with or without meta-analysis and psychometric evaluations (Definition after Knapp, 1998).

According to Burns and Grove (2003), nursing research is a process of systematic inquiry or study to build knowledge in a discipline. The purpose of research is to develop an empirical body of knowledge for a discipline or profession.

Nature of research may be observational and hypothesis-generation study (descriptive). It may be hypothesis testing study (observational analytical strategy). It may be based on animal and human experiments. Observation as time motion study is also one of the natures of research called operational strategy.

Conceptual idea of research involves a population (group of patients for study) and parameters (to describe characteristics of population). Since a representation of population is selected, it will always be a "sample" in research.

Let us study the formulation of a research question for a study.

No. 1: Is this a problem?
- It gives new knowledge.
- It clarifies our objectives when they are put forth.

No. 2: What are its characteristics?
- It is a clinical appraisal of existing information.
- It helps to formulate hypothesis.

No. 3: What seems to have caused it?
- It helps in further strengthening the formulated hypothesis.

No. 4: What must be done to prove the actual cause?
- This helps in verifying the hypothesis.

No. 5: How can it be stopped and how further occurrence of public health problem is prevented?

This will be a practical application.

Scope

Scopes of research are manifold. They are:
- Drawing conclusions
- Improving nursing care facility
- Order for new innovations
- Adopting science and technology
- Makes cost benefit
- Bring out cost-effective procedures
- Control of health problems
- Prevention of risks.

Characteristics
- It is attached with significance and relevance.
- They are made amenable to scientific study.
- Need facility, equipment and resources.
- It needs personal interest in researcher.
- Curiosity leads to research.

Source, Process and Evaluation

Research in nursing is to make judicious decisions in nursing care delivery at individual patient level, at group of patients level and also at large in community who are healthy. Indian Council of Medical Research and Indian Council of Nursing Research are supporting research on biologic and behavioral aspects of critical health problems.

Nursing as a discipline deals with variations of characteristics such as cholesterol level, lung function, and blood pressure, because of pathological variations. This again is determined by biological factors such as genetic constitution, age, sex and personality. In majority of cases, environmental factors, such as lifestyle, stress, strain, diet, etc., add to the process of research.

During the process of research, nurse has to undertake following steps:
1. Think scientifically, logically and critically about health problems
2. Assess the available evidence for decision making
3. Be aware of possible risk associated with nursing decisions
4. Identify decisions and conclusions that lack scientific and logical basis.

Evaluation of research is necessary in the following areas of nursing care:
- Handling of variations in nursing care
- Diagnosis of patient's ailments
- Diagnosis of community health problem
- Predictions of likely outcome of an intervention
- Selection of appropriate intervention measures
- Planning, administration in nursing
- Final reports for policy making in nursing profession.

Research Types

There are two types of research available in nursing profession. One is basic research and another is applied research.

1. Basic research: This is also called observational research seen as routine research activities. It may be pure observational type where nursing activities encompass, e.g., breastfeeding practices or delivery practices, etc. It may be observational and interview type when response is obtained from respondent and are recorded. Examples are study of sexual behavior, community participation in tubectomy camp, etc.

This may be observation and analysis where knowledge of analytical epidemiology is used as in **case control study** or **cohort study**.

2. Applied research: This is also called explorative research. Main objective is to get new insight or to standardize a procedure. Here, by exploratory applied research, nurse can augment her skills or procedures. For example, exploration for a better fetoscope, an instrument for a better infusion, a good gadget for an effective first-aid, etc.

Research Methods

Here researcher is able to modify the risk factors by giving drug, vaccine, nutrient, etc. Sometimes changes must have occurred as a coincidence in nature. Experimental research is undertaken with control group or without control group. They are of following types:

1. Randomized controlled trial **(Flowchart 7.1)**
   - Clinical trial
   - Field trial
   - Community study
2. Nonrandomized trial
   - Trial without control
   - Natural experiments with or without control
   - Before and after comparison studies

In clinical study, both diseased and healthy are selected. In preventive study, only healthy are selected. They may be for treatment, surgery (therapeutic) or protective such as— (a) for vaccine or contraceptive (prophylaxis), (b) for side effect of medicaments (safety studies), and can be, (c) efficiency studies, such as copper T efficiency, traditional birth attendant trained for efficient services, etc.

Steps taken in clinical trial are:
1. Informed consent of participants
2. Protocol is drawn
3. Reference population is selected

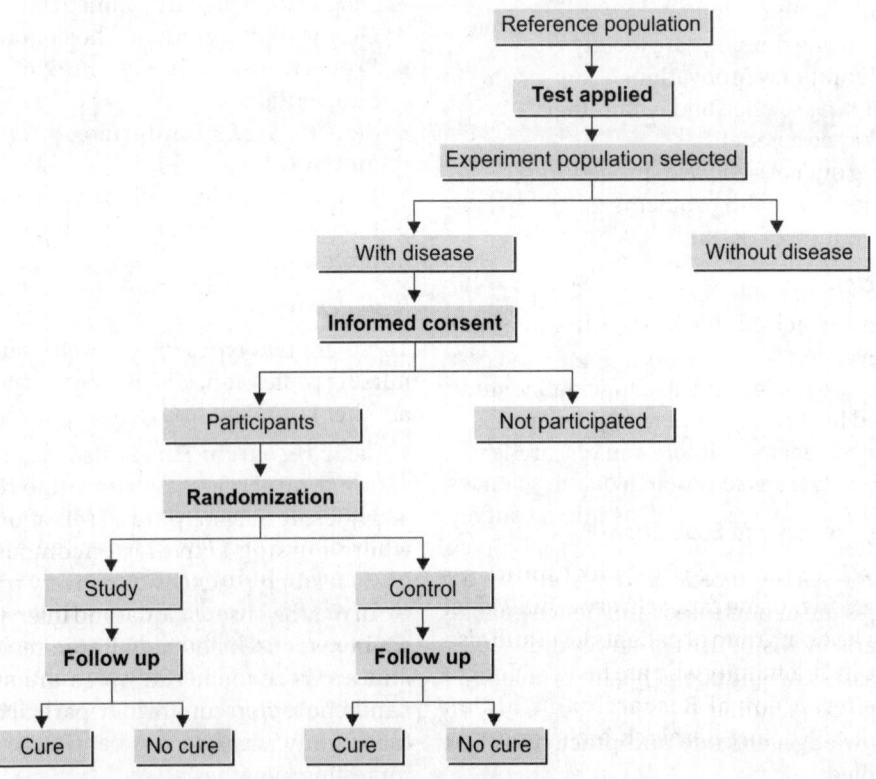

Flowchart 7.1: Randomized controlled trial.

Table 7.1: Types of blinding in research.

Single blinding	Patient do not know
Double blinding	Patient and nurse (researcher) do not know
Triple blinding	Patient, nurse and statistician all do not know

4. Study population is selected
5. Randomization done
6. Intervention done
7. Recorded and followed up
8. Data analyzed
9. Report prepared

To overcome bias, blinding is done which do not allow patient or nurse or data analyst to know about drug or placebo **(Table 7.1)**.

Historical Study

It is retrospective historical study which has already occurred before the start of the study. Here we do not select case or control. Exposed group is selected and studied.

Cohort Study

It is a prospective study where a cohort is selected which is a group of people experiencing common characteristics. They can be birth cohort, marriage cohort, treated cohort, exposure cohort, occupational cohort or insured cohort. The steps followed are:
1. Identification of reference population
2. Selection of study population
3. Formulation of cohorts
4. Follow up

This cohort study can be differentiated from case control study as shown in **Table 7.2**.

Survey

It is a basic tool of research in health sciences. There are many types such as impact survey, utilization survey, Gallup survey, social survey, morbidity survey, mortality survey, etc. Survey provides the denominator and hence enables comparison. Major uses of survey are:
* To assess magnitude of health problem
* To guide planning
* Knowledge, attitude and practice can be studied

Table 7.2: Difference between case control study and cohort study.

Case control study	Cohort study
Goes from effect to cause	Cause to effect
Starts with disease	Starts with risk
No risk group	There is a risk group
Cases are selected	Cases are involved
Odds ratio is available	Relative risk and attributable risk are available
Not expensive	Expensive
Small universe	Large universe
Suitable for rare problem	Not suitable for rare problem
No other information is available	Yields other information
Less attrition	More attrition

* To know the extent of service utilization
* Helps to test hypothesis on health related event

Meticulous planning is needed for a survey. Survey instruments can be Interview, Observation, Questionnaire, Schedules, Techniques and Investigations.

Field Study

A designed research undertaken at community level constitutes field study. This can be rural, urban, industrial or nutritional in nature. It is an active process by a researcher to visit, observe and collect data at family level or at social unit level. This involves understanding of local customs, culture and traditional value. Field study requires local dialect for information collection.

Case Study

This is extensively used in nursing science and in behavioural science. It involves in-depth study of one or a few cases as representative of a larger number of cases. The subject of investigations may be a few selected characteristics in individual and family. Case studies do not generate information which can be adopted on a wider scale. However "case study" method can be used as an area for testing hypothesis.

Ethical issues in Research

Since research involves human population, it has to be carefully reviewed at proposal level. Any research on human brings commands certain amount of service benefit may be in the form of cash or kind. So it is advisable to earmark a budget for it.

All examinations procedure should be harmless and noninvasive.

Outcome of research must be shared with the community for their welfare.

In interventions, informed consent should be obtained. Confidentiality should be ensured. Poorer section of society should not be exploited. Special care must be taken to take permission from ethical committees for drug trial, animal experiments and invasive procedures among human subjects.

Research Process

Overview: It is essential to have overview of the research process from the point of view of manpower, money and material. At the beginning, feasibility and applicability in nursing set up should be viewed. As far as possible, a research should be a need-based beneficial proposal where time and money are not wasted.

Steps: Following are the major steps in research process:
1. A good research topic of relevance is selected.
2. A research problem is selected from the topic. This leads to proper formulation of research hypothesis.
3. For further understanding, search for literature on related research work is undertaken.
4. Objectives of research proposal are formulated.
5. Variables that are needed to be measured are clearly spelled out. They are dependent, independent, confounding and background variables.
6. Strategies are drawn up for research study. They include descriptive, experimental and operational strategies.
7. Selection of appropriate sample is done.
8. Pilot study is undertaken for final preparation of protocol.
9. Plans for data analysis and interpretation are drawn.

Purpose: The main purpose is to fulfil the objectives of the study and proving the hypothesis by verification of hypothesis done at protocol.

Review of literature: Review of literature is done for information on related aspects of research process. This helps in:
- Further understanding of research
- Helps in identification of proper and appropriate variable
- Helps in drawing research hypothesis
- Helps to design the protocol based on what has been followed earlier
- Getting familiarity of methods used in the protocol.

The search can be undertaken by:
- Scan of literature, periodicals
- Discussion with experts
- Library index search such as:
  - International Nursing Index
  - Excerpta Medica
  - Index Medicus
- Computer search such as:
  - MEDLARS
  - MEDLINE
  - CATLINE
- Bibliographic
- Statistical reports

Research Topics

Research topic must be of current problem oriented. By using outcome of research, there must be benefit to patient, family or community. In other words, the topic must be need based. As far as possible, the topic should have relevance to the local area or region where it can stand as baseline data for therapy, management or intervention. When information on a particular topic is readily available, it needs not be repeated. In case of repetition, it can be taken after a lapse of 5–10 years for a study on secular changes of characteristics.

Broad area of topic can be study of rare occurrence, of common practical concern, for a need of comparing an alternative treatment modality or for additional information on a given illness.

Research Hypothesis

Let us study the following statements:
- "Tropical eosinophilia is associated with high absolute eosinophilic count"
- "Amoxycillin cures pharyngitis to the tune of 100%"
- "Dry ginger with fatty meal inhibits platelet aggregation"
- "Drug consumption and sleep disturbances increase with age"

Above statements are assumptions. They are called hypothesis. Testing the hypothesis involves making assumption about the parameter which can check our assumption.

There are two types of research procedures with reference to testing of hypothesis. They are:
1. Comparative study on two or more population or samples
2. Studying the relationship between two or more factors on the population.

In testing hypothesis, we have to deal with sampling variation because we make inferences on the basis of samples. If the observed sample difference is larger than that which the sampling variation would produce, we can conclude that differences exist in the population.

In the beginning, we assume "NH", which means that no difference exist between populations.

If an observed value is greater than expected value (which is table value) at a given degree of freedom and at minimum probability (it is called critical probability) of 0.05, we infer that it is significant meaning the occurrence is not by chance.

Research Design

True validity of research rely upon data analysis, planning and execution of research design. Appropriate design and careful execution are necessary to provide specific answer to hypothesis which also take care of complete use of men, material and money used in the research.

Following principles are followed for an effective research design:

Bias: They are overcome by appropriate sampling techniques and suitable randomizing procedures.

Precision of sensitivity: This is overcome by collection of data from (as far as possible) a large sample and quality control of instruments that are used in research.

Use of common research design: This is necessary to disallow unnecessary and harmful effects of treatment in research activity. Here, principle followed is to conduct research on population which show little variation, study of subgroups for separate studies and evidence-based activities are incorporated.

Following simple designs are advocated (**Table 7.3**):

Individual comparison: This helps in refinement of experiment on the knowledge of variation on group research. Depending on number of treatment, number of groups is made.

Group comparison: Valid conclusion can be drawn by research on group by random allocation of treatment or intervention.

Concurrent comparison: Here, many groups are simultaneously exposed for specified treatment. Simultaneous trial will reduce the cost of research.

When 60 subjects are used, response of 15 subjects each are available for treatment A, B, C and control. If results are not incoming in the simple design, then factorial design may help where comparison is possible as under: (where

Table 7.3: Simple design in research (simple allocation pattern).

Treatment A	15 subjects
Treatment B	15 subjects
Treatment C	15 subjects
Control	15 subjects
Total	**60 subjects**

Table 7.4: Factorial design in research (factorial allocation pattern).

Treatment A	10 subjects
Treatment B	10 subjects
Treatment C	10 subjects
Treatment A and B	10 subjects
Treatment B and C	10 subjects
Control	10 subjects
Total	**60 subjects**

again 60* subjects are sufficient in research design) (**Tables 7.4**).
* Comparison of A and B
* Comparison of B and C
* Comparison of A and A & B
* Comparison of B and B & C
* Comparison of A and control
* Comparison of B and control

Experimental design

The experimental design needs the fulfillment of requirement of procedure and good design. A statistician should be consulted before the experiment and not after the experiment. Avoiding postmortem analysis is the best for a good experimental design.

Following principles are followed in a good experimental design:
* Random allocation of individuals
* No arbitrary correction is allowed
* Whatever result comes that should be taken
* Use of control with similar characteristics but without the testing variable
* The controls can be:
  * Concurrent (simultaneously used)
  * Volunteer (not found effective)
  * Geographical (elsewhere done)
  * Historical (earlier done)
* Experimental errors should be measured by:
  * Randomization (no over estimation or no underestimation)
  * Replication (repetition)
* Reducing the errors due to working condition.

---

*In the consideration of number of cases to be studied with permissible error of 5%, 10% or, at the most, maximum 20% permissible error rate, prevalence of event or proportion of event will be helpful.

Common experimental designs:

One-way approach	Allocating patients at random to the various treatment
Two-way approach	Grouping patients according to known response on them
Latin square approach	For example, treatment can be started by four replication to four treatment: A D C B B A D C C B A D D C B A

Factorial design	When two or more factors are under investigation, this is found useful.
	Example of two factors at two level
	
	              Low Normal Total
	              dose dose dose
	Old treatment 15 15 30
	New treatment 15 15 30
	                   30 30 60

Split plot design	This design is used when we need precise information on one factor, on the interaction of this factor on the second factor. Actually, precision on second factor is ignored in this study design.
Use of analysis of covariance	

Nonexperimental design

These are observational studies. Depending on risk factor present or not, we get comparative group for observation. Nonexperimental design has an innate bias. Still, it is most feasible and community-conducted research design.

Following are the types of nonexperimental designs:
1. Cross-sectional study
2. Prospective study
3. Retrospective study

Bias in nonexperimental design is due to case selection type, information collection methods, confounding of variables. This bias of nonexperimental design can be overcome by:

Chapter 7: Basic Statistics and its Application

- Restricting people who are within narrow range to produce confounding
- Matching the cases for values which influence confounding
- Subgrouping of study individuals
- Use of standardized rates
- Use of analysis of covariance for adjustment

For establishing casual associations, "Hill's criteria" is used (after Bradford Hill):

- Study design
- Strength of association
- Consistency
- Correct temporal relationship
- Dose-response relationship
- Plausibility
- Specificity
- Analogy

Sample Size

In research, it is not possible to study the whole universe which is called population. So we restrict to a sample from that population which is representation of whole population.

Sample is minimum number of objects or individuals for a study which is statistically determined and which represent the population in their characteristics.

Student is directed to refer to biostatistics for sample size determination.

Types of Sampling

Random	• Simple random sampling (by lottery or random numbers) • Stratified random sampling (sample from each strata) • Systematic sampling (every 10th case) • Cluster sampling (selecting natural groups) • Multistage sampling (for HIV study, four states are selected as primary, four district are selected as secondary, four villages are selected as final)
Nonrandom	• Area sampling (a nonprobability sampling) • Quota sampling (a nonprobability sampling) • Incidental sampling (a nonprobability sampling) • Purposive sampling (a nonprobability sampling)

Tool for Data Collection

Proper training and pilot study before actual research is mandatory. The tools such as observation, interview, checklist, survey, case study, sociometry and sociogram, scaling methods such as nominal, ordinal, interval and ratio scales are worth mentioning in nursing research. Precision of measures used determines valid nature of data.

Item analysis: Measurement used in data collection will have scientific base when it follows set of rules and scientific basis.

Reliability: Reliable conclusion is possible by a large universe of study. It is dependent on individual variability and test variation. Common causes of poor reliability are—a) biological variation, b) technical variation, and c) intra- and interobserver variation.

Validity: It measures accuracy of a test. Indicators that are used to measure validity are sensitivity, specificity, and positive and negative predictive values.

- Extent of disease detection by a test is sensitiveness or true positiveness.
- Extent of normalcy detected by a test is specificity or true negativeness.
- Predictive values are probability of percentage of positive and negative result.

Let us put this information in a contingent table:

Test		Disease		
		+	−	
	+	a	b	= a+b
		True positive		
	−	c	d	= c+d
				True negative
		a+c	b+d	= a+b+c+d
				Prevalence

Example:

ECG	Heart attack		
	+	−	
+	23 (a)	4 (b)	= 27 (a+b)
−	7 (c)	66 (d)	= 73 (c+d)
	30 (a+c)	70 (b+d)	= 100

Sensitivity (true positive) = a/a+c × 100 = 76.7%

Specificity (true negative) = d/b+d × 100 = 94.3%

False positive = b/b+d × 100 = 5.7%

False negative = c/a+c × 100 = 23.3%

Predictive value of positive = a/a+b × 100 = 85.2%

Predictive value of negative = d/c+d × 100 = 90.4%

Source of Error

There are a few factors in data collection which cannot be eliminated. They are even controlled by the investigator. They are called experimental error because they are associated with random variation of the experiment. Randomization and replication make this error less important.

When we draw conclusion, we are likely to make two types of error, viz., type I error and type II error (they are called α and β errors, respectively).

Data Analysis

A research is considered very good if the kind of data processing that may be applicable is decided beforehand, even if the study is a small one.

Knowledge of elementary statistics is required and is found advantageous for the analysis of result. Personal involvement of investigator in analysis adds immensely to the reliability and value of nursing research. If the investigator is amateur, it has to be checked by a senior statistician. Association of statistician and senior faculty from the beginning brings best result out of the research. Application of appropriate statistical analysis is the secret of efficiency and success in research.

Manual data analysis and computer-assisted data analysis are common in research. Common significance test applied in the statistical inference of the result are:
- Standard error (SE) of the difference between two means
- SE of the difference between two proportions
- Chi-square test
- Student 't' test
- Z test.

Presentation of Findings

With formulated objective and postulated hypothesis, the nurse investigates and conducts research to arrive at validated hypothesis. When fruitful observation is arrived and is found useful and beneficial to nursing community, it has to be presented in the form of a report or dissertation or thesis. From this, the nursing community should get the benefit and research result should be a guide in nursing care, nursing management or nursing technique. The presentation made should be comprehensive in nature and a nurse should take care of the guidelines given for the scientific presentation or for submission of a dissertation.

This amounts to the publication of results of research. The publication can be in the form of project, thesis, study, case study, research, clinical trial or a dissertation. State and central Nursing Council and affiliated universities that embodies nursing colleges and nursing schools define the presentations of research.

Minimum standardized steps in reporting shall be:
- Title
- Introduction with aims and objectives
- Review of literature
- Material and methods
- Results and observations
- Discussion
- Summary
- References

In case of references, scientific nursing article commands Vancouver style (the list is at the order of appearance in the text). Nursing dissertation commands Harvard style (alphabetically arranged).

Time has come to prepare nursing profession to have an appreciation of research and to participate in research design implementation and evaluation at the level of their preparation. Administrators shall promote and support research efforts. The result of such research can be translated into policy.

Chapter 7: Basic Statistics and its Application

SOURCES OF STATISTICS

- Census (**Table 7.5**)
- Registration of vital events such as birth, death, marriage
- Sample registration system (SRS)
- Notification of diseases
- Hospital records
- Health center records
- Registration of diseases in National Registry
- Epidemiological studies
- Surveys by interview, examination, records and by post.

Sources of Vital Statistics

Vital statistics keeps a check on demographic changes. Legal registration help in the collection of data on vital statistics.

Vital statistics pertains to vital events namely births, deaths, fetal deaths, marriages, divorces, adaptations, legislations and legal separations. Thus, registration is the foundation of vital statistics.

In India, Birth, Death and Marriage Registration Act came into existence in 1873. This is influenced by illiteracy, ignorance, and lack of motivation of public. Even lack of uniformity in collection is seen because vital data are collected by Health Department, Zila Parishad, Police and Revenue.

Vital statistics calls for proper storage, proper processing and proper dissemination.

Vital statistics refers to data from all vital events.

Main sources are:

- *Census*: It is complete enumeration, involves more cost, more manpower. Time taken is more. Information will be available after 3-5 years.

Table 7.5: Difference between census and sample.

	Census	Sample
Enumeration	Complete	Fraction
Cost	More	Less
Manpower	More	Less
Time	More	Less
Error	More	Less
Information	After 3-5 years	Soon after study

- Registration of vital events such as births, deaths and marriages.
- Sample registration system
- Notification of diseases
- Hospital records
- Health center records
- Registration of diseases in National Registry
- Epidemiological studies
- Surveys by interview
- Surveys by examination
- Survey by records
- Data obtained by post.

SCOPE OF STATISTICS (USES)

- Helps in mapping health problem
- Helps in deciding about health care used
- Comparison is easy
- Efficiency of program is checked
- Assess health care utilization
- Help in planning, implementing and evaluating health services.

DATA COLLECTION, CLASSIFICATION, ANALYSIS, INTERPRETATION, AND PRESENTATION

Data Collection

- Study
- Experiment
- Survey
- Hospital record
- Clinical trial
- Census

Data Presentation (Tables 7.6 and 7.7)

This is required to bring out clear and striking points in the collected data. They are done through the following:

Uses of Data Presentation

- Easy for comparison
- Trend observation with time possible
- Lay people can understand
- Median, percentile, quartile can be calculated
- Inferences are drawn
- Conclusions are drawn
- Helps for further analysis

Table 7.6: Types of data presentation.

Tables	Charts	Diagrams
• Simple table • Cross table • Tables with multivariable	• Bar chart • Vertical chart • Horizontal chart • Multiple chart • Component chart • Histogram chart • Frequency polygon	• Line diagram • Pie diagram • Pictogram

Simple Table (Table 7.7)

Table 7.7: Distribution of GE cases taluk-wise.

Taluk	No.
Dharwad	39
Hubli	23
Kalghatgi	14
Kundgol	9
Navalgund	5
Total	90

Simple table gives frequency distribution. It will have title. Percentage may be added as another column.

Charts

See **Figures 7.1 to 7.9**.

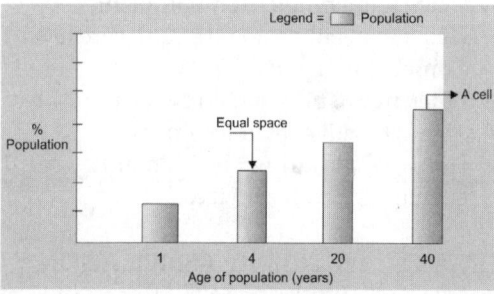

Fig. 7.1: Simple bar diagram.

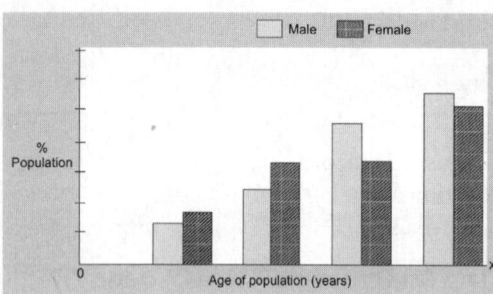

Fig. 7.2: Multiple bar diagram.

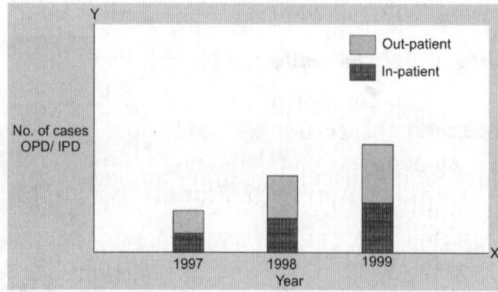

Fig. 7.3: Component bar diagram.

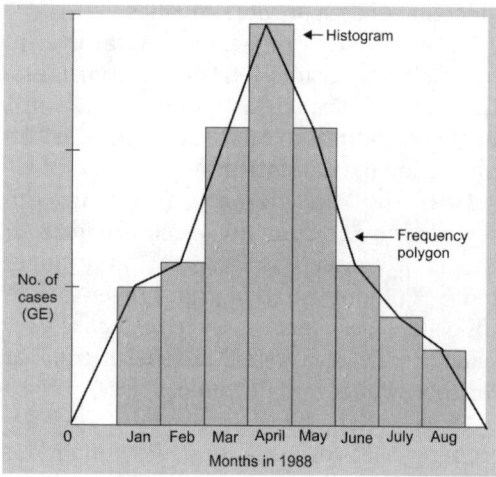

Fig. 7.4: Histogram and frequency polygon. GE cases at Hubli, January–August 1998.

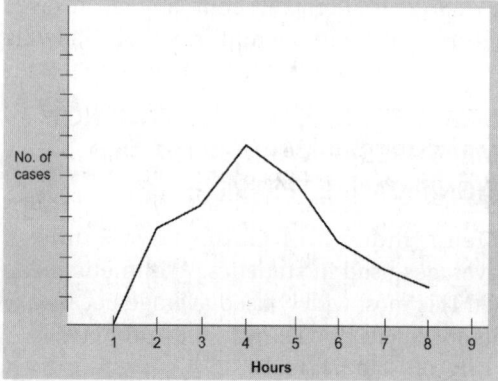

Fig. 7.5: Line diagram showing number of cases by hour of regain consciousness.

Chapter 7: Basic Statistics and its Application

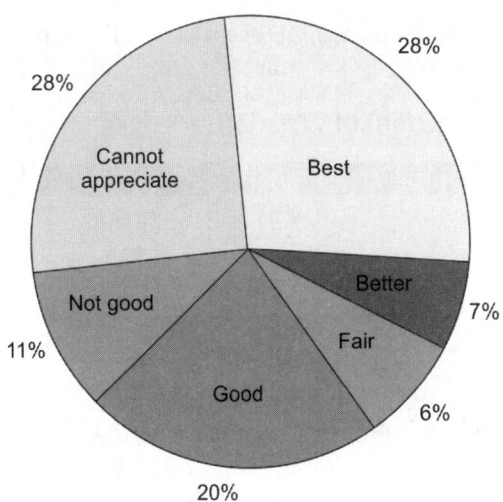

Fig. 7.6: Pie diagram showing duration of priming effect with pancuronium in clinical anesthesia.

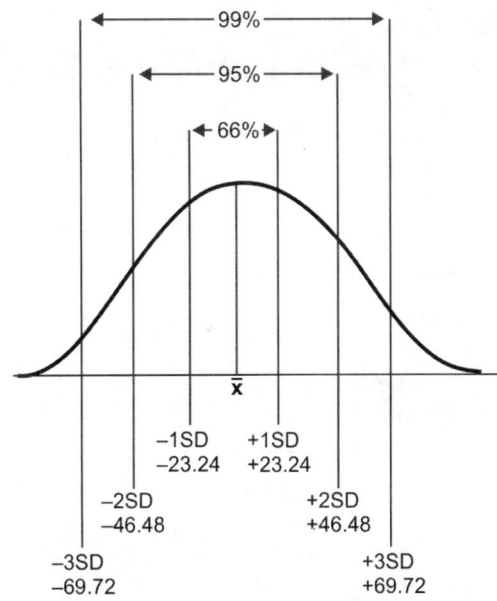

Fig. 7.8: Showing distance and coverage of values in a normal curve, in reference to SD ($\bar{x} \pm 1$ SD, $\bar{x} \pm 2$ SD, $\bar{x} \pm 3$ SD)

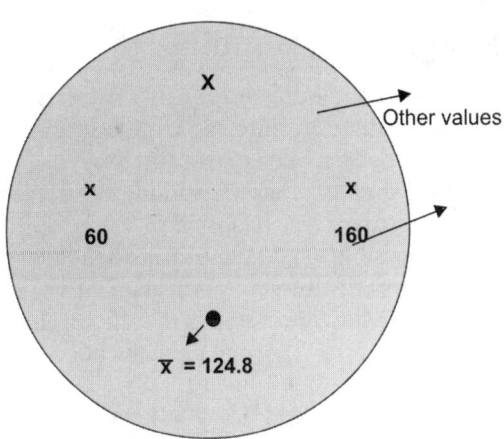

Fig. 7.7: To show the extent of deviation of values from mean.

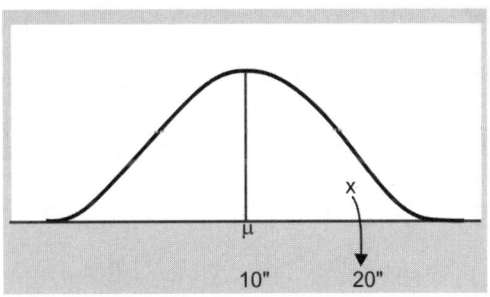

Fig. 7.9: Showing normal deviate.

Mean

Mean =

$$\frac{158+139+120+146+111+99+114+156+111+94}{10} = \frac{1{,}248}{10}$$

Arithmetic mean = 124.8

MEASURES OF CENTRAL TENDENCY, MEASURES OF VARIABILITY AND SIGNIFICANCE TESTS

Mean, mode and median are common averages used in statistics. Arithmetic mean (AM) is most widely used average because of its specificity and less variation property.

IQ of 10 individuals:
158, 139, 120, 146, 111, 99, 114, 156, 111, 94

Median

Arranged in ascending order and mid value is found out.

94, 99, 111, 111, 114, 120, 139, 146, 156, 158

234/2 = 117   Median = 117

Mode

Repeatedly occurring value (most fashionable number)
Mode also can be found out by:
Mode = 3 (Median) – 2 (Mean)
   Mode = 111

MEASURES OF VARIABILITY

They are:
- Range
- Mean deviation (MD)
- Standard deviation (SD)
- Coefficient of variation (CV)

Range: The value between minimum and maximum (Highest – Lowest)

IQ of above 10 individuals is taken and MD as well as SD is calculated:

x	$(x - \bar{x})$	$(x - \bar{x})^2$
158	33.2	1102.24
139	14.2	201.64
120	–4.8	23.04
146	21.2	449.44
111	–13.8	190.44
99	–25.8	665.64
114	–10.8	116.64
156	31.2	973.44
111	–13.8	190.44
94	–30.8	948.64
1248	199.6	4861.6

$\bar{x} = 1248$ $\Sigma \times - \bar{x}$ — $\Sigma (\times - \bar{x})^2$
AM = 124.8
$\Sigma | \times - \bar{x} |$

Mean deviation = 199.6 ÷ 10 = 19.96

$\text{Standard Deviation} = \sqrt{\dfrac{(x-\bar{x})^2}{n-1}} = \sqrt{\dfrac{4861.6}{9}} = 23.24$

Steps in calculating mean deviation:
- Find AM of IQ
- Find mean deviation of each and their sum $\Sigma | x - \bar{x} |$
- Divide $\Sigma | x - \bar{x} |$ by number of observations

Steps to calculate SD:
- Find AM of IQ
- Find MD of each $| x - \bar{x} |$
- Find square of MD of each $(x - \bar{x})^2$ and their sum $\Sigma (x - x)^2$. sum $\Sigma (x - \bar{x})^2$

Coefficient of Variation

	Height	Weight
Mean	160 cm	55 kg
SD	10 cm	5 kg

$CV = \dfrac{SD}{Mean} \times 100$

CV of height = $\dfrac{10}{160} \times 100 = 6.25\%$

CV of weight = $\dfrac{5}{55} \times 100 = 9.09\%$

Inference: Height is more consistent than weight or weight is more variable than height.

NORMAL DISTRIBUTION

It is smooth, bell shaped, symmetrical curve obtained by entering large number of observations between two ordinates.

Mean and standard deviation define area under normal curve (Gaussian).

It is possible to relate the distance between any observed value (x) and mean of curve (μ), i.e., (x-μ) distance to the SD of that curve. Thus, we get a standard normal deviate called 'Z'.

$Z = \dfrac{x - \mu}{SD}$

μ of height of population = 10"
X of height of observed population = 20"
SD of normal curve = 5"

$Z = \dfrac{x - \mu}{SD} = \dfrac{20-10}{5} = \dfrac{10}{5} = 2$

i.e., χ can be located at 2 SD distance from the center of curve.

SIGNIFICANCE TESTS

They are applied on qualitative or quantitative data (which are tabulated) to find out their relationship or association. It also tells us whether the outcome of the study has occurred by chance or not occurred by chance.

Chapter 7: Basic Statistics and its Application

Common significance tests used are:
- SE of the difference between two means
- SE of the difference between two proportions
- Chi-square test
- Z test
- t test

P value (probability) range from 0 to 1. It is the probable chance of occurrence of an event. It expresses the relative frequency of occurrence of an event.

Examples:
- Tossed coin head or tail
- Chance of male baby to new couple
- Chance of the drug A being better than B

Theory of probability (chance) may be binomial or multinomial. This is just distribution in nature.

Normally, critical probability P = 0.05 (one in 20) is selected.

Other P values are:
0.01 (1 in 100)
0.005 (5 in 1000)
0.001 (1 in 1000)

Level of Significance

It is adjusted as the limit at which point chance is operating. Normally, in biological science, P = 0.05 which is critical probability refers to limit of 5%. Accordingly, 1% (P = 0.01), 0.5% (P = 0.005), and 0.1% (P = 0.001) are the expression of chance limit in scientific studies.

If the calculated value is greater than table value for given P, it is unlikely to occur by chance.

If the calculated value is lesser than table value for given P, it is likely to occur by chance.

SE of the Difference between 2 Means

Illustration

A sample of 6,400 Englishmen has a mean height of 67.85 inches and a SD of 2.56 inches while another sample of 1,600 Australians have a mean height of 68.55 inches and a SD of 2.52 inches. Do the data indicate that Australians are taller than Englishmen on the average basis?

$$SE\,\bar{x}_1 - \bar{x}_2 = \sqrt{\frac{SD^2}{n1} + \frac{SD^2}{n2}} = \sqrt{\frac{2.56^2}{6400} + \frac{2.52^2}{1600}}$$

SE $x_1 - x_2$ = 0.071
Twice the $x_1 - x_2$ = 0.141322
Difference observed (0.7) is more than twice the SE $x_1 - x_2$ which is 0.14.

Inference: Hence, significant. The data indicate that Australians are taller than Englishmen on the average basis.

SE of the Difference between Two Proportions

Illustration (Table 7.8)

Mortality from peritonitis among dogs treated with two types of sulfa is as under:

Survival rate is 10% more in sulfanilamide. Is it significant?

$$SE_{p-p} = \sqrt{\frac{p_1\,q_1}{n_1} + \frac{p_2\,q_2}{n_2}}$$

Here $p_1 = 50$ $q_1 = 50$ $n_1 = 100$
$p_2 = 40$ $q_2 = 60$ $n_2 = 100$

$$SE_{p-p} = \sqrt{\frac{50 \times 50}{100} + \frac{40 \times 60}{100}} = 70$$

Twice the SE_{p-p} = 14.0

Difference observed in above illustration is 50 – 40 = 10.

Difference (10) is less than twice the SE_{p-p} (14). Hence, not significant. More survival rate seen with first drug is only by chance.

Inference: Not statistically significant.

Chi-square test (χ^2)

X = normal distribution, where x = 0, SD = 1
X^2 = follows X^2 distribution.

Table 7.8: Mortality from peritonitis.

Treatment	Death	Survival	Total
Sulfanilamide	50	50	100
Sulfathiazole	60	40	100

This significance test is used:
a. To test the goodness of fit (i.e., observed and expected difference is significant or not).
b. To find association of attribute (dependent or not).

Illustration (Table 7.9)

A cancer screening test was carried out by a team of oncologists at a cancer hospital in Mysore of Karnataka state. Total 300 people were screened for oral cancer and the findings were:
1. Oral cancer and related were 100, of whom 20 were found positive for chewing tobacco.
2. 200 people were without oral cancer, of whom 110 people were found positive for chewing tobacco.

What is your interpretation?

$$E = \frac{\text{Row total} \times \text{Column total}}{\text{Grand total}}$$

$$x^2 = \frac{\Sigma(O-E)^2}{E} = \frac{(20-43.3)^2}{43.3} + \frac{(80-56.7)^2}{56.7} + \frac{(110-86.7)^2}{86.7} + \frac{(90-113.3)^2}{113.3}$$

$$= 12.54 + 9.57 + 6.26 + 4.79 = 33.16$$

Degree of freedom (DF) = (c–1) (r–1), where c = column and r = row.

X^2 calculated (33.16) is greater than X^2 table value at DF = 1, and P = 0.001.

(Table value for DF = 1 at P = 0.05 is 3.84, at P = 0.01 is 6.64, at P = 0.001 is 10.83)

Hence, significant.

Inference: Oral cancer and chewing tobacco are dependent on each other.

Yate's Correction

It is a correction given for continuity to compensate for the application of continuous distribution to discrete or qualitative data, used in X^2 test with one degree of freedom. The correction is subtraction of ½ in each difference.

$$\text{Yate's correction} = X_c^2 = \frac{(|O-E|-1/2)^2}{E}$$

Student's 't' Test

With smaller number of sample, 't' test will allow us to interpret properly. The 't' curve is symmetrical, bell shaped but has more values farther away from the mean than does normal curve. It is found out by:

$$t = \frac{\bar{x} - \mu}{s/\sqrt{n}} \text{ where}$$

$\bar{x}$ = mean of the sample
μ = mean of the population
S = SD of sample mean
n = number of observation

ANOVA

A method of partitioning variance into parts (Between and within) so as to yield independent estimate of the population variance. This is tested with F distribution. It is a method of testing sample means significance.

F distribution is the distribution followed by the ratio of two independent sample estimates of a population variance. $F = S_1^2/S_2^2$

Uses

It is useful to test the assumption which underlines many statistical tests that two population variance are equal.

Steps

I. a. Calculation of sum of squares
   – Row total square
   – Ratio of row total square to row number
   b. Similarly to column numbers
II. Using correction factor, calculation of total sum of squares, between sum of squares, within sum of squares and error sum of squares

Table 7.9: Tobacco chewing and oral cancer.

Chewing		Not chewing	Total
Oral cancer	20 (43.3)	80 (56.7)	100
No cancer	110 (86.7)	90 (113.3)	200
	130	170	300

Note: Values in parenthesis are expected values (E)

III. Finding out F ratio.
IV. Statistical inference with the help of ANOVA table.

SAMPLING

When a portion of a group is taken for a study from large group (universe), it is called sample. Different methods of sampling are:
- Simple random sample (by random number or by lottery)
- Systematic random sample (every 10th value taken)
- Stratified random sample (to include each portion of the sample)

Sampling error—variation from one sample to another.

STANDARD ERROR

The average in a group is mean and the SD of mean is a measure of SE which is found out by:

$$SD/\sqrt{n}$$

SAMPLE SIZE

In research, in investigation or survey of number of cases/unit/patients is called sample size. This is influenced by—(a) prevalence of an event, (b) prevailing status of estimates of the characteristics, (c) predetermined desired accuracy of the estimate of characteristics, (d) the probability level considered, (e) availability of money, material and manpower, and (f) time bound.

This is found out by the formula $n = \dfrac{4pq}{L^2}$ where
p = prevalence/proportion of an event q = 1 − p
L^2 = permissible error in the estimate of p

Suppose we want to calculate sample size for diabetic survey, assuming that prevalence rate in the community is 22%. Then, with permissible error of 5%, the sample size works out to be;

$$n = \frac{4 \times pq}{L^2} = \frac{4 \times 22 \times 78}{(1.1)^2} = 5672$$

Note: 1.1 is 5% of 22.

SUMMARY

Data collection, data classification, data analysis, data interpretation and data presentation are described. Measures of central tendency, measures of variability, significant tests are described. Sampling is detailed.

VIVA VOCE

1. What is placebo?
2. What is triple blinding?
3. What are the differences between case control study and cohort study?
4. What is random sampling?
5. Mention source of statistics.
6. Mention measures of variability.
7. What is normal curve?
8. Define SE.

SECTION 3

Section Outline

Chapter 8. Epidemiology

Chapter 9. Epidemiology of Communicable Diseases

Chapter 10. Epidemiology of Noncommunicable Diseases

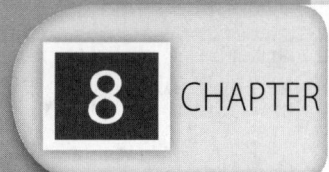

CHAPTER 8

Epidemiology

CHAPTER OUTLINE

- Milestones
- Definitions
- Terms Used in Epidemiology
- Types of Epidemiology
- Investigation of an Epidemic
- Quarantine
- Emporiatrics
- Desmotology
- Disinfection
- Dynamics of Disease Transmission
- Immunity
- Adverse Event Following Immunization (AEFI)
- Prevention and Control of Diseases
- Epidemiometrics Analysis
- Screening Tests

INTRODUCTION

Epidemiology is one of the developing areas over the last five decades, which covers all health-related events of man. We have many offshoots, such as clinical epidemiology, cancer epidemiology, neuroepidemiology, serological epidemiology, genetic epidemiology, etc.

MILESTONES IN EPIDEMIOLOGY

- ❖ Epidemiology is known since 3rd century BC
- ❖ Properly identified in 19th century
- ❖ In 1850, epidemiological society in London was established
- ❖ In 1920, lecture series on epidemiology by Winslow and Sedgwick in USA
- ❖ In 1927, Wade Hampton (WH) Frost was appointed as professor of epidemiology in USA
- ❖ In 1930, Major Greenwood was appointed as professor of epidemiology in London
- ❖ In 1948, Framingham Heart Study was initiated
- ❖ In 2000, firmly established subject in Medical Education. India declared guinea worm free. Declared National Population Policy (NPP) 2000
- ❖ In 2001, policy for empowerment of woman launched
- ❖ In 2002, National Acquired Immunodeficiency Syndrome (AIDS) Prevention and Control Policy declared. Severe Acute Respiratory Syndrome (SARS) Epidemic emerged
- ❖ In 2003, National Vector Borne Disease Control Programme approved. Cigarette and tobacco products prohibited
- ❖ In 2004, Integrated Disease Surveillance Projects launched
- ❖ In 2005, Reproductive and Child Health (RCH II)/Janani Suraksha Yojana launched. Leprosy Elimination Target implicated
- ❖ In 2006, Revised National Tuberculosis Control Programme (RNTCP) covers entire India
- ❖ In 2007, Senior Citizen Bill passed
- ❖ In 2009, H_1N_1 Pandemic
- ❖ In 2013, National Health Mission
- ❖ In 2014, Declared Polio Free
- ❖ In 2015, National Institution for Transforming India (NITI) Aayog replaced

Yojana Aayog. Swachh Bharat Abhiyan launched
- In 2016, Sustainable Development Goals came to force. Malaria eradication plan 2016–2013 launched
- In 2017, National Health Policy (NHP) 2017
- In 2018, National Health Protection Scheme.

DEFINITION

"The study of the distribution and determinants of health related states or events in specified populations, and the application of this study to the control of health problems."
—John M Last

The study of the distribution and determinants of disease frequency in man.
—MacMahon

Epidemiology is a science always treats epidemics and is related with mass phenomenon of infectious diseases.

Graphical representation of occurrence of cases of a disease with the passage of time is called epidemic curve.

Well known epidemiological studies in the history of public health are:
- Moses—leprosy.
- Fracastorius—syphilis.
- John Snow—cholera.
- William Budd—typhoid.

Epidemiological Triad

The causative factors of disease agent, host and environment are referred to as epidemiological triad.

Agents

Living or nonliving such as biological agents, nutrient agents, physical agents, chemical agents, mechanical agents, social agents.

Host

Biological and demographic characteristics of man, and animal reservoirs.

Nature of host

- Definitive host (sexual life-cycle of parasite +).
- Intermediate host (asexual life-cycle of parasite +).
- Transport host (carrier).
- Obligate host (when only infect man).

Environment

Macro- or microenvironment such as physical, biological, and psychosocial.

TERMS USED IN EPIDEMIOLOGY

Infection: Entry and multiplication of pathogens in human body which show inflammatory response in the form of disease.

Contamination: Pathogens on nonliving things which do not show any response.

Infestation: Surface (skin) infection and intestinal infections.

Communicable disease: Specific pathogen transmission directly or indirectly.

Noncommunicable disease (NCD):
- Nonspecific pathogen.
- No direct or indirect transmission.
- No vectors in transmission.

Infectious disease: Disease by an infectious agent, show SAR (secondary attack rate).

Contagious disease: By contact transmission.

Epidemic: Disease occurring more than our expectation.

Pandemic: Large populations are involved (all nations at a given point).

Sporadic: Cases occurring here and there.

Zoonoses: Mainly disease of animals, man gets the disease in the dynamic of transmission.

Epizootic: Epidemicity of zoonotic disease in animal population.

Enzootic: Endemicity of zoonotic disease in animal population.

Panzootic: Large section of animal involved by zoonoses at a point of time across the continent.

Exotic: Disease from other country which does not exist.

Epornithic: Epidemic in birds.

Incidence: Number of new cases in a defined population during 1 year.

Prevalence: Number of cases at a given point of time (prevailing cases).

Chapter 8: Epidemiology

Random: Selection of items without giving room for bias.

Risk: A determinant which is significantly associated with diseases.

Sample: Scientifically selected small group for a study.

Universe: Whole group of mankind or a big group selected for a study.

Validity (accuracy): Extent of accuracy of a test in epidemiology.

Association: Concurrence of two variables which is not by chance.

Bias: It is a systematically expressed error found out in the determination of the association between exposure and disease.

Nosocomial infection: Hospital acquired infection.

Iatrogenic disease: Adverse reaction by drug, vaccine, and diagnostic agents.

Surveillance: Watch over a disease or event.

Active surveillance: When profession goes to the community for surveillance.

Passive surveillance: When community comes to profession for surveillance.

Control: Measures to overcome emergency.

Eradicate: Absolute process to root out disease by terminating pathogen.

Mortality: Deaths occurring by disease or event in man.

Morbidity: Deviation from physiological basis in man.

Case: Person having disease or health disorder.

Case control: Two groups with same character one for study and the other for control.

Cohort: Group of people who share common characteristics.

Contact: Those who come in contact with a given disease or health conditions.

Confounding: If a factor is associated with both disease and a variable (third influencing factor).

Correlation: Extent of relationship between variables (degree of association).

Coverage: Coverage of all in a study, in an immunization session, and in sterilization operation which are expressed in percentage.

Prediction: Future forecast on epidemics.

Trend: Anticipated future occurrence.

Association: The concurrence of two variables more often than would be expected by chance.

Components

- *Frequency of disease* is measured by rate and ratio. Indirectly it is also measured by health-related events.
- *Distribution of disease* occurrence by time, place and person.
- *Determinants of disease* by risk factors.

Aims of Epidemiology

- Map out magnitude of health and disease.
- Risk factor identification.
- Plan for implementation and evaluation.

Concept of Epidemiology

- Universe of study is a defined population.
- Disease pattern in the community is studied.
- Both health and diseases are concerned.
- Source of infection is a clue to control measures.
- Should help national health programs.
- Investigation is done in community.
- Takes the help of clinical consideration in identification.

Approach in Epidemiology

- Six questions are asked on health-related *events.*
  1. What?
  2. Where?
  3. When?
  4. Who?
  5. Why?
  6. How?
- Six questions are asked on health-related *actions.*
  1. How to reduce?
  2. How to prevent?
  3. What is activity?
  4. Where resources?
  5. Possible difficulties?
  6. Immediate benefit.

- Comparative study done with laid down standard criteria, definition and procedure.

TYPES OF EPIDEMIOLOGY

Descriptive Epidemiology

Main aim is to investigate the characteristics of specific group of population. The components included are (7**D**s):
- **D**eaths
- **D**iseases
- **D**isabilities
- **D**iscomfort
- **D**issatisfaction
- **D**eviation from social norm
- **D**eviation from statistical norm.

It asks the question—When?, Where?, Who? It gets the answer—Time, place, and person.

Uses of Descriptive Study
- Gives morbidity
- Gives mortality
- Gives clue to the cause
- Gives ideas for hypothesis
- Help in health planning and evaluation
- Help in identifying the determinants of disease.

Characteristics in Descriptive Studies (Table 8.1)

Disease load in the community is found out or measured by the incidence and prevalence through cross-sectional and longitudinal studies.

Difference between Cross-sectional Study and Longitudinal Study

See **Table 8.2**.

Changing Concepts in Epidemiology

See **Table 8.3**.

Analytic Epidemiology

To test a hypothesis and to infer about the population analytical epidemiology is used. They can be case control study or cohort study.

Table 8.1: Time, place and person in disease distribution.

Time distribution	Place distribution	Person distribution
Long-term secular	**Local geographic pathology**	**Childhood**
• Upward trend of heart disease, lung cancer, diabetes	• Cholera cluster epidemic in London	• ARI
		• Measles
		Old age
	• Case cluster of AIDS in an area	• Atherosclerosis
		• Arteriosclerosis
• Downward trend of TB, typhoid, polio		**Women**
		• Obesity
	Rural geographic pathology	• Hyperthyroidism
Seasonal		• Diabetes
• Measles in early spring	• Helminthic infestation, skin infection, zoonotic diseases	**African race**
• URI in winter		• Sickle cell anemia
• GE in summer		**Coal miner**
Cyclic trend		• Silicosis
• Influenza once in 10 years	**Urban geographic pathology**	• Hookworm anemia
		Upper class
• Traffic accident on Saturday	• Accidents	• Diabetes
	• Lung cancer	• Hypertension
	• Heart diseases	• MI
• Rubella once in 9 years		**Mass movement**
• Measles once in 3 years	• Chronic bronchitis	• Cholera
Point source epidemic	**National geographic pathology**	**Sedentary life**
		• MI
• Food poisoning	• Malaria	**Migration workers**
Common source by repeated exposure	• Endemic goiter	• Malaria
		Stress
	• Guinea worm disease	• Migraine
		• Hypertension
• Gonorrhea	• Leprosy	**Marriage**
Propagated epidemic	**International geographic pathology**	• Longevity of life
• Polio epidemic	• Ca stomach in Japan	
• Hepatitis A epidemic	• Ca cervix in India	

(URI: upper respiratory tract infection; GE: gastroenteritis; TB: tuberculosis; Ca: cancer; AIDS: acquired immunodeficiency syndrome; MI: myocardial infarction; ARI: acute respiratory infection)

Table 8.2: Difference between cross-sectional and longitudinal study.

Cross-sectional study	Longitudinal study
Single examination at one point	Repeated over long time
Can be projected to the universe	It is a universal project
When repeated it can be serial survey description	Cannot be repeated easily
Fast approach	Slow approach
Inexpensive	Expensive
Study of NHD not possible	NHD study is possible
Study of risk factors is not possible	Possible to study risk factors
Gives prevalence	Gives incidence

Table 8.3: Changing concepts in epidemiology.

Concept of yesterday	Concept of today
Dispensing at dispensary (clinical concept)	Case management and follow-up (health center concept)
Only at hospital and dispensary	Subcenter, primary health center, district hospital, teaching hospital, regional hospital, super specialty hospital and national institutes
Based on symptoms and signs	Based on information system
Cure of illness	Improving health of community
Case examination	Community diagnosis
Case treatment	Community treatment
Case investigation	Community survey
Clinical case record	Epidemiological information and epidemiological investigation
Role of doctor and a compounder	Role of community health guide, medical social worker, Anganwadi worker, traditional birth attendant, MPW (M) and (F), health supervisor (M) and (F), and doctors
Only advice	Health education, primary health care, comprehensive health care, integrated health care, risk approach, total health care, health package, and cafeteria approach
Only medical component	Social component and behavior component
No association, correlation or validity of attributes and variables	Association + Correlation + Validity

(MPW: multipurpose workers)

Case Control Study (Table 8.4)

Starts at effect and goes back to cause.

Table 8.4: Difference between case and control.

Case	Control
Study group	Control group
Effect on health is seen	Effect on health not seen
Diagnostic criteria should prove disease	Not necessary
Inclusive criteria is important	Exclusive criteria is important

Design (Fig. 8.1)

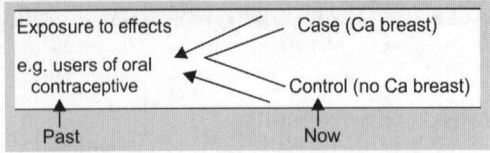

Fig. 8.1: Design for cross section study.

Analysis Used

Exposure: Smoking five cigarettes per day.

	Smoking		
	+	−	Total
Case (Ca lung)	a	b	a + b
Control (No Ca)	c	d	c + d
	a + c	b + d	a + b + c + d

$$\text{Cases} = \frac{1}{a+c} \quad \text{Control} = \frac{b}{b+d}$$

$$\text{Relative risk} = \frac{\text{Incidence among exposed}}{\text{Incidence among nonexposed}}$$

$$= \frac{a}{a+c} / \frac{b}{b+d}$$

$$\text{Attributable risk} = \frac{\text{Incidence among exposed} - \text{incidence among not exposed}}{\text{Incidence among exposed}} \times 100$$

Odds Ratio

This is the measure of the strength of the association between risk factor and outcome which is equivalent to relative risk. It is also called cross product ratio.

	Case	Control	Total
Exposed	a	b	a + b
	800	200	1000
Not exposed	c	d	c + d
	100	400	500
	a + c	b + d	a + b + c + d
	900	600	1,500

$$\text{Odds ratio} = \frac{a \times d}{b \times c} = \frac{800 \times 400}{200 \times 100} = \frac{32}{2} = 16.0$$

Inference

The risk for the exposed is 16 times that of nonexposed.

Use

- Frequently occurring health problem
- Less cost, small duration, and
- Identify risk factors.

Examples of case control study:
- Maternal smoking and birth defects
- Viral infection and Bell's palsy
- Exercise and myocardial infarction (MI)
- Occupation and carcinoma bladder
- X-ray and blood cancer.

Cohort Study

Group with similar characteristics constitutes a cohort, e.g., birth cohort, marriage cohort.

It proceeds forward from cause to effect.

Design

See **Figure 8.2**.

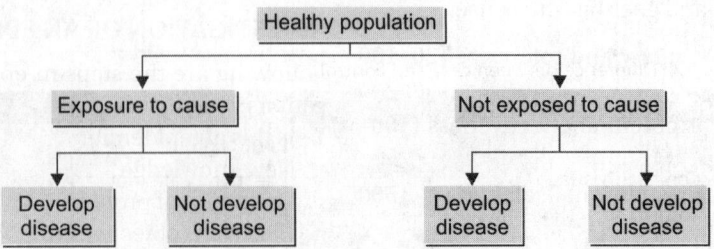

Fig. 8.2: Design for cohort study.

Analysis

	Developed	Disease not developed	Total
Exposed group	a	b	a + b
Not exposed group	c	d	c + d
Total	a + c	b + d	a + b + c + d

$$\text{Incidence among exposed} = \frac{a}{a+b} \times 100$$

$$\text{Incidence among not exposed} = \frac{c}{c+d} \times 100$$

$$\text{Relative risk} = \frac{a/(a+b)}{c/(c+d)}$$

$$\text{Attributable risk} = \frac{a/(a+b) - c/(c+d)}{a/(a+b)} \times 100$$

$$\text{Odds ratio} = \frac{ad}{bc}$$

Uses

* Relative and attributable risk available
* Multifactorial study possible, and
* Nocturnal hemodialysis (NHD) is identified.

Examples of cohort study:

* Risk factors in coronary heart disease (CHD)
* Oral contraceptive (OC) in cancer development
* Smoking in lung cancer.

Experimental Epidemiology

Clinical Trial

It is a controlled experimental study that is used to assess safety and efficacy of treatment for diseases or health problems.

Stages

1. Stage I—for safety and tolerance (20–100 cases).
2. Stage II—for potential effectiveness (100–200 cases).
3. Stage III—for additional safety (500–1500 cases).
4. Stage IV—for long-term effect (post-marketing study).

Design

1. Parallel design

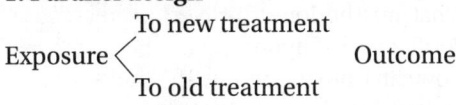

2. Crossover design

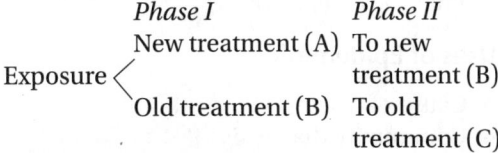

3. Drug change design

	Phase I	Phase II
Exposure	Drug (A)	Drug (B)
	Drug (B)	Drug (A)

Randomized Clinical Trial

Random selection helps in:

* Reducing bias
* For equal chance
* Comparability

Methods

* Assign alternatively
* Coin flipping
* Card shuffling
* Throwing dice
* Random table

Blinding

It is a method of reducing the bias in a clinical trial.

Types

* *Single blind:* Treatment is concealed from participants
* *Double blind:* Concealed from investigator and participants
* *Triple blind:* Concealed from investigator, participants and evaluators.

INVESTIGATION OF AN EPIDEMIC

Following are the steps in epidemic investigations:

1. Is this an epidemic?
   New knowledge.
   Definition of problem
   Clarifying objectives.
2. What are its characteristics?
   Critical appraisal of existing information.

3. What seems to have caused it?
   Formulation of hypothesis.
4. What must be done to prove the actual cause?
   Verification of hypothesis.
5. How can it be stopped and further epidemic be prevented?
   Practical application.

Uses of Epidemiology

- Cause of disease and health
- Community diagnosis
- Clinical picture
- Determinants and distribution
- General practice
- Investigation of an epidemic
- Mass survey
- Need and methods of control and prevention
- Operational research
- Risk chances
- Syndrome
- Social factors
- Temporal variation

Example of Use of Epidemiology

Framingham Heart Study through epidemiological studies, it could establish Natural History of Rheumatic Heart Disease (1956), Smoking and cardiovascular disease (CVS) risk was established (1960), Cholesterol and CVS risk was established (1961), low-density lipoprotein (LDL) (bad), high density lipoproteins (HDL) (good) were described (1977), new risk prediction formulated for CHD (1998).

QUARANTINE

It is the limitation of freedom of movement of such persons or domestic animals exposed to communicable disease for a period of time not longer than the longest incubation period to avoid transmission.

Quarantinable Diseases

- Cholera
- Yellow fever
- Relapsing fever
- Plague

EMPORIATRICS

It deals with science of health of travelers.

Causes

- Overcrowding
- Change in eating habit
- Change in climate
- Unaware of health facilities
- Exposure to local diseases

Prevention

- To avoid taking bath in polluted water
- Drinking safe and potable water
- Eating cooked hot food
- Be aware of oral rehydration salts (ORS)
- Chemoprophylaxis when required
- Immunoprophylaxis when required
- Compulsory international vaccination

DESMOTOLOGY

The word is derived from Greek word "Desmoterion" meaning "Prison". This deals with the epidemiology of Prison Health.

The discipline desmotology deals with health of inmates in Jails, Prisons and Juvenile Detention facilities. It is estimated that about 12% of inmates seek services.

DISINFECTION

Disinfectants (Table 8.5)

A method of killing pathogens outside human body by physical and chemical agents (through antiseptics and disinfectants).

Table 8.5: Difference between disinfection and antiseptic.

Disinfection	Antiseptic
Kills outright immediate action, short duration	Prevent growth, mild, prolonged
Can be antiseptic in weaker strength	–
Bactericidal	Bacteriostatic

Detergents

- Lower surface tension has cleansing property
- Anionic—soap
- Cationic—cetrimide.

Deodorant—agent which controls bad odor.

Disinfectant—agent killing vermin (lice, flea, bugs).

Types
Concurrent

- Course of illness
- Sputum, vomitus, stool, urine
- Linen, hand, cloth, apron, gown

Terminal

- Recovery—infective material, utensil
- Death—infective material and room, article.

Prophylactic

- Chemical—water purification
- Boiling water in cholera epidemic
- Milk pasteurization
- Cleaning hand before eating.

Test

$$\text{Rideal Walker coefficient (RWC)} = \frac{\text{Min. conc. of phenol which kills 24 h B typhosa}}{\text{Min. conc. of disinfectant which kills 24 h B typhosa}}$$

Natural Agents

- Sunlight
- Dry air.

Physical Agents

- Burning—swab, dressings
- Hot air—limited use
- Boiling—in 10 minutes bacteria are killed, in 30 minutes spores destroyed.
  Linen, utensil, instrument, glassware, rubber (contaminated linen—1% soap or 0.3% washing soda in 2 hours).
  Steam—at 100°C in 5 minutes kill spores.
  Flaming—use in laboratory only.
  Radiation—dressing, bandage, catgut.

Chemical Agents

- Solids
  - Lime—feces (2:1 for 4 hours), walls
  - $CaOCl_2$—stool 400 g/L, urine 5 g/L, 10 hours
    Sputum 200 g/L, 1 hour
  - $KMnO_4$—fruits, vegetable wash
- Liquid
  - Formalin—40%, 2-3% wall
  - Phenol—10% feces, 5% floor
  - Cresol—5-10% feces, room, sputum drain
  - Lysol—emulsion with cresol
- Gas
  - Formaldehyde—room (12 hours)

Public Health Importance

Ship Disinfection for Quarantine (By Fumigation)

- Cyanogas
- Sulfur dioxide

Operation Theater (OT) Disinfection

- Soap and water clean, aeration, sunlight,
- Wash with chlorinated lime (25 ppm),
- Wash with 1% formaldehyde solution,
- Wash with 2.5% cresol (4 hours contact),
- 500 mL formalin in 1 L per 30 cubic meters as fumigation, and
- 200 g $KMnO_4$ in 500 mL formalin in 1 L water—for 30 cubic meters (boiling liberates formaldehyde, allowed for 12 hours disinfection).

Hospital Disinfection

Fces, urine: 2 hours contact phenol 10%, formalin 10%, $CaOCl_2$ 8%, cresol 5%.

Sputum: Burning, autoclave (20 minutes, 20 lb) 5% cresol.

Room:

- Soap water—48 hours.
- 2.5% cresol, 5% phenol, 10% formalin—4 hours
- Formaldehyde vapor—6 hours
- Formalin + $KMnO_4$ (200 g/½ L) in water (for every 30 cubic meter)

- *Linen:* Bed-cloth, cover, towel—Boil, steam, cresol 2.5%—12 hours.
- *Dead body:* Covered bed sheet—10% formalin or 5% phenol.
- *Instruments:* Knife, scissor (lysol, phenol), syringe (boiling).
- *Dressing glove*—autoclave
- *Rubber or plastic catheter*—boiling
- *Gum elastic catheter*—formalin vapor
- *Cystoscope*—pasteurization
- *Facemask*—pasteurization
- *Suture (Catgut)*—Lugol's iodine
- *Other suture*—autoclave
- *Polythene tubing*—gamma radiation
- *Urinals*—hypochlorite solution
- *Bedpan*—lysol
- *Blanket*—hot formalin vapor.

DYNAMICS OF DISEASE TRANSMISSION

Components

1. Source
2. Transmission
3. Host.

Source
Case
A person having infection may be clinical or subclinical.

First case introduced = Primary case. First case noticed = Index case.

Subsequent contact cases = Secondary cases.

Carrier
Man or animal harboring pathogen but apparently healthy and serve as source of infection.

- *Healthy carriers:* Polio, cholera, diphtheria
- *Convalescent carriers:* Typhoid, amebic dysentery
- *Incubatory carriers:* Measles
- *Temporary carrier*
- *Chronic carrier* (excrete pathogen over 3 months)
- Urinary carrier
- Intestinal carrier
- Respiratory carrier
- Nasal carrier.

Reservoir
- *Animal reservoir:* Rabies, yellow fever, influenza.
- Nonliving reservoir soil (tetanus).

Transmission
Direct Transmission
- Contact—sexually transmitted disease (STD), leptospira, skin infection, eye infection.
- Droplet—whooping cough, tuberculosis (TB)
- Soil—hookworm, tetanus
- Inoculation—rabies, hepatitis B
- Transplacental
- Torch agent*, syphilis, AIDS (*Toxoplasma, Rubella, Cytomegalovirus, Herpes).

Indirect Transmission (Five Fs—Finger, Fomite, Fly, Food, Fluid).
- Food borne—gastroenteritis (GE), typhoid, food poisoning
- Waterborne—hepatitis A, cholera, polio
- Vector borne—malaria, plague, Japanese encephalitis (JE), dengue
- Soil borne—TB, influenza, chickenpox, measles
- Blood borne—hepatitis B, malaria, syphilis, human immunodeficiency virus (HIV)/AIDS.

Vector Transmission
- Mechanical—housefly
- Biological:
  - Propagative (multiplication)—plague bacilli in flea
  - Cyclopropagative (multiplication and development)—malaria parasite in mosquito
- Cyclodevelopment (Development)—Microfilaria in mosquito
- Transovarian—vertical transmission from infected female vector to her progeny (ticks)
- Transstadial—transmission of agent from 1 stage of life cycle to another, (e.g., nymph to adult).

Host

Successful parasitism (requisite of infection)
* Entry to host
* Select site for survival
* Find to exit from host
* Survival till finding new host.

Incubation period—agent entry till appearance of signs and symptoms [communicable disease (in CD)].

Latent period—disease initiation to disease detection [noncommunicable disease (NCD)].

Use of incubation period
* Source and contact detection
* Advice selective isolation.

Use of immunizing agents (active, passive)
* Identifies point source
* Track down propagated source, and
* Useful in prognosis.

Serial interval
* Period from onset of primary case to onset of secondary case.
* Generation time (roughly incubation period but different from incubation period).
* It indicates the peak of infection from onset of infection.

Communicable Period

Period of infectivity, measured by SAR

$$SAR = \frac{No. \, exposed \, in \, incubation \, period}{Total \, susceptible \, and \, exposed} \times 100$$

$$= \frac{No. \, exposed \, among \, contacts}{No. \, of \, person - weeks \, of \, exposure} \times 100$$

IMMUNITY (HOST DEFENSE)

* Active (humoral, cellular, both)
* Passive (human immunoglobulin (HIG), animal antitoxin, animal antisera).

Primary Immune Response

First time entry of antigen produces accelerated production of IgG and IgM.

Humoral immunity from bone marrow derived B lymphocytes.
* IgG (general immunity)
* IgM (intravascular)
* IgA (local immunity)
* IgD (undetermined)
* IgE (Allergy reaction).

Cellular immunity from thymus derived T lymphocytes.

Herd Immunity

Group immunity that affect limited disease occurrence. It is an immunological barrier.

Immunizing Agents

Vaccine: Immunobiological substance which produces specific protection.

Toxoid: Detoxicated toxin of organism.

Polyvalent: Prepared from many strains.

Vaccines

Live attenuated.

Bacterial: Bacillus Calmette-Guérin (BCG), oral typhoid, plague.

Viral: Oral poliovirus vaccine (OPV), yellow fever, measles, rubella, mumps, influenza.

Rickettsia: Epidemic typhus (killed)

Bacterial: Typhoid, cholera, whooping cough, meningitis, plague.

Viral: Rabies, injectable polio, influenza, hepatitis B, JE, Kyasanur Forest Disease (KFD).

Toxoid

Bacterial: Diphtheria toxoid (DT), tetanus toxoid (TT).

Immunoglobulin

Human normal: Measles, rabies, hepatitis A, tetanus, mumps.

Human specific: Hepatitis B, diphtheria, varicella.

Nonhuman: Antidiphtheric serum (ADS), antitetanus serum (ATS), gas gangrene. *bacterial (antisera):*

Nonhuman viral: Antirabies serum (ARS), botulism.

Difference between Killed and Attenuated Vaccines

See **Table 8.6**.

Common Immunoglobulin Used

Hepatitis B: Hepatitis B immunoglobulin (HBIG)—0.07 mL/kg for prevention (II dose after 30 days)

Table 8.6: Difference between killed and attenuated vaccine.

Killed	Attenuated
High dose	Small dose
Frequent booster needed	Not needed
Revaccination not possible	Can be done
Short protection	Long protection

Measles: Human immunoglobulin 0.25 mL/kg for prevention

Rabies: Rabies immunoglobulin (RIG) 20 IU/kg for prevention

Tetanus: Tetanus immune globulin (TIG)—250 units for prevention. 6000 units for therapy.

Common Antisera Used

Antirabies serum: 40 IU/kg IM

Antitetanus serum: 1,500 units subcutaneous (SC) or intramuscular (IM) ADS 1000 IU IM.

Gas gangrene 10,000 IU [clostridium (Cl) perfringens].

Botulism 10,000 units 4th hourly IM.

Immunization Schedule

Universal Immunization Programme (UIP) (1985)

1. Universal child immunization (UCI).

Age	Vaccine
• Birth	BCG, OPV
• 6 weeks	DPT, OPV
• 10 weeks	DPT, OPV
• 14 weeks	DPT, OPV
• 9 months	Measles

2. Universal mother immunization (UMI)

Early in pregnancy	TT I or booster
After 1 month	TT II

National Immunization Schedule (NIS)

In addition to UCI and UMI it includes:

• 16–24 months old child	DPT, OPV
• 5–6 years old child	DT (DPT primary doubtful)
• 10 years old child (school)	TT
• 16 years old child (school)	TT

Cold chain

It is a system of storage and transport of vaccine from manufacture to site of vaccination.

Freezer (-20°C): OPV, measles.

Fridge point: DPT, TT, DT, BCG, diluent.

Cold chain equipment

Deep freezer and ice lined refrigerator (DF and ILR) used in primary health center (PHC), postpartum center (PPC), family planning (FP) centers.

Deep freezer to prepare frozen ice packs, to store OPV, measles.

Ice lined refrigerator to store DPT, TT, DT, and BCG

Cold box—for the transport of vaccine in peripheral center.

Vaccine—for transport of vaccine in small

Carrier—quantity for outreach areas.

Day carrier—for transport of vaccines in small scale for nearby place.

Walk-in-cooler (WIC)—at regional centers.

Immunization hazards

Local reaction—pain, swelling, redness, nodule.

Faulty technique—hepatitis B, Staph infection.

Hypersensitivity—dyspnea, collapse (anaphylactic shock), fever, edema, joint pain (serum sickness).

Neuritic manifestation

Provocative reaction—latent infection to clinical attack.

ADVERSE EVENT FOLLOWING IMMUNIZATION

Standard operating procedure government of India 2006, mention cluster showing more than 2 cases of same adverse reaction, related in time.

This is a medical incident that takes place after an immunization causes concern and is believed to be caused by immunization.

Vaccine samples should be sent for testing to National Control Laboratory, Kasauli. They are sent at 2–8°C by fastest means. Used vials with remaining and diluents and unused vials of same batch are sent. Minimum quantity shall be 50 mL (e.g., twenty-five 2 mL vial, Five 10 mL vial, etc.). They are sent after packing in polythene and keeping upright.

PREVENTION AND CONTROL OF DISEASE IN MAN

See **Figure 8.3**, and **Table 8.7**.

EPIDEMIOMETRIC ANALYSIS

Rate

Occurrence of an event during a period over a given population (BR, DR).

Ratio

Occurrence of an event or proportion of one group over the other (doctor population ratio, sex ratio).

Table 8.7: Prevention and control of disease in man.

Attack source	Interrupt transmission	Protect susceptible
Treatment case carrier	Environment hygiene	Immunization
Isolate case	Personal hygiene	Chemo-prophylaxis
Surveillance of suspects	Vector control	Immuno-prophylaxis
Control animal reservoir	Disinfection	Personal protection
Notify disease	Sterilization Restrict population movement	Better nutrition

Proportion

Magnitude of occurrence of an event or proportion through ratio [protein energy malnutrition (PEM) among under 5 years age group in percentage].

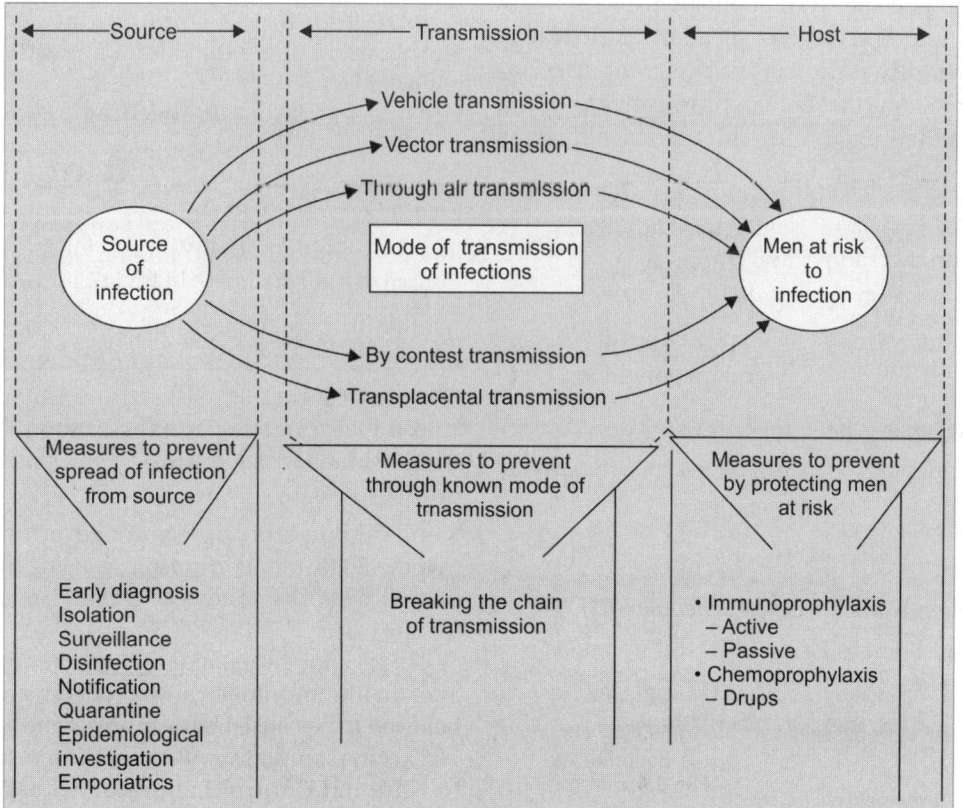

Fig. 8.3: Prevention and control of disease in man.

Mortality Rate

Death rate: (Death per 1000 MYP)

Specific death rate: (Cholera death per 1000 MYP).

Case fatality rate: (Deaths by cholera out of cholera cases) (in percentage).

Proportional mortality rate: (Number of specific disease death out of total death (%)).

Survival rate: Number of survival after 5 years out of total diagnosed (%).

Standardized rate: By direct and indirect methods.

With populations of different age or sex composition, we need to adjust or standardize the rate for comparison. In direct standardization, standard population is selected and applied to that selected standard population. Thus, expected deaths divided by standardized population give standardized death rate per 1000 population.

In indirect standardization, standardized mortality ratio studies the comparison of mortality in the study group with the group what would have had if they had experienced national mortality.

$$\text{Standardized mortality ratio} = \frac{\text{Deaths observed in the study}}{\text{Deaths expected in the group}} \times 100$$

$$\text{Standardized death rate} = \frac{\text{Expected deaths}}{\text{Standard population}} \times 1000$$

Morbidity rate

Incidence: New cases over a specified period.

$$\text{Incidence} = \frac{\text{Number of new cases of sepcific disease during a given time}}{\text{Population at risk during that period}} \times 1000$$

$$= \frac{\text{No. developing disease in 1 year}}{\text{Population exposed in 1 year}} \times 1000$$

Prevalence: All cases at a given point of time

$$\text{Prevalence} = \frac{\text{Current cases in a given time}}{\text{Population at that time}} \times 100$$

$$= \frac{\text{No. with diesease at a point of time}}{\text{Population exposed}} \times 100$$

$$\text{Prevalence ratio} = \frac{\text{Prevalence of exposed}}{\text{Prevalence of unexposed}} = \frac{P_1}{P_0}$$

Duration of illness: Duration influences prevalence. Longer the duration greater the prevalence.

$$\text{Duration of illness} = \frac{\text{Prevalence}}{\text{Incidence}}$$

Death Certificate (Fig. 8.4)

It is the basis of mortality data. It forms major source of information in epidemiology.

SCREENING TESTS

We come across small section of disease and a major portion is lying hidden. This phenomenon is called *Iceberg phenomenon*.

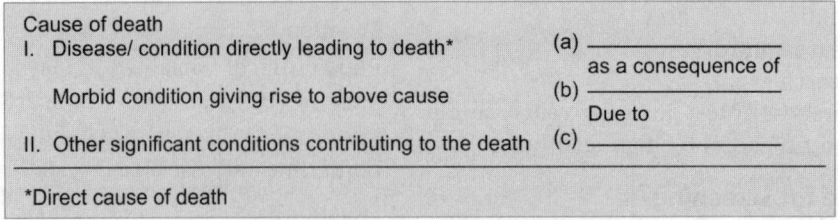

Cause of death
I. Disease/ condition directly leading to death* (a) _____
 as a consequence of
 Morbid condition giving rise to above cause (b) _____
 Due to
II. Other significant conditions contributing to the death (c) _____

*Direct cause of death

Fig. 8.4: International form of certificate of death.

Chapter 8: Epidemiology

Table 8.8: Difference between screening test and diagnostic test.

Screening	Diagnostic
• On healthy people	On sick people
• In groups	On single patient
• One cut-off point used	Sign, symptom, laboratory result used
• Not costly	Costly
• Not for treatment	For treatment
• Not demanded	Demanded by patient
• Once done is final	Repeated, other tests done
• Accuracy not justified	Is justified
• It is an epidemiological	It is a therapeutic tool procedure

Difference between Screening Test and Diagnostic Test (Table 8.8)

The search for unrecognized disease in the community are done through rapidly applied tests which form the basis of screening, which is more useful than annual health check-up or periodic health check-up.

(See difference between screening test and diagnostic test).

Lead Time

It is the time between screening result and diagnostic result. Earlier the screening higher the lead time. It has an impact on disease outcome.

Types

- Mass screening—leprosy, TB.
- High-risk screening—hypertension, diabetes.
- Multiphase screening—cancer cervix (Pap test I phase, biopsy II phase).

Uses

- Identification of cases
- Disease control
- Research
- Awareness at test gives high survival rate
- Good prognosis by high lead time.

Criteria for Screening

For Test

- Acceptable, and repeatable
- Minimum intraobserver variation
- Minimum interobserver variation
- Minimum biological variation
- Minimum technical variation.

For Disease

- Major pH problem
- Early detection possible
- Nocturnal hemodialysis known
- Further confirmation possible
- Benefit by early detection is present.

Disease			
Test	+	−	Total
+	a. TP	b. FP	(a + b)
−	c. FN	d. TN	(c + d)
	(a + c)	(b + d)	(a + b + c + d)

$$\text{Sensitivity} = \frac{a}{a+c} \times 100 = \frac{\text{True possitive}}{[TP/(TP+FN)]}$$

$$\text{Specificity} = \frac{d}{(b+d)} \times 100 = \frac{\text{True negative}}{[TP/(TP+FN)]}$$

$$\text{False positive} = \frac{b}{(b+d)} \times 100$$

$$\text{False negative} = \frac{c}{(a+c)} \times 100$$

$$\text{Predictive value of positive} = \frac{a}{(a+b)} \times 100$$

$$\text{Predictive value of negative} = \frac{d}{(c+d)} \times 100$$

Unimodal and Bimodal Distribution

When people are healthy at outlook but diseased (apparently healthy) are recognized, cut-off points between normal and diseases arise. There are two such situations.

Situation 1

Physiological variables like systolic blood pressure (BP) normal curve is fit, it is unimodal where criteria fixed help in identifying normal, borderline and diseased (**Fig. 8.5**).

Situation 2

In bimodal distribution of normal and diseased, level C is used as cut-off point, e.g., phenylketonuria (**Fig. 8.6**).

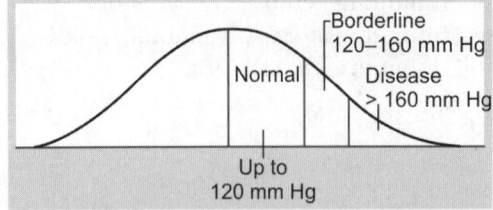

Fig. 8.5: Unimodal distribution (e.g., hypertension)

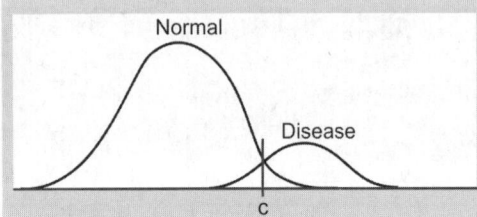

Fig. 8.6: Bimodal distribution (e.g., phenylketonuria)

Common Screening Tests

- Hemoglobin (Hb%) for anemia
- Blood pressure in population, in pregnancy
- Postprandial blood sugar (PPBS) in population
- Venereal disease research laboratory (VDRL) in pregnancy
- Human immunodeficiency virus in pregnancy
- Pap test in elderly women with cervical dysplasia
- Audiometry in children
- Mass miniature radiography (MMR) in TB
- Peak expiratory flow rate (PEFR) in lung diseases.

Future Hold of Epidemiology

Analytical epidemiology is a potential to integrate remote factors into a single factor of cause of health or disease.

Social position of a person and local environment can be predicted by the knowledge of epidemiology.

From epidemiology we can ascertain future indicators of advantage or of disadvantage.

Prediction of future physical and mental health can be ascertained.

Exposures and influences during a person's life are going to be life time epidemiology. Historical data by survey, records of schools, hospitals and other institutions will open up window for health and disease of a person, of a family or of a society.

Undergoing health transition with a shift away of disease pattern of a society can be predicted. When predicted, influencing mass scale health phenomena can be tackled.

Methods of Screening of High-risk Group

Identification of unrecognized disease among risk group which is selected on the basis of epidemiological research. Common example is cancer of cervix in low social group. High risk does not mean that absolutely positively develop disease. It means that when statistically compared to other women, chance is higher.

This is also called selective screening where people are at high state of a health problem, so that early treatment can be offered or information given to help them taking decision.

In case of risk group for screening off cancer breast, the risks in the population include age, personal history, family health history, nutritional level, level of physical activity, environmental exposure, and drug use are guidelines for high-risk screening. Factors which put the group into risk are:

- Breast cancer genetic situation
- First degree family member has breast cancer
- Strong family history of breast cancer
- Personal history of invasive ductal carcinoma
- Lobular carcinoma in situ.

Sharing of gene is

First degree relative	Second degree relative	Third degree relative
Mother	Grandparents	Great grandparents
Father	Grandchildren	First cousin
Full sibling	Half siblings	
Child	Aunt/uncle Niece/Nephew	
Share 50% gene	**Share 5% gene**	**Share 12.5% gene**

Other selective screening (High-risk) are:
- Similarly risk group for ovarian cancer
- High risk for papillomatous testing for cancer cervix
- Colorectal cancer
- Down's syndrome
- Lung cancer
- Diabetes
- Hypertension screening
- Screening high-risk elevated serum cholesterol that is prone for CHD.

SUMMARY

Definition and types of epidemiology are described. Investigation of epidemic is illustrated. Emporiatrics is highlighted. Disinfection in public health practice is described. Adverse effects of immunization is described.

VIVA VOCE

1. Define epidemiology.
2. What is triad of epidemiology?
3. Define pandemic. Give example.
4. What are differences between control and eradication?
5. Differentiate cross sectional study and longitudinal study.
6. What is odds ratio?
7. What is cohort Study?
8. Enumerate uses of epidemiology.
9. Name important quarantinable diseases
10. Differentiate antiseptic and disinfectant.
11. How OT is disinfected in your hospital?
12. What is the specific disinfection for catheters?
13. Name vector borne diseases.
14. Name water borne diseases.
15. State UIP immunization schedule.
16. Differentiate screening test with diagnostic test.

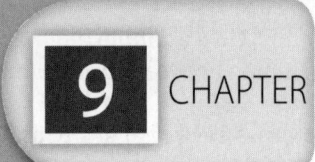

CHAPTER 9

Epidemiology of Communicable Diseases

CHAPTER OUTLINE

- Intestinal infections
  - Poliomyelitis
  - Viral hepatitis
  - Diarrhea
  - Cholera
  - Food poisoning
  - Amebiasis
  - Hookworm
  - Guineaworm
  - Round worm
  - Enteric fever
- Respiratory infections
  - Severe acute respiratory syndrome (SARS)
  - Acute respiratory infection (ARI)
  - Tuberculosis
  - Measles
  - Diphtheria
  - Whooping cough
  - Chickenpox
  - German measles
  - Influenza
  - Meningococcal meningitis
- Vector-borne infections
  - Malaria
  - Filaria
  - Kala azar
  - Dengue syndrome
  - Arboviral infection
  - Rickettsial infection
- Surface infection
  - Sexually transmitted infection (STD)
  - Tetanus
  - Leprosy
  - Trachoma
- Zoonotic infections
  - Rabies
  - Japanese encephalitis (JE)
  - Plague
  - Kyasanur forest disease (KFD)
  - Yellow fever
  - Brucellosis
  - Leptospirosis
  - Anthrax
- Emerging and re-emerging infections
- Hospital-acquired infections

INTESTINAL INFECTIONS

Poliomyelitis (Infantile Paralysis)

Acute viral infection is caused by ribonucleic acid (RNA) virus. Man being the only host, effective potent oral polio vaccine (OPV) and community participation have helped to launch intensified pulse polio immunization program (IPPI) to interrupt and eradicate wild poliovirus in the world. Now with annual event of IPPI polio cases are just countable in single digit.

Epidemiology: Mode of Transmission (Fig. 9.1)

Fecal, oral, and droplet infection.

Incubation Period

About 7–14 days

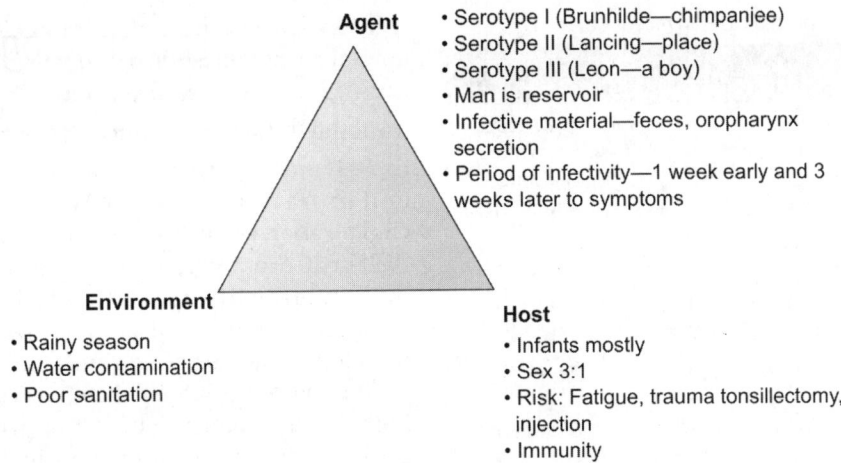

Fig. 9.1: Epidemiological triad in polio.

Clinical Aspects

Ninety-five percent are not apparent, 5% have fever, sore throat, vomiting, abdominal pain, and malaise. It could be abortive polio. In 0.5% paralytic polio (residual flaccid paralysis at 60 days), rarely bulbar polio which has the risk of death.

Differentiations needed for paralytic polio are:
- Guillain–Barré syndrome
- Transverse myelitis
- Traumatic neuritis
- Less commonly encephalitis, meningitis, and tumors.

Distinguishing features are:
- Asymptomatic flaccid paralysis
- Fever at onset
- Rapid progression
- Residual paralysis after 60 days
- Preservation of sensory nerve function.

Reported Cases in Recent Times (Table 9.1)

Epidemiology relevant to eradication
- Only human host and cannot survive in environment—suitable for eradication.
- One dose inactivated polio vaccine (IPV) introduced in all routine immunization.
- tOPV (Trivalent oral polio vaccine) is taken over in the place of bOPV (bivalent oral polio vaccine).
- This is an end-game strategic plan in polio eradication. This activity in immunization is called THE SWITCH.

Virus in stool up to 14 days

Isolation of wild poliovirus from stool is the recommended method for laboratory confirmation of paralytic poliomyelitis.

Intestinal immunity—OPV is choice.

Type-2 is first to disappear—indicates the progress toward eradication.

Prevention

Oral polio vaccine (OPV) (Sabin) use

Table 9.2 lists the difference between OPV and IPV.

Epidemiological investigation is done with the help of checklist.

Line listing is done to check duplication, to check residual paralysis existing, to identify high-risk pockets. In case of acute flaccid paralysis (AFP), details are collected as per national guidelines.

Mopping up

This involves door-to-door OPV to below 5-year-old children in the village or settlement where the case is detected. This is done in active and final stage of polio eradication.

Ring immunization

It is mopping up operation in cities where door to door OPV to below 5-year-old children, covering an area of the radius of 3 km.

Pulse immunization

Oral polio vaccine (OPV) is given to all 0–5-year children in a country on a single day

Table 9.1: Reported cases in recent times.

World	1988	125 countries	350,000 cases
Nigeria	2008 November	4 endemic countries	1,387 cases (from India, Pakistan, Afghanistan)
India	2003	87 districts	225 cases
	2004	43 districts	134 cases
	2005	35 districts	66 cases
	2006 May	10 districts	66 cases (from Bihar 30, UP 29, Jharkhand 2, Delhi 1, Gujarat 1, Haryana 1, Uttarakhand 1 and Punjab 1)
	2007	22 states	532 cases
Karnataka	1998		71 cases
	1999		21 cases
	2000		8 cases
	2001		Zero cases
	2002		Zero cases
	2003		36 cases
	2004		1 case (from Raichur case)
	2005		Zero cases
	2006		Zero cases
	2007		1 case
	2008		Zero cases

Table 9.2: Difference between OPV and IPV.

OPV	IPV
Live attenuated	Killed formolized
Oral	IM or SC
Humoral and intestinal immunity	Only humoral
Prevents reinfection	Does not prevent reinfection
Useful in epidemic	Not useful
Cheap	Costly
Cold chain required	Not stringent

(IPV: inactivated polio vaccine; OPV: oral polio vaccine; IM: intramuscular; SC: subcutaneous)

regardless of previous immunization. This is an annual event hence the name pulse. *For IPPI and AFP surveillance, refer chapter 36.*

National Polio Surveillance Project

In 1997, project was established as a joint collaboration between World Health Organization (WHO) and Health and Family Welfare, Government of India. The objective was to intensify surveillance for polio eradication through detection and investigation of childhood acute flaccid paralysis.

National Polio Surveillance Project (NPSP) comprises a central unit for providing guidance, support, coordination, monitoring, and data analysis of various activities related to surveillance of polio and NPSP field units headed by SMOs (Surveillance Medical Officers) who are deployed in all states and union territories. They are given responsibility for facilitating surveillance and immunization activities aimed at polio eradication.

Viral Hepatitis

It is an infection of liver by viruses belonging to hepatitis A virus (HAV) (RNA enterovirus) (50%), hepatitis B virus (HBV) [deoxyribonucleic acid (DNA) hepadna] (20%) and non-A non-B (NANB) (30%). Among non-A non-B, hepatitis C (RNA flavivirus), delta viral hepatitis (RNA incomplete virus), hepatitis-E (RNA calicivirus), hepatitis-G (RNA flavivirus), cytomegalovirus, Epstein-Barr virus, and rubella virus are identified.

Table 9.3 gives some common laboratory tests done in hepatitis infection.

Hepatitis A

It is the most common hepatitis with low case fatality rate (0.1%), 10 persons per 100,000 are affected annually.

Mode of transmission

Fecal oral route

Incubation period (Fig. 9.2)

About 15–45 days

Diagnosis

Hepatitis A virus (HAV) particle in stool, anti HAV titer and presence of immunoglobulin M (IgM) antibody.

Chapter 9: Epidemiology of Communicable Diseases

Table 9.3: Common laboratory tests for hepatitis infections.

Investigations	Reference range
Total protein	6.0–7.5 G%
Albumin	3.5–5.3 G%
Globulin	2.0–2.5 G%
Albumin globulin ratio	2:1
Serum bilirubin	0.1–1.0 mg%
Direct bilirubin	0.0–0.35 mg%
Indirect bilirubin	0.1–0.65 mg%
SGOT	0–40 IU per liter
SGPT	0–38 IU per liter
Serum alkaline phosphate	00–290 IU per liter
GGT	5–38 U per liter (male) 5–29 U per liter (female)

(SGOT: serum glutamic oxaloacetic transaminase; SGPT: serum glutamic pyruvic transaminase; GGT: gamma-glutamyl transferase)

Prevention and control

- Control of reservoir
- Control of transmission
- Protection of susceptible population
- Havrix vaccine is used, but not found to have absolute effectiveness.

Hepatitis B

It is associated with chronic active hepatitis and hepatocellular carcinoma. It is risky when HBV infection with delta virus infection is found together. Based on hepatitis B surface antigen (HBsAg) carrier rates regions are divided into high (5%), intermediate (2.5%) and low prevalence (<2%) areas. Chronic carrier state varies from 0.6 to 5.8%. This has three different antigens that are as under **(Fig. 9.3)**:

Surface Ag	=	HBsAg induces surface Ab anti-HBs
Core Ag	=	HBcAg induces Core Ab anti-HBc
E Ag	=	HBeAg induces e Ab anti-HBe

(HBsAg: hepatitis B surface antigen; HBcAg: hepatitis-B-core-antigen; HBeAg: hepatitis B e antigen)

Table 9.4 gives the WHO criteria for serological pattern in hepatitis B.

Dane particle

42-nm double-shelled DNA virus a morphological form of virus which is infectious form.

Mode of transmission

- Parenteral
- Perinatal
- Sexual
- Child to child (horizontal)

Incubation period

About 45–180 days

The epidemiology of hepatitis B is depicted in **Figures 9.4 and 9.5** which gives the natural history of hepatitis B viral infection.

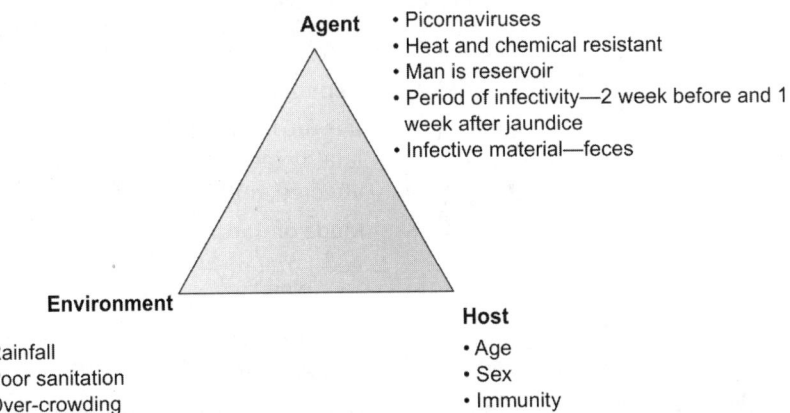

Fig. 9.2: Epidemiological triad in hepatitis A.

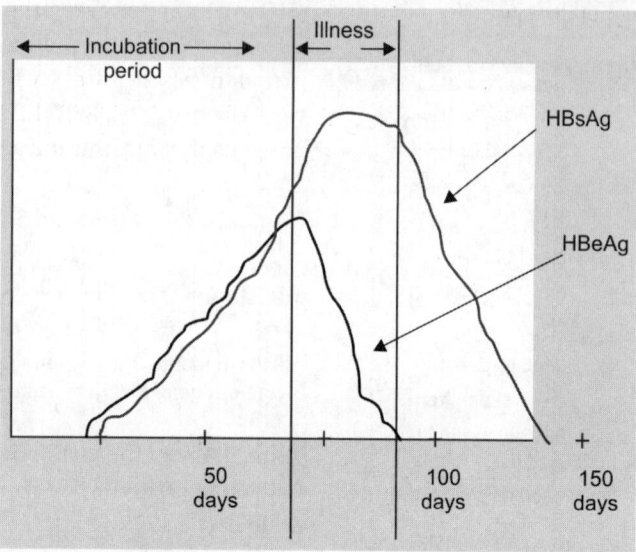

Fig. 9.3: Serum level of hepatitis B antigen.
(HBsAg: hepatitis B surface antigen; HBeAg: hepatitis B e antigen)

Table 9.4: WHO criteria for serological pattern in hepatitis B.

	Acute hepatitis	Recovery and developed immunity	Vaccination done
Anti HBc	+	–	–
HBs Ag	+	–	–

(WHO: World Health Organization; HBsAg: hepatitis B surface antigen)

Prevention

- Plasma derived surface antigen formalin inactivated subunit viral vaccine. Intramuscular 1 mL at 0, 1, and 6 months. Below 10 years 0.5 mL at 0, 1, and 6 months. It is avoided in previously infected person.
- Recombinant deoxyribonucleic acid (RDNA) yeast derived vaccine (genetically engineered dose of 10 µg). 1 mL at 0, 1, and 6 months. Below 10 years 0.5 mL at 0, 1, and 6 months.

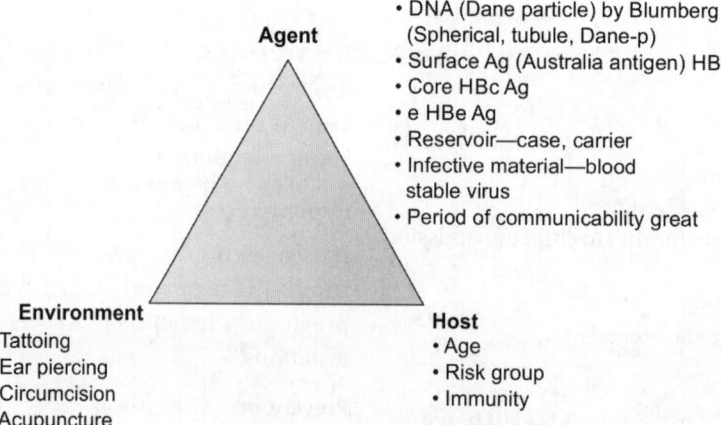

Fig. 9.4: Epidemiological triad in hepatitis B.
(DNA: deoxyribonucleic acid; HBcAg: hepatitis B core antigen; HBeAg: hepatitis B e antigen)

Chapter 9: Epidemiology of Communicable Diseases

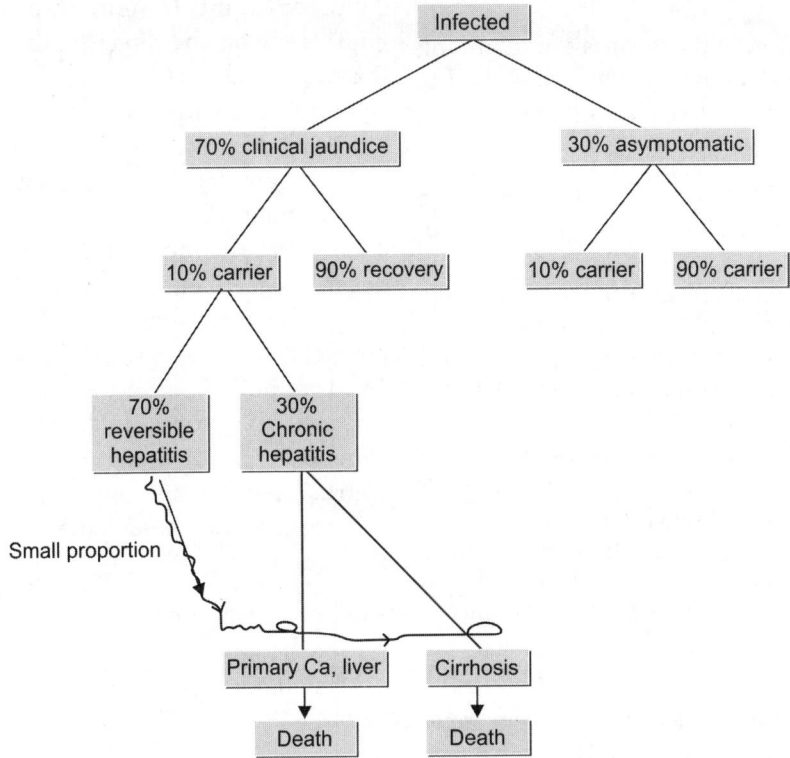

Fig. 9.5: Natural history of disease—hepatitis B viral infection.

- Hepatitis B immune globulin (HBIG) for acute exposure by surgeon, nurse, laboratory worker, newborn, and sex contact. Dose is 0.05 mL per kg body weight. This gives immediate protection with 2 doses 4 weeks apart. In case of accidental exposure HepB vaccine + HBIG given.
- Blood safety, hospital disinfection, and diagnosis of carrier status.

Health sector strategy at global level is initiated in 2016 to complete by 2021 has taken up following intervention:
- Hepatitis B vaccination
- HBV to prevent mother to child transmission
- Blood safety
- Injection safety
- Testing services

Hepatitis C

It is parenterally transmitted NANB hepatitis. It is RNA virus transmitted through blood transfusion of contaminated blood. Cirrhosis of liver and liver cancer are closely associated. Prevention is the compulsory test of blood donors for hepatitis C virus. Interferon has been found effective in the treatment. Vaccine is also available for this.

Delta Hepatitis

This is always in a combination with hepatitis B virus. Delta hepatitis very similar to HBV but it is not a public health problem in India. It is seen as predecessor to hepatitis E and causes super infection.

Hepatitis E

It is a water-borne RNA viral hepatitis. Incubation period is 2–9 weeks. During pregnancy, hepatitis E is severe in its manifestations.

Prevention

Water purification, sewage disposal and food hygiene are the preventive measures to be taken. No vaccine is available.

Hepatitis G

Recently, identified flavivirus found among IV drug users, among patients who undergo hemodialysis. This is found commonly in hemophilia patients.

Hepatitis Vaccines

- Hepatitis A vaccine (Havrix) intramuscular, deltoid
  Adult above 18 years 1.0 mL 0 and 6 months
  2–18 years 0.5 mL 0 and 6 months
- Hepatitis B vaccine (Engerix B). Adult 1 mL 0, 1, and 6 months children 0.5 mL. 0, 1, and 6 months
- Hepatitis-combined vaccines A + B (Comvax) 0–5 years 0.5 mL 2, 4, and 12 months A + B + Polio (Pediarix)
  Infanrix + Engerix B + Inactivated polio vaccine
  A + B (Twinrix) 1.0 mL 0, 1, and 6 months.

Diarrhea

This is a change in consistency and character of stool which is characterized by the passage of loose, watery stool more than three times in a day. It is dysentery if it is mixed with blood. Sudden onset of diarrhea in a community is called acute diarrhea or gastroenteritis.

An attack of sudden onset which usually lasts 3–7 days, but may last up to 10–14 days (WHO).

An epidemiological importance of community history directs to the etiology of diarrhea:
- Fever and bloody diarrhea suggest invasive dysenteric processes
- Incubation of below 18 hours suggests food poisoning
- Incubation above 4–5 days suggests protozoal or helminthic.

In India, it is prevalent among 17% of the people. Pediatrics prevalence is 20%. Among children below 5 year age group, it is 1.7 episodes per year per child (morbidity). Very commonly rotavirus and *E. coli* bacteria cause diarrhea in the community.

The pathogenesis of diarrhea is shown in **Figure 9.6**.

Mode of Transmission

Fecal oral route

The epidemiological triad is depicted in **Figure 9.7**.

Control

Diarrheal disease control (DDC) has the following program implementations:
- Clinical management
  - ORS

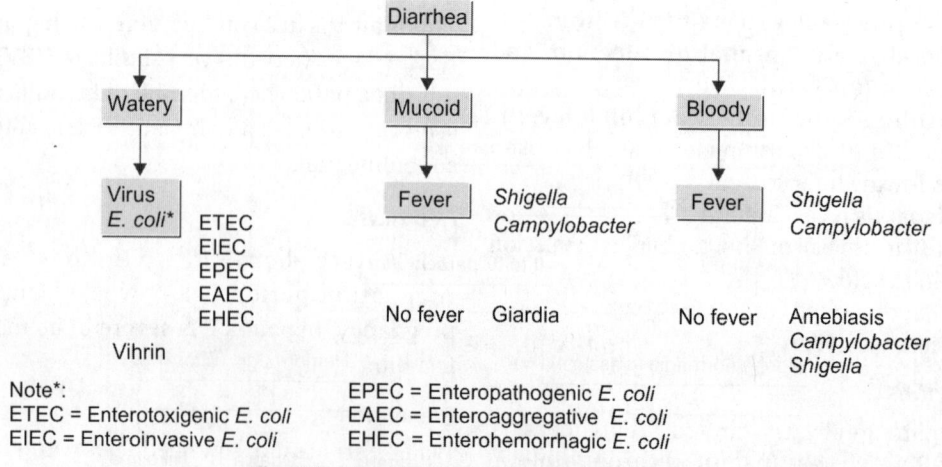

Fig. 9.6: Algorithm in diarrhea pathogenesis.

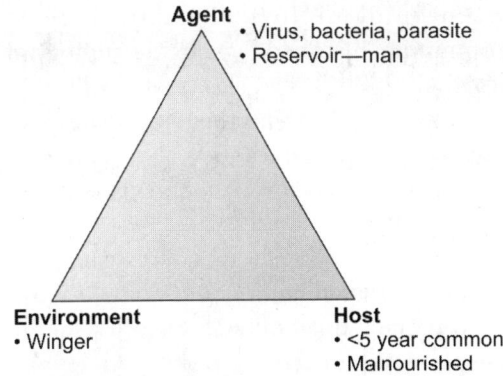

Fig. 9.7: Epidemiological triad in diarrhea.

Homemade fluids:

Finger measures	Spoon measures
2 finger pinch salt	1 flat spoonful salt
3 finger pinch sugar	8 flat spoonful sugar
In one glass of water	3 drops lemon juice in one liter of water

- Feeding
- Drugs when etiology is known.
❖ Good reproductive and child health (RCH) practice of safe motherhood and child survival
❖ Protected water supply, and sanitary disposal of night soil
❖ Health education
❖ Measles immunization under universal immunization program (UIP)
❖ Fly control measures
❖ Zink supplementation for reducing episode duration and severity prevention.

Diarrhea control started as Water and Sanitation (WATSAN) program in 1978, incorporated in oral rehydration therapy (ORT) in 1985, became part of child survival and safe motherhood (CSSM) in 1992 and it has now been part of RCH since 1997.

In the control of diarrhea, following vaccines are licensed for use:
❖ Rotarix (Monovalent human rotavirus vaccine)
❖ Rota Teq (Pentavalent bovine human reassorted vaccine).

Cholera

Cholera is an acute diarrheal disease caused by *Vibrio cholerae*. Endemicity and epidemicity are caused by:
❖ Carriers,
❖ Water contamination,
❖ Congregation of people leading to poor environmental sanitation
❖ Abundant flies which transmit by mechanical means.

Common types which cause cholera are (**Fig. 9.8**):
❖ Classical *Vibrio cholera*
❖ El Tor *Vibrio cholerae*
❖ 0139 new strain *Vibrio cholerae*.

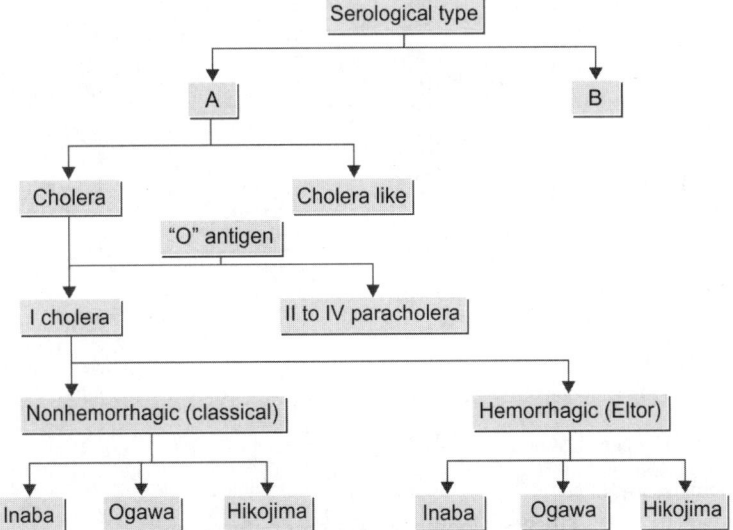

Fig. 9.8: Common types of cholera organism.

There are seven major pandemic recorded, and five of these originated in India.

First pandemic	1817–1823
Second pandemic	1826–1837
Third pandemic	1842–1862
Fourth pandemic	1865–1875
Fifth pandemic	1881–1896
Sixth pandemic	1899–1923
Seventh pandemic	1964–2003

Annual cases of 2,635 thousand and case fatality rate (CFR) of 0.11% is recorded in India (Health information of India, 2008, WHO). This is reduced to 494 cases in 2017.

Difference between Classical and El Tor

- Community diagnosis

Classical	El Tor
Severe cases more	Mild, asymptomatic more
Secondary cases more	Secondary cases less
Not resistant to physical environment	More resistant to physical environment
Carrier stage—none	Carrier stage ++++

- Laboratory diagnosis

	Classical	El Tor
Chicken, sheep RBC	No agglutination	Agglutinate
Phase IV	Not resistant	Resistant
Polymyxin B	Not resistant	Resistant
VP reaction	Positive	Negative

(RBC: red blood cell)

Incubation period
5 days (6 days quarantine)

Mode of transmission
Water, food, and contact.

The epidemiological triad in cholera is depicted in **Figure 9.9**.

Clinical stages
- Stages of evacuation
- Stage of collapse
- Stage of recovery

Laboratory diagnosis
Water, food sample, and rectal swab are collected, transported in VR media, direct examination and culture are done.

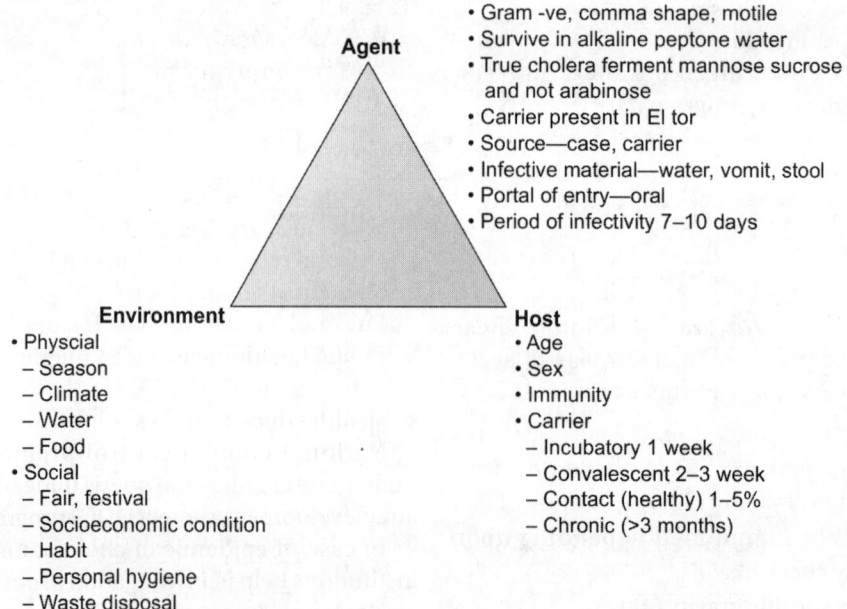

Fig. 9.9: Epidemiological triad in cholera.

Control of cholera

Early diagnosis and treatment are the major preventive measures for cholera.

Oral Rehydration

Assessment

	Mild dehydration	Severe dehydration
General condition	Thirsty, restlessness	Drowsy
Tachycardia	-	+
BP	Normal	Hypotension
Elasticity of skin	Retracts quickly	Retracts slowly
Tongue	Normal	Dry
Urine output	Normal	Low

Requirement

Weight (kg)	ORS requirement (mL)
Below 5	400
5–10	600
10–15	800
15–30	1,200
30+	2,400

(ORS: oral rehydration solution)

Composition

	ORS bicarbonate	ORS citrate
NaCl	3.5 g	3.5 g
$NaHCO_3$	2.5 g	-
Trisodium citrate	-	2.9 g
KCl	1.5 g	1.5 g
Glucose	20 g	20 g
Good water	1 liter	1 liter

Advantage

It reduces mortality among children, cheap and economical, is available easily and a housewife can prepare very easily.

Rehydration

5:4:1($NaCl:NaHCO_3:KCl$) alternated with ringer lactate. Initially 1 liter/15 minutes. Later on, it will be maintained depending upon laboratory check like:

- Plasma specific gravity (1,025)
- Urine output (1 cc/kg/hour).

Maintenance by oral rehydration

Mild

100 mL/kg per day

Severe

15 mL/kg per hour with laboratory monitoring

Antibiotics

Adult: 300 mg, doxycycline single dose

Child: Trimethoprim 5 mg/kg/day

Sulfamethoxazole 25 mg/kg/day for 3 days

Pregnant

Furazolidone 1.25 mg/kg/day for 3 days.

Prevention and control

- Selective isolation
- Notification within 24 hours
- Surveillance and epidemiological investigation
- Disinfection by cresol, boiling, soap (RW coefficient above 5)
- Quarantine 6 days
- Sanitation—food control, fly control, water control, and
- Vaccination

Cholera Vaccine

It is phenol killed containing classical *Ogawa*, and *Inaba* 6,000 million each per mL.

- 0.5 mL I dose and 4 week later 1.0 mL II dose produce immunity lasting for 3–6 months. 0.3 mL for 2–10 years of age 0.2 mL for 1–2 years of age No vaccine for below 1 year of age group.

Oral vaccines are available:
  Dukoral (monovalent injectable)
  Shanchol (serogroups 01 and 0139 oral)
  Euvichol (similar to shanchol oral)
- Public health measures in pilgrimage and congregations
- Health education.

National cholera control program has undergone changes and now is under disaster and development center (DDC) program.

In case of epidemic of cholera, following institutions help in investigation of outbreaks:

- National Institute of Communicable Diseases, New Delhi

- All India Institute of Hygiene and Public Health, Kolkata
- National Institute of Cholera and Enteric Disease, Kolkata

Food Poisoning (Gastroenteritis)

It is an acute gastroenteritis due to bacterial toxin or chemical toxicity which is secondary to food contamination.

Types

- Poisonous food (death cap, mushroom, fish)
- Chemicals
- Bacteria
- Toxin type (cholera, arsenic poisoning should be ruled out)
- Staphylococci (enterotoxin)
- Botulism (exotoxin—canned, bottled)
- *Clostridium (Cl) perfringens* (α, β toxin)
- Infective type, and
- *Salmonella* food poisoning.

Differential Diagnosis

- *Staphylococcal food poisoning:* Poor personal hygiene allows *Staphylococcus aureus* into dairy products, cheese, and cooked meat. This also can be by boils, furuncle and carbuncle. It produces enterotoxin A and B. Incubation period is 1–6 hours. Nausea and profuse vomiting develop within 1–6 hours after ingestion. Diarrhea is not marked. It is an intradietetic toxin that produces toxic effect. Antiemetics and fluid replacements are advocated. Suspected food is sent for laboratory examination. If food vending is involved, public health authorities are informed.
- *Bacillus cereus*: Preformed toxin of *B. cereus* produces rapid onset of vomiting within 1 hour of food consumption. It is commonly known as "Chinese Restaurant Syndrome". Fried rice and vanilla sauce are common source of toxin. Enterotoxin is liberated during storage. Significant enterocolitis occurs if viable bacteria are swallowed and toxin is liberated in the gut. Rapid and judicious fluid replacement and appropriate notification are mandatory.
- *Clostridium (Cl) perfringens:* This is common by contaminated meat, or incompletely cooked meat and when stored in anaerobic condition. Reheating causes sporulation of clostridia and enterotoxin liberation. Diarrhea and cramps are common. Incubation period is 6–12 hours. It is common in school, party and get-together eating. Usually, it is self-limiting.
- *Clostridium (Cl) botulinum:* It is due to neurotoxin of *Cl. botulinum* which is manifested in paralysis and neurological dysfunction. It is common in canned meat and preserved vegetables. Contaminated honey also can cause toxin production and symptoms. Ingestion of toxin produces difficulty in swallowing, blurred vision, ptosis, limb weakness and respiratory paralysis. Case management include assisted ventilation, and general supportive measures, which may take 2 months.
- *Plant toxin:* Beans and legumes produce oxidants which are toxic to man with G6PD deficiency. Headache, nausea, fever, hemolysis, hemoglobinuria and jaundice set in. Lectin content of red kidney beans cause acute abdomen, and diarrhea. In potato, alkaloids developed can cause toxic effect. Fungi and mushroom produce hallucinogens. Death head mushroom causes hepatorenal failure.
- *Chemical toxin:* Saxitoxin produced from shellfish and oysters can cause acute GE with gastrointestinal symptoms. It can cause respiratory paralysis within 30 minutes. Ciguatoxin from some fishes or histidine in some fishes cause acute gastroenteritis. Heavy metals, such as Thallium and Cadmium cause gastroenteritis.
- *Norwalk like agents:* These viruses are transmitted feco-orally transmitted cause nausea, vomiting, and diarrhea after 48 hours of incubation period. It is common in nurseries.
- *Salmonella poisoning: Salmonella typhimurium* from contaminated meat, milk and milk products produce symptoms with an incubation period of 12–24 hours. Fever, nausea, vomiting and watery diarrhea

are common. Reservoirs are poultry and farm animals.

Control

Following are the practical measures to be taken against food poisoning:
- Food sanitation
  - Meat hygiene
  - Personal hygiene
  - Proper handling of food
  - Milk pasteurization, and
  - Health education
- Food protection
- Refrigeration
- Care of canned foods
- Antitoxin in botulism
- Surveillance of food establishment by periodical laboratory analysis.

Investigation of an Epidemic of Gastroenteritis

- List of people involved is done.
- They are subjected for laboratory tests.
- Survey of eating places; kitchen and food handlers are done.
- Data is analyzed for time, place, and person distribution.
- In all epidemics of acute gastroenteritis, cholera is ruled out at investigation.

Food poisoning is differentiated from cholera as under:
- Involve group of persons and no epidemic
- One day incubation period
- No secondary cases
- Nausea and vomiting present
- Motion not rice watery
- Abdominal pain present
- Urine is not suppressed
- Blood examination normal.

Amebiasis

With/without clinical manifestation, if a person harbors *Entamoeba histolytica*, it is called amebiasis. It is estimated that 15% of population in India are affected with intestinal amebiasis.

It is transmitted by fecal-oral route and is more closely associated with poor sanitation and low socioeconomic condition. The incubation period is 2–4 weeks.

Difference between Amebic and Bacillary Dysentery

	Amebic	Bacillary
Number	6–8	10 or more
Amount	Copious	Small
Odor	Offensive	Odorless
Nature	Blood, mucous, feces	Blood, mucous
Consistency	Not adherent	Adherent
RBC	In clumps	Discrete
WBC	Scanty	Plenty
Specific microscopy	Entamoeba histolytica	Bacteria

(RBC: red blood cell; WBC: white blood cell; E: Entamoeba)

Amebiasis is severe in those who are on corticosteroids, malnourished individuals, and pregnant women and in very young children.

Specific Treatment of Intestinal Amebiasis

- Metronidazole 400 mg TDS for 10 days with diloxanide furoate 500 mg TDS for 10 days.
- Single dose of secnidazole 2 g therapy.

Prevention and Controls

Following are the preventive measures to be taken against amebic dysentery:
- Sanitation
- Protected water supply
- Food hygiene
- Health education
- Early diagnosis and prompt treatment of cases.

Usual chlorination does not kill amebic cysts. Contaminated water can be treated with 2% tincture iodine or 12.5 mL saturated aqueous solution of iodine crystals in 1 liter prepared and mixed.

Uncooked vegetables and fruits are treated with aqueous solution of iodine 200 ppm or with acetic acid 10%.

Hookworm Infection (Uncinariasis Fig. 9.10)

Infection caused by *Ancylostoma* (A). *duodenale* or *Necator* (N). *americanus* is the most common cause of anemia in our country. The latter is common in South India.

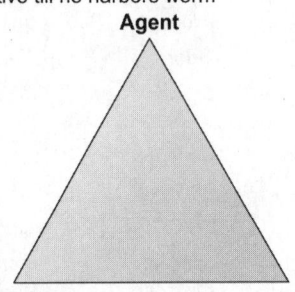

Agent
- Eggs are passed in stool
- Third stage larva is infective stage
- Infect by entering through skin
- Survive for 1–4 years
- Contaminated soil is infective material
- Person is infective till he harbors worm

Environment
- Sandy soil favors
- Damp, decaying vegetation
- 24 to 32 degree centigrade
- Rainfall
- Shaded area
- Open field defecation

Host
- Age and sex specificity not there
- Malnutrition predisposes infection
- Natural balance can create asymptomatic infestation
- Agricultural and mine workers susceptible

Fig. 9.10: Epidemiology of hookworm infestation.

Chandler Index (Endemic Index)

No. of eggs per 100 g stool	Remarks
<200	Not significant
200–250	Potential danger
250–300	Minor public health problems
300 +	Major public health problems

The disease is associated with open field defecation, walking barefoot in the area of open field defecation, and usage of untreated sewage for farming.

Chronic blood loss and depletion of body iron by hookworm infection is controlled by:
- Sanitary disposal of night soil and health awareness on open field defecation as well as use of foot wears while moving in open field defecation area.
- Chemotherapy for worm infestation. One tablet albendazole 400 mg single dose or tablet. Mebendazole 100 mg BD for 3 days.
- Anemia correction by ferrous sulfate (FS)
- Community health education.

Guinea Worm Infection (Medina Worm)

Predominant infection in Guinea and Medina has given the name to this nematode *Dracunculus medinensis*.

It is transmitted through drinking water from unsafe sources, such as step well, pond, etc. which contains Cyclops called water flea. Infection incapacitates man causing economic and productive loss to the family. When patient enters unsafe water, guinea worm emerges and discharge embryos to water which are taken up by Cyclops. When healthy man drinks this water he gets the disease after a period of 1 year.

Last case reported was in July 1996, in Aau village in Peelwa primary health center area of Jodhpur district in Rajasthan.

Eradication of guinea worm is made possible on following epidemiological basis:
- It is a simple life cycle.
- Cyclops is present only in unsafe water.
- Tools for control is available.
- No deaths are reported.

In 1983–1984, Government of India launched Guinea Worm Eradication Programme (GWEP) in the country. India

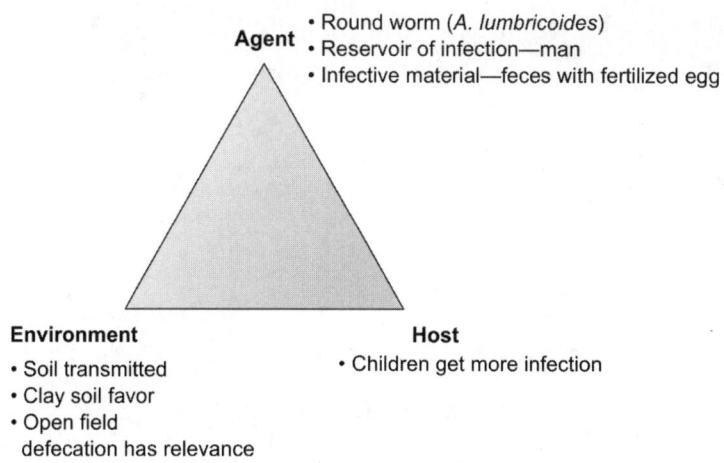

Fig. 9.11: Epidemiology of round worm.

did not record any case during July 1996 to July 1999 and became eligible for certification by the International Commission for Certification of dracunculiasis eradication.

Eradication of guinea worm Indian Scenario is detailed in Chapter 33.

Round Worm (*Ascaris lumbricoides*)

Round worm is one of the most common and most widespread human intestinal infection. It is estimated that 2 billion people are infected at a given point of time in the world (**Fig. 9.11**).

Mode of Transmission

Fecal oral route when the infective eggs are swallowed with food. Raw food convey infection readily. Water pollution also makes infection vulnerable.

Incubation Period

Incubation period is about 50 days. Course of larvae in man is showed in diagram.

Clinical Features

Mainly gastrointestinal manifestation in the form of vague abdominal pain form the main symptom. Extreme cases manifest as malnutrition. Migrating larvae produce (*Ascaris pneumonia*) fever, cough, dyspnea, and sputum examination show larvae. In 25% of cases, urticarial rash and eosinophilia are seen. Due to circulating larvae, functional disorders of brain, heart and kidney are unusual manifestations. Adult worm destroy nutrients and consume calories leading to subnutrition and malnutrition. Even vitamin A deficiency can also be seen, and ascarin in the body can also lead to edema of the face, conjunctivitis, urticaria and other toxic manifestations. Rarely, intussusception, obstruction and peritonitis (penetration through ulcers) are reported. Ectopic ascariasis can cause vomiting, suffocation, appendicitis, obstructive jaundice, pancreatitis and liver abscess.

Laboratory diagnosis is examination of ova by direct examination under microscope and concentration by floatation method. History of passing adult worms in the stool or vomitus and X-ray by barium examination are added pathognomonic investigations.

Specific Treatment

- Mebendazole 100 mg 12th hourly for 3 days
- Albendazole 400 mg as single dose
- Piperazine citrate 4 g as a single dose
- Pyrantel 10 mg/kg body weight (IG adult).

Surgical obstruction may need nasogastric suction for worms.

Improvement of sanitation eradicates round worm infestation. Mass treatment may be advocated in high incidence area.

Primary (First line) Treatment

Health education for the use of sanitary latrine, personal hygiene, and avoiding open field

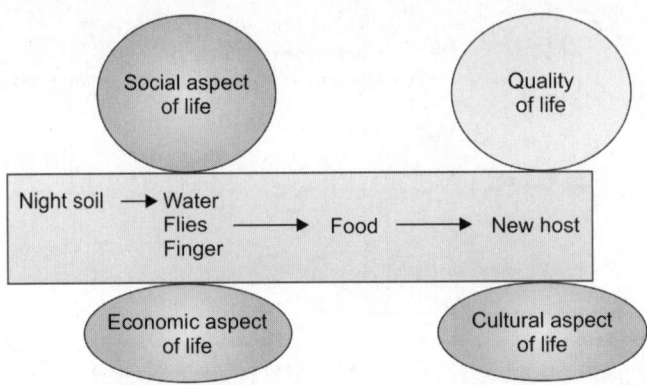

Fig. 9.12: Dynamics of typhoid transmission.

defecation play main role in prevention of round worm infection.

To reduce soil contamination, sanitary disposal of human excreta is very much needed. Food hygiene and provision of potable water (safe and wholesome) are basic needs in the prevention of ascariasis.

Enteric Fever

Typhoid, Paratyphoid A, B

Systemic infections by *Salmonella typhi, Salmonella paratyphi A, Salmonella paratyphi B are* occurring in sporadic, endemic and epidemic forms in our country. Paratyphoid C is not found in India. Typhoid and paratyphoid together are called "enteric fever". Prolonged fever (step-ladder type), relative bradycardia, transient rash called rose spots, splenomegaly and leukopenia with constitutional disturbances increase the morbidity status. Flies, fingers, feces, and water form vehicle and are the sources of infection (**Fig. 9.12**).

Incubation Period

- About 10–15 days
- *2017 reported 2*.22 million cases and 493 deaths.

Morbidity Pattern

- Indian picture morbidity—102–2,219 per 100,000
- Urban picture—110 per 100,000
- Relapse rate—15–20%
- Carrier rate—3.5%
- *Transmission:* Fecal oral route.

Carriers

Convalescent carriers, temporary carriers and permanent carriers are known types. About 2.5% of cases are permanent carriers. One permanent carrier—Mary Malon popularly called Typhoid Mary who was a cook to many families during 1901–1914, was found responsible in more than 200 secondary cases and transmitted to more than 1,300 cases in her life time.

The epidemiological triad in typhoid is depicted in **Figure 9.13**.

Prevention and Control

Vaccine

Monovalent *S. typhi* is generally chosen in India. Wherever bivalent vaccine (*S. typhi* + *S. paratyphi*) is advised, it can be given; but not commonly advocated. Typhoid-Paratyphoid A and B (TAB) vaccine is not advised because of its doubtful value.

- 0.5 mL subcutaneously (SC) with interval of 10 days and later booster dose after 1 year should give lasting immunity for 3 years.
- Vi polysaccharide vaccine is given to children above 18 months age as a single dose that can give 3 year immunity. Alternatively, 0.5 mL intramuscularly (IM) as I dose followed by 0.5 mL once in 2 years is advocated.
- Subunit vaccine Ty2S is used.
- Ty21a vaccine is licensed in 1983 is advised as capsule on every other day (1, 3, 5)

Oral vaccine

They are live vaccines prepared by *Ty21a* (Swiss) or *541 Ty* (USA). *Ty21a* oral vaccine available in enteric-coated capsule form

Chapter 9: Epidemiology of Communicable Diseases

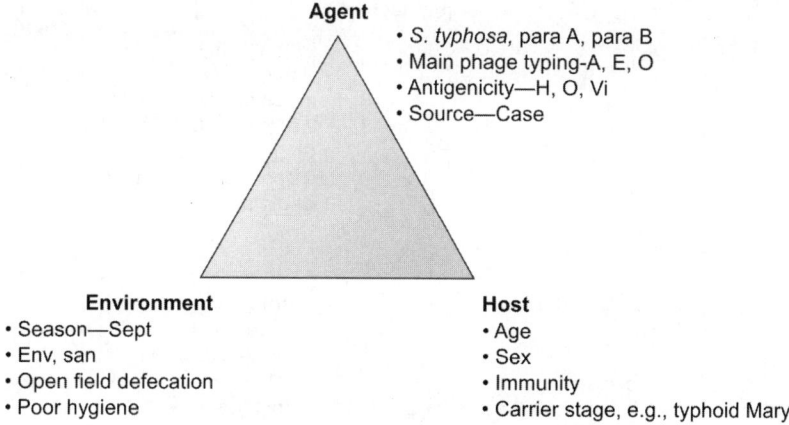

Fig. 9.13: Epidemiological triad in typhoid.

(Typhoral) is given to adults and children above 6 years on 1st, 3rd, and 5th day (1 hour before meal in pure water). Immunity commences from 15th day and lasts for 3 years.

Cases

- Early diagnosis (WBC count for leukopenia, blood culture in first week, stool culture in second week, and widal test in second week and prompt treatment (ciprofloxacin 500 mg 12 hourly, Cotrimoxazole 2 tablets 12 hourly, Amoxicillin 750 mg 6 hourly, and Chloramphenicol 500 mg 6 hourly)
- Elective isolation
- Disinfection
- Follow-up.

Contacts

- Immunization
- Surveillance
- Improved sanitation and improved living condition reduces the incidence. Travelers visiting endemic area are immunized to overcome the infection.

RESPIRATORY INFECTIONS

SARS (Severe Acute Respiratory Syndrome)

Severe acute respiratory syndrome (SARS) is a droplet infection by new coronavirus which is highly contagious and with high secondary attack rate and high case fatality rate. In early part of 2003, China, Hong Kong and Vietnam reported cases. Later the epidemic of SARS was reported from more than 20 countries. By April 2003, 2,671 cases and 103 deaths were reported around the world. This included the death of Dr Carlo Urbani, a WHO expert who found and worked on SARS virus (**Fig. 9.14**).

Ohio State University pointed out the relationship of SARS with cattle car-syndrome (shipping fever) where cough, pneumonia, drip mucous from eye and nose among cattles are seen.

It is known as "*shaheed haad Tanaffusi Alaiymia*" in unani. Herbal fumigation with neem, tulsi, loban, camphor, and sandal is advocated.

In India suspected cases are reported from Manipal, Kerala, Pune, and Goa. National Institute for Communicable Diseases (NICD) has observed 10 out of 12 are negative and that "all flu are not SARS."

Hong Kong study's observation has reported cockroaches spread SARS infection.

WHO has recommended infrared "Fever sensitizing system" for the diagnosis of SARS under "SARS surveillance".

Indian Council of Medical Research (ICMR) has stated that SARS is not a public health problem in India, since no single case fits to WHO criteria and as against this WHO declared India "SARS Free". India has only milder version of SARS since all cases are X-ray clear.

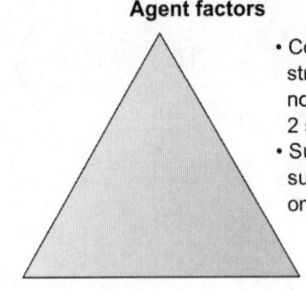

Fig. 9.14: Epidemiology of SARS.
(SARS: severe acute respiratory syndrome; RNA: ribonucleic acid)

National level screening committee is formed and Government of India has recommended "Watchdog Panel" in all the states.

WHO case definition:

Suspect Case

- High fever above 38°C
- Cough or breathing difficulty
- Close contact with a suspect or probable case of SARS
- History of travel to an affected area.

Probable Case

- A suspect case with X-ray finding
- Consistent pneumonia (Chest X-ray finding)
- Respiratory distress syndrome (RDS) (evidence of infiltrates)
- A suspect case with pathological findings of RDS.

Global Picture

Total of 8,422 cases were reported with 916 deaths by August 2003 (which include atypical pneumonia).

Clinical Features

- High fever above 38°C
- Dry cough
- Shortness of breath or breathing difficulties
- Changes in chest X-ray indicating pneumonia changes.
- Associated symptoms, such as headache, and muscular stiffness
- Loss of appetite, malaise, confusion, rash, and diarrhea.

Transmission

Severe acute respiratory syndrome (SARS) can be transmitted in any season; overcrowding precipitates the spread. Epidemic outbreak of SARS is influenced by population density and population movement. It is transmitted from person-to-person by droplet infection. Contact with aerosolized (exhaled) droplets and bodily secretions from infected persons appears to be important. Hospital workers, home contacts and nursing care personnel are high-risk group. Hence, for nursing care of SARS patient they are admitted in isolation hospitals. Robot to attend to SARS patient have been developed and are being tried.

Complications

- Severe pneumonia
- Respiratory failure
- Case fatality rate (CFR): Three percent

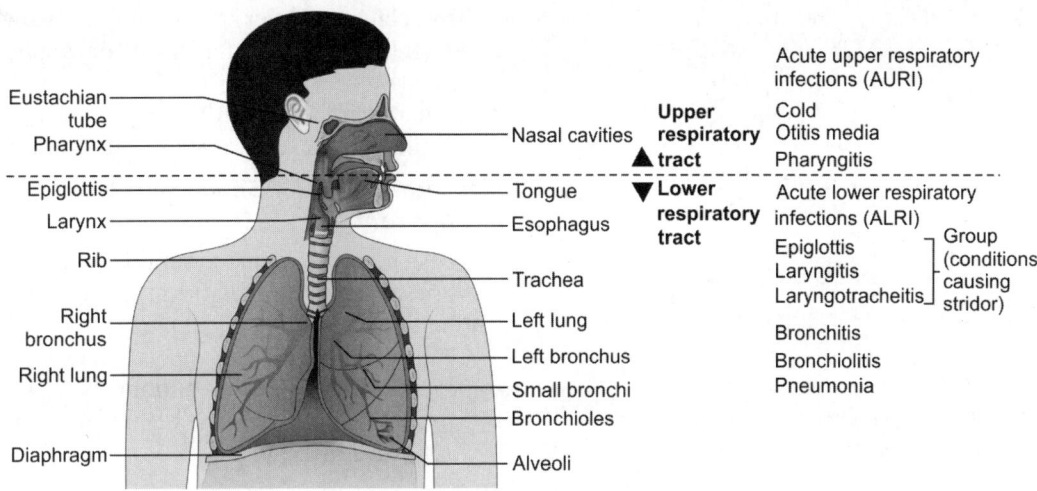

Fig. 9.15: Anatomical sites of acute respiratory infection: Clinical observation.

Acute Respiratory Infections (Fig. 9.15)

It is an episode of acute symptoms and signs resulting from infection of any part of respiratory tract or any related structures including paranasal sinuses, middle ear, and pleural cavity. They are the leading causes of morbidity in India. A complex and heterogenous group of illness with clinical outcome of: (a) bronchiolitis, (b) acute laryngitis, (c) pneumonia which are primarily responsible for under-five mortality.

Severe acute respiratory syndrome (SARS)-associated coronavirus has caused pandemic in June 2003.

Current influenza virus of public health importance are A/Shangdong/9/93(H3N2), A/Singapore/6/86/H1N1, B/Panama/45/90. Antigenic drift is seen with influenza A (H2N2). Antigenic shift is seen with influenza A (H1N1).

Indian Pattern

- 14.3% of deaths account infantile acute respiratory infection (ARI) (Urban hospital show 13% infant deaths by ARI).
- 15.9% of deaths accounts 1–5 years ARI (specific mortality rate 10 per 1,000 below 5 year age group)
- 5–8 episodes of ARI/year/child on an average 2–3 episodes per preschool per year in rural areas 5–7 episodes per preschool per year in urban areas.

Acute Respiratory Infections (ARI) Concepts

- **Fast breathing:** 60 breaths per minute in below 2 months child* (*to be repeated for successive reading since error is more) 50 breaths per minute in 2–12 months child 40 breaths per minute in 1–5 years child.
- **Chest in drawing:** Low chest wall goes in when child breaths in.
- **Stridor:** Harsh noise when breathing in.
- **Wheeze:** Soft whistling or difficulty in breathing out.

Risk Factors in Acute Respiratory Infection (ARI)

- Poor nutrition
- Smoke pollution
- Overcrowding
- Low birthweight

Epidemiology (Fig. 9.16)

Mode of transmission

Airborne

Acute Respiratory Infection (ARI) Control

Clinical assessment is done by noting cyanosis, malnutrition, wheeze, stridor, chest in drawing and fast breathing.

Following are WHO recent classification based on criteria for decision-making in case management in developing countries:

- Cough, cold, and fever present but no pneumonia, no fast breathing, no chest in-

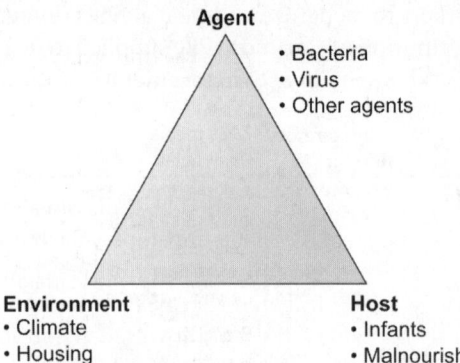

Fig. 9.16: Epidemiological triad in acute respiratory infection (ARI).

drawing—only supportive therapy and do not need penicillin.
- Cough and fast breathing is present suggests the treatment with cotrimoxazole*.
  - Below 2 months need ½ spoon syrup twice a day or 1 tablet twice a day
  - 2–12 months need 1 spoon syrup twice a day or 2 tablets twice a day
  - 1–5 years need 1.5 spoon syrup twice a day or 3 tablets twice a day.
  (*5 mL syrup contains 200 mg sulfamethoxazole + 40 mg trimethoprim. 1 tablet contains 100 mg sulfamethoxazole + 20 mg trimethoprim)
- When pneumonia present, antibiotic is needed + symptomatic treatment + fluid/food intake monitoring + home management on discharge for 2 months to 5 year age.
Benzylpenicillin 50,000 IU per kg 6 hourly IM.
Or
Ampicillin 50 mg per kg 6 hourly IM.
Or
Chloramphenicol 25 mg per kg 6 hourly IM.
- When pneumonia present, antibiotic is needed + hypothermia avoided + breastfeeding promoted for below 2 months child
Benzylpenicillin 50,000 IU per kg 12 hourly for below 7 days child and 6 hourly for above 7 days child
Or

Ampicillin 50 mg per kg 12 hourly for below 7 days child and 8 hourly for above 7 days child
Plus
Gentamicin 2.5 mg/kg 12 hourly for below 7 days child and 8 hourly for above 7 days child.

Classification (Table 9.5): Summary of Case Management

The case management is summarized as:
- Very severe—admit, and give chloramphenicol
  (25 mg/kg 6 hourly IM)
- Severe—admit, and give antibiotics.
- Moderate—antibiotics at home plus supportive therapy.

Table 9.5: Classification of ARI.

Etiological	Anatomical	Management-oriented
Viral bacterial other causes	URI (upper respiratory infection) LRI (lower respiratory infection) (sinusitis laryngitis bronchitis, etc.)	Below 2 months age • Very severe pneumonia stopped feeding • Well convulsions • Sleepy/difficult to wake • Stridor in calm child • Wheezing • Fever • Severe pneumonia • Severe chest indrawing • Fast breathing 60 and above • Simple cold and cough • No chest in drawing • No fast breathing (less than 60) 2 months to 5 years • Very severe pneumonia • Not able to drink • Convulsions • Sleepy/difficult to wake • Stridor in calm child • Severe malnutrition • Severe pneumonia • Chest indrawing pneumonia • No chest indrawing • Fast breathing (50 and above in 2–12 months) (40 and above in 12–60 months) Simple cold and cough • No chest indrawing • No fast breathing (<50 in 2–12 months) (<40 in 12–60 months)

❖ Mild—no antibiotics, only supportive therapy.

Supportive Therapy (Fig. 9.17)

It consists of:

❖ Continue breastfeeding
❖ Encourage the child to drink
❖ Encourage the child to eat
❖ A neutral thermal environment
❖ Paracetamol as antipyretic
❖ Clearing the nose
❖ Cough suppressant
❖ Oxygen.

Prevention and Control of ARI

❖ Improvement of living standard
❖ Better nutrition
❖ Reduction of air pollution
❖ Good RCH care
❖ Implementation of ARI control program.

Acute respiratory infection control program was taken up in 1990. It became part and parcel of CSSM in 1992. It is part of RCH program at National level since 1997. Training of health workers to recognize and treat at first contact, distribution of cotrimoxazole supplied to RCH drug kit are main activities under ARI control program.

Tuberculosis

Every year 1.8 million people in India develop tuberculosis (TB) (5,000 develop every day), 0.8 million develop new smear positive cases (40,000 newly infected cases every day) and nearly 4.17 lakhs die from it which accounts for 1,200 deaths every day. The incidence of tuberculosis has changed little in the past 30 years. Human immunodeficiency virus (HIV). associated TB and the emergence of multidrug resistant TB will increase the magnitude and severity of TB epidemic. It has become a major barrier to economic development.

Active culture positive TB is of the order of 15 per 10,000 population. It is estimated that 30% of population have TB infection and the annual risk of TB infection is around 0.6–2.3% among unvaccinated 0–9 years age children.

Feed the child
• Feed the child during illness
• Increase feeding after illness
• Clear the nose if it interferes with feeding

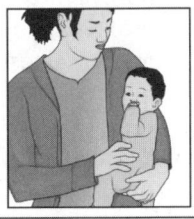

Increase fluids
• Offer the child extra to drink
• Increase breastfeeding

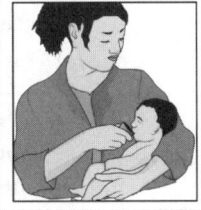

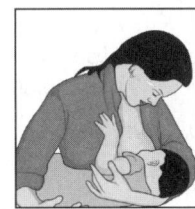

Soothe the throat and relieve the cough with a safe remedy

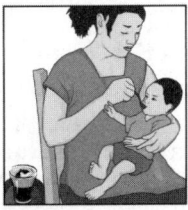

Most important
Watch for the following signs and return quickly if they occur

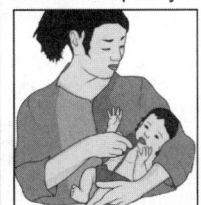

• Breathing becomes difficult
• Breathing becomes fast
• Child is not able to drink
• Child becomes sicker
This child may have pneumonia

Fig. 9.17: Home care instructions for children for acute respiratory infection (ARI).

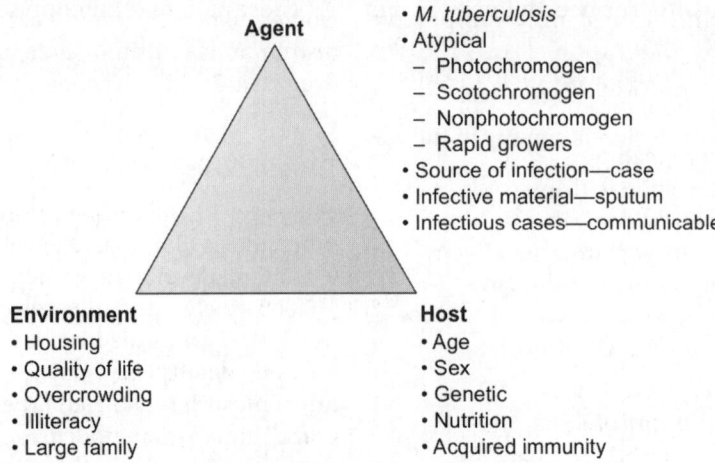

Fig. 9.18: Epidemiological triad in tuberculosis.
M. tuberculosis: Mycobacterium tuberculosis

Extrapulmonary tuberculosis comprises about 10–15% of all TB cases in India. Among them, 75% have lymph nodal or pleural TB.

The epidemiological triad in TB is give in **Figure 9.18**.

Community Parameters

- Prevalence of infection—tuberculin positive = 30.4%.
- Incidence of infection—newly infected (annual) (TB convention index) = 1–2%.
- Prevalence of disease = Acid-fast bacilli (AFB) positive = 0.4% (4/1,000).
- Prevalence of X-ray suspect = 2%.
- Prevalence of drug resistant = 10%.
- Mortality rate = 37 per 100,000.

Mode of Transmission

Droplet infection.

Incubation Period

Varies from weeks to years.

Concepts in Tuberculosis

New cases: Sputum positive pulmonary tuberculosis who has never taken treatment.

Failure cases: Sputum positive case, after 5 months treatment, still show positive.

Relapse: Sputum positive case declared cured, show again sputum positive.

Defaulter: One who left the treatment in-between.

Cured: Sputum positive case after treatment show sputum negative at least on two occasions.

Sputum positive: A case which shows two sputum positive for AFB. This also can be one AFB positive and one culture positive.

Sputum negative: Three negative smear positive for AFB in spite of TB symptoms, in spite of X-ray abnormalities or in spite of culture positive.

Tuberculin Test

It helps to map out prevalence of infection. There are three types of tests. These are:
1. Mantoux test (intradermal test)
2. Heaf test
3. Tine test

Mantoux is commonly done by injecting 0.1 mL PPD on flexor forearm. Result is read after 72 hours. Above 10 mm reaction is positive and below 6 mm is negative. Between 10 and 6 mm is not a decisive result.

Control of Tuberculosis

Reason for Failure of TB Control

- Quality of sputum examination in the field is not good.
- Case detection is not up to the mark.
- Annual yield of bacillary cases is not 100% (it is just 35%).
- Drug defaulter rate is increasing.

- General health service delivery is not satisfactory.
- Low socioeconomic status of the people of the country is not raised.
- Population explosion is coming in the way of achievement.

Case Finding (Fig. 9.19)

- Sputum examination of all cases who present with history of cough over 4 weeks (2 weeks as per the guidelines to primary health center by NTP). Continuous fever, chest pain and hemoptysis are the other major symptoms.

Three sputum specimens obtained over 2 days visit as under;
First visit—a spot specimen is collected; sputum container is given for early morning specimen.
Second visit—early morning specimen brought is collected and another spot specimen is collected.
- MMR (mass miniature radiography)
- Tuberculin test

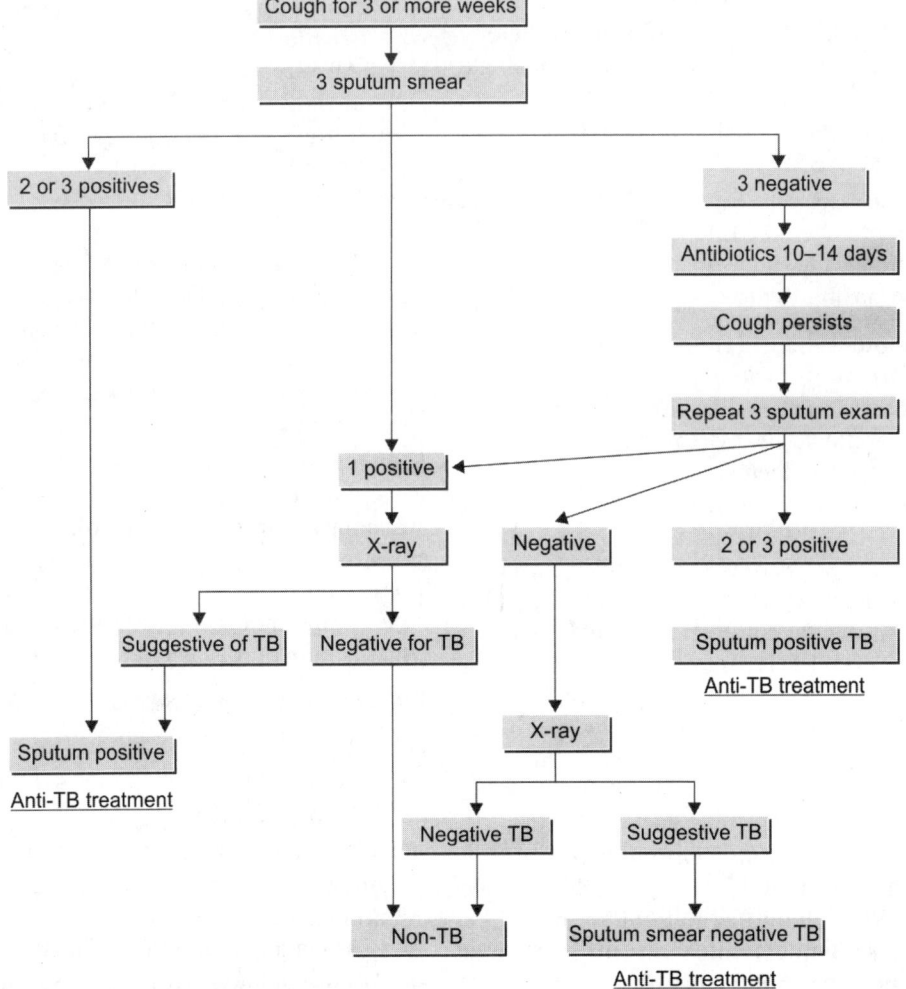

Fig. 9.19: Pulmonary tuberculosis–algorithm for diagnosis.
(TB: tuberculosis)

Chemotherapy

Common bactericidal drugs	Common bacteriostatic drugs
Streptomycin	Ethambutol
INH	Thiacetazone
Pyrazinamide	Ethionamide
Rifampicin	PAS
	Cycloserine
	Kanamycin
	Vancomycin

(PAS: para-aminosalicylic acid)

National Tuberculosis Institute (NTI) Bengaluru suggested classical *long course conventional* chemotherapeutic regimens:

Daily regimen: Not supervised chemotherapy
- 300 mg INH + thiacetazone 150 mg as single dose
- Streptomycin initially for first 2 months total duration is 1.5 years.

Bi-weekly regimen: Supervised chemotherapy
- Streptomycin 1 g IM
- INH 600 mg single dose
- Pyridoxine 10 mg.

Chemotherapeutic arrows

First arrow: Motivation
- Not to stop drugs on initial improvement.
- Side effects if any, the same should be reported to doctor.

Second arrow: Treatment

Option A: Standard regimen
- R_1: AFB negative, X-ray positive, toxic, new AFB positive, TB of lymph nodes, sputum positive after completion of treatment
  - 2STH/10TH for sputum positive or seriously ill patients of pulmonary TB.
  - First 2 months (intensive phase)
  - S—0.75 g—daily at PHC/hospital
  - H—300 mg + T.150 mg daily in single dose at home (to collect monthly)
  - Next 10 months (continuation phase)
  - H—300 mg + T.150 mg—daily in single dose at home (to collect monthly)
- R_2: AFB negative, X-ray positive, lost patients, irregular patients
  - 12TH for smear negative but radiologically active patients.
  - H—300 mg + T.150 mg both drugs in single dose should be given orally on daily wise at home (to collect monthly).

Option B: Short course regimen.
- R_A: All new cases
  - 2 EHRZ/6TH all smear positive patients or patients with serious forms of extrapulmonary TB (meningeal, spinal, and bony).
  - First 2 months (intensive phase).
  - H—300 mg; R—450 mg; E—800 mg and Z— 1.5 g daily, single dose at home (to collect once in 15 days).
  - Next 6 months (continuation phase)
  - H—300 mg; T—150 mg, daily single dose should be given at home (to collect once in a month).
- R_B: All retreatment cases
  - $2SHRZ/4S_2H_2R_2$: For patients remaining smear positive after treatment and relapses.
  - First 2 months (intensive phase).
  - S—0.75 g; H—300 mg; R—450 mg; Z—1.5 g daily at PHC/hospital/district tuberculosis centers (DTC).
  - Next 4 months (continuation phase)
  - H—600 mg; R—600 mg; S—0.75 g twice daily—all drugs together at PHC/hospital/DTC.

Note for option A and B: Ethambutol can be replaced by thiacetazone depending on availability of drugs or tolerance by the patient.
(S = streptomycin; R = rifampicin; T = thiacetazone; H = isoniazid or INH; Z = pyrazinamide; E = ethambutol)
Organization of NTP is given in **Figure 9.20**.

Follow-up in National TB Programme (NTP)

Patients on standard regimen (R_1 and R_2) are reviewed after 6 and 12 months from the initiation of treatment.

Patients on short course regimen (R_A and R_B) are reviewed after 3 and 6 months from the initiation of treatment.

District TB center (DTC) is a specialized center for diagnosis, case management of TB in a district. It is also responsible for training and supervising staff.

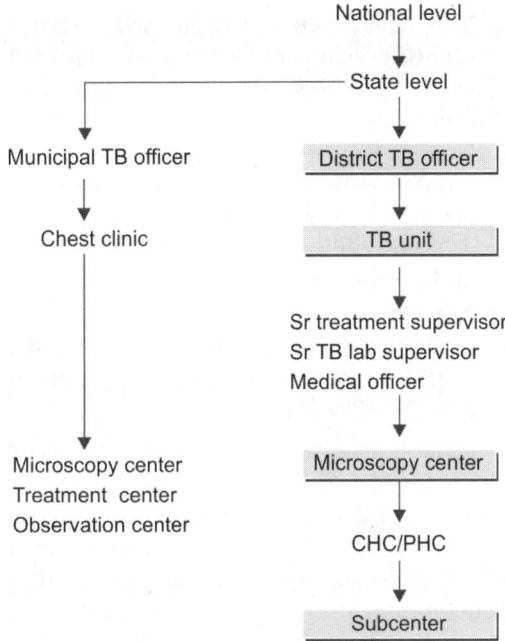

Fig. 9.20: Organization of NTP.
(CHC/PHC: community health center/primary health center; TB: tuberculosis; lab: laboratory; NTP: National TB Programme)

In RNTCP (Revised National TB Control Programme) subdistrict level TU (tuberculosis unit) is responsible for supervision of laboratories and treatment. TU covers 5 lakhs people. Microscopy center covers 1 lakh people.

Revised National TB Control Programme (RNTCP)

The district is the key level for the management of PHCs. The District Health and Family Welfare Officer (DH FWO) is responsible for all medical and public health activities including control of TB.

The DTC is the nodal point for TB control activities in the district. In RNTCP, the role of DTC has shifted from a clinical one to a managerial one. The District Tuberculosis Officer (DTO) has the overall responsibility of physical and financial management of RNTCP at the district level as per the guidelines of the DTCs. The DTO is also responsible for involvement of other sectors in RNTCP and is assisted by a medical officer (MO), statistical assistant and other paramedical staff. For each district, there should be a full time DTO, who is trained in RNTCP at a central level institution.

Unique features of RNTCP

- District TB Control Society called DTCS
- Subdistrict level supervisory staff for microscopy and treatment services [MOTC, senior treatment supervisor (STS) and senior tuberculosis laboratory supervisory (STLS)]—provision of two wheelers for supervision by STS/STLS
- Modular training for all staff
- Patient wise treatment boxes (PWB) patient wise box (PWB)—red for category I, blue for category II, and green for category III. Each PWB has 2 pouches; one for intensive phase called A (contains 1 day medication), one for continuous phase called B (contain 1 week supply). Each combipack contains 2 isoniazid, 1 rifampicin, 2 pyrazinamide, and 2 ethambutol.
- Robust recording and reporting system
- Quarterly review of performance at all levels.

The basis and treatment regimen of TB is outlined in **Table 9.6**.

Table 9.6: Basis and treatment through regimen.

Category	Patient	Regimen
I. This is generally prescribed to new sputum smear positive patients. They have a high bacillary population with higher chances of having naturally occurring drug resistant mutants. Therefore, four drugs are prescribed during the intensive phase	• New sputum positive • Seriously ill new sputum negative • Seriously ill new extrapulmonary	$2H_3R_3Z_3E_3 + 4H_3R_3$

Contd...

Contd...

II. This category includes patients who have had previous antituberculosis treatment. Therefore, the chances of harboring resistant bacilli are higher. Hence, a 5 drug regimen is prescribed in the intensive phase, and the total duration of treatment is 8 months	• Sputum positive relapse case • Sputum positive failure • Sputum positive after default • Extrapulmonary relapse who show sputum negative	$2H_3R_3Z_3E_3S_3$ + $1H_3R_3Z_3E_3$ + $5H_3R_3E_3$
III. This category includes sputum smear negative cases with a low bacillary population. There is a lower chance for drug resistant mutants. Therefore, a 3 drug regimen is prescribed	Not serious, new sputum negative, new extrapulmonary, not seriously ill	$2H_3R_3Z_3$ + $4H_3R_3$

Number before alphabet is months of treatment. Subscript after alphabet is the doses per week.

Symbols	Adult dose	Pediatric dose
H = INH	(600 mg)	(10–15 mg/kg)
R = Rifampicin	(450 mg)	(10 mg/kg)
Z = Pyrazinamide	(1,500 mg)	(30–35 mg/kg)
E = Ethambutol	(1,200 mg)	(30 mg/kg)
S = Streptomycin	(750 mg)	(15 mg/kg)

Line of management of TB patient who interrupt TB treatment

❖ Acid-fast bacilli (AFB) negative who interrupt after 1 month treatment, continue all doses by resuming treatment.
❖ Acid-fast bacilli (AFB) negative who interrupt after 2 months or 2 months more of treatment, begin category I treatment afresh.
❖ New AFB positive who interrupt after 1 month of category I treatment, continue category 1 treatment or start category I treatment
❖ New AFB positive who interrupt after 2 months or more than 2 months of category I treatment, start category II treatment
❖ AFB positive who interrupt after 1 month of his category II treatment, start category II treatment
❖ AFB positive who interrupt after 2 months of his category II treatment, start again category II treatment.

Directly observed treatment short course (DOTS) chemotherapy

Directly observed treatment short course is a strategy to ensure that by providing most effective drug and confirming that the drug is taken. It is the only documented effective program in the world and its strategies are:

❖ Political commitment
❖ Diagnosis by sputum smear microscopy
❖ Adequate supply of right drugs
❖ Directly observed treatment
❖ Accountability.

During intensive phase, health worker watches as patient swallow the drug in his or her presence. During continuation phase, patient is issued medicine for 1 week in multiblister combipack, of which the first dose is swallowed by patient in presence of a health worker. The pack is checked at return when patient comes to collect next pack. Drugs are packed in patient-wise boxes with good shelf-life. In DOTS, alternate day treatment is used.

Antituberculosis treatment for patients on ART

Treatment of tuberculosis, who are HIV positive, cannot be envisaged without rifampicin. In TB patients coinfected with HIV, treatment should be first administered for TB under the DOTS strategy and ART should be started after completion of TB treatment. In patients, with very low CD4 counts requiring concomitant administration of ART and anti-TB treatment the antiretroviral (ARV) regimen should be modified by replacing nevirapine with efavirenz. On completion of

TB treatment such patients can be switched back to nevirapine.

Case detection

Following are the ways to detect the case of tuberculosis:
- Spot, early morning and again spot—three samples AFB examination
- Promote TB awareness in community
- Evaluate contacts of AFB-positive cases, and
- Evaluate abnormal X-rays.

Diagnosis

There are three ways to diagnose the tuberculosis:
1. Three AFB tests
2. Clinical and radiological for AFB positive, and
3. Extrapulmonary diagnosis.

Case classification

The case of tuberculosis has been categorized as:
a. Pulmonary AFB positive
b. Pulmonary AFB negative, and
c. Extrapulmonary TB.

Treatment

Category I
- New pulmonary AFB positive
- Seriously ill AFB negative (pulmonary), and seriously ill (extrapulmonary)
- $2(HRZE)_3/4(HR)_3$ initial phase extended by 1 month if AFB positive after 2 months.

Category II
- Retreatment cases, $2(HRZSE)_3/1(HRZE)_3/5(HRE)_3$, and
- Initial phase extended by 1 month if AFB positive after 3 months.

Category III
- New nonseriously ill AFB negative and extrapulmonary cases
- $2(HRZ)_3/4(HR)_3$
- If smear is positive at 2 months categorized as failure case and treated afresh.

(H = INH, R = rifampicin, Z = pyrazinamide, E = ethambutol, S = streptomycin, Prefix = duration in months, Subscript = number of dose per week).

In 2016, Bedaquiline is made available for drug-resistant cases (DR-TB) through revised guideline. Under regimen type, first and second line of drugs were included.

During intensive phase of treatment, every dose of medicine is to be taken under direct observation. This is called DOTS (directly observed treatment short course). DOTS is a strategy to ensure cure by providing the most effective medicine and confirming that it is taken.

Treatment evaluation: By 2AFB/patient/course.

Result
- Cured
- Completed
- Defaulted
- Failed
- Died, and
- Transferred.

The main records and forms in NTP are:
- Tuberculosis identification card
- Tuberculosis treatment card
- Tuberculosis register
- Laboratory register
- Quarterly report on new and retreatment cases
- Quarterly report on sputum conversion
- Quarterly report on results of treatment
- Quarterly report on program management.

Key recommendations of RNTCP are as following:
- Increase effective political commitment
- Expand the RNTCP
- Decentralization in a phased manner
- Increase intra- and inter-sectoral coordination.
- Optimization of diagnosis and treatment of TB in areas not yet covered by RNTCP.

Measles

It is an RNA paramyxovirus, acute highly infectious disease of childhood associated with high morbidity and mortality. The illness predisposes grade I and II malnutrition to severe (grade III and IV) malnutrition.

The CFR is 2–15% in developing countries and is 1.8–7.6% in India among hospitalized cases. CFR is gradually declining as a result of

Universal Immunization Programme in the country.

The epidemiological triad is given in **Figure 9.21**.

Koplik's Spot

On 3rd day of fever, cluster of bluish white pinpoints surrounded by erythema called "Koplik's Spots" are seen when oral mucosa is inspected. This is due to the action of virus on capillaries of mucosa which disappear within a day of its appearance.

Mode of transmission—droplet infection

Incubation period—10 days

Complications

Diarrhea, pneumonia, otitis media and neurological complications, such as subacute sclerosing panencephalitis (SSPE).

Control

There are four ways to control the disease:
1. Isolation of case for 7 days from rash
2. Immunization of contacts within 2 days of exposure
3. Routine immunization
4. Community measures against malnutrition.

Bidar Integrated Rural Development (BIRD) Project

Bidar integrated rural development project where measles prevention was introduced as a project for the first time in Karnataka state. It helped to develop media, methods and vaccine trial during 1982–1984.

Prevention

Tissue cultured measles vaccine (freeze dried) is given during 9–12 months 0.5 mL subcutaneously. Immunity develops 10 days later and persists throughout life. Vaccine is contraindicated in pregnancy. Measles vaccine is also available as combined vaccine measles, mumps, rubella (MMR) which is advocated and given to 1–1.5 year age group.

In case of prevention, during early incubation period 0.25 mL per kg immunoglobulin is given. The dose of human immunoglobulin is 1 g for adults. For below 1 year it is 250 mg, for 1–2 year age, it is 500 mg and for above 3 years age it is 750 mg.

Measles Elimination Strategy

All countries are going through stage of:
1. Control
2. Outbreak prevention
3. Elimination
   - *Catch-up vaccination:* One time nationwide vaccination of children 9–12 months of age under UIP.
   - *Keep-up vaccination:* Vaccinating above 95% of each successive birth cohort.
   - *Follow-up vaccination:* Nation-wide vaccination of all children born after catch-up vaccination once in 4 years.

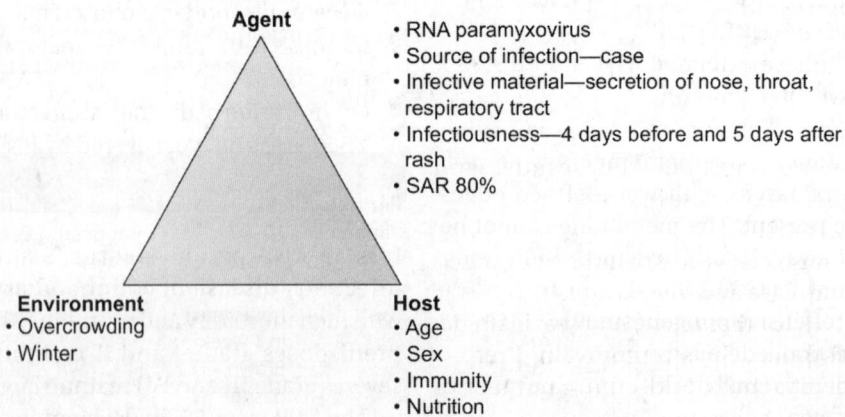

Fig. 9.21: Epidemiological triad in measles.
(RNA: ribonucleic acid; SAR: severe acute respiratory)

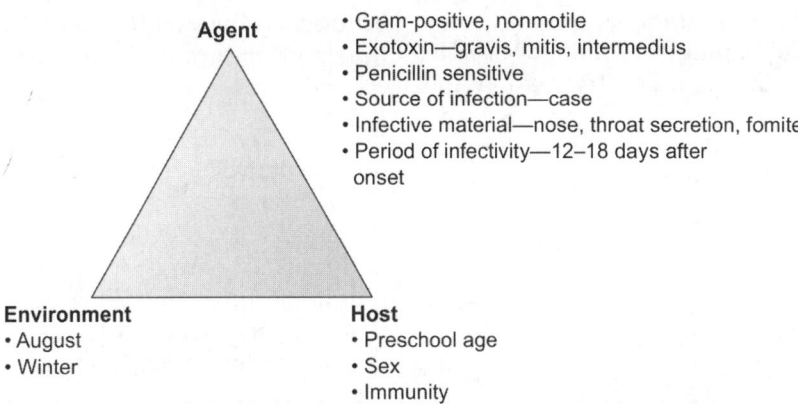

Fig. 9.22: Epidemiological triad in diphtheria.

Diphtheria

It is an acute communicable vaccine preventable disease. *Corynebacterium diphtheriae* attack nose, throat, and tonsil by membrane formation at the site of implantation. Toxemia is produced by toxin. Eradication is possible by active immunization. Both morbidity and mortality have come down to negligible level. Myocarditis in second week is common and hence electrocardiogram (ECG)/observation are advised.

Case fatality rate is 5% in treated cases. In India, the incidence has come down from thousands to negligible cases.

The epidemiological triad is shown in **Figure 9.22**.

Mode of transmission—droplet infection.

Incubation period—2–6 days

Pathogenesis

Local

- Exudates (false membrane); Grayish membrane, "False membrane" over tonsil, pharynx, larynx with well-defined edges will be present. The membrane cannot be wiped away. (It can be wiped off in other bacterial acute tonsillitis).
- Fetor (offensive pungent smell)
- Congestion, edema
- Periadenitis (bull neck).

General

Schick test—a skin test to find out susceptibility to infection and success in immunization. 0.2 mL of Schick test toxin intradermally is administered and control in other forearm. The Schick results are given in **Table 9.7**.

Control Measures

Cases

- Early diagnosis, prompt treatment, isolation 4 weeks,
- Disinfection, and
- Follow-up, carriers are given erythromycin 250 mg qid follow-up.

Contacts

- Swab test Schick test
- Antidiphtheritic serum (ADS) to Schick test-positive contacts surveillance and bacteriological examination.

Prevention

Active

- Alum-precipitated toxoid (APT) 0.5 mL PTAP (purified toxoid adsorbed on Al_2PO_4) mL

Table 9.7: Schick results.

Negative	Positive	Pseudo-positive	Combined
"Immune"	10–50 mm red flush in 24 hours max in 1 week Brown, desquamates "Susceptible"	Disappear in 4 days "Allergy"	Control is pseudo-positive test is positive "Susceptible"

- FT (Formal toxoid) 1.0 mL
- TAF (Toxoid antitoxin floccule) 1.0 mL DPT (Diphtheria, Pertussis, Tetanus) (Triple antigen—0.5 mL)
- DPT is as per UIP schedule under National Immunization Programme.

Passive

ADS 500—1,000 IU (lasts for 3–4 weeks).

Preference

Combine vaccines preferred

- DPT as primary immunization to infants and children below 12 years 0.5 mL
- Diphtheria and tetanus toxoids (DT) as booster immunization to infants and children below 12 years.
- T as primary immunization to children above 12 years and adults.

Single vaccines preferred

FT 0.1 mL for primary immunization of adults
TAF 0.1 mL for primary immunization for adults.

Not preferred

- Formal toxoid (FT)
- Purified toxoid aluminum phosphate (PTAP)
- Purified toxoid aluminum hydroxide (PTAH)

Not used

Alum precipitated toxoid (APT) 0.5 mL.

Whooping Cough (Pertussis, 100 days Cough)

It is an acute highly communicable respiratory disease caused by *Bordetella (B) pertussis*. The name is derived from severe cough ending in a whoop.

Remarkable reduction of cases, morbidity and mortality are observed in India. The incidence has come down from lakhs to thousands in recent times.

The epidemiological triad is shown in **Figure 9.23**.

Mode of transmission: Droplet, direct, fomite

Incubation period: 7–14 days

Complications: Bronchitis, bronchopneumonia, bronchiectasis.

Control: Following are the control measures against the disease.

- Early diagnosis and prompt treatment of cases
- Isolation
- Disinfection.

Prevention

- Vaccine in triple antigen under UIP.
- Vaccine in monoantigen as an alternative, 0.5 mL IM starting at 3 months of age, in 3 doses at 6 weeks interval is given.
- Complications of persistent screaming and collapse are seen.

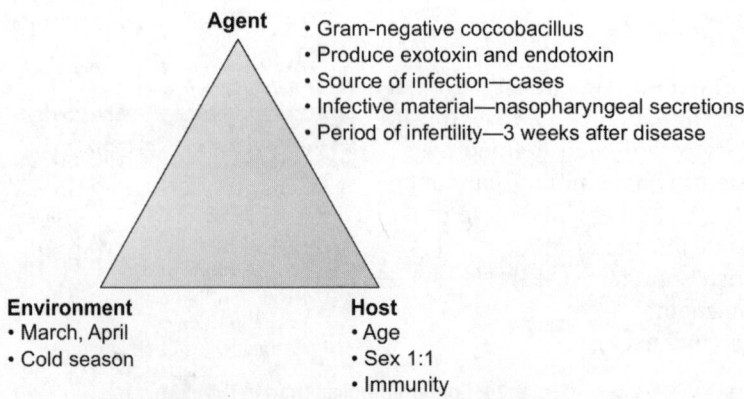

Fig. 9.23: Epidemiological triad in whooping cough.

- Vaccine is contraindicated in epilepsy.
- Hyperimmune globulin is not found useful as passive immunizing agent.

Chickenpox (Varicella)

This is an acute infectious disease caused by varicella zoster virus. Historically chickenpox had great importance because of its resemblance to mild smallpox. Mortality is practically nil in chickenpox.

Characteristics

Following are the characteristics of the disease:

Incubation period	15 days
Prodromal stage	Mild
Evolution	Rapid
Rash	Simultaneously, start with fever centripetal in distribution, no rashes on palm or sole pleomorphic in nature (all stages are present.)
Scab	Start from 4th day of rash

Treatment—Not specific

Prevention

No active immunizing agent is available for satisfactory results. Live attenuated OKA vaccine from Japan available, but not found practicable.

Immunoglobulin [varicella-zoster immune globulin (VZIG)] is given within 72 hours of exposure, 1.25–5.00 mL IM to modify the severity of the illness.

German Measles (Rubella, Three Day Measles)

German measles infection is ubiquitous in its distribution. Its relation with congenital defects was reported as early as 1941 by Norman Gregg from Australia. Infection in first 3 months of pregnancy can cause damage to the fetus and is 100%.

Rubella is usually mild and unnoticed childhood infection caused by RNA virus of Toga virus family, which become prominent when its infection showed teratogenic potential in early pregnancy. About 35–40% of women in India of child-bearing age are susceptible to rubella. German measles is associated with congenital cataract, deafness and cardiac malformations.

Congenital rubella is a chronic infection while acquired rubella is an acute infection. Infection in first trimester leads to fetal anomaly, abortion, and stillbirth.

The epidemiological triad is given in **Figure 9.24**.

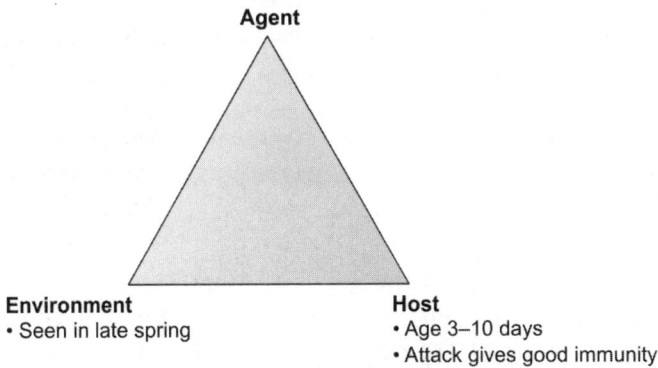

Fig. 9.24: Epidemiological triad in rubella.
(RNA: ribonucleic acid)

Mode of transmission: Droplet infection

Incubation period: 2–3 weeks.

Diagnosis

By HAI (Hemagglutination Inhibition Test) by paired sera, first within 5 days after the onset of illness and the second 2 weeks later. In paired sera 4 times rise in HI antibody titer after 2 weeks is diagnostic.

Prevention

Vaccine R_A 27/3, 0.5 mL subcutaneous route in single dose show 95% seroconversion.

Rubella vaccine in MMR. Vaccine is also equally effective.

Vaccination strategy advocated:
- Protecting women of child-bearing age
- Vaccinating all children of 1–14 years of age, and
- Vaccinating all children at 1 year of age by live attenuated vaccine (R_A 27/3).

Mumps

Infection of parotid gland by RNA myxovirus causes nonsuppurative enlargement and tenderness of the gland. The disease shows secondary attack rate of 80%. When parotid gland swelling subsides, it is not infectious. Overcrowding predisposes epidemic.

Complications of mumps have been orchitis, pancreatitis, ovaritis, and myocarditis.

Mode of transmission

It is through droplet infection.

Incubation period: 2–3 weeks

The measures to control the diseases are:
- Selective isolation up to 9 days after the onset of parotid swelling is advocated.
- Concurrent disinfection of handkerchief and articles soiled with nose and throat secretions are advisable.
- Surveillance of contacts.

Prevention

Attenuated mumps live vaccine 0.5 mL single dose through intramuscular route produces effective antibody titer among 95% of cases. Apart from monoantigen, we have double antigen (Rubella-Mumps) and Triple antigen (Measles-Mumps-Rubella) for the use.

Immunoglobulin for passive immunity is not found practicable.

Influenza

An acute respiratory infection caused by influenza virus has caused many pandemics cutting across the countries.

Antigenetically distinct strains (according to hemagglutinin and neuraminidase) are A, B and C that cause clinical illness as under:

A H_1N_1
A H_3N_2
A H_5N_1
B

At a given point of time, a community would have had exposure to influenza and about 20–25% of community would have had infection in their life time.

Antigenic variation is very common in influenza virus. Sudden, complete and major changes in antigenicity is called *antigenic shift*. Gradual, mild, minor and incomplete changes in antigenicity over a long period are called *antigenic drift*.

First epidemic in the history of medicine was seen in 1,173 and subsequently another 80 epidemics are recorded. To mention some of the epidemics, they are:

1918–1919	Epidemic 20 million cases and 2 million deaths
1934	Epidemic
1947	Epidemic
1957–1958	Epidemic by A/Japan/305/57 (H_2N_2)
1968	Epidemic by A/Hong Kong/1/68 (H_3N_2)
1977	Epidemic
1979	Epidemic by B/Singapore/222/79
2009	Pandemic by Influenza A (H_1N_1) pdm09

Epidemiologically, winter season and overcrowding have been found to influence the disease.

Incubation Period

About 1–3 days.

Virological confirmation is possible in the following Institutions in India:
- Pasteur Institute, Coonoor
- Haffkine Institute, Mumbai
- School of Tropical Medicine, Kolkata AIIMS, New Delhi
- Armed Forces Medical College (AFMC), Pune
- Vallabhbhai Patel (VP) Chest Institute, Delhi

H_1N_1 Swine Flu Pandemic 2009

This rapidly spreads to declare pandemic. Local pandemics are also occurring. In India, epidemic of 2014 is known where 937 cases and a fatality of 218 cases. Here, CFR has been 23.2%. New name of virus came to usage as influenza A (H_1N_1)pdm09. Neuraminidase inhibitors, such as oseltamivir and zanamivir are used in the treatment of pandemic influenza A.

Drugs

Amantadine and rimantadine therapy (100 mg twice daily for 3 days) found effective for treatment.

Control Measures

Control measures are not available and not useful because of antigenic shift.

Being a notifiable disease, it is obligatory to report to Government of India.

Vaccines

Killed vaccine
- Chick embryo harvested, formalin killed vaccine 0.5 mL
- Subcutaneous single dose.

Live attenuated
Administered as nasal drops.

Newer vaccines
- Split virus vaccine
- Neuraminidase specific vaccine
- Recombinant vaccine.

International measures
- Prompt notification to WHO
- Identification of virus type and reporting
- Continued epidemiological studies and exchange of information
- Continuing attempt to mobilize development and production facilities to permit rapid shipment and use of an appropriate vaccine when a new strain appears or when it threatens to become pandemic.

Please *see* Chapter 33 for Avian Influenza.

Meningococcal Meningitis (Cerebrospinal Fever)

It is cerebrospinal fever caused by *Neisseria (N). meningitidis*. Cases and deaths have been reported in India by meningococcal meningitis. In India, Delhi epidemic of 1985 is well known in public health practice.

Acute infection of meningococcal meningitis is characterized by pyrexia, headache, and meningism. This is associated with neck stiffness and meningeal irritation which is demonstrated by the following signs:

Kernig's Sign

With the hip joint flexed, extension at the knee causes spasm in the hamstring muscles.

Brudzinski's Sign

Passive flexion of the neck causes flexion of the thighs and knees.

Several serotypes have been identified which predominantly attack children. Disease occurs more frequently in dry and cold seasons. Common serotypes are:

A, B, C, D, X, Y, 29E and W 135.

Schools, refugee camps, and religious congregations have always been the areas for epidemics.

Case fatality rate of untreated cases is about 75–80% and of treated cases is about 5–10%.

On an average, about 8–10 thousand cases are occurring with 800–900 deaths in a year.

Mode of Transmission

Droplet infection

Incubation period

About 3–4 days

Control

Cases: Penicillin is the drug of choice. Next alternative is Chloramphenicol.

Carrier: Rifampicin

Contact: Rifampicin 600 mg BD for 2 days or sulfadiazine 1 g BD for 2 days.

Mass prophylaxis of selected community in an epidemiological approach is suggested under medical supervision.

Vaccine

- Meningococcal vaccine A (single antigen)
- Meningococcal vaccine C (single vaccine)
- Meningococcal A and C (Double antigen)
- Meningococcal vaccine A, C and Y (Triple antigen).

Vaccine is administered to adults and children above 2 years of age. It is contraindicated in pregnancy. The vaccine gives immunity for 3 years.

High-risk group who visit Mecca, Medina in Saudi Arabia are given polyvalent (A and C) vaccine 2 weeks earlier to the date of their departure.

VECTOR-BORNE INFECTIONS

Malaria

Malaria is one of the most serious diseases to affect people in developing countries with tropical and subtropical climates. It is particularly dangerous for young children and for pregnant women and their unborn children, besides others who may be seriously affected in some circumstances.

Chronic Malaria

In endemic areas, repeated malaria infection causes malaria immune response with parasitic tolerance. Clinically anemia, cachexia, splenomegaly, butterfly pigmentation of face, and low grade fever are manifested.

Major events in the history of malaria

- Ayurvedic period: Vivid picture of disease related with mosquito bite in Charaka period
- Fifth century: Hippocrates has given
- BC: Description of malaria
- Ancient Italy: Malaria in bad air described
- 1880 Laveran: A French army surgeon discovered malaria parasite
- 1891 Romanowsky: Developed staining method
- 1894 Manson: Described mosquito transmission of malaria
- 1897: Ronald Ross discovered malaria parasite (in India) on the stomach wall of anopheles mosquito.
- 1898 Ronald Ross: Outlined (in India) the life cycle of malaria parasite.
- 1898 Bignami, Bastianelli Grassi: (Italian scientists) demonstrated the presence of sporozoites of human malaria in salivary glands of anopheles mosquito.
- 1939: Paul Muller discovered dichlorodiphenyltrichloroethane (DDT).
- 1948: Shortt and Garnham discovered pre-erythrocytic phase.
- 1953: National Malaria Control Programme (NMCP)
- 1958: National Malaria Eradication Programme (NMEP)
- 1961: Focal outbreak
- 1976: Resurgence of malaria
- 1977: Modified Plan of Action
- 1995: Malaria Action Program
- 1998: Roll Back Malaria Initiative
- 1999: National Anti-Malaria Programme
- 2001: Focus on epidemiological types
- 2007: National Drug Policy on Malaria
- 2007–2012,
- 2012–17,
- 2017–2022: Strategic Action Plan for Malaria Control
- 2016–2030: Global Technical Strategy

Malaria is curable and preventable. Main causes of mortality in developing countries are:
- They do not realize, they have malaria (think they have cold, influenza or other infection).
- People living far from health service will often go to local vendors (sellers) for advice (not appropriate) and buy medicine (not effective).
- Many do not know what causes malaria, how it spreads, so they are not able to protect themselves from the disease.

Malaria is caused by *Plasmodium* group of parasites.

Table 9.8: Vector bionomics.

Rural malaria	Urban malaria	Project area malaria	Border malaria
• In irrigated areas	• In cosmopolitan cities	• In construction place and in labor place	• In mixed population
• Transmitted by *Anopheles culicifacies*	• It covers 50 million population	• These are Chloroquine resistant areas	• Poor administration is seen
• Caused by *Plasmodium vivax*	• Transmitted by *A. culicifacies* • Caused by *Plasmodium vivax*		

Vector Bionomics

Refer **Table 9.8**.

Rural area
Anopheles (A). culicifacies, breeds in gentle flowing and stagnant water; flight range 1 mile. It causes epidemic malaria in project and irrigation areas.

Hilly area
A. fluviatilis breeds in slow running water; flight range ½ mile.

Urban area
A. stephensi, breeds in used well and cistern overhead tank; causes epidemic malaria.

Sea coast area
A. sundaicus breeds in salt water.

Tea garden area
A. minimus breeds in slow running water.

Water logging area
A. philippinensis breeds where subsoil water level is high and also in water stagnation between the cracks of soil.

Major Elements of Malaria Transmission

$$Z_0 = \frac{ma^2 bp^a}{-r \log_e P} \text{(MacDonald)}$$

Where Z_0 = (The basic reproduction rate) denotes the number of cases resulting from the seed case in a nonimmunes, i.e., fully susceptible population.

- m = the density of vector mosquitoes
- a = their daily number of bites of man
- b = the proportion of mosquitoes with gland infections having viable sporozoites
- p = the probability of mosquito survival through 1 day
- n = the number of days required for sporogony.
- r = the proportion of infected persons who revert to the uninfected state in a day.

Values of m, a, p, n and $\log_e p$ are given by the bionomics of the vector and the environment conditions.

Vector control measures are used to modify m, p and $\log_e p$ (plus some impact on "a" also). Immunity has major bearing on "b" and r while "b" is, so far, outside the reach of antimalaria measures, a modification of "r" can be achieved through radical and gametocytocidal treatment.

Malarial Parasite (MP) Smear

a. **Making blood films**
   1. *Thin film:* Finger-tip is cleaned with alcohol. After allowing the skin to dry, punctured with sterile blood lancet or needle with a firm quick stab. The first drop which appears is wiped off. A small drop of blood on a clean slide (about 1/2" from the end) is taken, using care that the slide does not touch the skin. Edge of an another slide is placed against first slide with an angle of 35° and drawn up against the blood drop which will immediately run across the end filling the angle between the slides. The upper slide is pushed back along the other slowly to get a thin film. The film is dried in air.
   2. *Thick film:* Three drops of blood close together on the slide is taken with the corner of another slide and it is spread out (enough to show hands of watch through the film). The film is dried in air.

3. *Fixation*: Blood films are dried rapidly in air and fixed by immersing in methyl alcohol for 3 minutes (or ethyl alcohol for 15 minutes).

b. **Staining of blood films**
1. *Original Romanowsky stain:* This depends on action on the compounds formed by the interaction of methylene blue and eosin. The stain gives a reddish purple color to the chromatin of malaria and other parasites. This color is due to a substance which forms when methylene blue is ripened either by age as in polychrome methylene blue or by heating with sodium carbonate.
2. *Modified Romanowsky stain:* (Giemsa stain)
   Leishman stain is prepared as under:
   Leishman powder   1.5 g
   Methanol   to 1,000 mL
   Rinse out a clean staining bottle with methanol. Add a few clean dry glass beads. Add the staining powder and methanol and mix well. The stain is ready to use for the following day.
   Undiluted Leishman stain is poured on dry unfixed blood film and allowed for 3 minutes (methyl alcohol in the stain fixes the film).
   By means of a pipette with rubber teat, buffer solution (equal in quantity) is added. Mixed by gentle blowing allowed for 7 minutes.
   The film is washed in distilled water allowing the preparation to differentiate until the film appears bright pink in color (it takes usually half minute), dried in air.
3. *Modified Romanowsky stain:* (Leishman stain)
   Rapid Method
   Blood films fixed in methyl alcohol for 3 minutes. Diluted Giemsa stain (1:2) is poured and allowed to act for 3 minutes, washed with water for 5 minutes, dried in air.
   Slow Method
   The film is fixed in methyl alcohol for 3 minutes. Diluted Giemsa stain (1:10) is taken in a dish. A piece of glass rod is placed in it. Slide is placed with film downward in the fluid with one end of the slide resting on the rod. After 24 hours, the slide is washed and dried. This method is also useful in staining spirochetes.

c. Malarial parasite (MP) smear by Field Stain
   1. Field stain A from prepared powders
   2. Field stain A powder 5 g
   3. Distilled water heated to 80°C to 600 mL
   4. Field stain B from prepared powders
   5. Field stain B powder 4.8 g
   Distilled water heated to 80°C to 600 mL.
   This is a method which is done in short time and without fixation. Field stain contains solution A and solution B.

Solution A

Methylene blue:	0.8 g
Azure I (Azure B):	0.5 g
Disodium hydrogen phosphate:	5 g (anhydrous)
Potassium dihydrogen phosphate:	6.25 g (anhydrous)
Distilled water:	500 mL

Solution B

Eosin (Yellow and water soluble):	1 g
Disodium hydrogen phosphate:	5 g (anhydrous)
Potassium dihydrogen phosphate:	6.25 g (anhydrous)
Distilled water:	500 mL

Preparation
The phosphate salts are first dissolved, and then the stain is added. Solution of Azure I granules may be facilitated by grinding in a mortar with the phosphate solvent. Each of the prepared solution is set aside for 24 hours and after filtration is ready for use. If precipitate or scum is formed, then again it needs refiltration.

Caution
Eosin solution should be renewed as soon as it becomes greenish.

Procedure
Field stain A and B are kept in separate jars with wide neck which permits the insertion of

Table 9.9: Identification of malaria parasite.

P. vivax	P. malariae	P. ovale	P. falciparum
Increase in size	No increase in size	Oval shape	No increase in size
Schuffner dots+	No Schuffner's dots	irregular	No Schuffner's dots
30–40 merozoites	Band form + 10–15 merozoites	Schuffner's dots + 8–10 merozoites	8–10 merozoites Ring stage +

(P: *Plasmodium*)

slide. The depth of field stain solution should be of 3 inches. This level should be maintained by adding fresh solution from time to time.

Steps

1. Thick film is placed in field stain A for 2 seconds.
2. Then removed and rinsed in clean water for few seconds till glass slide is free from stain.
3. Then placed in field stain B for 1 second.
4. Rinsed in clean water for 3 seconds.
5. Allowed to dry in vertical position.

Identification of Malaria Parasite (Table 9.9)

Malarial parasite smear differentials are illustrated in **Figure 9.25**.

Present picture

World

Every year 500,000,000 cases are occurring, 3,000,000 deaths are occurring that include 1,000,000 child deaths. DALYS lost is 46.48 million annually.

India

- Incidence—8–10 cases per 100,000 population
- Mortality—3–4 deaths per 100,000 population
- 4–6 deaths per 100,000 population in 0–4 age group.

Malaria Statistics during 2005–2007 in India

Total cases = 3.79 million

Total severe malaria cases = 1.7 million

Malaria Statistics during 2016 in India

Total cases = 1.09 million

Total severe malaria cases = 66%

Total deaths due to malaria = 2,762 average annual parasite incidence (API) = 1.62.

Mode of transmission: From the bite of infected female anopheles mosquito.

Incubation period: 10 days.

Clinical stages: Cold stage, hot stage, and sweating stage.

Malariometric Values

- Spleen rate,
- Parasite rate,
- Infant parasite rate,
- Proportional case rate, and
- Annual parasite incidence = (API)

$$= \frac{\text{Confirmed cases}}{\text{Population under surveillance}} \times 1000$$

- Annual blood examination rate = (ABER)

$$= \frac{\text{No. of slides examined}}{\text{Population}} \times 100$$

- Vector indices include sporozoites rate, mosquito density, man biting rate, and inoculation rate.

The epidemiology of malaria is depicted in **Figure 9.26**.

Malaria Control

Case management

Case detection: All fever cases are subjected to laboratory examination under surveillance.

Active surveillance: Fortnightly visit by health worker, who detects fever case or history of fever, collects blood smear for malaria parasite.

Passive surveillance: All health care institutions detect fever case or history of fever, collect blood smear for malaria parasite.

Treatment

Presumptive treatment with chloroquine (in low risk area) (**Table 9.10**).

Presumptive treatment with chloroquine and primaquine (in high risk area) (**Table 9.11**).

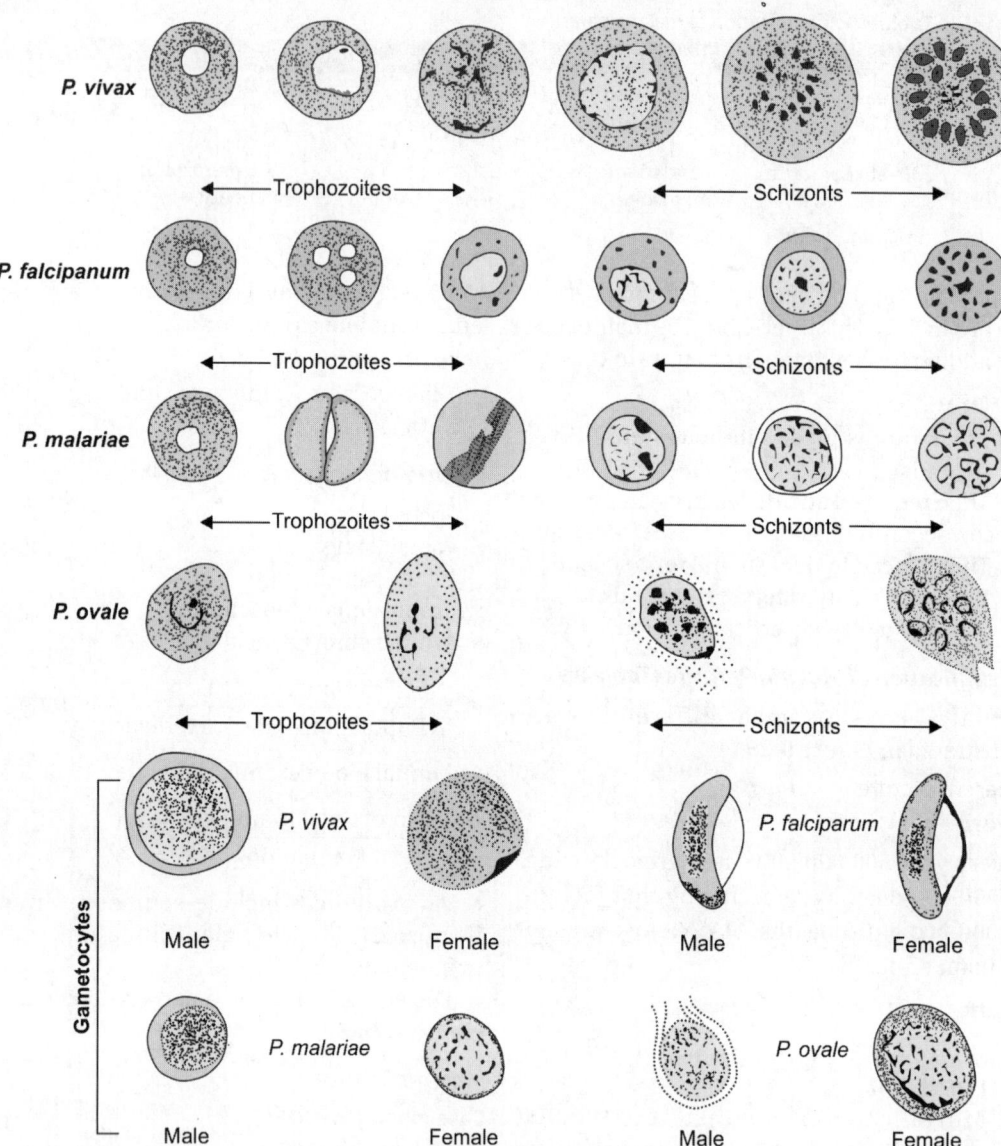

Fig. 9.25: Malaria parasite (MP) smear differentials.

Table 9.10: Presumptive treatment with chloroquine.

Age	Chloroquine	Remarks
Below 1 year	75 mg (½)	Blood smear taken
1–4 years	150 mg (1)	PT given to all
4–8 years	300 mg (2)	After food
8–14 years	450 mg (3)	
Above 14 years	600 mg (4)	

Note: Tablet in parenthesis
(PT: presumptive treatment)

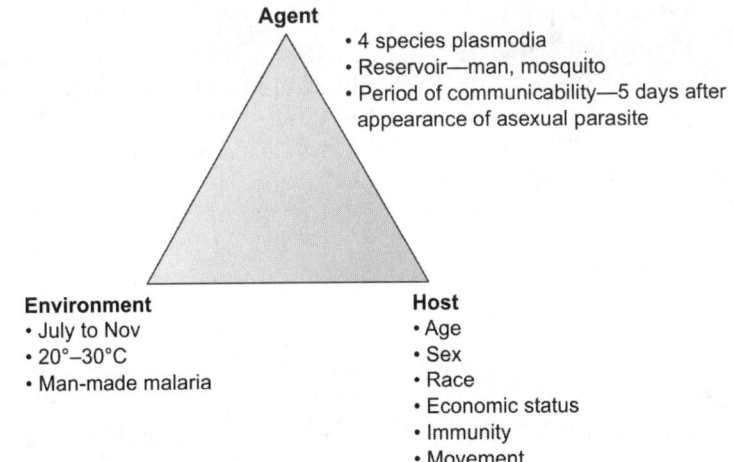

Fig. 9.26: Epidemiological triad in malaria.

Table 9.11: Presumptive treatment with chloroquine and primaquine.

Age	Chloroquine			Primaquine	Remarks
	I day	II day	III day	I day	
Below 1 year	75 mg	75 mg	37.5 mg	-	Blood smear taken
1–4 years	150 mg	150 mg	75 mg	7.5 mg	PT given to all
4–8 years	300 mg	300 mg	150 mg	15 mg	After food
8–14 years	450 mg	450 mg	225 mg	30 mg	No primaquine for pregnant and infant
Above 14 years	600 mg	600 mg	300 mg	45 mg	

Radical Treatment (Tables 9.12 and 9.13)

Table 9.12: Radical treatment in *P. vivax, P. malariae, P. ovale* cases.

Age	Chloroquine	Primaquine	Remarks
Below 1 year	75 mg	-	
1–4 years	150 mg	2.5 mg	
4–8 years	300 mg	5 mg	No primaquine for pregnant, infants
8–14 years	450 mg	10 mg	
Above 14 years	600 mg	15 mg	

(P: *Plasmodium*)

Table 9.13: Radical treatment in *P. falciparum* case.

Age	Chloroquine (mg)			Primaquine (mg)	Remarks
	I day	II day	III day	I day	
Below 1 year	75 mg	75 mg	37.5 mg	-	
1–4 years	150 mg	150 mg	75 mg	7.5 mg	
4–8 years	300 mg	300 mg	150 mg	15 mg	No primaquine for pregnant infant
8–14 years	450 mg	450 mg	225 mg	30 mg	
14 years +	600 mg	600 mg	300 mg	45 mg	

Chloroquine resistant cases (adult dose)
- Presumptive treatment amodiaquine 600 mg or sulfalene 1,000 mg pyrimethamine 50 mg
- Radical treatment
  Sulfalene 1,000 mg pyrimethamine 50 mg single dose primaquine 45 mg
  Chemoprophylaxis (for protection of healthy individuals)
  - Chloroquine 500 mg weekly,
  - Chloroquine 300 mg weekly + proguanil 200 mg daily.
  - Chloroquine 300 mg weekly + pyrimethamine 50 mg daily.

Any one of above regimen till they move about in endemic areas.

Malaria Drug Resistance

Ability of a parasite strain to survive or multiply despite the administration and absorption of a drug in doses equal to the recommended but within the limits of tolerance of the subject. The resistance is tested by administering drug for 7 days results are abbreviated as under:

S = Sensitive: clearance of asexual parasitemia within 7 days

R_1 = Mild resistant: clearance of asexual parasitemia within 7 days followed by recurrence

R_2 = Moderate resistant: only reduction but no clearance of asexual parasitemia within 7 days

R_3 = Severe resistant: No reduction in asexual parasitemia within 7 days.

Public Health Measures

Following public health measures are undertaken:

Area with API above 2:
- Spraying two rounds DDT/three rounds of HCH
- Entomological assessment
- Surveillance
- Case management.

Area with API below 2 should be taken following measures:
- Spraying (focal); if *Plasmodium falciparum* occurs
- Surveillance
- Case management
- Follow-up
- Epidemiological investigations.

Integrated Vector Control

Following measures are undertaken through integrated vector control:
- Residual spray
- Antilarval measures
- Personal protection
- Control of breeding places (intermittent irrigation) (source reduction).

Vaccines

All stages of parasite are used in the preparation and testing of immunity in experimental animals. Research is ongoing with SPf66, PfS25 vaccines for their immunological effect. But the vaccines are not available for community prevention.

Asexual blood stage vaccines and vaccines to arrest the development of the parasite in mosquito are common types under trial funded by United Nations Development Programme (UNDP) and World Bank.

National Level Control Programs

Following programs are observed in the control of malaria in different periods of time:
- 1953 NMCP initiated
- 1958 NMEP initiated
- 1961 Focal outbreaks started
- 1976 Resurgence malaria because of:
  - Administrative failure: Shortage of insecticides, drugs, inadequate budget, diversion of funds, and lack of commitment by health workers
  - Technical failure: DDT resistance, and chloroquine resistance
  - Operational failure: Epidemiological knowledge not properly used, poor surveillance, poor coverage by insecticide spray, and premature take off to succeeding phase.
- 1977 modified plan of operation launched
- 1995 malaria action program initiated:
  - To create awareness among community about cause
  - To encourage community participation
  - To continue control with effective diagnosis and treatment as the main thrust area of the antimalarial month.

Chapter 9: Epidemiology of Communicable Diseases

- 1998 Roll back malaria initiative launched with World Bank Assistance through WHO, UNICEF and UNDP with the following main strategies:
  - To strengthen district malaria activities
  - To motivate for insecticide treated mosquito nets
  - To make health care facility available to all
  - To train health worker in healthcare activities
  - To prepare local community ready (such as mothers, teachers, postman, village *panchayat* member, village health guide, village accountant, etc.)
  - To encourage research on malaria drug and vaccine
- 2001 Focus on epidemiological types of malaria: (a) Urban malaria, (b) Rural malaria, (c) Tribal malaria, (d) Border malaria, and (e) Project area malaria.
  - 2008 National malaria control project
  - 2016 Global technical strategy
  - 2016 National framework for malaria elimination
  - 2017 National strategic plan for elimination by 2022.

National Anti-malaria Program

Government of India dropped the term NMEP and renamed the program as National Anti-Malaria Programme (NAMP) in the year 1999.

The anti-malaria activities were intensified with additional inputs in selected districts of Madhya Pradesh, Rajasthan, Orissa, Gujarat, Maharashtra, Bihar, and Andhra Pradesh. Total intensification of activities in cities of Karnataka, West Bengal and Tamil Nadu World Bank supported this enhanced malaria control project. Components strengthened were:
- Case detection and treatment
- Use of insecticide treated mosquito nets
- Integrated vector control
- Use of larvivorous fish
- Intersectoral coordination.

Information education and communication (IEC) activities were enhanced with more funds. Blister packs for RT were provided. Other provisions in NAMP were synthetic pyrethroids, bed nets, rapid diagnostic kits, and arteether injections.

Tenth five year plan (2002–2007) has the goals of:
- Annual blood examination rate to more than 10%
- Annual parasite index to 1.3
- About 25% reduction of morbidity and mortality due to malaria by 2007
- About 50% reduction of morbidity and mortality due to malaria by 2010.

Activities under National Malaria Surveillance
- Health worker male covers 5,000 population in subcenter area
- Visits all houses once in 15 days
- Collects MP smear for fever cases and gives PT
- Gets MP smear tested at PHC and collects the results
- All positive cases are given RT
- Collects information on all fever cases, all immigrated fever cases, all emigrated fever cases from concerned houses where fever cases detected.
- If MP smear positive for plasmodium falciparum, he collects blood smear of neighboring 20 houses and gives PT to all such cases.
- If MP positive in contacts, he screens the whole village.

Please *refer* Chapter 33 for Severe Malaria.

Algorithm for Malarial Parasite (MP) Slide Preparation

Algorithm is a procedure to solve the problem of MP slide preparation. Manpower and time is reduced by using automated computational techniques. This involves check in morphology, check on analysis of colors.

Algorithm has higher predictive rate. Algorithm can identify malaria parasite in less perfect dirty slides. Hence, it is powerful and robust method in MP slide preparation.

Algorithm has higher prediction rate.

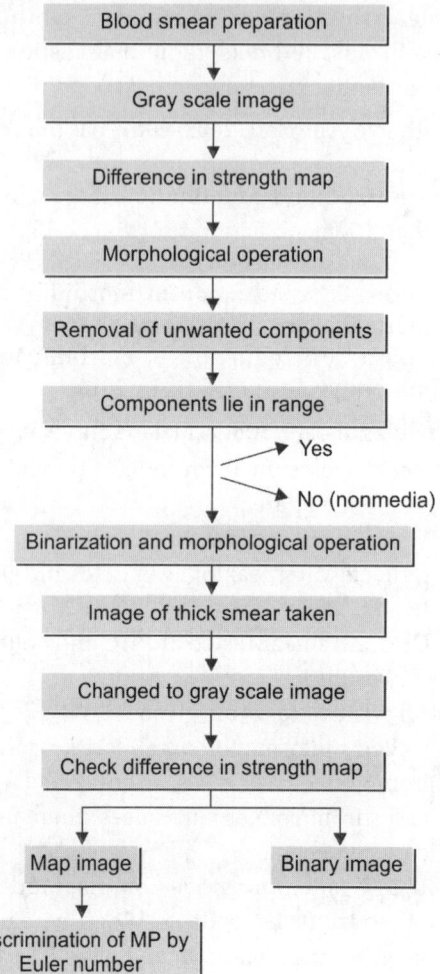

Filaria

Filaria is the major public health problem in India caused by *Wuchereria (W). bancrofti, Brugia (B). malayi* and *Brugia (B). timori* and is transmitted by mosquitoes. Filaria is manifested in the form of lymphangitis, lymphadenitis, elephantiasis of leg, arm, genital, tropical pulmonary eosinophilia (occult filaria) and arthritis.

Type	Caused by	Transmitted by
Urban filarial	*W. bancrofti*	*Culex* mosquito
Rural filarial	*B. malayi*	*Mansonia* mosquito

Nocturnal periodicity is a predominant character of filaria. Third stage larva in mosquito is infective form with an extrinsic incubation period of 10–14 days.

Periodicity

It is the biological adaptation to the nocturnal biting habits of mosquitoes. Maximum microfilariae are present during 10 PM to 2 AM.

Problem

World load of filaria is about 140 million population.

India load is about 20 million cases. High endemic states are Tamil Nadu, Orissa, Andhra Pradesh, Uttar Pradesh, Bihar, Jharkhand, Kerala, and Gujarat.

The epidemiological triad in filaria is depicted in **Figure 9.27**.

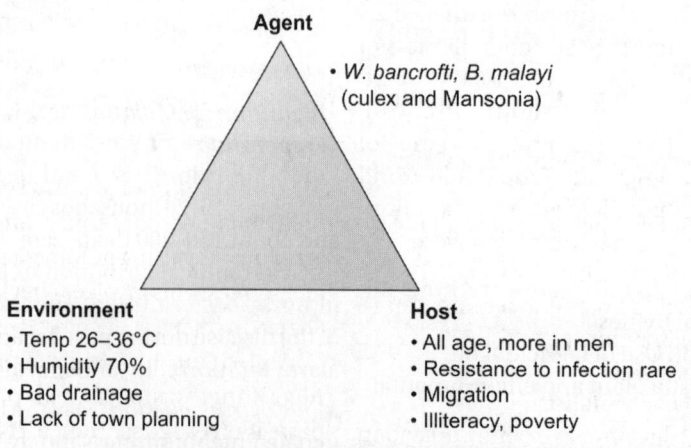

Fig. 9.27: Epidemiological triad in filaria.
(*W. bancrofti: Wuchereria bancrofti; B. malayi: Brugia malayi*)

Filaria Survey

- Clinical examination of cases
- Mass blood survey with thick film, 5% population for screening and 20% for evaluation survey
- Mass blood survey with membrane filter concentration method and diethylcarbamazine (DEC) provocative test (100 mg oral is given and blood smear is taken after 1 hour) in selected samples. DEC provocated microfilariae appear in ¼ hour and decrease in 2 hours
- Parasite antigen detection tests
- Mosquito dissection and examination (Xenodiagnosis) after entomological survey.

Filariometric values

- Prevalence of chronic filaria (elephantiasis, hydrocele, etc.)
- Microfilaria rate,
- Filaria endemicity rate,
- Microfilaria density (vector density)
- Average infestation rate.

Filaria control

The major ways to control filaria are:

- Case detection by clinical and laboratory tests.
- **Treatment:**
  Diethylcarbamazine (DEC) 6 mg/kg for 12 days in divided doses after food.
  Ivermectin 200 µg per kg body weight (200–400 µg range), single dose, clears microfilaria.
  In highly endemic areas, following community approach is undertaken:
  - DEC mass therapy to all in highly endemic areas
  - DEC selective treatment to microfilaria positive cases
  - DEC salt 1 g DEC per 1 kg of salt (1–4 g range)
  - Community health guide training in antifilaria activities
- **Vector control:** Use of larvicidal oil.
- Removal of pistia plant and environmental measures.

Now, filaria control has become simple by the available approaches, such as:

- Safe single dose annual treatment with DEC
- Single dose Ivermectin
- Hygiene of affected limb or part
- DEC medicated table salt
- Sealing of water seals or water tank with polystyrene beads.

Indicators of Filaria Control

- Below 5% microfilaria rate in the community
- Zero prevalence of microfilaria among children aged 1–10 years in the community
- National Filaria Control Programme is detailed in Chapter 21.

Kala-azar

Kala-azar is a protozoal infection caused by *Leishmania (L). donovani, L. tropica* and *L. braziliensis* causing visceral, cutaneous and mucocutaneous leishmaniasis. These clinical manifestations are known as kala-azar, oriental sore and espundia which are common infections in man.

Depending upon the manifestation, lesions are abbreviated as under:

VL	Visceral leishmaniasis
CL	Cutaneous leishmaniasis
MCL	Mucocutaneous leishmaniasis
ACL	Anthroponotic cutaneous leishmaniasis
ZCL	Zoonotic cutaneous leishmaniasis
PKDL	Postkala-azar dermal leishmaniasis.

World Picture

The disease is endemic in 88 countries.

Indian Picture

The disease is endemic and epidemic in the states of Assam, West Bengal, Bihar, Uttar Pradesh, Sikkim, Orissa, and Tamil Nadu. Every year about 15–20 thousands cases are occurring and about 150–200 deaths are occurring.

Geographic distribution in India is mainly in north-eastern India. The increasing trend of the disease during past decade has given an alarm for morbidity and mortality (**Fig. 9.28**).

Mode of transmission: May the bite of infected female Phlebotomine 'sand fly'.

Incubation Period: 1–4 months.

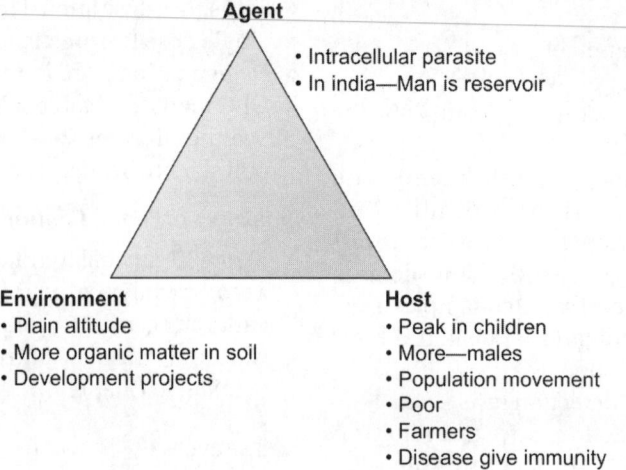

Fig. 9.28: Epidemiological triad in kala-azar.

Diagnosis

Demonstration of Donovan bodies in the aspirations.
- Leukopenia and increased erythrocyte sedimentation rate (ESR)
- Serum tests **(Fig. 9.29)**
- Culture NNN media (Novy-MacNeal-Nicolle) and staining (Giemsa).

Kala-azar Control

- **Treatment of cases:** Sodium stibogluconate (pentavalent antimony compound).
    - 10 mg/kg for 20 days or pentamidine isethionate (diamidine compound)
    - 3 mg/kg for 10 days
- Identification of human reservoir and treatment (no animal reservoir is reported in India).
- Vector control combined with sanitation measures.
- Protection from sand fly bites by specified measures.

Dengue Syndrome

Dengue syndrome constitutes:
- Undifferentiated dengue fever
- Actual dengue fever
- Dengue hemorrhagic fever (DHF) without shock
- DHF with shock.

The natural history of dengue syndrome is given in **Figure 9.30.**

In India, epidemics are occurring and creating public health problem. Major epidemic is recorded in 1996. Another epidemic is recorded in 1998 when pandemic of dengue syndrome was seen across the countries. In India every year, on an average 12,000 cases are occurring and about 200 deaths are occurring. In 2006 epidemic of India, total cases recorded are 8,180 and death count to 144. In Delhi, epidemic alone total cases were 2,458 with 55 deaths in the year 2006. Classical dengue known as *break bone fever* is caused by four serotypes. *Aedes aegypti* mosquito is the main vector. DHF is clinically differentiated into four grades depending upon bleeding and shock. Hemoconcentration and thrombocytopenia help in diagnosis.

Common breeding places of vectors are found to be discarded tin, broken bottle, fire bucket, flower pot, earthen pot, tree hole, tyer, overhead tank, water cooler, flower vase, and defreeze container of fridge.

Diagnosis is done by clinical examination for fever, hemorrhage, positive tourniquet test (above 20 petechiae per square inch).

Incubation period is commonly 5–6 days.

Dengue Control

- Preventive measures to be taken to control dengue:

Chapter 9: Epidemiology of Communicable Diseases

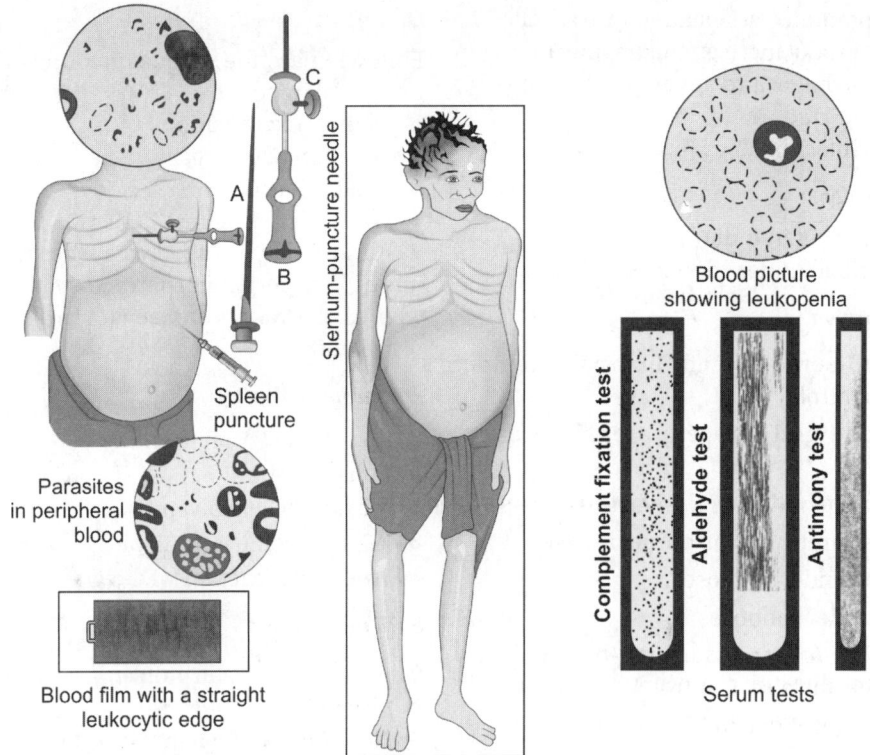

Fig. 9.29: Organs involvement and laboratory tests in kala-azar.

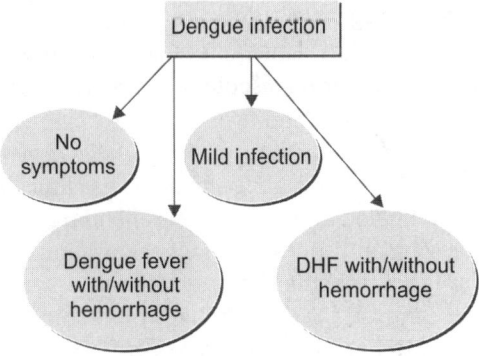

Fig. 9.30: Natural history of dengue syndrome.
(DHF: dengue hemorrhagic fever)

- Control of vector breeding places
- Screening of rooms
- Use of mosquito repellent
❖ Control of patient, contact and environment:
  - Obligatory reporting
  - 5 days selective isolation of case
  - Contact investigation, search of undiagnosed cases
❖ Epidemic measures:
  - Vector density determination and elimination
  - Mosquito control
  - Repellents use by people who are occupationally exposed
❖ International measures:
  Enforcement of provisions of international agreement in ship, airplane and land transport.

Arboviral Infections

Arboviral infections are viral infections always occurring in nature, transmitted by arthropods. There are more than 40 arboviral infections recorded in India. Many of them are named after places such as Japanese encephalitis (JE), West Nile fever, Kyasanur forest disease (KFD), Chittur fever, Ganjam fever, Vellore fever, etc.

Other common classifications are as follows:
- Fever producing, e.g., chikungunya, dengue
- Hemorrhage and fever producing, e.g., DHF, KFD
- Brain infection, e.g., JE.

Yellow Fever
- Not present in India
- Described under zoonoses.

Chikungunya
Mosquito-borne fever and limb pain. Control: Vector control.

Described under recent area of interest, Chapter 33.

Dengue: See under vector-borne diseases.

DHF: See under vector-borne disease.

KFD: See under zoonoses.

JE: See under zoonoses.

West Nile fever: Mosquito-borne fever, headache, malaise. Control: Vector control.

Sand fly fever: Seen in Maharashtra. Control: Vector control.

Epidemic hemorrhagic fever: Also called hemorrhagic fever with renal syndrome probably transmitted by tick.

Others
- O' nyong nyong (mosquito)
- Semliki Forest disease (mosquito)
- St Louis encephalitis (mosquito)
- Murray valley fever (mosquito), and
- Russian spring summer fever (tick)
- Omsk hemorrhagic fever (tick).

Rickettsial Infections
These are diseases by rickettsiae organisms transmitted by arthropods.

Common Pathology
- Parasites attack vascular endothelium [Heart, central nervous system (CNS), lung, kidney, and muscle]
- Produce perivascular reaction (nodule of Fraenkel)
- Cause thrombosis and hemorrhage. Incubation period: 10–12 days.

Diagnosis
Following are the diagnostic procedures for rickettsial infections:
- Clinical examination
- Isolation of organism
- Agglutination
- Weil-Felix (proteins OX19, OXk).

Almost all types produce rashes which are more in the peripheral part, except tick typhus where more rashes are seen toward the center of the body.

Epidemic Typhus
- *Rickettsia (R). prowazekii*
- Louse-borne
- Mostly CNS involvement
- Killed vaccine is available
- Weil-Felix reaction (OX_{19}, OX_2).

Endemic Typhus
- *R. mooseri*
- Flea-borne
- Neill-Mooser Reaction (scrotal swelling +)
- Weil-Felix reaction (OX_{19}, OX_2).

Scrub Typhus
- *R. tsutsugamushi*
- Infective larval mite (Trombicula akamushi)
- Usually, cardiovascular system (CVS) and lung are involved.

Other Typhus
- *R. conori*
- *R. australis*
- Transmitted by ticks
- Weil-Felix reaction (OX_{19}, OX_2, OXk).

Rocky Mountain Spotted Fever
- *R. rickettsii*
- Tick-borne
- Neill-Mooser reaction (scrotal necrosis +)
- Weil-Felix reaction (OX_{19}, OX_2, OXk).

Query (Q) fever
- *R. burnetii*
- Vector (not specific).

Rickettsial pox
- *R. akari*
- Mite-borne.

Trench fever
- Rochalimaea quintana
- Louse-borne.

Prevention and Control
- **Treatment:** General specific
- **Prophylaxis:** Vector control
- Health education.

Zika Viral Infection
See Chapter 33.

SURFACE INFECTIONS

Sexually Transmitted Diseases

They are group of classical venereal diseases and other of late inclusion of sexually transmitted diseases (STD). They are called social diseases because stigma is attached to them. The word venereal disease has come from Venus, the Goddess of Love. Of late, it is replaced by the word sexually transmitted diseases due to the mode of transmission. The epidemiological triad in STD is given in **Figure 9.31** and **Table 9.14**.

Incubation Period

Syphilis—10–90 days—10 weeks.
Gonorrhea—2–10 days—1 week
Chancroid—1–5 days—5 days.
LGI—3–20 days—2 weeks
Granuloma inguinale 10–60 days—8 weeks.

Major public health relevance
- Not socially acceptable
- Attached with low morale
- Traditional remedy masks STD
- Not fatal, and
- Signs and symptoms not visible.

Misconceptions in STD
- Sign of growing adolescence
- Signs of maturity
- By eating betel leaves
- Intercourse with menstruating women
- Sin committed in past life.

Major social factors in STD
- Broken home
- Prostitution
- Emotional immaturity.

Laboratory Tests

Following are the laboratory tests:
- Direct examination
- Culture
- Venereal disease research laboratory (VDRL)
- Biopsy.

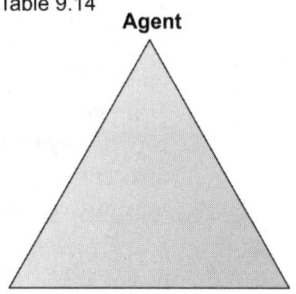

Important causatives agents are listed in Table 9.14

Agent

Environment
Prostitution
Broken home
Easy money
Travel
Social stigma
Alcoholism
Independent personality

Host
Age 20–30 years
Morbidity is high
Single, divorced, separated
Low socioeconomic group
Urban migration

Fig. 9.31: Epidemiological triad in STDs.
(STDs: sexually transmitted diseases)

Table 9.14: Important causative agents of STD.

Sexually transmitted	World	India	Non-STD
First generation STD			
Syphilis	12 million	1–2%	Pinta (Skin infection)
Gonorrhea	62 million	-	Bejel (No primary lesion and no severe manifestations)
Chancroid	2 million	-	
LGV	-	5% of STD	
Granuloma inguinale	-	7% of STD	Yaws endemic, 50 million
Second generation STD			
Scabies genitalia	-	-	
T. vaginalis	170 million	-	
Thrush	-	-	
Herpes simplex	-	-	
Genital warts	-	-	
Hepatitis B	-	-	
Genital Molluscum	-	-	
Vaginitis by Candida albicans	-	-	
Third generation STD			
HIV/AIDS	46 million	5 million	

(HIV/AIDS: human immunodeficiency virus/acquired immunodeficiency syndrome; STD: sexually transmitted diseases; LGV: lymphogranuloma venereum; T. vaginalis: Trichomonas vaginalis)

Lymphogranuloma venereum (LGV) Frei test, 0.1 mL intradermal 48 hours result >6 m positive.

Syndrome-based Approach

Syndrome approach is a method of management and control of STDs where diagnosis and treatment is based on a group of symptoms and signs. Treatment is targeted toward all diseases that could cause that syndrome. It allows diagnosis without extensive laboratory tests and treatment within a single visit. This approach is relevant in the context of Indian condition where laboratory facilities for diagnosis are limited. Syndrome-based approach for five field approach is:

- Genital ulcers
- Vaginal discharge (no speculum examination)
- Vaginal discharge (with speculum examination)
- Urethral discharge
- Lower abdominal pain in the female called pelvic inflammatory disease (PID).

Control

- Diagnosis and treatment through syndrome approach and etiological approach. Clinical facility provides effective case management.
- Follow-up.
- Social therapy (health and sex education counseling).
- AIDS surveillance where STD data is collected, compiled, analyzed and disseminated for necessary action.
- Plan to define problem, to identify priorities, to set objectives and plan out intervention strategies.
- Strategies include case detection by screening, contact tracing, cluster testing, case holding and treatment, contact treatment, personal prophylaxis by mechanical barriers and creating health awareness by health education.
- Supportive therapy with the following:
  - Establishment of STD clinic for all possible STD services
  - Laboratory tests for diagnosis
  - Integration into public health care system
  - Notification
  - Surveillance
  - Legal Immoral Traffic (Prevention) Act 1986
  - Good living conditions
  - Rehabilitation of prostitutes.

Yaws

About 400 million people are at risk in the world and about 100 million active yaws are present in the world.

Yaws is endemic in Andhra Pradesh, Chhattisgarh and Odisha states of our country.

Mother yaw
It is primary lesion appearing after incubation of 3–5 weeks which is extragenital.

Crab Yaw
It is the destructive lesion on sole and palm.

Gangosa
It is the destructive lesion of nose and palate.

Goundu
Osteoperiostitis of superior maxillary bone. The epidemiological triad in Yaws is shown in **Figure 9.32**.

Incubation period: **3–5 weeks**

Differentiated from syphilis by the following:
- Not congenital
- No CNS involvement

Yaws eradication program with survey and treatment:
Total mass treatment: Above 10% prevalence.
Juvenile mass treatment: 5–10%.
Specific mass treatment: Below 5%.

Human Immunodeficiency Virus/Acquired Immunodeficiency Syndrome (HIV/AIDS)

Introduction

Acquired immunodeficiency syndrome is caused by human immunodeficiency virus. It is a serious disorder of the immune system in which the body's normal defenses against infection break down, leaving it vulnerable to a host of life-threatening infections, including unusual malignancies. Once infected by HIV/AIDS, man will have infection for life. Last stage of HIV infection is AIDS.

Human immunodeficiency virus-1 causes acquired immunodeficiency syndrome that was first recognized in 1981. Less aggressive illness is caused by HIV-2.

In case of HIV/AIDS, opportunistic infections seen in the order of highest number of cases are as under:
- Tuberculosis
- Candidiasis
- PCP (*Pneumocystis carinii* pneumonia)
- Herpes
- Para infections
- Cryptosporidiosis
- Toxoplasmosis
- Kaposi sarcoma
- Others.

Significant clinical findings are anemia, neutropenia and thrombocytopenia in most of the cases.

HIV/AIDS is a big social problem which inhibits patients to be nearer to society; people and health workers do not touch them and even patients lose their job when once they are known to be HIV/AIDS.

Also, known as "Slim Disease" because of huge weight loss.

Window Period

During window period diagnostic tests give negative result. Commonly window period is 6–24 weeks during which period no antibodies develop. Correctly to define, it is the period from infection to appearance of detectable HIV antibody in blood.

Global Picture

Out of 369.2 million people living with HIV/AIDS 43% are women. South-East Asia accounts for 4.06 million cases.

Indian Picture

HIV has crossed 5 million and about 86,000 AIDS cases are reported. Cumulative

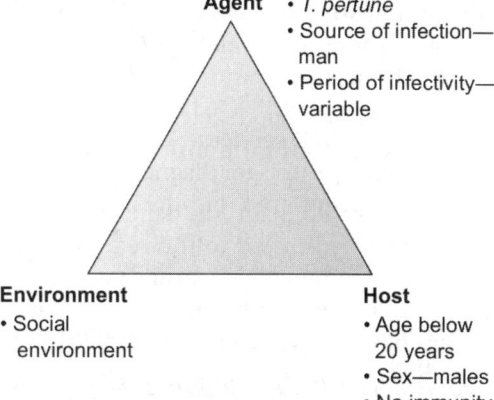

Fig. 9.32: Epidemiological triad in yaws.

seropositivity is 20.0%. Among AIDS cases, 72.1% are males.

The distribution of HIV cases in India is given in **Table 9.15**. HIV prevalence among antenatal clinic (ANC) is high in Northern and Southern states of the country (**Fig. 9.33**).

National AIDS Control Organization, Ministry of Health and Family Welfare (FW), Government of India use following formula to estimate HIV infection among adult population.

Table 9.15: The distribution of HIV cases in India.

High prevalence Above 5% HIV Above 1% ANC positive	Moderate prevalence Above 5% HIV Below 1% ANC positive	Low prevalence Below 5% HIV Below 1% ANC positive
Maharashtra Tamil Nadu Karnataka Andhra Pradesh Nagaland	Gujarat Goa Puducherry	Arunachal Pradesh Assam Bihar Chhattisgarh Haryana Himachal Pradesh Jammu and Kashmir Jharkhand Kerala Madhya Pradesh Manipur Meghalaya Mizoram Odisha Punjab Rajasthan Sikkim Tripura Uttaranchal Uttar Pradesh West Bengal Andaman and Nicobar Chandigarh Dadra and Nagar Haveli Daman and Diu Delhi Lakshadweep

(HIV: human immunodeficiency virus; ANC: antenatal clinic)

$$V = \frac{P}{T} \times R$$

Where,
V = Estimate of burden of HIV P = HIV positive cases
T = Tested sample number R = Population size.

The distribution of HIV in Indian territory is given in **Table 9.15**.

Determinants: Described in **Figure 9.34**.

Distribution
- **World:** 33.2 million
- **South-East Asia:** 4.06 million
- **India:** 2.4 million
- **Seroprevalence rate India:** 20.0%
- **ANC HIV:** 1–2%
- Females are prone for seropositive (HIV)
- Males are prone for disease (AIDS)
- Number of healthcare workers with documented HIV/AIDS = 59
- Number of possible occupationally acquired HIV/AIDS = 164.

Risk groups (Fig. 9.35)
- Presence of STD, frequency of unprotected sex
- Drug users, lymphopenia.

Natural History of HIV/AIDS

Stage 1: Primary infection (normal CD_4 count) Infection with HIV results in rapid proliferation of the virus in blood and lymph nodes. The infected person may experience a seroconversion illness, which usually resolves within weeks. The CD_4 cell count declines rapidly before virus is controlled by the immune system, whereupon the count returns to near normal.

Stage 2: Early immunodeficiency (CD_4 >500) During stage 2, the immune system has controlled the virus, which is largely restricted to lymphoid tissue. In this, the damage inflicted by the virus is limited to the regenerative capacity of the immune system and people with HIV are usually without symptoms. CD_4 count will be above 500 per microliter in this stage.

Stage 3: Intermediate immunodeficiency (200–500)

Chapter 9: Epidemiology of Communicable Diseases

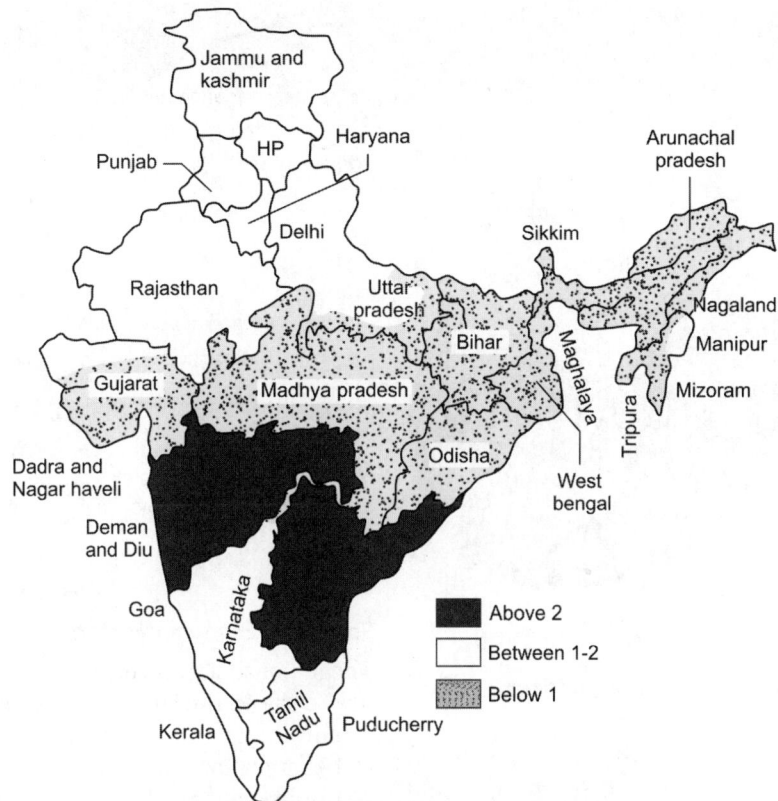

Fig. 9.33: HIV prevalence among ANC cases.
(HIV: human immunodeficiency virus; ANC: antenatal clinic)

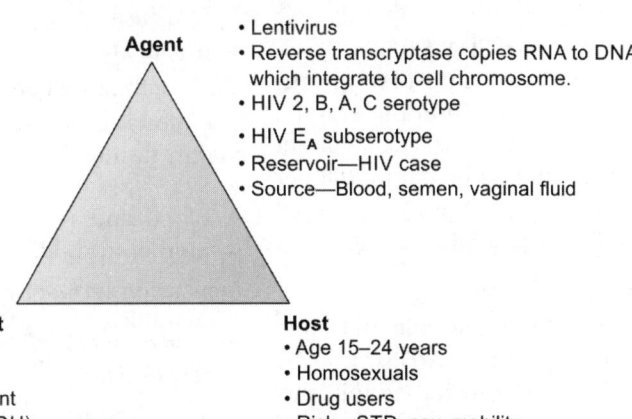

Agent
- Lentivirus
- Reverse transcryptase copies RNA to DNA which integrate to cell chromosome.
- HIV 2, B, A, C serotype
- HIV E_A subserotype
- Reservoir—HIV case
- Source—Blood, semen, vaginal fluid

Environment
- Literacy
- Urban
- Imprisonment
- Drug use (IDU)
- Alcohol use
- Economic
- Sex practice (MSM)
- War
- Civil unrest
- No intervention
- Condom acceptance
- Culture, Taboo, Scar

Host
- Age 15–24 years
- Homosexuals
- Drug users
- Risk—STD, sex, mobility
- Immunity

Fig. 9.34: Epidemiological triad in HIV/AIDS.
(HIV: human immunodeficiency virus; STD: sexually transmitted disease; RNA: ribonucleic acid; DNA: deoxyribonucleic acid; AIDS: acquired immunodeficiency syndrome)

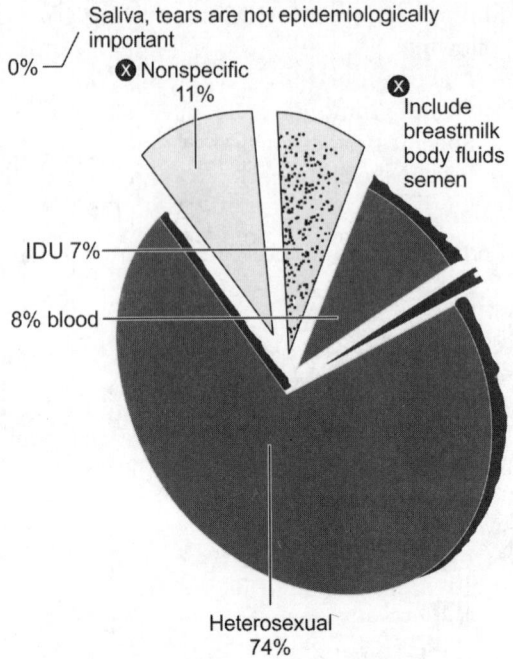

Fig. 9.35: Source of infection.

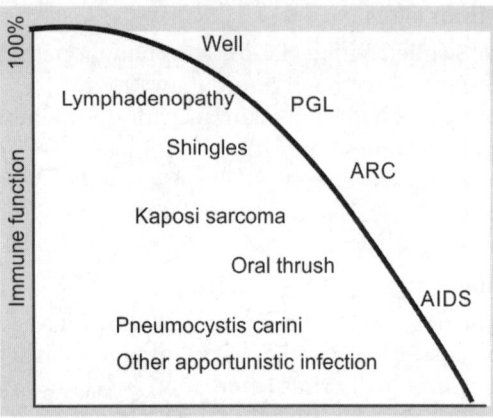

Fig. 9.36: Immune function observed in NHD. (ARC: aids-related complex; PGL: persistent generalized lymphadenopathy; AIDS: acquired immunodeficiency syndrome)

In this stage, viral replication is very high and CD4 cell turnover is rapid. Subtle signs and symptoms indicating compromise of immune system begin to appear. CD4 cell count will be 200–500 per microliter.

Stage 4: Terminal (below CD4 200)

The virus which proliferate throughout the body, overcomes the immune system. Major opportunistic infections take an upper hand. CD4 cell count will be below 200 per microliter. This is the stage of advanced immunodeficiency (**Fig. 9.36**).

Political and Cultural Factors

Following are the political and cultural factors which have a bearing on HIV/AIDS:
- Acceptability of certain indigenous sex practice
- War and civil disturbances
- Limitation on intervention
- Social nonacceptance of condom
- Women status
- National policies
- Norms and practices
- Culture and ethnic practices
- Marginalized population.

Social and Economic Factors

The major social and economic factors which have a say on the HIV/AIDS are as following:
- Low literacy
- Urbanization
- Imprisonment
- High mobility
- Migration and separation from families
- Drug use
- Alcohol use.

Mode of transmission

The modes of transmission of HIV/AIDS are mainly through:
- Sex
- Blood, and
- Mother to child.

Incubation period: Not certain

Human Immunodeficiency Virus (HIV) and Tuberculosis

In India, where most people are susceptible to tuberculosis infection, people with HIV often develop resistant strains of TB. These two interact in several ways.

Clinical diagnosis of acquired immunodeficiency syndrome (AIDS)

If a person above 12 years has 2 major signs and 1 minor sign is defined as CASE for AIDS surveillance.

Minor signs
- Swollen lymph glands (lymphadenopathy)
- Persistent cough (more than 1 month)
- Generalized itchy skin (pruritic dermatitis)
- Recurrent herpes zoster
- Chronic, generalized herpes simplex
- Candidiasis in mouth and throat
- Progressive disseminated herpes simplex.

Major signs
The major signs of AIDS are as following:
- Loss of weight (below 10% of body weight)
- Chronic diarrhea (more than 1 month)
- Prolonged fever (more than 1 month).

Case
Following conditions if present in a person who is HIV positive, then also it is a CASE for AIDS surveillance:
- Cachexia, diarrhea or fever or both for over a month
- Cryptococcal meningitis
- Pulmonary or nonpulmonary TB
- Kaposi sarcoma
- Neurological impairment by trauma or cerebrovascular accident
- Candidiasis of esophagus
- Life-threatening pneumonia
- Invasive cancer (Ca) cervix.

Laboratory tests
Following are the laboratory test available for AIDS:
a. Sensitive test to detect HIV antibody—enzyme-linked immunosorbent assay (ELISA)
b. Confirmatory test to detect specific antibody (p24, gp 41)—western blot
c. Absolute CD4 lymphocyte count, below 200 cells per microliter
d. Virus isolation is costly and not practiced.

Preventive measures
The major preventive measures against AIDS are as given below:
A. AIDS education on nature, transmission and prevention of AIDS.
B. Counseling in HIV infection and face to face communication to help person to make decision and act according to them.

Main functions of AIDS counseling are as following:
- Prevention
- Health promotion
- Specific protection, and
- Psychosocial support.

Counseling
Requirement of AIDS counseling are:
- Rapport
- Acceptance
- Accessibility
- Consistency and accuracy, and
- Confidentiality.

Pretest counseling consists of: (a) personal history and assessment of risk, (b) assessment of factors and knowledge.
- It explores patient's knowledge about HIV
- It helps to cope with HIV positive status if the test turns out to be positive.
- We can tell about test procedure, about HIV result.
- It helps to get informed consent.

Post-test counseling for both negative and positive cases.
- There may not be any problem where test is negative.
- If positive, it helps to provide emotional support.
- It helps to adopt treatment modalities.
- Overcomes fear of disclosure
- Overcomes fear of discrimination
- Help in telling about safer sex
- Convey message about needle exchange
- Help to modify sex behavior
- Can protect uninfected partners.

Treatment
Antiretroviral treatment by:
- **Nucleoside analogs:**
  - Zidovudine (AZT) 100 mg tablet oral 2 TDS
  - Lamivudine (3TC) 150 mg in 2 divided doses oral
  - Didanosine (ddl) 300 mg in 2 divided doses oral
  - Abacavir 300 mg in 2 divided doses oral
  - Stavudine (d4T) 40 mg in 2 divided doses oral
  - Zalcitabine (ddC) 0.75 mg in 3 divided doses oral.

- **Nucleotide analog:** Tenofovir 300 mg once a day oral.
- **Protease inhibitors:**
  - Saquinavir 600 mg in 3 divided doses oral
  - Lopinavir 400 mg in 2 divided doses oral
  - Amprenavir 1.2 g in 2 divided doses oral
  - Nelfinavir 750 mg in 3 divided doses oral
  - Ritonavir 600 mg in 2 divided doses oral
  - Indinavir 0.8 g in 3 divided doses oral.
- **Nonnucleoside reverse transcriptase inhibitors (NNRTI):**
  - Nevirapine 200 mg once a day for 15 days followed by 100 mg BD oral
  - Efavirenz 0.6 g daily oral
  - Delavirdine 400 mg in 3 divided doses oral.

Approach to Antiretroviral Combination Therapy

- **First line of treatment:**
  - Zidovudine with Lamivudine
  - Zidovudine with Didanosine
  - Zidovudine with Zalcitabine
- **Second line of treatment:**
  - Saquinavir with Zidovudine
  - Indinavir with Zidovudine
  - Stavudine with Lamivudine
  - Stavudine with Didanosine
- **Third line of treatment:**
  - Saquinavir with Indinavir with Zidovudine
  - Nevirapine with Didanosine with Zidovudine
  - Nelfinavir with Zidovudine.

Human Immunodeficiency Virus (HIV) Vaccine

Candidate vaccines have been tried which of course gave some promising results. But none of the vaccine is found effective against HIV- IC strains found in India. World Health Organization has given priority for the development of preventive vaccine. Other types of vaccines that are under trial are perinatal vaccine and therapeutic or postinfectious vaccine.

The National Institute of Allergy and Infectious Diseases have supported all clinical trial of HIV vaccine. Since 1987, about 31 different preventive vaccine candidates in National Institute of Allergy and Infectious Diseases (NIAID) funded clinical trials have been conducted. Types of experimental vaccines are Subunit vaccine, Live vaccine, Peptide vaccine, Killed vaccine, and Live attenuated vaccine.

Needle Prick Injury

Immediate blood testing for core antigen.

Azidothymidine (AZT) monotherapy started within 2 hours of exposure.

National AIDS Control Organization (NACO) guideline is followed for postexposure treatment free of cost to health workers.

Further action is based on the test result.

Accidental exposures to HIV are 0.3%. Prevention is the main strategy to avoid occupational exposure to HIV. Use of protective barrier, such as latex or vinyl gloves, heavy duty rubber glove at cleaning, gloves and apron at surgery, protective eye wear and safe handling of sharps. In case of needle prick or an injury where the person is exposed, steps taken are:

To wash the injury with soap and water splash to the nose, mouth skin should be flushed with water.

- Eyes are irrigated with clean water
- One should not put pricked finger into mouth
- One should report to authorities
- Postexposure prophylaxis is recommended.

When source material are blood, bloody fluid or other potentially infectious material, determination of the exposure code (EC) and determination of HIV status code (HIVSC) as EC1, EC2, EC3, EC4 and HIVSC1, HIVSC2, HIVSC unknown, will help in case management with recommended prophylaxis.

Specific prophylaxis: Against opportunistic infections sterilization to ensure protection. By steam and by dry heat:

High level infection by boiling 20 minutes Sodium hypochlorite (0.5%):

Advantages	Disadvantages
Bactericidal	Corrodes metal
Virucidal	Deteriorate rapidly
Inexpensive	
Easily available	

Chemical disinfectants are:
  Ethanol/propanol/alcohol/spirit (70%)
  Polyvidone iodine (2.5%)
  Formaldehyde/Formalin (4%)
  Chloramine (2%),
  Gluteral/Glutaraldehyde (2%)
  Hydrogen peroxide (6%).

Surface and spills: Sodium hypochlorite solution (0.5–1.0%).

HIV/AIDS Surveillance

Collection of epidemiological information of sufficient accuracy and completeness regarding the distribution and spread of HIV to be relevant to the planning, implementation, and monitoring with following steps:
- Collection of data
- Compilation of data
- Analysis of data
- Action
- Feedback.

The methods of HIV testing are as follows:
- Voluntary confidential testing
- Voluntary anonymous testing
- Unlinked anonymous testing, and
- Mandatory testing.

National AIDS Control Program

1987 National AIDS Control Programme started with the following objectives:
- To reduce the HIV spread
- To decrease morbidity and mortality rate, and
- To minimize socioeconomic impact.

1992 National AIDS Control Organization was set up. As 100% centrally sponsored project HIV/AIDS Control Project was launched from 1992 to 1999.

1999 Phase II National AIDS Control Programme was launched to reduce HIV infection spread, to strengthen long-term measures against HIV/AIDS, to reduce prevalence rate in stages, to reduce blood transmission to less than 1%, to create AIDS awareness and to promote condom use among high-risk categories.

2001 Prevention of HIV transmission from mother to child by using nevirapine single dose each to the mother and the child and was taken up as project in selected centers.

2002 National AIDS Prevention and Control Policy was approved by Government of India, to achieve zero transmission rates by 2007. Main components included blood safety program, counseling and HIV testing, STD control program, condom promotion, HIV surveillance, AIDS education through IEC activities, targeted interventions and family health awareness campaign.

2003 HIV/AIDS prevention initiative through prevention, care, and surveillance.

2003 WHO and UNAIDS launched in December 2003 to provide ART to 3 million out of 5 million by 2005, called 3 by 5 Target.

2002–2007 Tenth five year plan with the goals of:
- Targeted interventions to high-risk groups covering up to 80%
- AIDS education of schools and colleges covering up to 90%
- AIDS awareness of public covering up to 80%
- Blood transmission to reduce to less than 1%
- Voluntary Counseling and Testing Center (VCTC) in every district
- District level project to reduce mother to child transmission (MTCT) of HIV/AIDS
- AIDS prevalence of zero by 2007.

2007–2012 National AIDS Control Programme III launched.

2012–2017 National AIDS Control Programme IV launched.

2017–2024 National Strategic Plan launched.

Achievements
- Sixty-five serosurveillance centers
- There are 180 sentinel surveillance system centers
- There are also 504 STD clinics
- Five regional STD research training centers
- National and state blood transfusion councils started
- About 815 blood banks modernized
- About 40 blood component separation units
- Complete ban on professional blood donation with effect from 1st January 1998.
- Mandatory screening of blood units for HIV, HBV, syphilis, malaria.

- Social mobilization and university involvement
- Targeting intervention projects on high risk (commercial sex worker, trucker, drug user)
- Now, NACP II is started by behavioral change intervention with following objectives:
  - To reduce spread of HIV in India, and
  - To strengthen India's capacity to respond to HIV/AIDS on long-term basis

AIDS Day Theme is detailed in Chapter 33.

Tetanus

A bacterial disease by *Clostridium tetani* exotoxin inducing lockjaw, risus sardonicus, opisthotonus with 40–80% mortality and 80–90% case fatality rate. The disease results from infection with *Clostridium tetani* that are found present in gut of man and animals, in soil. Injury, gardening and farming can be occupational source. Tetanus neonatorum occur at childbirth by unhygienic conditions where mortality is 100%.

Clinically painless lockjaw, rigid muscles of face, neck and trunk are observed. Muscles of angles of mouth and frontalis contracts to give appearance of *risus sardonicus*. Arched back produce opisthotonus. The word teino meaning to stretch has come from Greek has given rise to the term "Tetanus".

Global Picture

Puerperal cause	5%
Others like tattooing, burns, injection, postoperative	4%
Others	11%

It is much lesser in developed countries than in developing and underdeveloped countries.

Neonatal tetanus is predominant in developing countries.

Earlier mortality of 3/1,000 live births in urban and 13/100 live births in rural have come down to a considerable extent. However, road accident, cultural practice in delivery and contaminated instruments at hospital practice, postoperative conditions, puerperal conditions, otogenic conditions and crude termination of pregnancy in underdeveloped countries still seem to be source of infection.

Child survival and safe motherhood (CSSM), Government of India classified three categories of districts according to neonatal tetanus rates. This is as under:

Neonatal tetanus rate above high-risk situation 1/1,000 LB
or
2 doses tetanus toxoid (TT) coverage in RCH is below 70%
or
attended deliveries by trained are below 50%
Neonatal tetanus rate below situation is under control 1/1,000 LB
or
2 doses TT coverage in RCH is above 70%
or
attended deliveries by trained are above 50%
Neonatal tetanus rate below eliminated from the area 0.1/1,000 LB
or
2 doses TT coverage in RCH is above 90%
or
attended deliveries by trained are above 75%

Various studies have shown that estimated sources have been as under:

Injury	50%
Ear infection	20%
Cord infection	10%
Puerperal cause	5%
Others, such as tattooing, burns, injection, postoperative	4%
Others	11%

In India, tetanus is still a public health problem. The epidemiology is as given in **Figure 9.37**.

Mode of Transmission

The disease is transmitted through contaminated wound.

Incubation period: 6–10 days. The major types are:

- Traumatic
- Puerperal
- Otogenic
- Idiopathic, and
- Neonatal.

Chapter 9: Epidemiology of Communicable Diseases

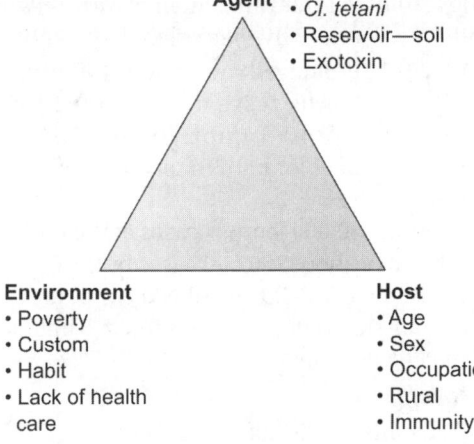

Fig. 9.37: Epidemiological triad in tetanus.

Treatment

1,200 mg penicillin is given immediately; followed by 7-days course of oral penicillin. When the case is at risk, 250 units of human tetanus antitoxin is given in 2 doses at interval of 10–12 weeks. Booster for already immunized is advocated.

Prevention

The preventive measures against tetanus are:

Neonatal tetanus

Clean delivery precautions such as clean hands, clean delivery surfaces, clean cord care (clean blade, clean tie for cord and no cord stump)
 Training of TBA
 TT pregnant women
 I dose as soon as pregnancy is diagnosed second dose 4 weeks later
 Booster for previously immunized.

Postinjury tetanus

- Local care of injury
- Wound categorization for treatment.

Wound Treatment Strategy

	Less than 6 hours	Other wounds
TT taken 5 years earlier	No treatment	No treatment
TT taken 5–10 years	TT (1) dose	TT (1) dose
TT taken 10 years above	TT (1) dose	Active +
TT unknown	TT one course	TT one course and immunoglobulin

Active immunization

- Diphtheria, pertussis, tetanus (DPT) active immunization
- Tetanus toxoid (TT) immunization (frequent booster TT is not advocated to avoid risk of hyperimmunization and risk of side-effects).

Passive immunization

- Immunoglobulin 250–500 IU
- Antitetanus serum (ATS) 1,500 units.

Active and passive

- Active and passive immunization

Antibiotics

- Antibiotics (penicillin 1.2 mega units of long acting penicillin IM that gives 4 weeks concentration or erythromycin for penicillin sensitive person, 7 day course 500 mg 6th hourly oral).

Disinfective Procedures

Operation theater (OT) is disinfected with formaldehyde fumigation. After closing the doors and windows, formalin filled in large jar is kept on high table in operation theater. $KMnO_4$ is added and the OT is closed. Formaldehyde liberated spreads and acts. After 12 hours, OT door and windows are opened, OT is aired for 24 hours. Later OT is prepared for recommissioning. For every 30 CC of space 500 mL of formalin and 200 g of potassium permanganate are required.

Other Effective Disinfection Procedures are:

- 5% phenol for 15 minutes
- Autoclaving at 105°; dry heat at 160° for 1 hour
- 2–5% tincture iodine for 6 hours.

Tetanus spores can be destroyed by:

- Steam in pressure at 120° for 20 minutes
- Gamma irradiation.

Leprosy (Hansen's Disease)

It is a chronic infectious disease caused by *Mycobacterium (M). leprae,* with cardinal features of:
- Hypopigmented patches
- Partial or total loss of cutaneous sensation in the affected areas
- Presence of thickened nerves
- Presence of AFB in skin and nasal smears.

Prominent History in Leprosy

1873:	*M. leprae* identified
1943:	Dapsone was invented
1955:	National Leprosy Control Programme (NLCP)
1960	Shepard experiment with footpads of mice
1971	Kirchheimer experiment with armadillos
1980	Resulted to eradicate leprosy by 2000
1981–1982	Multidrug therapy (MDT) under National Leprosy Eradication Program (NLEP)
1983	NLEP with a goal for 1/10,000 case load
1996	Special action projects for the elimination of leprosy (SAPEL) was initiated
1997	Modification of 1981 MDT. Multibacillary (MB) cases on 12 months MDT. Paucibacillary (PB) cases on 6 months MDT. Single skin lesion without nerve involvement. Single dose ROM (rifampicin, ofloxacin, minocycline)
1998	Modified leprosy elimination campaign (MLEC) and leprosy elimination campaign (LEC) elimination strategies adopted
2000	Target prevalence of leprosy is 1/10,000 population.
2005	Total elimination targeted. 2006–2007 National Action Plan
2012–2017	Program implementation program under five year plan
2016–2017	Prolonged strategy for NMEP with leprosy case detection focused leprosy campaign, and special plan for hard to reach areas

World picture:
- Around 550,000 leprosy cases at the end of 2002. It is about 200,000 cases by 2017
- Prevalence 0.4–5.0 per 10,000 population
- Overall steady decline is observed (5 million to 200,000 cases).

India's picture:
- Accounts for 75% of World Cases
- Prevalence 2.3 per 10,000 population
- Annual new case detection rate 2.7 per 10,000 population. Single skin lesion among new cases = 4.1%.
- Proportion of MB and PB cases: MB = 49.2%, PB = 50.8%
- New case rate is 55 per 100,000.
- Annual new case detection rate is 1.02 per 10,000 population.
- Prevalence rate is 0.66 per 10,000 population.

Mode of Transmission via Aerosols, Close Contact

The epidemiology is shown in **Figure 9.38**.

Incubation Period: (Average 2–5 years) 2–40 years.

Types (Fig. 9.39)

Lepromatous:
Infectious, generalized, bad prognosis, Lepromin negative, Bacilli positive.

Tuberculoid:
Noninfectious, localized Lepromin positive, Bacilli negative.

Borderline:
Same as lepromatous type

Indeterminate:
Early cases with vague symptoms

Pure neuritic:
Show nerve involvement

Histoid leproma:
Cutaneous nodule, red, oval, shiny, and resistant to sulfones.

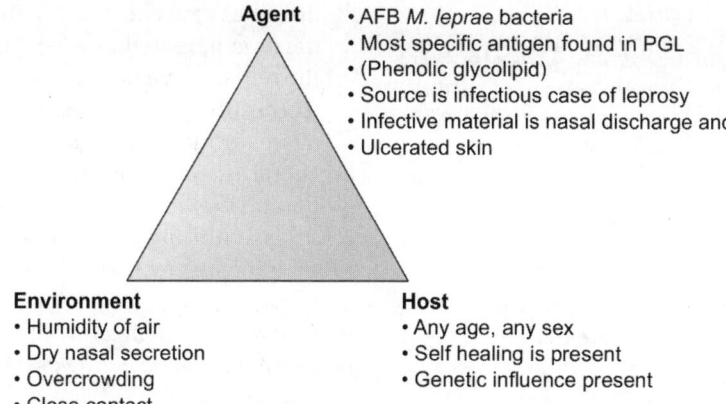

Fig. 9.38: Epidemiological triad in leprosy.
(AFB: acid-fast bacilli)

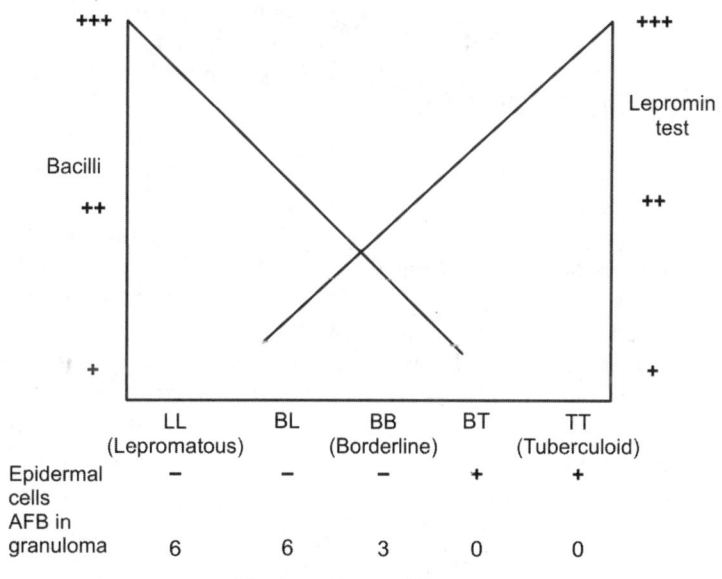

Fig. 9.39: Types of leprosy.

Diagnosis

Clinical examination for hypopigmented patch with loss of sensation, thickened nerve.

Bacteriological examination of skin smear, nasal smear, nasal scraping
Footpad culture
Biopsy
Histamine test

Lepromin test
Not diagnostic
0.1 mL intradermal injection of suspension of triturated lepromatous tissue rich in *M. leprae* in an isotonic solution of NaCl.

Early reaction (Fernandez) appears 24–48 hours—disappear in 3–4 days positive = erythema induration 10 mm and above.

Delayed reaction (Mitsuda) appear after 1 week, maximum in 3–4 weeks positive = induration 5 mm and above.

Bacteriological index
Refer **Table 9.16**

Table 9.16: Bacteriological index.

Negative	+	++	+++	++++
No bacilli in 100 fields	1 or less in each field	Present in all fields	Many in each field	Abundant* in all fields

*in case of Globi, entry as "G" is done

Morphological index
- Solid and nonsolid
- Has therapeutic effectiveness.

Lepra Reaction

Reactions during the course of leprosy type I and type II are known. Type I is reversal and type II is erythema nodosum leprosum.

Deformities

See **Table 9.17**.

Strategies of National Leprosy Eradication Program (NLEP)

Following are the major strategies for NLEP:
- **Early case detection:**
  - Ask for symptoms, such as numbness, tingling, stuffiness of nose, and nasal bleeding
  - Skin of whole body scanned for patches
  - If patch is present, test for touch, pain and heat
  - Nose is checked for ulcer and thickening
  - Earlobe is checked for thickening.

Nerve thickness for ulnar nerve, lateral popliteal nerve, median nerve, radial nerve, posterior tibial nerve, anterior tibial nerve, great auricular nerve, supraorbital nerve, and cutaneous branch of radial nerve are commonly tested in clinical examination.

Ulnar nerve is palpated immediately above the ulnar groove, the site being the groove behind the medial epicondyle at the posterior part of elbow. (The forearm is kept flexed at examination). Lateral popliteal nerve is palpated around the knee to feel the nerve in the popliteal fossa just medial to the biceps femoris tendon and as it passes around the neck of fibula, i.e., on the lateral aspect of the knee (A finger is hooked behind the head of fibula at examination).

Case finding methods adopted are (a) contact survey, (b) group survey and (c) mass survey.
- *Prompt treatment with MDT*
- *Prevention of disability among patients.*

The total elimination of the disease can be achieved by following ways:
- MDT is made accessible to all communities and areas.
- Treatment of all registered cases with MDT is undertaken.
- Diagnosis and prompt treatment of all new cases is encouraged.
- Improving quality of patient care including disability, prevention and management is advocated.
- Ensuring regularity and completion of treatment.
- Enlisting community support for the program.

Accelerated approach for elimination of leprosy is brought out through leprosy elimination campaign (LEC) and special action projects for elimination of leprosy (SAPEL).

Modified Leprosy Elimination Campaign (MLEC)

1997	I round detected	4.63 lakh cases
2000	II round detected	2.13 lakh cases
2001–2002	III round detected	1.65 lakh cases
2002–2003	IV round detected	1.04 lakh cases
2003–2004	V round urban 2 lakh population VRC and slums LELLC	

Table 9.17: Grades of deformities.

	Hand and feet	Eye
Grade 0	No change	No change
Grade I	Anesthesia +	Eye problem +
Grade II	Damage +	Vision impaired

Chapter 9: Epidemiology of Communicable Diseases

- Rural prevalence rate below 5/10,000 VRC and active search
- Rural prevalence rate 3/10,000 SAPEL
- **NLEP projects:**
  - I Project ended in 2000
  - II Project 2001–2004

Leprosy Elimination Monitoring is a WHO assisted National Project.

Leprosy Elimination Campaign (LEC)

An initiative aiming to detect leprosy (MB) that remained undetected and to cure them. Elements involved are:
- Capacity building measures for local health workers to improve MDT
- Increasing community participation, and
- Diagnosis and curing leprosy patients.

Special Action Projects for the Elimination of Leprosy (SAPEL)

It is an initiative aimed at providing MDT services to patients living in special difficult to access areas or situation or to those belonging to neglected population groups.

Tenth Five-Year Plan Leprosy Goals

Attain prevalence rate of leprosy to less than 1/10,000 population.

Horizontal program to be converted to vertical program by 2007 and personnel employed under leprosy to be transferred to the states.

Leprosy Work

Teachers and technicians are deployed for future integration into primary healthcare system.
- Training of health personnel in case detection and management of leprosy.
- Reconstructive surgery for rehabilitation
- Nongovernment organization involvement.

Program Implementation under five-year plan
- To bring down the prevalence to less than 1 per 10,000 population
- To strengthen the disability prevention steps
- Reduction of level of stigma in the society.

World Health Organization (WHO) multidrug therapy (MDT) regimens

A. Clinical Grouping (PB = 1–5 skin lesion, MB = more than 5 skin lesions)			
Lesion	PB single skin lesion (patch)	PB (Paucibacillary)	MB (Multibacillary)
Skin lesion	1	2–5	6 and 6+
Nerve involvement	No	Only one trunk	>1 nerve trunk
Skin smear	–	–	+

B. Treatment (Adult)				
	Drug	Dose	Frequency	Criteria for cure
MB	Rifampicin	600 mg	Once monthly	Completion of 12 monthly
	Dapsone	100 mg	Daily	
	Clofazimine	300 mg	Once monthly	Pulses within 18 months
		50 mg	Daily	
PB	Rifampicin	600 mg	Once monthly	Completion of 6 monthly
	Dapsone pulses within 9 months	100 mg	Daily	
Single skin lesion	Rifampicin, ofloxacin, minocycline	600 mg 400 mg 100 mg	Single dose	Single dose treatment

Contd...

Contd...

C. Treatment (Child) 10–14 years given. Below 10 years should receive appropriately reduced dose.			
Drug	Dose	Frequency	Criteria for cure
MB rifampicin	450 mg	Once a month	Under supervision
Dapsone	50 mg	Daily	Self-administration
Clofazimine	150 mg	Once a month	
	50 mg	Every other day	
PB rifampicin	450 mg	Once a day	Supervised
Dapsone	50 mg	Daily	Self-administration

Proposed Strategy Beyond 2000
- Leprosy services to integrate with general health services.
- All new cases will be brought under MDT with probably better regimen than the current one.
- **The old cases:** Disabled will continue to receive health care service especially for their disabilities.

Vaccine
- No definite role
- Bacillus calmette-guérin (BCG) vaccine by trial has shown 30–90% protection
- Killed Indian Cancer Research Centre (ICRC) bacillus as candidate vaccine is tried.

Chemoprophylaxis
- Dapsone 1–4 mg per kg per week
- Acedapsone one injection IM every 10 week.

Surveillance
- Single patch/1–5 patch once in a year up to 2 years, after complete treatment
- 6 and 6+ patches once in a year up to 5 years, after complete treatment.

Following are the summary of control/elimination/eradication:
- Case finding
- Chemotherapy **(Figs. 9.40 and 9.41)**
- Selective isolation
- Follow-up
- Chemoprophylaxis
- Rehabilitation
- Health education
- Segregation of children and FP of cases.

In the elimination programme, about 778 leprosy control units (LCU), 5,744 survey education and treatment (SET) centers and 150 voluntary agencies are working for the cause. Major voluntary organizations are

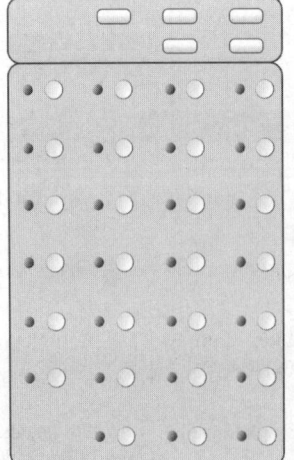

Detachable portion contains 3 caps clofazimine, 2 rifampicin and 1 dapsone to be given by health worker

Lower portion contains 27 clofazimine and 27 tablet of dapsone for 27 days treatment at home by the patient

Fig. 9.40: Blister pack for multibacillary treatment (12 packs for total treatment).

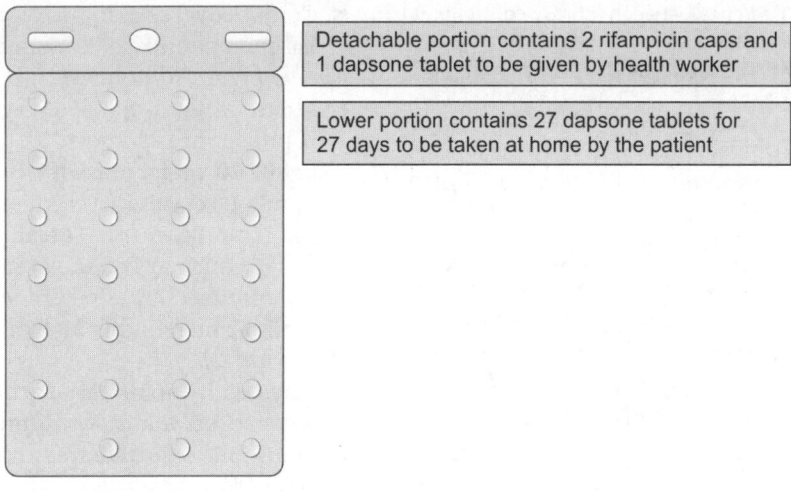

Fig. 9.41: Blister pack for paucibacillary treatment (6 packs for total treatment).

Hind Kusht Nivaran Sangh, Gandhi Memorial Leprosy Foundation and Japan Leprosy Mission for Asia (JALMA).

Trachoma

(Inclusion conjunctivitis) (Communicable keratoconjunctivitis)

Surface infection caused by an obligatory intracellular bacteria, *Chlamydia trachomatis*. It causes conjunctival scarring, trichiasis, entropion and corneal ulceration. Common clinical manifestations are conjunctival irritation and blepharospasm. It is one of the causes for preventable blindness.

World Picture

190 million are at risk of infection in the world, 1.2 million are economically blind. 1 million have irreversible blindness, and 152 million are suffering from trachoma.

Indian Picture (Fig. 9.42)

125 million cases in India, 5 million are economically blind. 5% of visual impairment and blindness is by trachoma.

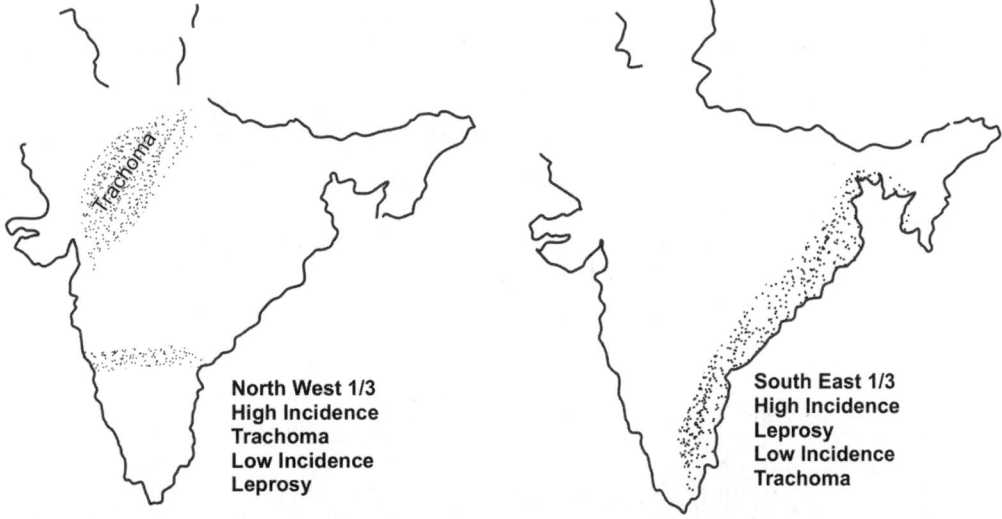

Fig. 9.42: Geographic pathology related to ecological barrier (Trachoma is reversal to leprosy).

Table 9.18: Difference between leprosy control unit (LCU) and survey education training (SET) unit.

	LCU	SET
Prevalence It is	1% A control unit	0.5–1.0% A subcenter
Staff	One medical officer Two paramedical workers	One nonmedical supervisor, 5 paramedical workers PHC MO looks after
Coverage	150,000 population	10,000 populations

(PHC: primary health center; MO: medical officer)

Difference between LCU and SET
See **Table 9.18**.

Mode of Transmission (Fig. 9.43)
Modes of transmission are both direct and indirect. Kajal or Surma, towel and infected fingers communicate the infection.
Incubation Period: 5–12 days.

Laboratory Diagnosis
- Conjunctival scraping by staining with iodine
- Culture in Chick embryo.

Control
- *Avoidable blindness assessment in the field*
  - Field survey for trachoma diagnosis is undertaken
  - Follicle on upper tarsal conjunctiva limbal follicles
  - Conjunctival scarring
  - Vascular pannus at the superior limbus
- *Chemotherapy (ointment)*
  - About 1% tetracycline or erythromycin. If prevalence is above 5% in children below 10 years, mass treatment called blanket treatment is given to all in the community. Tetracycline 1% for 5 consecutive days each month (*Intermittent:* 1% tetracycline BD 5 days/month, and monthly for 6 months)
  Or
  - Once daily for 10 days each month for 6 consecutive months. If prevalence is below 5%, selective treatment to all at risk is undertaken.
- *Surveillance of the community*
- *Health education.*
- *Evaluation at frequent interval.*

Prevention
- Personal hygiene
- Care of eye in newborn
- Population survey
- Trachoma clinic in endemic areas.

Control Program
National Trachoma Control Programme started in 1968. It got incorporated into National Programme for the control of blindness in 1976. Main strategy has been to reduce the prevalence to 0.3%. Target for Tenth-five year plan, Vision 2020, and National Programme for the Control of Blindness are dealt in Chapter 20.

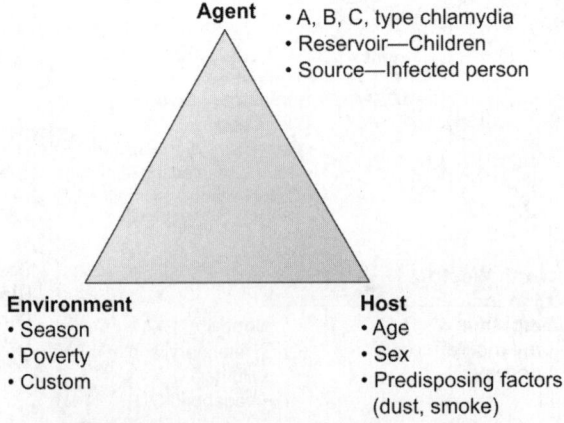

Fig. 9.43: Epidemiological triad in trachoma.

ZOONOTIC INFECTIONS

Rabies (Hydrophobia)

It is an acute fatal viral disease caused by (Rhabdovirus) Lyssavirus type 1. Clinically with the history of rabid dog bite, patient develops fever, paresthesia at the site of bite. In about 10 days patient develops hydrophobia. Later delusions and hallucinations may develop with maniac symptoms. Terminal hyperpyrexia is common. Mortality is 100% which occurs within 10 days of the onset of clinical manifestations.

Global Picture

Australia, Taiwan, Japan, Malta, New Zealand, United Kingdom (UK), Cyprus, Iceland, Western Pacific Island, Finland and the Liberian Peninsula are *Rabies free*.

About 10 million are bitten and need antirabies vaccine (ARV) every year. It is estimated that around 60,000 human deaths are occurring due to Rabies.

Indian Picture

History of dog or animal bite is occurring every 10 minutes and annual incidence of dog bite is around 3 million (2–3 per 1,000 population animal bite cases). 50% of them, i.e., 1.5 million are receiving postexposure treatment with ARV. Every year 30,000 deaths are occurring. Dog population in India is estimated to be around 40 million and only 9% of them are protected against rabies. It is prevalent in the entire country except Andaman, Nicobar and Lakshadweep islands.

Mode of transmission: Infected (dog) animal bite.

Incubation period (IP): 3–8 weeks.

Epidemiology depicted in **Figure 9.44**

Difference between Street Virus and Fixed Virus

Street virus	Fixed virus
Natural virus	Modified virus by intracerebral passages
Incubation period 10–12 days	Incubation period 5 days
Causes disease	Does not cause disease
Gives rise to formation of Negri bodies	No Negri bodies

Rabies in Man

Prodromal: Fever, headache, malaise, sore throat.

Sensory change: Intolerance to light, cold, heat.

Motor change: Hyperreflexia, hypertonia.

Sympathetic change: Pupillary dilatation, perspiration, salivation, lacrimation.

Mental change: Fear, anger, irritability, depression.

Hydrophobia: Advanced symptom

Diagnosis

* History of rabid dog bite
* Clinical signs and symptoms
* Laboratory
  * Virus isolation from saliva
  * Antigen detection using immunofluorescence of skin biopsy or corneal impression smears
  * Negri body demonstration from brain.

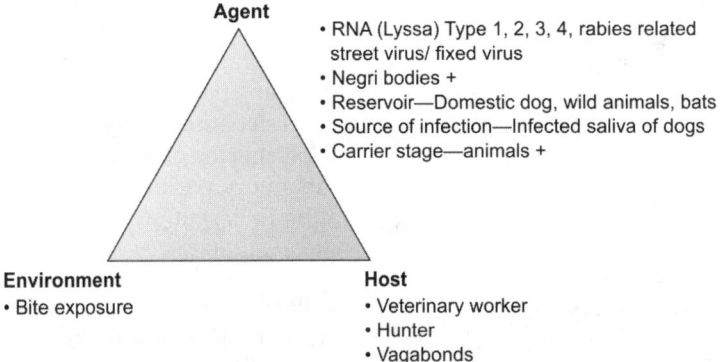

Fig. 9.44: Epidemiological triad in rabies.
(RNA: ribonucleic acid)

Case Management

Following are the ways to manage the disease:
- Isolation in dark, silent room
- Should be heavily sedated with diazepam 10 mg 6th hourly
- Muscle relaxants
- Later supportive therapy with nutrition and fluids by intravenous (IV) or through gastrostomy.

Disinfection

The virus can be killed by sunlight, by acids, by alkalis and soap. Virus is killed in 30 minutes at 58°C.

Vaccines

Following are in use:
- Nervous tissue vaccine (sheep brain or mice brain used)
  - Sheep (semple) beta propiolactone (BPL) vaccine
  - Mouse (less neuroparalysis)
- Duck embryo vaccine (has risk of allergy)
- Cell culture
  - Human diploid cell vaccine (HDCV) (human-fibroblast cell)
  - Nonhuman tissue culture vaccine (dog kidney, chick embryo fibroblast, fetal rhesus cells, fetal bovine kidney cells, hamster kidney cell).

Postexposure Treatment

General

- Treated as emergency
- All need active and passive immunization.

Local

- Wound wash
- Chemical treatment of wound (alcohol, povidone-iodine, tincture)
  - No immediate suturing
  - Local ARS
  - Antibiotic treatment
  - Antitetanus treatment, and
  - Observation of dog for risk estimation.

Wound Classification

Class I: Licks, suspected not boiled milk consumption, scratches

Class II: Fresh cut, oozing blood, minor wounds

Class III: Wound on neck, face, palm, lacerated wound

A. BPL inactivated vaccine schedule (Pasteur Institute, Coonoor).

Give ARV before 5 days of bite. Abdominal wall is selected and the area is divided into quadrants and different site is used for injection.

Wound	Adult	Child	Duration
I	2 mL	1 mL	7 days
II	3 mL	3 mL	10 days
III	5 mL	3 mL	10 days

B. Cell culture vaccine schedule (Give ARV before 5 days of bite)

Intramuscular schedule

6 doses (IM) 1 mL each on 0, 3, 7, 14, and 28 days with booster at 90th day. Except cost, advantageous by safety, potency and practicability.

Intradermal schedule

Two site intradermal schedule involves 0.2 mL given intradermal at each of two sites on days 0, 3, and 7 followed by one site injection on 28th day and on 90th day. It is called 2-2-2-0-1-1 schedule.

Eight site intradermal schedules involve 0.1 mL given intradermal at each of four sites over deltoid and thighs. This is followed by one site injection on 28th day and 90th day. It is called 8-0-4-0-1-1- schedule.

C. ARS (Horse) 40 IU/kg (maximum 3,000)

Pre-exposure treatment (to high-risk group) Cell culture vaccine 1 mL IM on days 0, 7, 28 and booster once in 2 years.

Rabies in Dog

Clinically, manifestation of rabies in dog observed are of two types:
1. Furious type with behavioral change, running amok, voice paralysis
2. Dumb type with quite nature and spending in sleepiness stage.

Suspected or died dog's head can be sent to laboratory, packing in ice, in air tight container. If brain is sent, it should be sent with 50% of glycerol saline.

Dog Vaccine

Beta-propiolactone (BPL)

Single dose 5 mL II dose at 6th month, revaccination once a year.

Modified Live Viral Vaccine

Single dose 3 mL revaccination once in 3 years.

Oral Vaccines

Used as oral vaccine baits to foxes is being tried on dogs and this is showing promise in immunization against rabies on dogs.

Public Health Measures

Following are the public health measures:
- Elimination of stray dogs
- Registration, licensing of domestic dogs
- Owner of dogs can cover dog's mouth with a muzzle in public places
- Destruction of animals, bitten by dogs
- Six months quarantine for imported dogs, and
- Rabies awareness in the community.

Japanese B Encephalitis (Brain Fever)

One of the zoonotic diseases of public health importance, JE is caused by flavivirus and transmitted by *Culex* mosquitoes. It was in the year 1870 first case was recorded in Japan and hence, the name Japanese encephalitis. Japan witnessed severe epidemic in 1924.

Global Picture

Ubiquitous in distribution with annual cases of 43,000 and deaths of 11,000. Case fatality rate is about 25%. About 50% of survivors are left with neurological sequelae.

Indian Picture

India had no record of this disease till 1955, when first case was identified. From 1955 to 1972 outbreaks of epidemics are recorded. There was a major outbreak from 1973 onward in the nation. Each year 2–3 thousand cases with 500–600 deaths are occurring.

Mode of Transmission (Fig. 9.45)

By bite of infected female *Culex vishnui*, *Culex tritaeniorhynchus*, *Culex pseudovishnui* mosquitoes.

Epidemiology is depicted in **Figure 9.46**.

Reservoir of Infection

Pigs are amplifier host and common reservoirs. Birds are also found to be the reservoirs.

Incubation Period: 5–15 days.

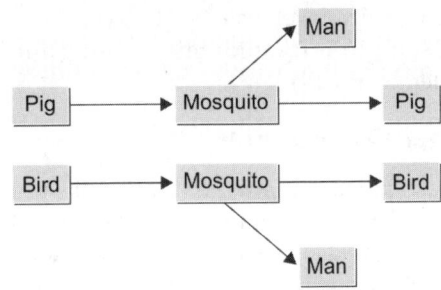

Fig. 9.45: Mode of transmission of Japanese encephalitis (transovarian transmission in mosquitoes is possible).

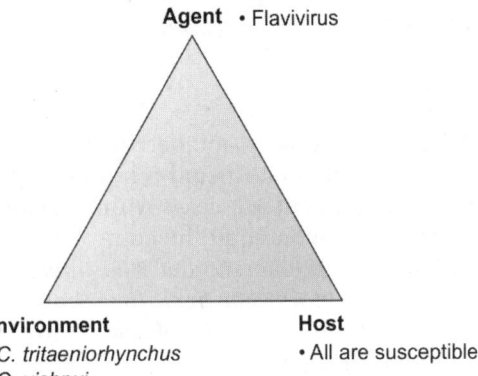

Fig. 9.46: Epidemiological triad in Japanese encephalitis.

Clinical Picture

Prodromal stage, succeeded by acute encephalitic stage (brain fever).

Treatment

There is no specific treatment. There is only supportive treatment and treatment of complications.

Control Measures

Vector control: Integrated vector control.

Air fogging and ground fogging by Malathion or Fenitrothion by Ultra-low-volume methods (ULV).

Vaccination of risk group by mouse brain vaccine: JE vaccine—2 doses of 1 mL each subcutaneous 2 weeks apart. 0.5 mL for children below 3 years of age. Booster is given before the completion of 1 year from primary course of injection at 1 year.

Immunity develops after 30 days.

Useful in interepidemic period (not in epidemic period).

Plague (Black Death)

Known killer of mankind, plague has many epidemics with millions of deaths recorded in history of medicine. Plague bacilli was isolated in 1894. Plague is an important notifiable and quarantinable disease.

Global Picture

Case fatality rate (CFR) is around 7%. Global epidemic have been recorded in 6th century, in 14th century, and in 1860.

Indian Picture

Maharashtra, Gujarat, and Karnataka are still with endemic foci. Recent Surat endemic has a recording of 910 cases with 52 deaths in 1994. Of late, it could be controlled at a short time. WHO has recorded it as *supportive of plague and not confirmatory*. Later in 1995, Government of India declared through committee that it is plague.

Up to 1966 plague epidemic was present. From 1966 to 1994 *nil* cases were reported. In 1994, Surat epidemic and in 2002 Himachal Pradesh epidemic are recorded. Last recorded cases of human plague was in 2002.

Terminology

Domestic plague

"Plague that is intimately associated with man has a definite potential for producing episodes".

Wild plague

"Plague existing in nature independent of human populations and their activities".

Clinical type (**Table 9.19**)
- Bubonic plague
- Pneumonic plague and septicemic plague

Vector

- Rat flea X cheopis
- Blocked flea—dangerous because of obstruction of its intestine by fleas by a bolus of plague organism.
- Flea index.
- **General flea index:** This is GFI, SFI, specious percentage.

Table 9.19: Clinical manifestations.

Bubonic plague	Septicemic plague	Pneumonic plague
Rigor, high fever, dry skin, severe headache, lymph node enlargement in groin, rapid pulse, hypotension, mental confusion, and splenomegaly	Meningitis, pneumonia, and blood stained sputum	Sudden onset, cough, dyspnea, copious sputum (blood stained), cyanosis, lobar opacity in X-ray, and death common

Dead rat examination

Autopsy and collection of material/smear for pathological changes.

Animal inoculation of guinea pig/mouse (guinea pig dies in 7 days and mouse in 2 days).

Mode of Transmission

Biological, mechanical, droplet

Incubation Period (IP)

- Six days (pneumonic 4 days).
- Epidemiology is depicted in **Figure 9.47**.

Diagnosis

Sputum examination for organism and culture aspiration of Bubo for organism and culture. Clinical manifestation is given in **Table 9.19**.

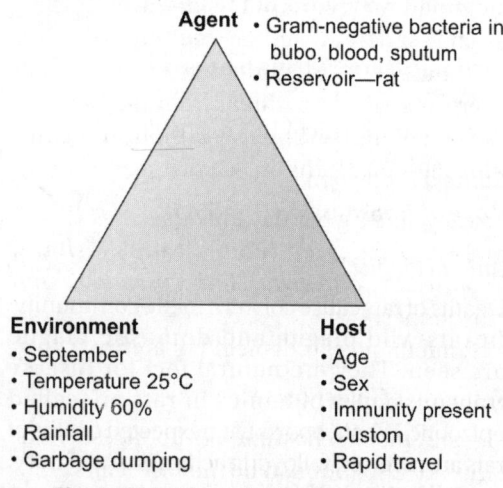

Fig. 9.47: Epidemiological triad in plague.

Chapter 9: Epidemiology of Communicable Diseases

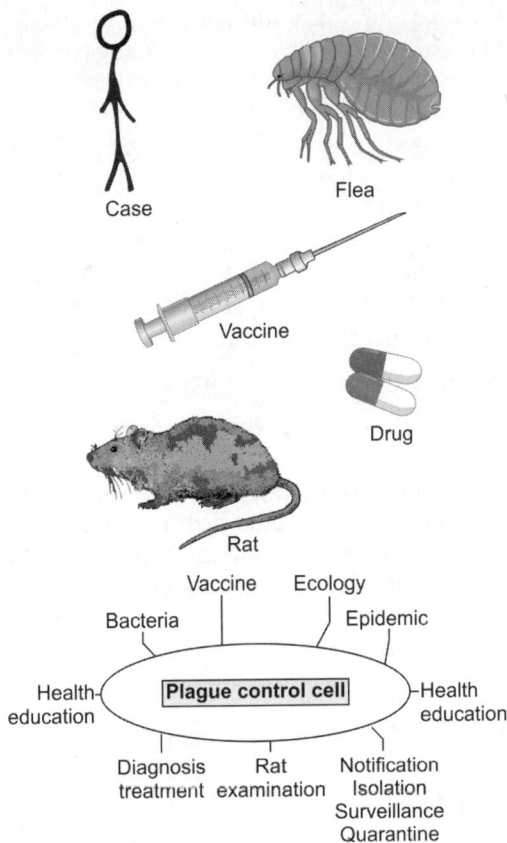

Fig. 9.48: Plague prevention and control.

Prevention and Control (Fig. 9.48) Treatment

Streptomycin 1 g 12 hourly
  Or
Gentamicin 1 mg/kg 8th hourly
  Or
Tetracycline 500 mg 6 hourly
  Or
Chloramphenicol 12.5 mg per kg 6th hourly.

Contact Protection

Tetracycline 2 g per day for 7 days.

Animal Plague

Deaths of rats cause concern in the community. In rats wild plague and domestic plague are seen. They are natural foci for disease transmission. Epidemics in rats are called epizootic. When reports of unexpected deaths of rats are received following action is mandatory.

- Collection and forwarding rats to nearest laboratory
- Autopsy of rats is done
- Plague bacilli in them are demonstrated
- Appropriate public health measures are taken.

Experience from plague control cell

Following are the negative aspects the plague control cell found with ordinary practices to control the plague.

- Rodent control activity in connection with plague usually ceases when the disease is brought under control and no more human cases occur.
- Trapping and poisoning demand large investments in terms of personnel, equipment, pesticides that are neither available nor justified.
- Elimination of rats leads to faster reproduction among survivors, infiltrate from outlets. Then density becomes more than one existed early.

Effective methods: The effective methods to control plague are:

- Improve sanitation
- Proper waste disposal
- Proper storage of grain food/food stuff, and
- Rat proofing of structure.

Control

- **Bubonic:** Interrupt rodent/flea/man transmission.
- **Pneumonic:** Interrupt man/man transmission.

The other practical methods to control the plague are:

- Preventive measures: Investigate dead rat/man, autopsy, smear from spleen, liver, lung and glands.
  - *Rat control*—sanitation, housing, quality of life.
  - *Patient*—tetracycline 500 mg, 6 hourly for 5 days.
  - *Risk group*—tetracycline 500 mg 12 hourly for 5 days.
  - Take care of docks, warehouse, harbor and ship.
- Patient, contact, environment:
  - Reporting, isolation and concurrent disinfection.

- Terminal disinfection and quarantine. Vaccine 0.5 mL/1.0 mL at 1 week interval subcutaneously
- Rodent, rat flea check
- Waste disposal in sanitary way
❖ During epidemic the measures to be taken are:
- Death investigations, autopsy, and laboratory examination
- Intensive flea control
- Supplement rat destruction
- Prophylactic use of tetracycline capsule for 5 days
- Personal protection from flea bite and from inhalation of patient breath by proper use of mask
❖ International measures:
- The internationally accepted measures to be taken against plagues are:
  - Telegraphic notification to the concerned authorities of ship, aircraft and land transport are considered to be checked/under surveillance.
  - Rat proof building in port and airport. Check on international travelers.

Kyasanur Forest Disease (KFD) (Monkey Fever)

One of the viral hemorrhagic fevers, Kyasanur Forest disease (KFD) is Tick-borne fever confined to 4 districts (Shimoga, North Canara, Chikmagalur and South Canara) of Karnataka State in India. This flavivirus of Togaviruses group of infections in monkeys and cattle, seen only in Karnataka state (found in Kyasanur Forest and hence the name for the disease). There was a large epidemic in 1983–1984 that involved 2,167 cases and 69 deaths. Every year 400–500 cases are occurring in the endemic area.

In the history of KFD, first case was detected in 1957 in Sagar of Shimoga district of Karnataka state in India.

Present Picture

Now, it has spread over to adjoining districts of Shimoga. Every year seasonal epidemics are occurring. Now, annual cases has been around 100 and annual deaths is around 3. Epidemics are associated with heavy mortality of monkeys in the forest. Case fatality rate has been 5–10%.

Epidemiology is depicted in **Figure 9.49**.

Mode of Transmission

Bite of infected hard tick. The disease does not spread from man to man. It is dead end with him.

Hot Spots

Areas where monkey deaths are reported which cover 50 meters around. This is important for insecticide spray to control ticks.

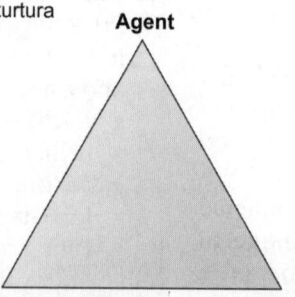

Agent
B group togavirus
Amplifying host is monkey
Natural hosts are rats, squirrels
Vectors are haemaphysalis apingera
And haemaphysalis turtura

Environment
More in jan to june
Human activity in forest has been found related

Host
20–30 years
More in men
Cultivators and forest visitors

Fig. 9.49: Epidemiological triad in KFD.
(KFD: kyasanur forest disease)

Chapter 9: Epidemiology of Communicable Diseases

Incubation Period
About 3–8 days.

Clinical Picture
Usually, bradycardia, conjunctival congestion and generalized lymphadenopathy are common

Abortive type: Headache, fever, myalgia, and prostration

Gastrointestinal (GI) type: Nausea, vomiting, diarrhea, and bleeding

Central nervous system (CNS) type: Encephalitis type

Prevention and Control
The major preventive and controlling measures are:
- **Vaccine:** Formalin killed and inactivated KFD vaccine (chick embryo fibroblasts vaccine) to risk group,
  Vaccine 1 mL subcutaneous followed by 1 mL subcutaneous after 4 weeks. 0.5 mL is the dose for children below 6 years. Immunity starts 4 weeks after II dose and lasts for 3 years.
- Personal protection from bite of hard tick
- Insecticide sprays for hard tick control, by any of the following:
  - About 5% Dichlorodiphenyltrichloroethane (DDT)
  - 0.5% Lindane
  - 5% Carbaryl
  - 0.5% Diazinon
  - 2% Malathion
- Forest tick control by aircraft mounted spray with carbaryl.
- Health education to the local community on KFD.

Yellow Fever

It is not present in India, but we are frightened of its entry as it causes fatal damage to the community. An arboviral zoonotic international quarantinable disease usually manifests with hepatic or renal manifestations viz., Jaundice, hematuria and intense albuminuria. This disease has high case fatality rate which is preceded by anuria, shock and coma.

Patient is infectious during viremic phase, i.e., 3–6 days after the bite of infected mosquito and lasts for 4–5 days.

Global Picture
Africa and South America.

Mode of Transmission
- Commonly, it is transmitted by bite of infected mosquito
- **Urban area:** *Aedes (A). aegypti*
- **Jungle area:** *Hemogogus*

Incubation Period
About 3–6 days.

Indices

Aedes aegypti index (House index)

$$= \frac{\text{No.} + \text{ve}}{\text{House examined}} \times 100$$

(In half a mile, it should be <1%)

Others
- Container index
- Breteau index
- Biting rate
- Epidemiology is depicted in **Figure 9.50**.

Treatment
Supportive therapy by:
- Fluid and electrolyte balance
- Blood transfusion
- Plasma expander's peritoneal dialysis

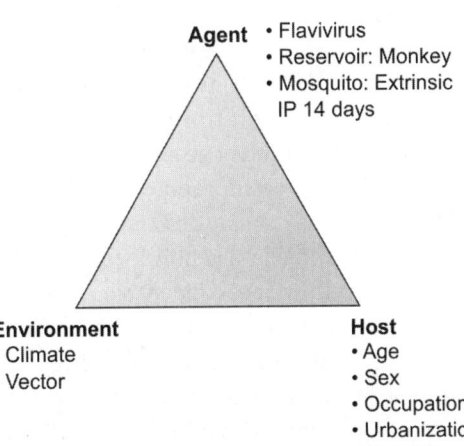

Fig. 9.50: Epidemiological triad in yellow fever.

Prevention and Control

Preventive and controlling measures are as given below:

Mosquito control

- Reducing mosquito bite particularly as per International Aircraft Regulation 1950 is implemented. These include:
  - Airport should be half kilometer away from residential area.
  - No mosquito zone up to 300 meters of airports.
  - Airport staff be actively immunized.
  - Strict policy for yellow fever vaccination certificate.

Aircraft Disinfection

Spray of 0.4% *Pyrethrum* (minimum 300 mg per cubic meter) is done. Doors are closed for 5 minutes. Aircraft disinfection is advised
a. Before passengers embark
b. After luggage is stored.

Vaccine

- 17D stain (chick embryo) 0.5 mL subcutaneous immunity starts on 10th day lasts for 10 years
- French neurotropic vaccine (FNV) (Dakar) (mouse brain).

India and Yellow Fever

- Quarantine (airport and Seaport regulations), strict vigilance on International Vaccination Certificate is kept.
- Ecological barrier unanswered; cross immunity with viral infections, such as KFD, Dengue, JE may protect Indians from yellow fever. Development of antibody by *Aedes aegyptie* mosquito bite may show deleterious effect on yellow fever virus.
- India is yellow fever receptive area, and requires valid vaccination certificate from people (including infants) coming from yellow fever endemic areas.
- Care to be taken with other vaccine.
- Two reference centers are at Pune and Kasauli available for all queries.

Brucellosis (Undulant Fever) (Malta fever) (Mediterranean fever)

Common enzootic infection in which infected animals excrete *Brucella* organisms in their milk.

One of the economic consequences producing zoonotic disease by *Brucella* organism is characterized by fever, sweating, arthritis splenomegaly and hepatomegaly. It was identified in Malta for the first time in 1906 and hence the name Malta Fever. Seropositive in urban population is about 2% and among milk samples it is about 3%.

Immunoglobulin M is decreased within few months of infection.

Common clinical manifestations can be grouped under four heads:

Musculoskeletal	CNS	Ocular	Heart
Psoas abscess	Meningitis	Uveitis	Myocarditis
Arthritis	Myelopathy		
Bursitis			
Osteomyelitis			

Global and India's Picture

Endemic all over. But cases are reported from Middle East countries. (**Fig. 9.51**).

Mode of Transmission

Following are the ways through which the disease is transmitted:
- Animal contact
- Consuming contaminated milk, and

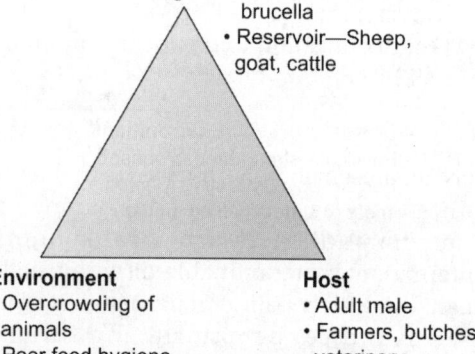

Fig. 9.51: Epidemiological triad in brucellosis.

- Occupational—dust with *brucella* inhalation.

Incubation period: About 1–3 weeks

Treatment

Doxycycline 100 mg 12 hourly for 6 weeks along with streptomycin 1 g intramuscular daily for 2 weeks for complications.

Acute stage (adults) tetracycline 500 mg 6 hourly for 3 weeks.

Control

- Animal control in herds, slaughterhouse
- **Human control by:**
  - Diagnosis, treatment
  - Milk pasteurization
  - Personal protection when moving with animals
- Human live vaccine of *Brucella (B). abortus* 19BA is available in limited quantity.

Indian Veterinary Research Institute, Uttar Pradesh is helping in research, survey and surveillance activities in the country.

Leptospirosis

See Chapter 33. Check

Anthrax (Woolsorter's Disease) (Malignant Pustule)

For centuries, it is known as disease of livestock. It is caused by *Bacillus anthracis*. Historically, we know that grazing lands remaining infective and elders advising to bury infected carcasses deeply to avoid soil contamination.

Mode of Transmission (Fig. 9.52)

- Through cut or abrasion of skin
- Through contaminated meat
- Through inhalation of spores.

Incubation Period

- In animals, 3–6 days.
- In man, 1–7 days.

Case Definition (WHO)

Suspect

A case that is compatible with the clinical description and has an epidemiological link to confirmed or suspected animal cases or contaminated animal products.

Probable

A suspected case that has a positive reaction to allergic skin test (in nonvaccinated).

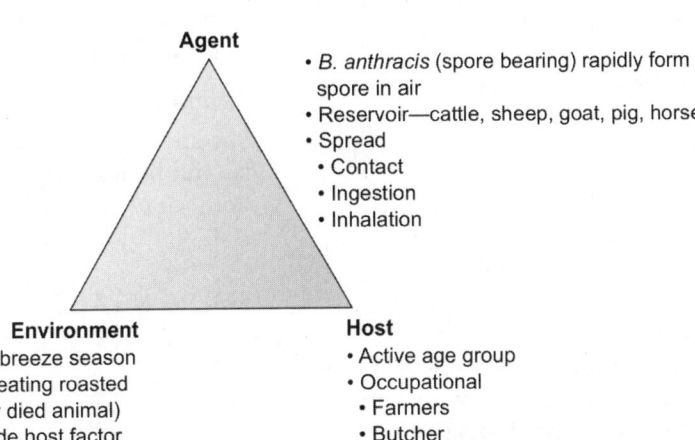

Fig. 9.52: Epidemiological triad in anthrax.

Confirmed

A suspected case that is confirmed by laboratory procedure, such as
a. Isolation of *B. anthracis* from specimen of blood, lesions, discharges
b. Direct examination of bacteria in smear
c. Positive ELISA, western blot, toxin detection, chromatographic assay, FAT

Case Fatality Rates

- Inhalation type: 100%
- Ingestion type: 25-60%
- Cutaneous type; 20% (treated) 80% (untreated).

Manifestations

Cutaneous type

Begins as painless pruritic papule (such as insect bite) form vesicle and later ulcer with black necrosis in the middle.

Malaise, lymphadenopathy, local edema, induration, and toxemia.

Ingestion type

a. Oropharyngeal—sore throat, dysphagia, fever, lymphadenopathy, and toxemia
b. Intestinal—nausea, vomiting, fever, abdominal pain, hematemesis, bloody diarrhea, ascites, and toxemia.

Inhalation type

Common cold, such as symptoms leads to breathlessness, shock, and death.

Complications

- Acute pneumonia
- Meningitis

Laboratory Diagnosis

- Smear from skin lesion, respiratory secretion or blood to demonstrate *B. anthracis* by direct polychrome methylene blue stain.
- Culture in sheep blood agar (large, rough, gray white with irregular tapered, and curving outgrowths of colonies).
- Serological tests, such as ELISA, Western blot, and chromatography assay.

Susceptibility

Not certain

Period of Communicability

- Uncertain in normal conditions.
- Contaminated article and soil remain infective for years.

Prevention and Control

- Treatment of suspected cases
  - First line of drug—ciprofloxacin
  - Second line of drugs—penicillin, streptomycin, amoxicillin, and doxycycline
- Notification
- Surveillance
- Compulsory postmortem of suddenly died animals
- Preprocessing disinfection of hair, wool, hides and bone meal
- Ban on sale of infected animal carcasses.

Present Problem in Prevention and Control of Anthrax

- Custom of butchering and eating roasted meat of suddenly dead animal is prevailing
- No reporting over sudden death of animal exist
- Poor communication and poor laboratory facility delays in diagnosis
- Policy on disposal of suspected carcass is not specific
- Anthrax has become weapon as aerosol spread by terrorists (Bioterrorism similar to chemical and nuclear terrorism).

Disposal of the Dead

Specific recommendations of Municipal Act should be followed in the disposal of dead body (animal and human).

Bioterrorism is detailed in Chapter 33.

EMERGING AND RE-EMERGING INFECTIONS

Many infectious diseases once thought to be fully controlled and conquered have come back.

WHO under United Nations visualized this and took a note on the issue through 1997 WHO day theme "Emerging Infectious

Diseases—Global alert: Global response" to give solutions to the health problems.

We also notice the related factors, such as poor sanitation, over population (density of human population), poor health manpower, drug resistance (antibiotics not judiciously used), increased food catering establishments and rapid international communications in predisposing emerging and re-emerging diseases.

We are facing with reappearance or resurgence of controlled infections and also by appearance of new infections which were unheard of.

Prevention and Control

Following are the major preventive and controlling measures of emerging infections:
- Diagnosis and treatment (good laboratory services)
- Efficient surveillance system
- International health regulation (global surveillance)
- Personal and environmental hygiene
- Vaccination/immunization
- Health education.

Following are the major reappeared infections that are differentiated:

Emerging diseases	Re-emerging diseases
They are newly discovered diseases	They are diseases which were public health problem
Diseases by a variant of known agent	But later controlled and now have appeared as recent
This will be a public health problem	Public health problem
It can be a new problem by new disease	They can be diseases of one geographical areas spread to other areas
	They are problems by old diseases
Legionellosis	Malaria
Ebola hemorrhagic fever	Plague
AIDS	Leptospirosis
Rota virus diarrhea	Dengue

Monkeypox		
KFD		
Mad cow disease (Creutzfeldt-Jakob disease)		
New variant vibrio 0139 cholera		
New variant H5N1 1996 influenza		
Kaposi sarcoma by human herpes virus		
SARS		

Major newly appeared infections:

Bacterial	Campylobacter jejuni: E. coli 0157:H7: Vibrio 0139:	Enteropathogenic Colitis, uremia Epidemic cholera
Viral	Rota: Ebola: HTLV I and II: HIV B, A, C serotype HIV, EA Subserotype Hepatitis E and C Sabia virus Nipah virus	Infantile diarrhea Hemorrhagic fever Cancer HIV/AIDS epidemic Hepatitis Hemorrhagic fever Viral epidemic
Indirect (viral)	Mad cow disease	Spongiform encephalopathy (Creutzfeldt-Jakob disease in man)

Vision for the millennium (to control emerging and re-emerging infections):
- Strong National Disease Surveillance and Control Programs.
- Global networks of centers, organizations and individuals to monitor disease (medical informatics).
- Rapid information exchange through electronic links to guide policies, international collaboration, trade and travel.
- Effective national and international preparedness, and rapid response to contain epidemics of international importance.
- Undertaking research activities on the issues.

HOSPITAL ACQUIRED INFECTIONS (NOSOCOMIAL INFECTION) (HOSPITAL CROSS INFECTION)

Over-crowding, unhygienic methods and resistant strains of organisms are common causes of Hospital Acquired Infections.

Global and Indian Pictures

- About 10–12% of hospital admission.
- Marginal allowance is given up to 1%.

Source

- Patients in hospitals, e.g., urinary tract infections, skin infections, viral infections, respiratory infections.
- Hospital staff, such as doctors, nurses, ward boys who can harbor pathogens in their noses, skin surfaces and mobiles.
- Hospital environment, e.g., dust, furniture, any facilities.

Various types of infections are:

- Viral infections
- Skin infections
- Respiratory infections
- Urinary tract infections.

Routes of the infections are:

- Droplet
- Direct, and
- Hospital procedure.

Prevention

The major preventive measures are:

- Isolation of cases
- Judicious use of antibiotics
- Hospital disinfection procedures including CSSD strengthening
- Isolation and treatment of hospital staff who are source of infection
- Universal precautions at hospital
- Notification (periodic)
- Hospital auditing procedure maintenance
- Hospital infection control committee for policies.

Educate and train health workers in disease surveillance control and treatment and HE and the principles of management of information system

By quantitative methods, management of information system is made possible to reach health manpower on one side and the community on the other side.

Most of the information system is managed by computers and digital system. With this, feedback is very good with health planners.

Good information systems help in monitoring health problems. Further it will also help in evaluation of health programs.

For everyday life and every system of Health and Family Welfare (H & FW), formal information and informal information are major sources to plan and to execute to manage the health situation.

Information system is one of the methods which is based on behavioral sciences.

Management is for getting things for effective use of manpower, material and money.

a. Preplanning and planning about course of action
b. How to go about is determined. Selected groups are allotted to do assigned course
c. Public are motivated by way of good communication
d. Progress of work started is monitored for satisfactory progress.

To bring the change in desirable community behavior, health education is imparted through education. It is justifiable to maintain and restore positive health.

Health education has teaching activities and learning activities for health manpower and the public to bring about change in healthy behavior.

As part of health care, knowledge is imparted to public which certainly bring about positive change in the community.

Training and deduction programs are planned in training of medical staff, paramedical staff and nonmedical staff.

Chapter 9: Epidemiology of Communicable Diseases

Various approaches followed in training health workers:
A. Regulations existing in PHC training programs through manual supplied by government
B. At the time of provision of Health and Family Welfare services.

Emphasis is made young health workers who are recruited are deputed for training through manual guide provided by government. Contents are usually—personal hygiene, better nutrition, small family norm, disease control and good mental health.

Training in disease surveillance include:
- Drug for treatment
- Awareness of natural history of diseases
- Social and behavioral components in illness control and control of recurrence of illness
- Educate the mass/community/public on eradication and or control of illness
- Training shall emphasize malaria, tuberculosis, leprosy, filaria, and goiter.

Health worker male	Health worker female
• Survey of families	• Notification diarrhea/dysentery/fever/rash
• Immunization	• Jaundice
• Control of vector-borne malaria	• Fever inform HW male for blood smear/presumptive treatment
• Spraying operation	• Skin patch survey
• Training of field spraying staff	• Record maintenance—malaria/TB/leprosy
• Kala-azar	• ORS
• JE	• STD/HIV awareness
• Filaria	• Help in filarial endemic
• Leprosy	
• Tuberculosis	
• EPI vaccination	
• Communicable disease—diarrhea dysentery	
• Rash identification	
• Jaundice	
• Eye infection	
• General control measures	
• ORS	
• Health education	
• Record keeping	

Health workers training is scheduled at PHC, using training manual supplied by government.

SUMMARY

Intestinal infection, respiratory infection, vector-borne infection, surface infection and zoonotic infection are detailed. Note on emerging and re-emerging infection are highlighted. Hospital acquired infection importance is highlighted.

VIVA VOCE

1. Difference between OPV and IPV.
2. What is IPPI?
3. How homemade fluid is made for diarrhea?
4. Mention differences between classical *Vibrio* and *El Tor Vibrio*.
5. Clinical difference between food poison and cholera poison.
6. What is the use of Chandler's index?
7. Mention preventive steps for corona virus infection.
8. What is DOTS chemotherapy?
9. Mention distinctive strain that cause influenza.
10. Mention malariometric values.
11. Give examples for Arboviral infection.
12. What is lepra reaction?
13. Mention differences between LCU and SET centers in leprosy.
14. What is fixed virus? How does it differ from street virus?
15. Name some emerging diseases.

Chapter 10: Epidemiology of Noncommunicable Diseases

CHAPTER OUTLINE

- Epidemiological Findings
- General Measures in Prevention
- Selected Noncommunicable Diseases
  - Cancer
  - Coronary Heart Disease (CHD)
  - Hypertension
  - Diabetes
  - Blindness
  - Stroke
  - Rheumatic Heart Disease (RHD)
  - Obesity
  - Accidents

INTRODUCTION

Diseases which are not communicable, associated with specific risk factor, take longer time to get manifested and which necessitate modification of normal life are called noncommunicable diseases (NCDs).

Noncommunicable diseases are called *white plague*. Day by day the incidence is increasing even in developing countries like India.

Noncommunicable diseases are also being called *chronic disabling conditions* because of their characteristics like:

- Cause permanent damage
- Disability is known to occur
- All noncommunicable diseases need rehabilitation
- Health care of noncommunicable diseases is life long
- Dependency is a definite stage in the natural history.

COMMON NONCOMMUNICABLE DISEASES (TABLE 10.1)

- Cancer
- Coronary heart disease
- Hypertension

Table 10.1: Source of white plague.

Hypernutrition	Obesity
Serum cholesterol (LDL)	Coronary heart disease
Stress	High blood pressure
High blood pressure	Stroke
Heavy traffic	Accident
Smoking	Cancer

(LDL: low-density lipoprotein)

- Renal and urinary tract disease
- Diabetes
- Respiratory diseases
- Gastrointestinal diseases
- Musculoskeletal diseases
- Neurological diseases
- Blindness
- Psychiatric diseases
- Stroke
- Rheumatic heart disease
- Obesity
- Accidents.

EPIDEMIOLOGICAL FINDINGS IN NONCOMMUNICABLE DISEASE

- Early diagnosis and specific treatment cannot be provided to the entire sector of

population. Failure to obtain preventive care exists.
- Lifestyle is changing due to civilization, urbanization and sophistication.
- Modern society is facing stress in all walks of life such as domestic, office, industry, and business, social and political systems.
- We are faced with atmospheric pollution such as air pollution, water pollution, and soil pollution.
- Habits or customs make a necessity or sometimes tradition to use certain nonessential substances such as cigarette, cigar, snuff, *beedi* and alcohol.
- Periodic health check-up is neither feasible nor accepted in developing countries.

Unknown of Known Noncommunicable Diseases (NCDs)

- When starts? When develops and when manifests are uncertain.
- Latent period between exposure to cause (or risk) and manifestation is uncertain.
- Identified and evaluated causative factor is uncertain.
- In the triad of epidemiology of NCD, agent is uncertain.

GENERAL MEASURES IN PREVENTION OF NONCOMMUNICABLE DISEASE

Political approach: Smoking, alcoholism, and drug abuse.

Behavioral approach: Lifestyle.

Educational approach: Cancer education.

Screening approach: Pap smear, biopsy, and laboratory test

Hi-tech approach: Cardiac surgery, neurosurgery, and eye surgery.

Rehabilitation approach: Stroke, and Alzheimer's.

SELECTED NONCOMMUNICABLE DISEASES

Cancer

The disease is characterized by unlimited growth, invasion to organs and organ failure and ultimately death (carcinoma, sarcoma, lymphoma, myeloma). Leukemia are major categories seen in clinical practice. Tumor is colloquial word used for cancer which may be primary or secondary as per cited occurrence.

Earlier, cancer used to be 6th leading cause of deaths and now it has occupied 2nd place.

World Picture

Millions of cases are occurring with 12 percent of deaths by cancer. Lung cancer is about 48/100,000 in occurrence. 25% of cancer is Ca breast in UK and its occurrence is 60/100,000. 50% of cancers are among people above 65 years of age.

- About 12 million patients are identified per year
- About 6 million cancer patients are dying per year
- About 25 million people are at risk of cancer
- About 20% is the incidence of cancer
- About 18% is the specific mortality for cancer.

Epidemiological aspects of specific cancers (**Fig. 10.1**).

2018 data shows incidence and deaths are 9.5 million and 5.4 million respectively among men.

The same data among women is 8.6 million and 4.2 million respectively.

Lung cancer

In India, 7.5% of cancers are lung cancers. Smoking, air pollution, and asbestos occupation are significantly related with cancer of lung.

Cancer of stomach

About 684,000 cases are occurring annually in the world. *Helicobacter (H) pylori* infection and spicy food are significantly related with cancer of stomach.

Cancer of cervix

About 570,000 new cases are occurring in a year around the world.

Genital warts, marital status and oral contraceptives are significantly related with cancer of cervix.

Cancer of breast

About 2,100,000 lakhs cases are occurring in a year.

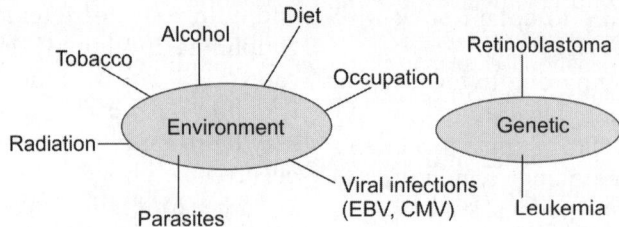

Fig. 10.1: Attributable causes of cancer by environment and genetic origin. (EBV: Epstein-Barr virus; CMV: cytomegalovirus)

Women aged above 35 years of age, parity, late menopause and radiation are significantly related with cancer cervix.

Oral cancer

About 6 lakh cases and 3 lakh deaths are occurring every year around the world.

About 50% of oral cancers are found in India.

Tobacco use, leukoplakia and indigenous way of smoking are significantly related with oral cancer.

Indian Picture

About 3 million cases are occurring and about 1 million are new among them. Every year about 3.5 lakh patients are dying due to cancer. Lung cancer is about 14 per 100,000 occurrences; 25% of cancer is breast cancer.

Incident of cancer both in rural or urban area is about 100–140 per 100,000.

Sociocultural factors associated with cancers

Smoking, alcoholism, tobacco use, low fiber diet, polyandry, sunbath are significantly related with cancer.

Cancer control approach

- Primary prevention
  - Tobacco
  - Diet
  - Alcohol
  - Occupation, environment
  - Infection and cancer
  - Sunlight
  - Sexual and reproductive factor.
- Early detection
  - Education for early diagnosis, and
  - Screening for cancer.
- Treatment for cancer
  - Chemical therapy: *Common cytotoxic drugs:*

Most common cancers in India are:

Men	Women
Lung cancer	Breast
Prostate	Colorectal
Colorectal	Lung
Stomach cancer	Cervical cancer
Liver	Thyroid

- Melphalan an alkylating agent
- Methotrexate an antimetabolite
- Vincristine a mitotic spindle poison
- Mitomycin an antibiotic combinations
- Carboplatin + Paclitaxel
- Cisplatin + 5 fluorouracil
- Radiotherapy
- Surgical intervention
- Palliative care for pain relief
- Research
  - Cancer control research.

National cancer control program (NCCP)

Started in 1975–1976

- 1984: Revised NCCP
- 1990: District cancer control program cobalt therapy installations
  - Assistance to mammography
  - Finance aid to nongovernment organizations (NGOs) oncology wing in medical colleges
- 2000: Revised district cancer control program women awareness about cancer and awareness on health facilities.
- 2004: The program was revised.
- 2010: Integrated under national program on prevention and control of diabetes, cardiovascular disease, and stroke. Cancer awareness day started observing

Chapter 10: Epidemiology of Noncommunicable Diseases

Basic steps for preventing cancer according to NCCP:
- Assess magnitude of national cancer problem
- Setting measurable cancer control objectives
- Evaluating possible strategies, and
- Choosing priority of action.

Goals of NCCP (Table 10.2)

The major goals of NCCP are as following:
- To prevent future cancers
- To diagnose cancer early
- To provide curative therapy (prompt treatment)
- To ensure freedom from suffering (palliative care)
- To reach all in population (cancer education).

District cancer control program
- Cancer education
- Cancer screening camps
- Ca cervix—Pap test
- Referrals
- Ca breast
  - Self examination
  - Clinical examination
  - Thermography
  - Mammography

Table 10.2: Specific objectives in NCCP.

Objectives	Strategy
Prevention of 1/3 cancer	Tobacco
	Diet
Palliative care	Alcohol
	Occupation/environment
	HBV immunization
	Solar radiation
Early diagnosis	Ca cervix
	Ca breast
	Ca oral cavity
Cure of curable cancer	Treatment policy
	Oral morphine
	Training of health professionals
Use of resource	Low cost high benefit strategy

(Ca: cancer; HBV: hepatitis B vaccination; NCCP: national cancer control program)

- Ca lung
  - MMR
  - Sputum cytology.

Warning signs of cancer

Following are the common symptoms of cancer:
- A lump in breast
- Change in bowel habit
- Change in mole
  - A change in the wart
  - Persistent cough
- Hoarseness of voice
- History of bleeding rectal, vaginal, and oral unless otherwise proved
- Loss of weight, and
- Difficulty in swallowing

Screening test in oncology

See **Table 10.3**.

Tests to detect stages of cancer:
- *Prostate and breast cancer:* Bone scan.
- *Colon cancer:* Ultrasonography (USG).
- *Lung cancer:* Chest X-ray and computed tomography (CT).

Cancer registry

Hospital-based as well as population-based cancer registrations are done, which are found useful for operational activities.

They are established in Mumbai, Chennai and Bengaluru.

Coronary Heart Disease (CHD)

Coronary heart disease (CHD) is impairment of heart function due to inadequate blood flow to the heart compared to its needs caused by coronary artery obstruction. It is also defined as progressive disorder of arteries by atherosclerosis where blockage of artery occurs. Common among people above the age of 35

Table 10.3: Screening test in oncology.

Cancer cervix	Pap smear
Cancer stomach	Endoscopy
Cancer colon	Sigmoidoscopy
Cancer prostate	Serum prostate specific antigen (PSA)
Cancer breast	Mammography

Tumor markers
See **Table 10.4**.

Table 10.4: Tumor markers.

PSA	Cancer prostate, Ca. breast
LDH	All types of cancers
α fp strain	Ca. liver, Ca. breast, Ca. GI tract
CA125	Ca. ovary
CEA	Ca. lung, Ca. breast, Ca. GI tract
hCG	Teratoma, Choriocarcinoma

(PSA: prostate specific antigen; LDH: lactate dehydrogenase; GI: gastrointestinal tract; CEA: carcinoembryonic antigen; hCG: human chorionic gonadotropin)

years. CHD is common form of heart disease and common cause of premature death also.

Atheromatous stenosis of coronary arteries, myocardial necrosis, myocardial dysfunction, altered conduction, ventricular arrhythmia, asystole, and massive myocardial infarction (MI) are manifestations in the course of the disease.

Usual presentations are as given below:
- Angina pectoris
- Myocardial infarction (MI)
- Heart fibrillation
- Cardiac failure
- Sudden death.

Community Index of Coronary Heart Disease (CHD)
- Proportional mortality ratio for CHD.
- Age-specific death rate due to CHD.
- Case fatality rate (CFR) of CHD.

Global Picture
Epidemiological transition has occurred due to urbanization and civilization with degenerative changes and with man made illnesses. About 8 million deaths are occurring due to cardiovascular diseases form 12.8% of total deaths. General incidence is 2/10,000. Among 25–64 age groups it is 3/10,000.

Proportional mortality ratio is around 25–30%. Life expectation lost by this chronic condition is 4–10 years. Regarding case fatality rates; 25% sudden deaths and 55% deaths in 1 hour are observed.

High in developed countries. Urban and civilized show 5 times more incidence than other places.

Age standardized death rate of CHD is highest in Scotland, and lowest in Japan.

Indian Picture
Out of 3 million deaths occurring in a year, 1 million is due to CHD.

Prevalence
- Male in urban areas 65 per 1000
- Rural areas 22 per 1000
- Female in urban areas 47 per 1000
- Rural areas 17 per 1000.

Peak incidence is seen in the age group of 50–60 years of age. Men are more prone to CHD than women. Hypertension, diabetes account for 40% of CHD cases in the country. Heavy smoking is found related with CHD.

Exposure to inappropriate nutrition, Lack of physical activities, Increased tobacco consumption → Log time → Mortality

In community, the manifestations such as angina, MI, heart irregularities, heart failure, and sudden death are specific entities in clinical practice.

Risk factors
Following are the major risk factors:

Nonmodifiable
- Age
- Sex, and
- Genetic.

Modifiable
- Smoking
- Blood pressure (BP)
- Serum cholesterol [low-density lipoprotein (LDL)]
- Diabetes
- Obesity
- Sedentary habits
- Stress condition
- Type A personality
- Consumption of soft water
- High serum level of homocysteine
- Drugs such as phentermine, fenfluramine
- Alcohol
- Oral contraceptives.

Long-term measures in the community

Saturated fat should be 10% of total calories (Diet control)

Cholesterol level 200 mg

Cholesterol intake 300 mg/head/day

Salt intake 5 g per day per head, Smoking is prohibited, Active aging (maintaining physical activities). Early diagnosis and treatment of hypertension (BP Control) and diabetes. Health education (maintaining traditional life-style), LDL level control.

Normal blood level suggested.

- High-density lipoprotein (HDL) 30–70 mg%
- Low-density lipoprotein (LDL) 90–150 mg%
- Triglycerides 60–170 mg%
- Total cholesterol 150–250 mg%

Prevention of CHD

- Population strategy
  - Smoking
  - Physical activity
  - Diet
  - Blood pressure, and
  - Lifestyle changes (primordial)
- High-risk strategy
- Secondary prevention.

Field trials in cardiovascular disease (risk factor intervention studies)

1. Framingham study
2. The Stanford Study of California
3. The North Karelia Project in Finland
4. The Multiple Risk Factors Interventional Trial in the USA
5. The Oslo study in Norway.

Hypertension (Table 10.5)

A systolic BP equal to or greater than 130 mm Hg and a diastolic BP equal to or greater than 85 mm Hg is treated as hypertension [World Health Organization (WHO)] (**Table 10.5**). Hypertension is a trait rather than a disease where target organs are blood vessels, central nervous system (CNS), retina, heart, and kidneys (**Fig. 10.2**).

Types

- Primary hypertension (essential)
- Secondary hypertension.

Table 10.5: WHO criteria for hypertension.

Range	Status
Below 130/85	Normal
130–139 / 85–90	High normal
149–159 / 90–99	Mild hypertension
160–179 / 100–109	Moderate hypertension
Above 180/110	Severe hypertension

(WHO: World Health Organization)

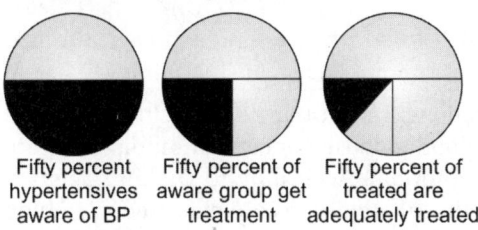

Fifty percent hypertensives aware of BP   Fifty percent of aware group get treatment   Fifty percent of treated are adequately treated

Fig. 10.2: Rule of half (halves).

Global Picture

About 10–20 percent prevalence in developed countries (WHO).

Indian Picture

- 6–7 per 10,000 urban population
- 3–4 per 10,000 rural population
  "Tracking" of blood pressure (persistence of rank order of BP).
- Low BP level tend to remain low
- High BP level tend to remain high, and
- This gives us risk group.

Risk factors

- Nonmodifiable
  - Age, and
  - Genetic.
- Modifiable risk factors
  - Overweight
  - High salt and high fat intake
  - Alcohol
  - Physical activity, and
  - Tension and stress.

Prevention of hypertension

- Primary hypertension
  - Population strategy

- Weight control
- Strict diet
- Physical activity
- Meditation
- Awareness
- Participation, and
- High-risk strategy.
  ❖ Secondary hypertension.

Government of India project

Control of cardiovascular diseases and stroke in organized sectors such as Railways, Central Government Health Scheme (CGHS) and industries was undertaken by Government of India in 1995–1996.

Diabetes

It is a metabolic disorder with many manifestations. It is not a single entity. In a community, blood glucose concentration distribution is unimodal. According to Diabetologists the clinical conditions are expected to treble by 2020.

Types

1. Gestational diabetes mellitus (GDM)
2. Impaired glucose tolerance (IGT)
3. Diabetes mellitus (DM)
   a. Insulin dependent (IDDM type I)
   b. Noninsulin dependent (NIDDM type II)
   c. Malnutrition related (MRDM)
   d. Pancreatic, hormonal and drug-induced diabetes.

Major differences between Type I and Type II diabetes mellitus (**Table 10.6**).

Global Picture

Fifty percent of diabetes are in developed countries, whereas, 10 percent of diabetes are in developing countries. The disease affects 1–2 percent population and the prevalence has risen to 15% in most of the community. Social stress seems to predominate in Type II diabetes. USA and UK have reported 1.4% and 1.13% respectively.

Indian Picture

Urban prevalence   4 percent
Rural prevalence   2 percent

Table 10.6: Differences between Type I and Type II diabetes mellitus.

	Type I	Type II
Age	Below 40	Above 50
Symptoms duration	In weeks	In years
Weight	Normal	Obese
Ketonuria	+	–
Complications	–	+
Family history	–	+

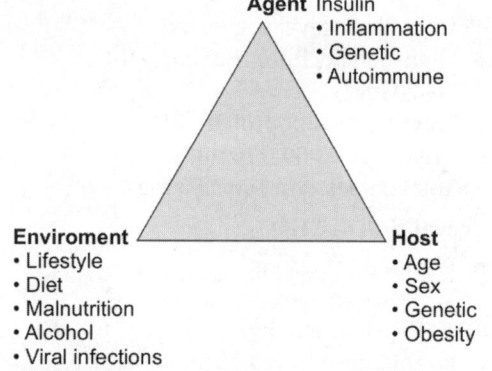

Fig. 10.3: Epidemiological triad in diabetes.

Indian Council of Medical Research (ICMR) has recorded 2.1% in urban and 1.5% rural population.

Epidemiology: See **Figure 10.3**

Influencing factors in diabetes:
Type I diabetes: Environment, virus, diet, stress, immunity, and pancreas pathology
Type II diabetes: Genetic, and environment.

Screening test (high-risk group is preferred)
- Urine test, and
- Blood sugar, fasting blood sugar (FBS), and postprandial blood sugar (PPBS).

Diagnostic test FBS if more than 140 (normal range is 70–120) and glucose tolerance (GT) 2 hours postprandial if more than 200 (normal is 140). In case of pregnant woman, the FBS value criteria is taken at 105 and GT 2 hours postprondial as 165 (If GT in pregnant woman is 3 hours postprondial the value taken is 145).

Criteria as per diabetes expert committee for the diagnosis of diabetes:

Chapter 10: Epidemiology of Noncommunicable Diseases

	Normal	Impaired	Diabetes
FBS	<110	110–126	>126
PPBS after 2 hours	<140	140–200	>200

Epidemiological triad is depicted in **Figure 10.3**.

Common and usual complications of diabetes

Organs	Complications
Eye	Cataract, and retinopathy
Kidney	Nephropathy
Nerve	Peripheral neuropathy, and autonomic neuropathy
Foot	Foot diseases
CHD	MI
Cerebrum	TIA, and stroke
Circulation	Claudication, and ischemia

(CHD: coronary heart disease; MI: myocardial infarction; TIA: transient ischemic attack)

Prevention

- Population strategy (primordial)
  - Weight control
  - Good nutrition habit, and
  - Physical exercise.
  Self-care is advised on diet, urine examination, weight reduction, and self-injection of insulin after guidance from physician, eye care, to avoid stress and about feet care.
- High-risk strategy
  - Treatment, diet, drug, and exercise
  - Periodic examination, and
  - Half yearly glycosylated hemoglobin (Hb%) estimation
- Tertiary strategy
  - Care of blindness, kidney failure, gangrene of lower extremities and coronary thrombosis.

Insulin resistance syndrome is seen with Type II obese and is associated with a genetic defect producing insulin resistance. It is also called syndrome X.

National diabetic control program

This program was started in Seventh Five year Plan in selected states. The main activities included:

- Identification of risk people
- Information, education and communication (IEC) activities
- Diagnosis and treatment
- Prevention of complication
- Rehabilitation.

Blindness

This is a condition with visual acuity of less than 3/60 (Snellen chart) or its equivalent (WHO). This is also equivalent to inability to count fingers in daylight at a distance of 3 meters.

Prevalence of above 1% of blindness is considered as public health problem.

WHO criteria for categorization of avoidable blindness:

Category 01	Below 6/18–6/60 or up to 3/60
Category 02	Below 6/60–3/60
Category 03	Below 3/60–1/60 or up to finger counting at 1 meter
Category 04	Below 1/60 to light perception
Category 05	No light perception
Category 06	Not specified conditions of vision defects.

Global Picture

Forty-five million of global population is blind and among them 80% is preventable blindness. 180 million are disabled due to blindness. Among causes of blindness; cataract cases are about 20 million, glaucoma cases are about 7 million and trachoma cases are about 6 million and about 10 million due to other causes.

Indian Picture

In India it is estimated that about 0.5% of population are having visual impairment and blindness at a given point of time. 0.7 percent of total population is blind. About 7 million people are blind in the country which is due to cataract (prevalence of blind due to cataract is 77%). Cataract surgery rate in India is about 3,500 per 1 million per year. Intraocular lens rate is about 34 per every 100 cataract surgery operations. Other causes are refractive errors, childhood blindness, and corneal blindness.

National survey has observed that the proportion of cataract is 62.6%, refractive error 19.7%, glaucoma 5.8%, and corneal opacity 0.9%.

Very high category (above 2% prevalence) is present in Madhya Pradesh (MP), Rajasthan, and Jammu and Kashmir (J & K) states.

According to National Program for the Control of Blindness in India, three categorization is done about avoidable blindness. They are:

Low vision	Below 6/18–6/60 in better eye
Economic blindness	Below 6/60–3/60 in better eye
Social blindness	Below 3/60 in better eye.

Survey findings by WHO and ICMR

Major conditions	WHO	ICMR
Cataract	81%	55%
Trachoma	0.2%	5.0%
Vitamin A deficiency	0.04%	2.0%

Epidemiology is depicted in **Figure 10.4**.

Eye health care (primary eye care)

The main objective of the primary eye care is to reduce blindness to the level of less than 0.3%.

1. Initial assessment of avoidable blindness. Area mapping according to prevalence:
   * Category I 1% prevalence
   * Category II 0.5% prevalence
   * Category III 0.2% prevalence
2. Intervention
   * I level (primary)
     – Foreign body removal
     – Infection control, and
     – Vitamin A prophylaxis.
   * II level (secondary)
     – Management of cataract, and
     – Management of glaucoma.
   * III level (tertiary)
     – Corneal graft, and
     – Retinal surgery
3. Special program
   * Trachoma control
     One percent tetracycline ointment BD 5 days a month and monthly for 6 months. Blanket treatment to all below 10 years.
   * School eye health service.
   * Vitamin A prophylaxis.
     Two lakh IU by oral route, at 6 monthly interval to children 9 months to 3 years.
   * Occupational eye care
4. Long-term measures
   * Water supply
   * Vitamin A supplementation
   * Social upliftment
5. Evaluation
6. Eye bank facility and service
7. Mobile ophthalmic unit for camp and service.
8. National control through training, laboratory facility, and district blindness control society establishment.
9. Voluntary contributory service by:
   * National Association for the Blind (NAB)
   * Danish International Development Agency (DANIDA).

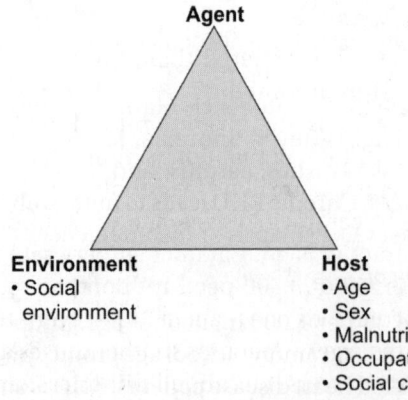

Fig. 10.4: Epidemiological triad in blindness.

Vision 2020

Vision 2000 was launched in 1999 with slogan "The Right to Sight" to eliminate avoidable blindness by 2020 AD. It is incorporated in National Program for the Control of Blindness. Main activities in the program are:

❖ To improve ophthalmic structure for high quality eye care [OT constructions, equipment and financial assistance of ₹ 150/- per operation for drugs and consumables, 75/- per case for spectacles, 75/- per case for transport, provision of sutures and intraocular lenses (IOLs)], cost for the equipment repair.
❖ To develop cost effective measures at rural areas

- To create awareness on the preventable blindness
- To give training to ophthalmologists, to ophthalmic assistants, and refractionists in the country
- To supply spectacles and IOL
- Arrangement of mega eye camps
- Arrangement for school screening.

Global eye health action plan 2014–2019 aims to reduce avoidable visual impairment.

Stroke (Apoplexy)

This is rapidly developed clinical sign of focal disturbance of cerebral function lasting more than 24 hours or leading to death with no apparent cause other than vascular origin (WHO). Thrombosis, embolism and hemorrhage of cerebrum lead to stroke which give rise to sudden dramatic neurological deficit (dysfunction of the brain) in the body.

Cerebral hemorrhage and cerebral thrombosis constitute major causes of stroke.

Types of stroke have been:
a. Transient (recovery within 24 hours)
b. Completed (focal deficit, not worsening)
c. Evolving (continued deficient, worsens).

Global Picture

- Two per 1,000 population per year is recorded.
- Highest morbidity has been in Japan.
- Sex preference to male is observed.
- Fatal stroke incidence has been 0.5 per 1,000 population.

Epidemiological factors in disease process:
- Above 40 years of age
- Men succumb twice than women
- Hemorrhagic stroke usually occurs in day time, and ischemic in early morning times
- Hypertension, coronary artery disease (CAD), RHD, and diabetes have their influence in the disease process.
- Oral contraceptives are found to be a risk factor.

Prestroke Warning

Presence of microemboli causing sudden focal reversible neurological deficit which is less than 24 hours duration which is called transient ischemic attack (TIA) form warning signals of recurrence of stroke.

Risk Factors

- High BP
- Left ventricular hypertrophy
- Diabetes mellitus
- Hypercholesterolemia.

Diagnosis

CT, lipoprotein (LP), echocardiography (ECG), Doppler USG, total cholesterol (TC) DC, cholesterol, clotting time and blood glucose.

Community Level Stroke Control Program

- Stroke awareness by cardiac education [prevention of atherosclerosis, maintenance of HDL 50, LDL 140, very-low-density lipoproteins (VLDL 10), total plasma cholesterol 200 and triglyceride below 50]
- Measures for control of arterial hypertension (BP control, no over sedation in elderly, no rapid diuresis)
- Diabetes control activities
- Elimination of smoking, and
- Health personnel training as an integral part of stroke control program.

Rheumatic Heart Disease (RHD)

Rheumatic heart disease (RHD) is one of the preventable heart diseases and manifested RHD is a crippling disease resulting in damage of the heart and causing disability. It is an acquired heart disease with multi system diseases found among 5–15 year children.

Rheumatic heart disease (RHD) is preceded by rheumatic fever (RF), a connective tissue disease from infection with group A beta hemolytic streptococci. Manifestations are pharyngitis, fever, anorexia, lethargy, joint pain, skin rashes, carditis, and neurological changes. Chronic RHD leads to mitral valvular diseases like stenosis or incompetence.

World Picture

Six to 33 per 1,000 in alcohol age group and 100/100,000 among school age group. Among admitted heart disease patients, RHD is about 30%.

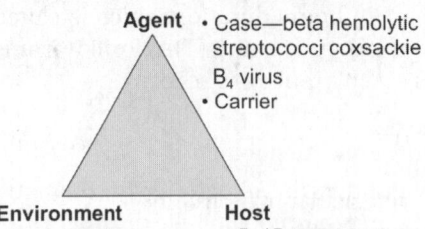

Fig. 10.5: Epidemiological triad in rheumatic heart disease (RHD).

Indian Picture (Fig. 10.5)

- 2–3 per 1,000 population
- 6–10 per 1,000 school age group.

Community Diagnostic Tool

- Jones criteria
  - Two major
  - One major + two minor
- Throat culture, and
- ASO antibody titer.

Revised Jones Criteria (WHO)

Major	Minor
Carditis	Fever
Polyarthritis	Arthralgia
Chorea	Past history of RF
Erythema marginatum	Abnormal ESR
Subcutaneous nodule	C-reactive protein
	Leukocytosis
	Prolonged PR interval

(ESR: erythrocyte sedimentation rate; RF: rheumatic fever)

Prevention

Primary level

a. Prevention of attack of RF by throat infection identification, single dose penicillin therapy (with 3 lakh units crystalline + 3 lakh units procaine, and 6 lakh unit benzathine).
b. Surveillance of high-risk prevalence group of children.
c. Improving living condition secondary prevention.

Secondary level

a. Prevention of recurrence of RF by long acting penicillin.

Prevention Chart of Rheumatic Fever

1. *Primary prevention*
   Benzathine penicillin 1 M single dose (crystalline 3 lakh + Procaine 3 lakh + Benzathine 6 lakh).
   a. Penicillin V oral 10 days 250 mg TDS
   b. For penicillin allergic erythromycin oral 10 days 40 mg/kg four times daily
   c. Increase standard of living
   d. Improve environmental sanitation
   e. Decrease overcrowding
   f. Sore throat screening procedures.
2. *Secondary prevention*
   a. Monthly injection of 6 lakh unit benzathine penicillin for 5 years or till attains 18 years.
   b. Early diagnosis and prompt treatment of rheumatic fever.

Obesity

It is a pathological stage of overweight for the given situation such as age, sex and height of individual. Body mass indexes (Quetelet's index) of above 30 in men and above 28.6 in women indicate obesity. Excessive adipose tissue is reflected by increased body weight.

Consumption of high fat diet, energy dense foods and alcohol are associated with obesity. Generalized and abdominal obesity are common which are called *pear-shaped* and *apple-shaped* obesity.

Types

- Hypertrophic obesity
- Hyperplastic obesity, and
- Both hypertrophic and hyperplastic obesity.

Global Picture

About 50% of adult are overweight and 20% are obese in developed countries.

Indian Picture

Urban picture is similar to global picture. Overall picture in India is less than 6% in the population.

The difference between overweight and obese are:

Overweight

Body weight is more than 110% that of acceptable range.

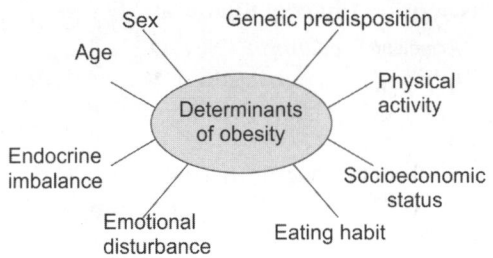

Fig. 10.6: Determinants of obesity.

Obese
Body weight is more than 120% that of acceptable range.
Determinants are depicted in **Figure 10.6**.

Community assessment of obesity
Weight recording and body mass index (BMI) are common measures for obesity.

Normal	<120% weight	<26 kg/m²
Mild	120–140% weight	27–30 kg/m²
Moderate	140–200% weight	30–40 kg/m²
Severe	>200% weight	>40 kg/m²

- **Harpenden skin caliper method:** Skin fold thickness of midtriceps, biceps, subscapular and suprailiac regions are obtained (sum of measurement 40 mm in boys and 50 mm in girls are acceptable levels).
- Quetelet index (body mass index) is found out by weight/height²
  - Below 0.140 normal
  - 0.140–0.144 sub-nutrition
  - 0.145–0.149 under-nutrition
  - Above 0.150 malnutrition
- Broca index is found out by height (cm) minus 100 for weight (kg)
- Ponderal index is found out by:

$$\frac{\text{Height (cm)}}{\text{Weight}^3 \text{ (kg)}}$$

- Corpulence index is found out by:

$$\frac{\text{Actual weight}}{\text{Desirable weight}}$$

(Acceptable level 1.2)
- Lorentz index is found out by men: (cm)

$$(Ht - 100) - \frac{Ht - 150}{4}$$

Women: (cm)

$$(Ht - 100) - \frac{Ht - 150}{2}$$

Obesity consequences
- Development of hypertension, diabetes, CHD, and thromboembolic disorders
- Development of varicose veins, hernia, and arthritis
- Increased mortality, and
- Increased morbidity.

Prevention
- Diet
- Exercise
- Regulation of over feeding behavior.

Accidents
It is defined as unexpected event involving injury, disability or death. Problems due to accidents are measured by disability, morbidity and mortality. Every year about 1.5 million are dying due to road traffic accidents. Morbidity is 19 per 100,000 population.

It is also defined an event against human will caused by external force on individual to cause physical and mental injury (**Fig. 10.7**).

Types
- Vehicular accidents
  - Road traffic
  - Aircraft
  - Railway and
  - Sea traffic
- Self-inflicted accidents
- Accidental falls
- Industry accidents
- Drowning
- Poisoning
- Fire accidents
- Disaster accidents.

According to WHO study (2016) following types are seen:
- Unintentional injuries
  - Road injury
  - Poisoning
  - Falls
  - Fire, heat, and hot substance
  - Drowning

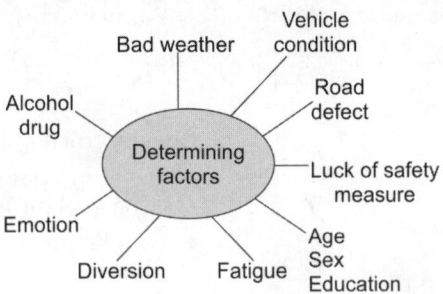

Fig. 10.7: Determining factors in accident.

- Exposure to mechanical forces
- Natural disasters
- Other intentional injuries
- Intentional injuries
  - Self-harm
  - Inter-personal violence
  - Collective violence and legal intervention.

This study also show that 8.6% of total deaths is from injuries.

Global Picture

Nine percent of all deaths are by accidents. Death by accident, poisoning, and violence has been about 64 per 100,000 population (WHO).

Suicide incidence in the world:
40/100,000   Hungary, Austria, West Berlin
3/100,000   Nigeria, Nicaragua, Middle East
8.8/100,000 India

Commonly, 5–45 age group individuals are involved in accidents. Motor vehicle and suicide are major causes of deaths among accidents.

Indian Picture

Now, set at four percent of all deaths slowly rising to global picture.

Two lakh people are dying annually by traffic accident alone.

Prevention of accidents

- Development of basic reporting system
- Development of safety education in public
- License withholding against drugs, and alcohol
- Trauma care center establishment in susceptible zones
- Road development programs
- New technology in vehicle, airway, railway, and sea travel
- Fire brigade development action force
- Safe storage of poisons.
  Law enforcement for:
  - Medical fitness among drivers of roadway, airway, seaway
  - Seat belts
  - Helmets
  - Factory safety
  - Industry safety

Accident Research (Accidentology)

Safety education

- Traffic regulation
- No alcohol at driving
- No smoking in bed
- Reading label before taking medicine
- Earthing of electrical equipment
- Visible light in vehicles
- Use of proper glass in vehicles
- Use of pneumatic doors in vehicles
- Curbing bad parking on roads
- Prohibiting alcohol while driving
- Use of low beam headlight
- Curbing the use of mobile at driving.

Personal protection

- Helmet for two wheelers
- Lead apron for radiologist and image technologists
- Rubber glove for electricians

- Steel clapped shoe for weight lifting occupation placement
- Life jacket for crew of ship
- Rug for gymnasts.

SUMMARY

Epidemiology of selected NCD namely cancer, coronary heart disease, hypertension, diabetes, blindness, stroke, RHD, obesity and accidents are detailed.

VIVA VOCE

1. Which are the warning signs of cancer?
2. Mention "rule of halves" in hypertension.
3. What are the complications of diabetes?
4. Briefly outline vision 2020-09-02.
5. What is Jones criteria in RHD?
6. What is quetelet index?
7. Mention prevention of accidents.

SECTION 4

Section Outline

Chapter 11. Demography and Vital Statistics
Chapter 12. Reproductive Maternal and Child Health
Chapter 13. School Health

CHAPTER 11: Demography and Vital Statistics

Chapter Outline

- Terminology
- Process
- Estimates of Demographic Values
- Demography and Genetics
- Demographic Cycle
- Major Sources of Data
- Population Dynamics
- Improvident Maternity
- Family Planning—Concept, Methods and Unmet Needs
- Population Education
- National Family Welfare (NFW) Program
- National Population Policy (NPP)

DEMOGRAPHY

Demography is a scientific study which deals with size, composition, and distribution of population.

TERMINOLOGY

Demography

This is the study of human population with respect to its size, type, composition, pattern and distribution.

Demographic Gap

It is the difference between births and deaths. It helps to know the rapid growth of a given population.

Population Dynamics

This is the study of mode of change of population and the factors responsible for such changes.

Population Education

A Health Education Program which provides for a study of population situation in the community, in a country and in the world with the purpose of developing rational and responsible attitude among present generation toward family planning behavior.

PROCESS IN DEMOGRAPHY

a. Migration
b. Social mobility
c. Marriage
d. Fertility, and
e. Mortality

Migration

Movement of people with any of the following reasons:
- Employment
- Calamity
- Industrialization
- Glamour of cities, and
- Educational purpose.

Social Mobility

Movement of people with the purpose of family settlement, occupational placement, temporary stay on account of religious, philanthropic and national purposes.

Marriages

The term marriage can well be defined as the socially accepted bondage in the process of family formation. Marriage rate is that the number of marriages in a year per 1000 population. Pregnancy rate is that the number of pregnancies in a year to married women in the age group of 15–44 years.

Fertility

It is the child-bearing process in the reproductive age group. It is determined by:
* Duration of marriage
* Education
* Socio-economic status
* Religion, and
* Awareness of family planning.

Fertility-related Rates are as given below:
* Birth rate (births per 1000 MYP)
* General fertility rate (GFR) [low birth (LB) per 1000 women of 15–44 ages]
* Age specific fertility rate (ASFR) (LB per 1000 women of given age group)
* Total fertility rate (TFR) (number of child-bearing in her reproductive years)
* Gross reproduction rate (GRR) (number of girls born to 15–44 age groups)
* Net reproduction rate (NRR) (number of female births to an woman in her lifetime)
* Child woman ratio (CWR) (0–4 age children per 1,000 women)
* General marital fertility rate (GMFR) (LB per 1,000 married women of 15–44 age groups).

Mortality

Death experienced in the community:
* Death rate—number of death per 1000 MYP
* Infant mortality rate (IMR)—number of infant death per 1,000 LB
* Maternal mortality ratio (MMR)—number of maternal death per 1,000 LB.

Age Sex Pyramid

When age and sex are represented inordinately, it gives wide base and narrow tapering tip in case of developing countries (narrow base and wide tapering tip in developed countries) (**Fig. 11.1**).

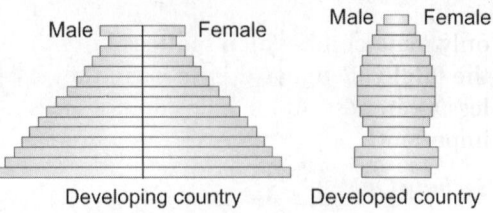

Fig. 11.1: Showing age sex pyramid.

Causes of Declining Sex Ratio and its Social and Health Implications

Recent census give sex ratio in India as 940 females per 1000 males. This is still poor in Haryana, Union Territory like Diu and Daman. Traditionally, first male child born is OK but first female child born, make parents go for another child. Still in tribal India, if girl child born, they kill girl child. In many occasion, infanticide used to be common.

All society, people prefer male child. In urban area, people knew neonatal test and about girl child. Sex determination followed by abortion; in spite of legal binding is existing. Domestic violence, dowry deaths and less attention on female medical illness do harm in the society.

Social Causes

Patriarchal society where more male centric thoughts force the family to have male child with old belief that male child is must for eternal peace or MOKSHA, lack of education leads to not following right attitude. Females are thought to be subject of pleasure. Nagar Vadhu system and Devadasi system existed made more harm. Normally, female child is under nourished succumbs to disease and death.

Technological Cause

Availability and accessibility of ultrasound examination for sex determination, leads to lowering sex ratio.

Economic Cause

Dowry system has led to economic burden. Male child earning source influences to have only male child, which reduces burden for the family. Females do not earn, they have less awareness and females do not feel it as important.

Security Cause

Females are more harassed. They are considered as weak sex, hence public feels they need security and protection.

Other Causes

- Sex ratio at birth
- Sex selective abortion
- Sex ratio of children
- Sex differentials in mortality
- Under enumeration of female births
- Son preference
- Daughter neglect.

Implications

- Imbalance in population structure
- Low status of women in society
- High incidence of crime against women.

Overcoming Declining Sex Ratio

- Provide benefits to the family with one girl child
- Free education to all girls
- Create awareness on Medical Termination of Pregnancy (MTP)
- Create awareness on Prenatal Diagnostic Technique (PNDT) Act
- Ban on clinics which carry sex determination
- Create positive value toward girl child
- Schemes such as universal education, Sukanya Samridhi, Beti Bachao Beti Padhao.

Demographic Gap

It is the difference between births and deaths. This indicates the rapid growth of population in a community.

ESTIMATES OF DEMOGRAPHIC VALUES OF INDIA 2019

Population: 1359.8 million (as per 2011 census = 1210.8 million)
- Birth Rate (BR): 20
- Death Rate (DR): 6.
- Growth Rate (GR): 1.2%

Most densely populated states are UP, Maharashtra and Bihar.
- 0–4 age group: 8.5%
- 0–14: 27.00%
- 65+: 5.40%
- Sex ratio: 1000:898
  [Societal dependency ratio 32.4% (0–14 age and 65+) age]
- Density of population: 876/sq km
- Family size: 2.3
- Urbanization: 31.8%
- Urbanrural ratio 32:68
- General fertility rate: 74.4
- General marital fertility rate: 113.3
- Total fertility rate: 2.3
- Total marital fertility rate: 4.8
- Gross reproduction rate: 1.1
- Literacy status: 74.04%
- Life expectancy: Males 64 years
- (Lifespan): Females 67 years
- Average age at marriage: 22.3 years.

DEMOGRAPHY AND GENETICS

The study of behavior of genes in a given population is also called population genetics.

Let us take the proportion of tallness and proportion of shortness in a population. If "AA" is very tall, "Aa" is moderate and "aa" is short, the total unit of the proportion shall be 100. Marriage and offspring make proportion through sperms and eggs contact and the possible gametic combinations could be as under;

$$AA + 2Aa + aa$$

This is represented by the formula $P^2 + 2Pq + q^2$.

Hardy-Weinberg postulated a law which states "the relative frequencies of each gene allele tend to remain constant from generation to generation in the absence of external forces." Mutation rate per million genes per generation is estimated and some of the examples are:
- Polyposis coli an autosomal dominant disease: 20
- Albinism an autosomal recessive disease: 28
- Hemophilia, a sex-linked recessive disease: 30.

Bad genes in a population cannot be eliminated. Instead affected persons might be persuaded not to have children.

DEMOGRAPHIC CYCLE

The reason behind change of population pattern over a period of time is distinguished by five cycles.

Cycles

1. High stationary (high growth and high death).
2. Early expanding (high growth and moderate death).
3. Late expanding (declining growth and declining death).
4. Low stationary (low growth and low death).
5. Declining (lower rate of births than deaths).

India is in a transition period between late expanding and low stationary period.

MAJOR SOURCES OF DEMOGRAPHIC DATA

- Registration of vital events,
- Census,
- Records of hospitals and health centers, and
- Notification of diseases.

Impacts of overpopulation on the society are:
- Hindrance in country's development,
- Unemployment,
- Illiteracy,
- Poor housing,
- Limited health care,
- Poor sanitation,
- Environmental pollution, and
- Problem of slum and shanty town.

Malthusian Theory of Population Explosion

This theory postulates that overpopulation is controlled by natural calamities such as volcano, earthquake, floods, epidemics, etc. This is not a scientific version. It is only an antithesis of population.

POPULATION ESTIMATION/DYNAMICS

In India de facto basis census is done. Estimation is done by mainly three methods:
1. Natural increase method
   = Census population + (births − deaths) + (immigrants − emigrants).
2. Arithmetic progression method

$$P = P_2 + \frac{P_2 - P_1}{n} \times d$$

Where, n = Number of years
d = years between census and required year

3. Geometric progression method

$$\text{Log} P = \text{Log} P_2 = \frac{\text{Log} P_2 - \text{Log} P_1}{n} \times d$$

IMPROVIDENT MATERNITY

It refers to childbirth occurring to women "who has already given birth to three children of whom one is alive". It is estimated at 44.8%.

FAMILY PLANNING (FAMILY WELFARE PLANNING)

Family planning (FP) is an adopted practice based on knowledge and attitude to avoid unwanted births, to have wanted births, to space pregnancy, to control births and to choose their own family size. **Table 11.1** depicts target and eligible couple.

Components

- Birth control
- Sterility and infertility management
- Sex education
- Marriage counseling
- Preparation for pregnancy, lactation and parenthood
- Management of unmarried mothers, and
- Care of reproductive health.

Present Concept of Family Planning

1. Inverted red triangle, a symbol of health and Family Welfare (FW) services available, seen from a distance by the primary red color.

Table 11.1: Difference between target couple and eligible couple.

Target couple	Eligible couple
Age group of 15–45 years	Following are deducted from target couple: • Primary sterility, • Secondary sterility, • Early menopause

Chapter 11: Demography and Vital Statistics

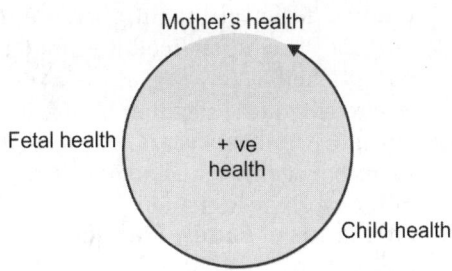

Fig. 11.2: Showing relationship between health and family planning.

2. Family planning is voluntary and not compulsory.
3. It is a cafeteria method; choice is left to the consumer.
4. It is not just FP but family welfare planning (**Fig. 11.2**).

Incentive and Disincentive in Family Planning

See **Table 11.2**.

Family Planning Methods

Temporary Methods

❖ Condom—barrier methods, pregnancy rate = 2–3 per 1000 women year, *Types:* Dry, deluxe, super deluxe.

Table 11.2: Incentive and disincentive in family planning (FP).

Incentives	Rupees (₹)
Tubectomy	1,400.00
Laparoscopy	1,000.00
Vasectomy	2,000.00
Motivation of tubectomy	200.00
Motivation of vasectomy	300.00
One special increment • 14 days of leave to women • 7 days of leave to men • Green card to individual acceptances for special attention **Disincentives:** • Improvident maternity • No housing loan • No subsidized medical treatment	

❖ Diaphragm—called Dutch cap, barrier method, trained person should insert.
❖ Vaginal sponge called *"Today"* barrier method, less advantage.
❖ Foams, creams, suppositories, soluble films are chemical methods. They are surface acting spermicides.
❖ Lippes loop—not used in the FP program
❖ Copper T—Copper T 200 and multiload 250 are commonly used which have 3.0 and 0.5 pregnancy rate. Have an effective life of 5 years. Mode of action is reducing chance of fertilization by foreign body reaction in uterus. Contraindications are pregnancy, undiagnosed bleeding, pelvic inflammatory disease (PID) and cancer.

Side effects are:
- Pain,
- Pelvic inflammatory disease,
- Bleeding,
- Expulsion, and
- Rarely ectopic, perforation and pregnancy.

❖ Oral pills—they are combined pill, progestogen-only pill (POP), postcoital pill, once a month pill and male pill.
- Mala D and Mala N [low dose oral contraceptives (OC)]
- Norgestrel 0.3 mg
- Ethinyl estradiol 0.03 mg
- Mala D is a packet of 28 pill containing 21 pills and 7 ferrous pills
- It is ₹ 2.00 under social marketing. Mala N is freely supplied under FP program. They prevent release of ovum from ovary. They are 100% effective.

Side effects:
- Effects on cardiovascular system (CVS),
- Carcinogenic effect
- Decrease in high-density lipoproteins (HDL)
- Effect on liver, and
- Unwanted effect like weight gain, migraine, bleeding, and breast pain.

❖ Postcoital contraceptive 50 mg. Diethylstilbestrol within 48 hours of unprotected intercourse.

- Gossypol derived from cotton seed oil which is not in wide use (male pill).
- Injectable contraceptives:
  - Depot-medroxy progesterone acetate (DMPA)
  - Norethisterone enanthate (NET-EN).
- Norplant for subdermal implant.
- Vaginal ring with levonorgestrel.

Permanent Methods

- Male sterilization (vasectomy).
- Female sterilization (tubectomy).

Family Planning Measures

- Raising age at marriage.
- Incentive (**Table 11.2**).
- Disincentive.

Medical Termination of Pregnancy (MTP) (1971)

Indications

- Medical
- Eugenic
- Humanitarian
- Socio-economic and
- Failure of contraception.

Authorized Person

- Registered Medical Practitioner (RMP) with Obstetrics and Gynecology (OBG) experience
- Two RMP when MTP done for case above 12–20 weeks, and above 20 weeks not indicated
- Place of MTP: Hospital, clinic, nursing home approved by government.

Medical Termination of Pregnancy (MTP) Rule (1975)

Following changes are made in MTP Act of 1971.
- District health authority can certify as to the qualification of doctor.
- Registered Medical Practitioner who assisted 25 cases in authorized place—eligible.
- 6 months housemanship in OBG—eligible.
- Diploma in Gynecology and Obstetrics (DGO) or MD in OBG—eligible.
- Registered Medical Practitioners before 1971 if they have practiced 3 years OBG practice—eligible.
- Registered Medical Practitioners after 1971 if they have practiced 1 year OBG practice—eligible.

Other Methods of Family Planning

- Abstinence
- Coitus interruptus
- Rhythm method (safe period)
- Basal body temperature (BBT) method of natural FP method
- Cervical mucous method of FP method
- Symptothermic method of natural FP method
- Continued lactation, and
- Beta subunit of human chorionic gonadotropin (hCG) as vaccine.

Present Status

- 197.4 million total eligible couple are there. 45.3% of eligible couple unprotected.
- The rest 53.5% are protected
  - 7.7% OC,
  - 6.5% *Nirodh,*
  - 9.3% intrauterine devices (IUD), and
  - 31.2% sterilization.

Unmet Need of Family Planning

- It is recent concept in FP
- It targets those who are not using contraceptives
- It is mainly by fear, lack of knowledge and poor (availability) of FP service, and
- It is met by good knowledge, attitude and practice (KAP) to cover the gap between child-bearing and FP behavior.

Prenatal and Postpartum Care (PPC) Postpartum Program

More than 550 medical institutions at national, state and district levels are covered under PPC. All medical colleges have PPC wing attached to OBG partum and postpartum period (time of delivery and later lying-in period). Mother is more receptive and we get direct acceptors and indirect acceptors. It has the package of antenatal care (ANC), INC, postnatal care

Chapter 11: Demography and Vital Statistics

(PNC), anemia correction and blindness control. There are 1,012 centers are working in India for the program.

POPULATION EDUCATION

It is a health education program which provides for a study of population situation in the community, country and world with the purpose of developing rational and responsible attitude among present generation toward FP behaviors.

Voluntary Organizations in Family Planning

- Family Planning Association of India (FPAI)
- Indian Medical Association (IMA)
- International Planned Parenthood Association (IPPA)
- United Nations Fund for Population Activities (UNFPA)
- United States Agency for International Development (USAID)
- The Population Council.

Population Control

Family planning is an adopted practice based on knowledge and attitude to avoid unwanted births, to have wanted births, to space pregnancy, to control births and to choose their own family size.

Components

- Birth control
- Sterility and infertility management
- Sex education
- Marriage counseling
- Preparation for pregnancy, lactation and parenthood
- Management of unmarried mothers, and
- Care of reproductive health.

Present Concept of Family Planning

1. Inverted red triangle, a symbol of health and family welfare services available, seen from a distance by the primary red color.
2. Family planning is voluntary and not compulsory.
3. It is a cafeteria method; choice is left to the consumer.
4. It is not just FP but family welfare planning.

Incentive and Disincentive in Family Planning

Incentives:	Rs.
Tubectomy	200.00
Laparoscopy	145.00
Vasectomy	180.00
Motivation of tubectomy	10.00
Motivation of vasectomy	40.00

One special increment
14 days of leave to women
7 days of leave to men
Green card to individual acceptances for special attention.

Disincentives:
Improvident maternity
No housing loan
No subsidized medical treatment

Family Planning Methods

Temporary Methods

- Condom—barrier methods, pregnancy rate = 2-3 per 1000 women year, *Types:* Dry, deluxe, super deluxe.
- Diaphragm—called Dutch cap, barrier method, trained person should insert
- Vaginal sponge called *"Today"* barrier method, less advantage.
- Foams, creams, suppositories, soluble films are chemical methods. They are surface acting spermicides.
- Lippes loop—not used in the FP program
- Copper T—Copper T 200 and Multiload 250 are commonly used which have 3.0 and 0.5 pregnancy rate. Have an effective life of 5 years. Mode of action is reducing chance of fertilization by foreign body reaction in uterus. Contraindications are pregnancy, undiagnosed bleeding, PID and cancer.

Side effects are:
- Pain,
- PID,
- Bleeding,
- Expulsion, and
- Rarely ectopic, perforation and pregnancy.

g. Oral pills—they are combined pill, POP, postcoital pill, once a month pill and male pill.
Mala D and Mala N (Low dose OC)
- Norgestrel 0.3 mg
- Ethinyl estradiol 0.03 mg

Mala D is a packet of 28 pill containing 21 pills and 7 ferrous pills.
It is Rupees 2.00 under social marketing.
Mala N is freely supplied under FP program.
They prevent release of ovum from ovary.
They are 100% effective.

Side effects:
- Effects on CVS,
- Carcinogenic effect,
- Decrease in HDL,
- Effect on liver, and
- Unwanted effect like weight gain, migraine, bleeding, breast pain.

h. Postcoital contraceptive 50 mg. Diethylstilbestrol within 48 hours of unprotected intercourse.
i. Gossypol derived from cotton seed oil which is not in wide use (male pill).
j. Injectable contraceptives
   - Depot-medroxy progesterone acetate (DMPA)
   - Norethisterone enanthate (NET-EN).
k. Norplant for subdermal implant.
l. Vaginal ring with levonorgestrel.

Permanent Methods
- Male sterilization (vasectomy).
- Female sterilization (tubectomy).

Family Planning Measures

- Raising age at marriage.
- Incentive.
- Disincentive.

Medical Termination of Pregnancy (MTP) (1971)

Indications
- Medical,
- Eugenic,
- Humanitarian,
- Socio-economic, and
- Failure of contraception.

Authorized Person
- Registered Medical Practitioner with OBG experience,
- Two RMP when MTP done for case above 12-20 weeks, and above 20 weeks not indicated.
- Place of MTP: Hospital, clinic, nursing home approved by government.

Medical Termination of Pregnancy (MTP) Rule (1975)

Following changes are made in MTP Act of 1971.
- District health authority can certify as to the qualification of doctor.
- Registered Medical Practitioner who assisted 25 cases in authorized place—eligible.
- Six months housemanship in OBG—eligible.
- Diploma in Gynecology and Obstetrics (DGO) or MD in OBG—eligible.
- Registered Medical Practitioners before 1971 if they have practiced 3 years OBG practice—eligible.
- Registered Medical Practitioners after 1971 if they have practiced 1 year OBG practice—eligible.

Other Methods of Family Planning

- Abstinence
- Coitus interruptus
- Rhythm method (safe period)
- Basal body temperature method of natural FP method
- Cervical mucous method of FP method
- Symptothermic method of natural FP method
- Continued lactation, and
- Beta subunit of HCG as vaccine.

Present Status
- 56% of eligible couple unprotected.
- The rest 44% are protected:
- 3.3% OC
- 4.2% *Nirodh*
- 7.4% IUD, and
- 29.1% sterilization.

Chapter 11: Demography and Vital Statistics

Unmet Need of Family Planning
- It is recent concept in FP
- It targets those who are not using contraceptives
- It is mainly by fear, lack of knowledge and poor (availability) of FP service, and
- It is met by good KAP to cover the gap between child-bearing and FP behavior.

Prenatal and Postpartum Care (PPC) Postpartum Program

More than 550 medical institutions at national, state and district levels are covered under PPC. All medical colleges have PPC wing attached to OBG partuml and postpartum period (time of delivery and later lying-in period). Mother is more receptive and we get direct acceptors and indirect acceptors. It has the package of ANC, INC, PNC, anemia correction and blindness control.

Population Education

It is a health education program which provides for a study of population situation in the community, country and world with the purpose of developing rational and responsible attitude among present generation toward FP behaviors.

NATIONAL FAMILY WELFARE PROGRAM

Started in 1952, now during 12th 5-year plan (2012–2017) with 371,600 crore of allocation it is an integral part of reproductive and child health (RCH) program, evolving a comprehensive National Population Policy (NPP) of 2000 to promote family welfare program (FWP). India Newborn Action Plan came to existence in 2014 with a goal to attain single digit neonatal mortality rate by 2030 and single digit neonatal mortality rate by 2030 Fund allocation for FP which was 0.65 crore in 1951 is seen to reach to 3,71,600 crore by 2017.

Family planning administration is depicted in **Figure 11.3**.

Family Planning (FP) Evaluation

It is done on following sectors:
- Need evaluation.

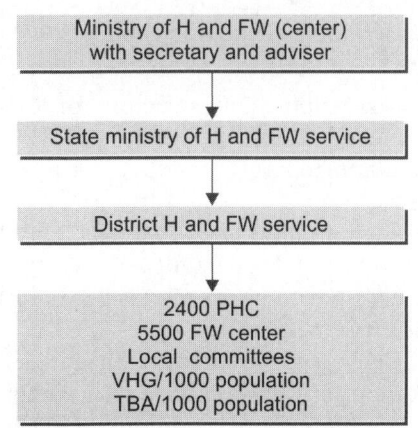

Fig. 11.3: Family planning (FP) administration. (PHC: primary health care; H: health; FW: family welfare; VHG: village health guide; TBA: traditional birth attendance)

- Family planning program plan evaluation.
- Performance evaluation.
- Knowledge, attitude and practice evaluation.
- Impact evaluation.

NATIONAL POPULATION POLICY (NPP)—2000

It is a national policy to check growth rate.

National Population Policy (NPP) 1976

- Age of boy to be married is 21 years and girl 18 years.
- No compulsion.
- Small FP norm.
- Incentive and disincentive.
- Cafeteria method.

National Population Policy (NPP) 1977: Modified guideline on 1976 issue. *NPP 1983* long-term goals are put forth, NRR by one was fixed.

National Population Policy (NPP) 2000

- Government's commitment is stressed.
- Target-free approach.
- Informed choice of FP methods.
- Voluntary approach.
- Women education, child survival, slum clearance.
- Now it is at Panchayat level and Nagar Palika level.

Goals of National Population Policy (NPP) 2000

- Service, supply, infrastructure for RCH to unmet need group.
- Free and compulsory education up to 14 years.
- Infant mortality rate to 60/1000 LB by 2010 MMR to 3/1000 LB by 2010.
- Age for boy to be married is 21 years and girl 18 years.
- All deliveries by trained health workers.
- Compulsory registration of vital events.
- Reproductive tract infections (RTI) and sexually transmitted infections (STI) component.
- To bring TFR to replacement level by the year 2010 (to 2.1)
- Birth rate (BR) to 24/1000 MYP and death rate (DR) to 9/1000 MYP,
  - Lifespan—male: 62, female: 63
  - Couple protection rate 60% and Annual growth rate 1.5%.
- Universal Immunization Program (UIP) coverage.
- Antenatal care 90%, delivery by trained 45%, institutional delivery by 35%.

NPP aims to stabilize population by 2045.

SUMMARY

Terminology and process are described. Giving the sources of data, population dynamics is described. Concepts, methods and unmet needs of family planning are described. Population education is stressed. This is concluded with national programs.

VIVA VOCE

1. What is population education?
2. Mention fertility-related rates.
3. What is demographic gap?
4. Mention five cycles of demography.
5. What are the sources of demographic data?
6. Define improvident maternity.
7. Differentiate eligible couple and target couple.
8. Mention family planning measures.

CHAPTER 12: Reproductive Maternal and Child Health

CHAPTER OUTLINE

- Elements
- Child Survival and Safe Motherhood (CSSM)
- Delivery Services at Primary Health Care (PHC)
- Emergency Care
- Empowered Action Group (EAG)
- Reproductive and Child Health (RCH) Indicators
- Handicap Child
- Growth
- Feeding Practices
- Social Welfare Scheme
- Integrated Child and Development Services (ICDS)
- Key Indicators

INTRODUCTION

Pregnant women, lactating mothers and children below 14 years have been the vulnerable group in a community. Their health indicates and determines the community health. Total women population of India as per 2011 census is 586,469,174 which constitutes 48% of the total population. Among them 15–45 years age group women constitute 22% of total population and 45–49 years age group women constitute 1.67% of total population. Thus, total of women 15–49 age group form 23.67% of total population. Children below 14 years form 42% of the total population; thereby together they constitute 65.67% of total population. This highlights the magnitude of maternal and child health (MCH) problems which the country has to encounter. Estimate for 2018 also corresponds to same proportions. 2018 population estimate is 1,359.8 million.

Government of India launched reproductive and child health (RCH) in December 1997. It was meant for integrating the following:

a. Fertility regulation.
b. Maternal health with reproductive health services.
c. Child health with reproductive health services.

Objectives of Reproductive and Child Health

Following are the major objectives of RCH:
- To reduce infant mortality rate (IMR) and maternal mortality rate (MMR)
- To reduce morbidity of mothers and children
- To reduce unwanted fertility
- To stabilize population growth, and
- To improve health of women and children.

Definition

World Health Organization (WHO) Definition

A state of complete physical, mental and social well-being and not merely the absence of disease of infirmity in all matters relating to the reproductive system, its function and process.

Government of India (GOI) Definition

People will be able to have the ability to reproduce and regulate their fertility, women are able to go through pregnancy and childbirth safely, the outcome of pregnancy is successful in terms of maternal and infant survival and well-being and couples are able to have sexual relations free of fear of pregnancy and of contracting disease.

BASIC ELEMENTS OF REPRODUCTIVE AND CHILD HEALTH

- Family planning
- Maternal and child health
- Safe abortion services
- Effective control of sexually transmitted disease (STD) and reproductive tract infection (RTI)
- Management of infertility
- Detection, treatment and prevention of reproductive tract malignancies.

Factors affecting RCH: The major factors affecting reproductive and child health are as following:
- Socioeconomic condition
- Status of women
- Educational opportunities
- Family environment
- Nutrition
- Gender relationship, and
- Traditional and legal structure of society.

Extrinsic factors affecting RCH care services are:
a. Adolescent health
b. Maternal mortality
c. Unsafe abortion
d. Reproductive tract infections (RTIs)
e. Sexually transmitted infections (STIs)
f. Acquired immunodeficiency syndrome (AIDS)
g. Infertility
h. Cancer
i. Empowerment of women.

RCH Administration

See **Fig. 12.1**.

Gender Communication and Decision-making

Gender is a powerful force in RCH; reproductive health in man is given equal emphasis for quality and progress of RCH.

Reproductive and Child Health Interventions

- For child survival
- For safe motherhood
- Information education and communication (IEC) activities
- Reproductive tract infection (RTI) and STI clinics
- Safe abortions,
- Laboratory facilities for RTI and STI
- Essential obstetric care
- Essential newborn care.

Reproductive and Child Health Differential Approach

More support is provided to weaker district. ABC categorization of districts is done by the criterion of birth rate and female literacy rate. The districts are covered in a phased manner. (58 districts under A, 184 districts under B and 265 districts under C). Sophisticated facility is proposed to advanced districts.

Recent Area of Interest in Reproductive and Child Health

Preventive obstetrics and pediatrics: Use of primary health care (PHC) concept.
Social obstetrics and pediatrics: Use of social and environmental concept.

CHILD SURVIVAL AND SAFE MOTHERHOOD

Child survival and safe motherhood program (CSSM) initiated in 1992, which later got integrated to RCH in 1997 has major public health interventions such as essential obstetric care, 24 hours delivery services at PHC, emergency obstetric care, medical termination of pregnancy (MTP), prevention of RTI and

Chapter 12: Reproductive Maternal and Child Health

STD and survey of districts. Following services are specified in RCH program:
* Registration of all pregnancies, as early as possible.
* Providing minimum 3 antenatal care (ANC) checkups.
* 100% coverage of tetanus toxoid (TT) to pregnant women.
* Nutrition education and advice.
* Detection of high-risk pregnancies
* Immediate and prompt referral of high-risk cases.
* Training of all indigenous untrained Dais.
* Safe delivery by trained Dai, multipurpose worker (MPW) in the community.
* Advice on birth spacing
* Provision of institutional deliveries.

DELIVERY SERVICE AT PRIMARY HEALTH CARE

To promote and provide institutional deliveries, 24 hours delivery facility at PHC and provision for additional honorarium to attending staff are provided at primary health center.

MTP (Medical Termination of Pregnancy)

Women opt MTP for unintended and unwanted pregnancies which is allowed and conducted at PHC on fixed days. Manpower training and provision of MTP equipment are attended under the scheme. This is mainly to reduce morbidity and mortality due to unsafe abortions.

Control of Reproductive Tract Infection/ Sexually Transmitted Disease (RTI/STD)

With the collaboration of NACO (National AIDS Control Organization) which provides assistance to set up clinics, a link with human immunodeficiency virus (HIV)/AIDS control is an ongoing program. Training of manpower, supply of drug kit is attended under the scheme. This scheme provides provision of contract technician (two) to each district.

Universal Immunization Program (UIP)

This was earlier a part of CSSM and is now under RCH. Since 1997, provides immunization against 6 preventable diseases. Supply of diphtheria, pertussis and tetanus (DPT), diphtheria and tetanus (DT), oral polio vaccine (OPV), measles, bacillus calmette-guérin (BCG) and cold chain establishment and additional items supporting UIP.

Drug and Equipment Kits

Drug kit and equipment kit to subcenter, PHC under RCH activities are given in appendix.

ORT

Under the RCH program ORS packets are supplied by the Central Government every

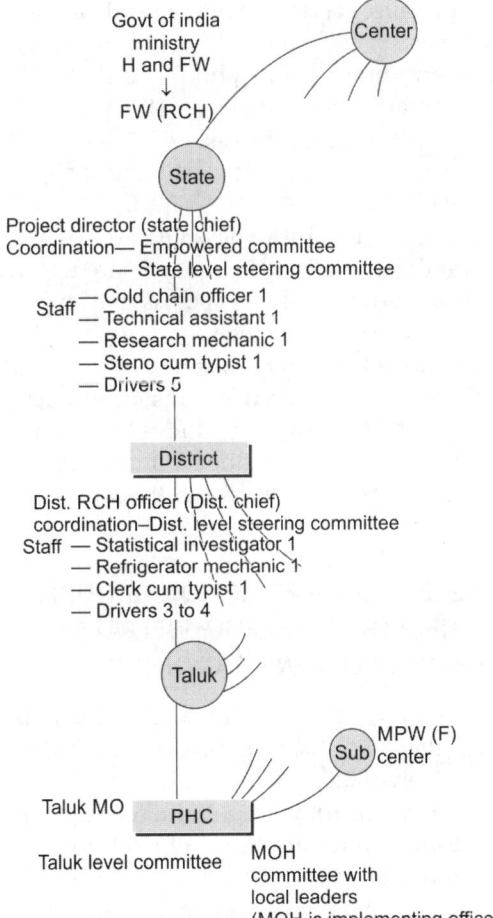

Fig. 12.1: RCH administration.
(H&FW: Health and Family Welfare; RCH: reproductive and child health; MOH: Ministry of Health; PHC: primary health care; MPW: multipurpose worker)

year, 300 pockets per year in two lots along with drug kit. Rational use of drug, nutritional care and preventive ORT are motivated to reduce child mortality.

Acute Respiratory Infections (ARI) Control

Acute respiratory infections are to be prevented to prevent deaths due to pneumonia. Health Workers are trained for the diagnosis and treatment through drug kit. Cotrimoxazole is supplied under the scheme.

Vitamin A Prophylaxis

Five doses of vitamin A to all children below the age of 3 years, is provided each with specified dose.

9 months	–	I dose 1 lakh units
18 months	–	II dose 2 lakh units
24 months	–	III dose 2 lakh units
30 months	–	IV dose 2 lakh units
36 months	–	V dose 2 lakh units

EMERGENCY CARE

Emergency Obstetric Care

Many deliveries are home deliveries and if they are associated with complications, maternal morbidity and mortality rate will go up. Thousands of referral units are identified under RCH program. They are strengthened with emergency obstetric kit, equipment kit, and skilled health professional. Involvement of nongovernment organization (NGO) for decentralizing activities is another novel idea under RCH scheme.

Essential Obstetric Care

This refers to basic maternity service to all pregnant women in the country. This ensures the following:
- Registration of pregnancy at 16 week or as early as possible.
- 3 ANC checkups by [auxiliary nurse midwife (ANM)] MPW
- Safe delivery (home or health center)
- Three postnatal care (PNC) checkups.

This component is greatly intended at home visiting and hence a specific criteria of domiciliary care.

Essential Newborn Care

This component reduces the perinatal and neonatal mortality in the community. Services extended under following areas are:
- Resuscitation of newborn with birth asphyxia
- Prevention of hypothermia
- Prevention of infection
- Exclusive breastfeeding
- Referral of sick newborn
- Care of low birth-weight (LBW) babies.

Other Initiatives of RCH Activity

- Reproductive and child health (RCH) camps with obstetricians and pediatricians for specialist's service to remote and outreach areas.
- Reproductive and child health (RCH) outreach activity to cover UIP and MCH services to remote areas.
- Neonatal care unit establishment at district level hospitals.
- Indian Council of Medical Research (ICMR) model home-based neonatal care unit to provide neonatal care at grass root level.
- Priority service to high mortality districts by focused interventions. It is called BDCS (Border District Cluster Strategy). This priority also includes integrated management of childhood illness (IMCI).
- Introduction of hepatitis B vaccination project in selected districts.

EAG (EMPOWERED ACTION GROUP) OF HEALTH AND FAMILY WELFARE SERVICE, GOVERNMENT OF INDIA

This scheme gives priority to UP, Bihar, MP, Rajasthan, Odisha, Chhattisgarh, Jharkhand, and Uttaranchal.

As per Government of India report based on district survey till the end of 1999 has given key indicators.

Maternal and Child Health Problem

- Malnutrition
- Infection, and
- Uncontrolled reproduction.

Chapter 12: Reproductive Maternal and Child Health

Malnutrition

Pregnant woman, lactating mothers and children are affected by malnutrition in developing countries. They cause LBW, anemia, toxemia, postpartum hemorrhage (PPH). Intrauterine period influence fetal growth and weaning period influence childhood malnutrition. Direct interventions like supplementation, indirect interventions like environmental sanitation prove effective anchor in the prevention of malnutrition.

Infection

Fetal growth retardation, puerperal sepsis and LBW are due to maternal infections. Women infected with toxoplasmosis and cytomegaloviruses are increasing. On the other hand, diarrhea, acute respiratory infection (ARI), skin infections of infants are seen to a great extent. Malaria and tuberculosis are serious infection of childhood. Programs under RCH are aimed at the prevention of those infections.

Uncontrolled Reproduction

Repeated childbirths have seen their association with anemia, abortion, LBW and antepartum hemorrhage (APH). There is a need for small family norm to safeguard mother and child health. High birth rate is associated with high IMR and under five death rate (**Table 12.1**) as per observations by UNICEF and UNDP.

Table 12.1: Factors influencing IMR.

Biological	Economical	Sociocultural
Birth weight	Income of family	Early marriage
Mother's age	Standard of living	Sex of child
Birth order	Purchasing power of family	Breastfeeding
Multiple pregnancy	Affordability	Planned motherhood
Family size	Possessions	Mother's education
High fertility		Broken family
		Unwed mother
		Overcrowding

SAFE MOTHERHOOD

Antenatal Care

Good ANC includes:
- Minimum of three visits from the time of pregnancy diagnosis; 20 weeks, 32 weeks, and 36 weeks.
- Urine examination, weight recording and BP recording.
- Hb% estimation.
- 100 iron and folic acid (IFA) tablets during pregnancy.
- Tetanus toxoid (TT) immunization two doses or booster dose.

Risk pregnancy: This comprises of:
- Elderly primigravida
- Short stature primigravida
- Malpresentations
- APH
- Preeclamptic toxemia (PET)
- Eclampsia
- Severe anemia
- Previous cesarean
- Pregnancy associated with systemic disease.

Antenatal Advice

- Personal hygiene
- Balanced diet
- Use of only essential drugs
- Avoidance of unnecessary exposure to radiation
- Reporting when warning signs such as pedal edema, convulsion, blurring of vision, and bleeding per vagina occur
- Mother craft education.

Specific Protection during Pregnancy

- TT two doses or booster doses
- Treatment of venereal disease research laboratory (VDRL) positive cases
- Preventive care for Rh incompatibility
- Anemic correction by IFA prophylaxis
- Periodic check-up for PET or eclampsia.

Intranatal Care

About 1–4% of deliveries require institutional delivery which is usually abnormal labor, difficult labor or high-risk pregnancy. This fulfils the requirement of services of doctors.

Domiciliary Care

Confinement at home by trained traditional birth attendant (TBA) or HW female in majority of cases where normal obstetric history is ideal. Outreach domiciliary care is an extension of good intranatal care to the community. There is a need of referral in cases of:
a. High temperature during labor
b. Heavy bleeding and collapse
c. Placenta not separated within 30 minutes after delivery (retained placenta)
d. Cord prolapse
e. Prolonged labor.

Rooming-in

Avoiding separate cradle and allowing newborn with mother is called rooming-in. Contact, affection, and breastfeeding are stabilized by way of rooming-in.
Prevention of maternal and neonatal sepsis by:
a. Application of five clean practices, which are:
   - Clean surface for delivery
   - Clean hands of attendant
   - New blade for cutting cord
   - Clean tie for cord, and
   - No application on cord stump.
b. Issue of disposable delivery kits (DDK) containing:
   - A piece of soap
   - A new razor blade
   - Two pieces of thread, and
   - Two cotton swabs.

Postnatal Care

This area needs the combined responsibility of obstetrician and pediatrician.

Common postnatal complications are as follows:
- Puerperal sepsis
- Thrombophlebitis
- Secondary hemorrhage
- Mastitis, and
- Urinary tract infection.

Early recognition and prompt treatment brings down morbidity and mortality.

Follow-up

- Twice a day for 3 days
- Once a day till cord stump drops off
- Once a week for 6 weeks
- Once a month for 6 months, and
- Once in 3 months for 12 months.

During postnatal follow-up, anemia corrections, nutrition advice, and advice for postnatal exercise are advocated. Counseling for emotional stress of childbirth is required to nearly 50% of cases.

Exclusive breastfeeding followed by weaning and supplementation is utmost important in PN care.

Postpartum period is highly receptive phase for an advice on family welfare planning. Basic health education for awareness regarding hygiene, feeding and check-up curtails morbidity.

Safe Motherhood Program has the following major components under CSSM.
- Early registration of pregnancy
- Minimum three ANC check-up provided
- Universal coverage with TT immunization
- Advice on balanced diet
- High-risk detection and referral
- Delivery by trained TBA
- Birth spacing, and
- Promotion of institutional delivery.

Child Survival

Care of child during infancy, preschool age, and school age from childhood care period under child survival. Child survival strategies include:
- Strengthening of essential newborn care
- Diarrhea management
- Acute respiratory infection (ARI) management
- High level immunization coverage
- Vitamin A prophylaxis
- Improving maternity care
- Promoting birth spacing.

Child survival is influenced by many cultural practices. Following are major harmful practices that influence child survival.
- Giving prelacteal feeds,
- Delay in initiating breastfeeding
- Discarding colostrum, and
- Giving water between feeds.

Essential Newborn Care

Prevention of birth asphyxia, hypothermia and infection from major task of essential newborn care.

i. Antenatal care to all to prevent anemia, undernutrition and obstetrical complication	Registration check-up, nutrition advice, anemia treatment, and TT
ii. Safe delivery practice ➢ Clean hand, surface, razor, cord tie, and cord stump ➢ Keeping newborn warm ➢ Care of the umbilical cord ➢ Care of the eyes, and by using disposable delivery kit ➢ No bath (immediately and till 1 week) ➢ Assessment of birth weight by spring balance	

Color code	Range	Place to manage
Green	2500–4000 G	Home
Yellow	2000–2500 G	Home
Red	Below 2000 G	Referral

- Exclusive breastfeeding and no prelacteal feed such as glucose, honey, *gur, janamgutti*, and
- Prevention of hypothermia.
  The measures to be taken to overcome poor thermal control mechanism are:
  - Contact with mother
  - Wrapping with cotton towel
  - Keeping room warm
  - Keeping 200 W lamp 45 cm above the baby
- Prevention of infection
- Resuscitation of newborn who do not cry soon after birth, and
- Advice to mother on danger signal in baby like refusal to feed, drowsiness, cold to touch, difficult and rapid breathing, abdominal distension, convulsion, persistent vomiting or deep jaundice.

Diarrhea Management

Diarrhea in children has been about three episodes per year causing considerable morbidity and mortality.

Danger signs are:
- Blood in stool
- Increased thirst
- Many watery stools
- Repeated vomiting
- Unable to drink
- Refusal to breastfeed
- Floppy, difficult to wake, unconsciousness
- Increased respiratory rate or chest indrawing, and
- Diarrhea within 6 weeks of measles.

Advice to Mother
- To give increased quantity of fluid
- To continue feed in diarrhea phase also
- To know early signs of dehydration and
- To know when to seek medical advice.

Specific advices are:
- Whole oral rehydration salt (ORS) packet in 1 liter of water.
- One teaspoon every 2 minutes and to give extraspoon at each vomiting or diarrhea, and
- Continue normal diet (kichari, sooji, rice in milk, idli, etc.)

Acute Respiratory Infections (ARI)

This includes infection of respiratory tract, sinuses, ear and pleural cavity.

Acute upper respiratory infections (AURI) constitute common cold, pharyngitis, and otitis media.

Acute lower respiratory infection (ALRI) constitutes epiglottitis, laryngitis, bronchitis, bronchiolitis, and pneumonia.

Pneumonia is considered if:
a. Fast breathing and chest indrawing are seen.
b. Even only with chest indrawing.

Criteria for fast breathing:
- 60 or above 60—0-2 months age child.
- 50 or above 50—2-12 months age child.
- 40 or above 40—12 months to 5 years.

Child with ARI, is checked for any malnutrition before putting on suggested line of treatment.

Pneumonia	Therapy	Where to treat
Fast breathing (as cited above)	Cotrimoxazole Oral	Home
Severe pneumonia Chest indrawing	IM antibiotic	IPD
Very severe illness	IM chloramphenicol	IPD

(IPD: invasive pneumococcal disease; IM: intramuscular)

- Cannot drink
- Drowsy
- Stridor
- Respiratory grunting
- Apnea, cyanosis, convulsion
- Severe malnutrition, and
- Hypothermia

Below 2 months, fast breathing is considered as severe pneumonia. Irrational drugs should not be used for a child (including cough, cold). Five-day treatment for ARI:

Age	Weight	Dose
Below 2 months	3–5 kg	1 tab/day or 2.5 mL/day
2–12 months	6–9 kg	2 tab/day or 5 mL/day
1–5 years	10–19 kg	3 tab/day or 7.5 mL/day

Note: 1 tab: Sulfamethizole 100 mg Trimethoprim 20 mg
5 mL syrup: Sulfamethizole 200 mg Trimethoprim 40 mg

High Level Immunization Coverage

National immunization schedule is followed for 100 percentage coverage. Specific care is taken (under RCH) on the following:
a. Reconstituted measles vaccine should be used within 4 hours.
b. Vaccine vial monitor (VVM) are checked for OPV.

(VVM are made of heat sensitive material which change color if the vaccine vials are exposed to high temperature than recommended) (**Fig. 12.2**).

Vitamin A Prophylaxis

Vitamin A deficiency is greatly associated with measles, intestinal worm infestations, ARI and tuberculosis. Inability of a child to see after it is dark (night blindness) form early sign of vitamin A deficiency.

Under RCH Program, vitamin A supplementation from 9 months to 3 years at 6 months interval is advocated.

Therapeutic dose of 200,000 IU after diagnosis followed by 200,000 IU 4 weeks later is advocated (Infants 100,000 IU). Food rich in vitamin A such as spinach, *methi*, capsicum, carrot, pumpkin, papaya, mango and yam are advised to the community.

Improving Maternity Care

a. Drug kits and equipment kits are supplied to subcenters and PHCs.
b. Control of RTI and STI.
c. Round the clock delivery facility at PHCs and community health centers (CHCs).
d. Provision of emergency obstetrical care.
e. Provision of essential obstetric care.

Promoting Birth Spacing

Under national FW planning Program condom, oral pills, and IUD are advocated for promoting birth spacing. It is a health measure to reduce maternal and perinatal mortality and morbidity. The use rate of measures is to be raised by giving information about contraceptive use to the mothers (to overcome myth).

Myth	Reality
Cancer is produced	OC prevent cancer of ovary, endometrium. There is no risk of ca breast
Infertility is induced	No permanent infertility
Harmful to health	No harm No complication Safe for mother and child
Deformed baby is born	No risk of fetal abnormality
Should stop in-between	Should be continuous to avoid unwanted pregnancy

(OC: oral contraceptive)

MATERNAL AND CHILD HEALTH (MCH) INDICATORS (RCH INDICATORS)

Maternal and child health is assessed by morbidity, mortality, growth and development, and achieving national targets in RCH

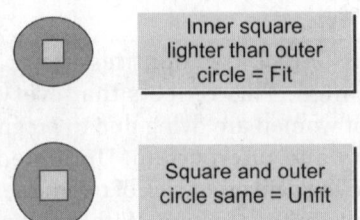

Fig. 12.2: Vaccine vial monitor (VVM) readings.

Chapter 12: Reproductive Maternal and Child Health

activities. Commonly used MCH indicators are:

Growth and development of child indicates the care given to a mother during her reproductive age. Similarly, illness of mothers and children reflect RCH status. But of late mortality rates are taken as indicators of the extent of RCH care in the community.

- Perinatal mortality rate
- Maternal mortality rate, and
- Infant mortality rate.

Other indicators are:
- Stillbirth rate
- Neonatal mortality rate
- Postneonatal mortality rate
- 1–4 years age mortality rate
- Under 5-year mortality rate, and
- Child survival rate.

Perinatal Mortality Rate

- Elderly mothers
- Young mother
- Parity 5 and above
- Heavy smoking
- Severe anemia
- Multiple pregnancies.

Causes of perinatal mortality can be grouped under three categories:
1. *Antenatal causes:* Maternal diseases, pelvic diseases, birth defects of reproductive organs, Rh incompatibility, toxemia of pregnancy, and APH.
2. *Intranatal causes:* Birth injury, asphyxia, and obstetric complications.
3. *Postnatal causes:* Premature baby, respiratory distress syndrome, and congenital anomalies.

Definition

It is late fetal and early neonatal deaths weighing over 1,000 G at birth expressed as ratio per 1,000 live births weighing over 1,000 g at birth.

$$= \frac{\text{Late fetal deaths and early neonatal death weighing over 1000 g, at birth}}{\text{Total live births weighting over 1000 g, at birth}} \times 100$$

= 44 per 1000 live births in India (Rural 47/1000 LB and urban 30/1000 LB).

Preventive Steps

Tackling causes of perinatal mortality at appropriate time and existing RCH program include catering TT, IFA, essential obstetric care, emergency obstetric care, safe delivery practice, and essential newborn care.

Maternal Mortality Rate

Definition

World Health Organization (WHO) has defined MMR as "the death of woman while pregnant or within 42 days of termination of pregnancy irrespective of duration and site of pregnancy from any cause related to or aggravated by the pregnancy or its management but not from accidental or incidental causes."

$$= \frac{\text{No. of mothers dying due to complications of pregnancy, childbirth or within 42 days of delivery in 1 year}}{\text{Total number of live births in 1 year}} \times 1000$$

= 4 per 1000 LB in India.

Infection and bleeding are common causes of maternal mortality. While hepatitis, heart diseases and endocrine causes are more in developed countries, in developing countries the causes are mostly infection, anemia, jaundice, and malaria.

Other influencing causes of maternal mortality have been:
- Women's age
- Birth interval
- Parity
- Socioeconomic status
- Cultural practices
- Nutritional status
- Environmental conditions.

Indian Picture

India is one of the countries where MMR is still high. This reflects that every year lakhs of women are dying due to pregnancy, delivery and puerperium. Untrained dais conducting deliveries, lack of referral services are contributory factors. Within India each state show variable rates with respect to MMR.

Infant Mortality Rate

It is the ratio of infant deaths to the total live births in 1 year.

$$= \frac{\text{No. of deaths of children } 0-1 \text{ year of age}}{\text{No. of live births in 1 year}} \times 1000$$

= 68 per 1000 live birth in India.

It is one of the most important and sensitive indicator of RCH. It is a unique rate because it covers a large 1 year age population, when they suffer from diseases or conditions which are specific to that age and intervention brings out *remarkable decline in IMR*.

IMR of India is estimated, at present, at 32 per 1,000 live births. Most of urban studies have shown a declined rate of IMR when compared to rural areas.

IMR is greatly related and influenced by female literacy rate and birth rate. Statistically, significant relation (r) is established by taking values of 15 states.

Causes of IMR
- *Neonatal causes*
  - Low birth rate (LBW)
  - Birth injury-birth defects
  - Rh incompatibility diarrhea
  - ARI NNT
- *Postneonatal causes*
  - Diarrhea ARI
  - Malnutrition
  - Birth defects
  - Other infections.

IMR is influenced by following factors (*See* **Table 12.1**):

Stillbirth Rate

Definition
Death of fetus weighing 1,000 g or more out of 1,000 live births and stillbirths.

$$= \frac{\text{Fetal deaths weighing 1000 g}}{\text{Total live births + stillbirths}} \times 1000$$

= 4/1,000 all births in India (rural 5/1,000 LB and urban 3/1,000 live births).

Causes
- Developmental anomalies of cord, placenta.
- Rh incompatibility, and
- Maternal diseases.

Prevention and Control
- Provision of essential maternity care.

Neonatal Mortality Rate

It is the death of newborn from 0 to 28 days out of 1,000 live births.

$$= \frac{\text{No. of deaths of children } 0-28 \text{ days}}{\text{Total live births of 1 year}} \times 1000$$

= 24/1,000 live births in India (rural 27/1,000 LB urban 14/1,000 LB).

Neonatal mortality reflects endogenous factors such as LBW, birth injury, etc., which affect newborn. It is directly related to gestational age and birth weight. In India 60% of infant deaths are occurring before 28 days after birth of newborn babies. It is approximately, estimated at present as 24 per 1,000 live births.

Causes
- Prematurity
- ARI
- Diarrhea
- Cord infection
- Birth injury, and
- Congenital anomalies.

Prevention and Control
By child survival strategies.

Postneonatal Mortality Rate

Definition
It is the death occurring in children from 28 days to 1 year out of 1,000 live births.

$$= \frac{\text{No. of deaths of children } 28 \text{ days to 1 year}}{\text{Total live births of one year}} \times 1000$$

= 11.0 per 1,000 live births in India (rural 11/1,000 LB and urban 9/1,000 LB).

Causes

- Diarrhea
- ARI
- Malnutrition, and
- Congenital anomalies.

Prevention and Control

Child survival strategies are the ways to prevent and control the increasing rate of postneonatal mortality.

1–4 Years Mortality Rate

Definition

It is the child death from 1 to 4 years per 1,000.

$$= \frac{\text{No. of deaths of children 1-4 years}}{\text{Total No. of 1-4 child population in 1 year}} \times 1000$$

= 30 per 1000 (1–4) child population in India (1.4% of total deaths in India is 1-4 years mortality). 1-4 mortality rate is 1.4% of total death).

Causes

- Diarrhea
- ARI
- Malnutrition
- Measles, and
- Accidents and injuries.

Prevention and Control

Child survival strategies are the major preventive and controlling measures.

Under-five Mortality Rate

Definition

It is the death of children under 5 years per 1,000 live births.
Live births in 1 year

$$= \frac{\text{No. of deaths of 0-5 years}}{\text{Total live birth in 1 year}} \times 1000$$

= 39.4 per 1,000 live births in India.

Causes

- Prematurity
- ARI
- Diarrhea
- Cord infection
- Birth injury
- Congenital anomalies, and
- Malnutrition.

Prevention and Control

Child survival strategy is the most effective preventive and controlling measures.

Child Survival Rate

It is the number obtained by subtracting under-five mortality from 1,000.

Child survival rate = 1,000 – under-five mortality (90.7% in India)

$$\text{To get \%} = \frac{1000 - \text{under five mortality}}{10}$$

$$= \frac{1000 - 90}{10} = \frac{910}{10} = 91\%$$

Congenital Malformations

It is anatomical defect, molecular defect, and cellular defect present at birth. Incidence of congenital malformation is around 30–70 per 1,000 live births.

Most common congenital malformations are:
- Congenital heart defects
- Cleft lip
- Cleft palate
- Spina bifida, and
- Anencephaly.

Causes

- Chromosomal abnormalities
- Genetically inherited disorders
- Intrauterine infections by rubella, cytomegalovirus, toxoplasmosis
- Drug (Thalidomide), and
- Irradiation.

Risk factors

- Advanced maternal age, and
- Consanguineous marriages.

Prevention and control
- Prenatal diagnosis by ultrasound and amniocentesis,
- Discouraging reproduction after a birth defect,
- Removal of teratogens,
- Rubella control, and
- Judicious use of radiation.

HANDICAPPED CHILDREN

It is defined as reduction in child capacity to fulfill a social role because of an impairment. Common types are:

Physical handicap	Deaf, blind, harelip, lame, cerebral palsy
Mental handicap	Mental retardation
Social handicap	Orphan, and destitute.

Prevention
- Genetic counseling
- Immunization
- At risk approach
- Good RCH program, and
- Early diagnosis and prompt treatment.

Juvenile Delinquency

It is defined as a boy child below 16 years and a girl child below 18 years who have committed some offenses. These are associated with behavioral problem and antisocial practices. In developing countries it is two percent of children who attend juvenile courts. In India juvenile delinquency is common between 15 and 18 years of age and five times more among boys.

Causes
- Hereditary disease (e.g. XYY chromosomes),
- Poverty, and
- Orphan and destitute.

Prevention
- Social welfare services
- Compulsory schooling
- Improvement of family life
- Implementation of Juvenile Justice Act (1986), and
- Child guidance clinic.

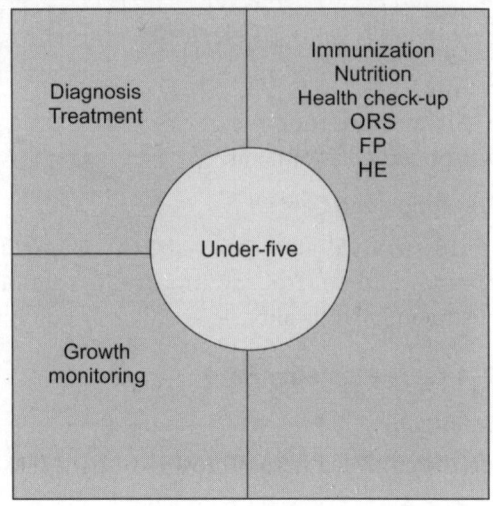

Fig. 12.3: Functions of under-five clinics.

Child Guidance Clinic

It was started in 1909 with an intention to deal juvenile delinquent child. Now, apart from juvenile delinquency all forms of child maladjustments are tackled through child guidance clinic.

Child guidance clinics are run in team spirit by child psychologists, psychiatrists, psychosocial workers, pediatricians, speech therapists, neurologists, and occupational therapists. Common methods employed in child guidance clinics are child counseling, play therapy and parental counseling.

Under-five Clinic

Earlier years well-baby clinic existed which took preventive care services. Now, of late under-five clinics have taken up the task of integrating treatment, prevention and surveillance activity in the community (**Fig. 12.3**).

THE GROWTH

The Growth Chart

This is also called road to health chart originally designed by Dr David Morley. The chart gives a visual display of child's physical growth, which is used as a tool in growth monitoring (**Fig. 12.4**).

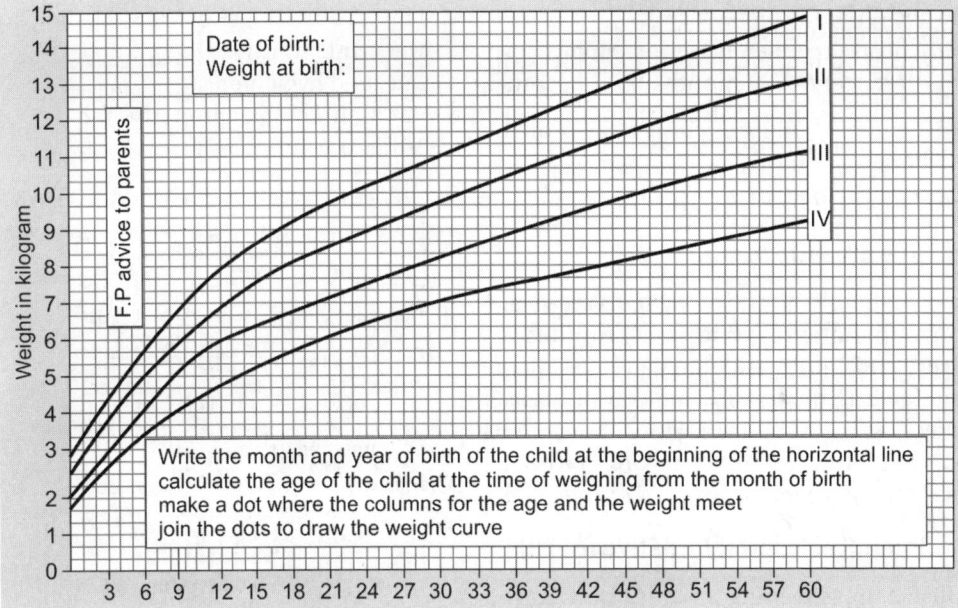

Fig. 12.4: Growth chart used in India.

Age in months versus weight in kg give a point located in the chart. The location can correspond and tell the following:
* Normal
* Grade I malnutrition
* Grade II malnutrition
* Grade III malnutrition, and
* Grade IV malnutrition.

Growth chart is a standard method of child's health monitoring. Growth monitoring identifies a risk child which further is used in following circumstances:
* Mother to visualize the need for health care.
* Health worker to give nutritional therapy.
* Administrator to evaluate nutrition program.
* Teachers to use for training people.
* Policy maker to take decision in planning.

Growth and Development

Growth is increasing in physical size of the body and development is increasing in skills and functions.

The main factors influencing growth and development are:
* Genetic inheritance
* Adequate nutrition
* Social factors
* Economic factors
* Psychological factors, and
* Physical environment.

Normal Growth

Maximum growth of brain after birth is noticed from 1 to 6 years. Maximum general growth is observed during 6–12 years. Reproductive growth is observed during 13–18 years.

Reference values that are considered for national and international comparisons are:
* Harvard standard
* WHO reference value
* ICMR values.

Weight

Usually, 1 kg per month in first 3 months:
* Doubling by 5 months
* Treble by 1 year
* Quadruple by 2 years.

Height

Usually, 25 cm during first year.
* 12 cm during second year.
* Maximum height reaches at 17 years for girls.
* Maximum height reaches at 18 years for boys.
* Weight for height is considered more important in growth monitoring.

Head and Chest Circumference

At birth head circumference is more than chest circumference. At 6-8 months both become equal. After 9 months chest circumference is more than head circumference.

INFANT FEEDING PRACTICES

Exclusive Breastfeeding

Except for breast milk no other items are given in birth to 4 months. Within 30 minutes of delivery and within 4-6 hours after cesarean breastfeeding must start. Refusal of breast means that the child is ill. Since, bottle-fed infant has 14 times higher risk of diarrhea, breastfeeding is panacea for child's protection.

Baby Friendly Hospital Initiative (BFHI)

Exclusive breastfeeding provides best nutrition and protects the child from infections, hypothermia and malnutrition. This initiative is created by WHO and UNICEF; and is supported by professional bodies in India and abroad.

Except for breast milk no other food or fluids, including prelacteal feeds and water should be given to a child from birth till 4 months of age. Breastfeeding should be initiated within the first hour of birth, after cesarean baby should be allowed to suck the breast as soon as mother comes to stable in 4-6 hours.

Hospitals where exclusive breastfeeding is the norm are called "Baby Friendly" hospitals.

Ten steps are given that all "BF" hospitals are expected to follow which are depicted under Chapter 36.

Development of child is gauged by milestone:

Age	Development
3 months	Holds head erect
5 months	Recognizes mother
8 months	Sits without support
10 months	Crawling
11 months	Stands with support, and tells word
14 months	Walks wide base
20 months	Walks narrow base and joins word
24 months	Full development in terms of motor, language, adaptation, and sociopersonal development

The major advantages of breastfeeding are:
* Meets the nutritional requirements
* Safe, and hygienic
* Has antimicrobial property, and
* Brings down IMR.

Difference between Breast Milk and Cow's Milk

	Breast milk	Cow's milk
Lactalbumin	More	Less
Immunoglobulin	More	Less
Lysozyme	More	Less
Lactose	More	Less
Calcium, phosphorus, iron	Less	More
Vitamin C	More	Less
Vitamin D	More	Less
Energy	Both are almost same	

Local Customs and Practices during Pregnancy, Child Birth, Lactation and Child Feeding Practices

Without sociological aspect and social content, health is almost incomplete. Diagnosis, investigation and treatment are influenced by social factors and economic factors. Literacy, sanitation, nutrition, culture and behavior predispose to diseases and disorders.

Culture

Learned behavior which has been socially acquired.

Cultural Factor

Religion, custom, habit, attitude, tradition, and belief.

Common examples of cultural practices:

Belief

Definition

Things derived from parents, grandparents and other people which are accepted without trying them to prove they are true.

Examples
1. Certain diseases are due to wrath of God and Goddess and administration of drugs is harmful, e.g., chickenpox, measles, and mumps.

2. Sexually transmitted diseases (STD) [venereal disease (VD)] is due to sex with women of lower caste or during menses.
3. Due to the sin committed in the past life, e.g., tuberculosis, and leprosy.
4. Spirit of ghost, e.g., hysteria, and epilepsy.
5. Impure blood e.g., skin diseases, boils, which need purification by taking castor oil or eating *neem* leaves.
6. Effect of cold and heat e.g., running in the nose, reddening of eyes, fisherman foot, angular stomatitis, burning during micturition, and heart burn.
7. God is present and he is watching all of us over our bad deeds.
8. Addition of little water to milk before boiling allow good yield of milk in cows.
9. Eating papaya during pregnancy causes abortion.
10. Eating green leafy vegetables cause dark skin in growing fetus, if eaten during pregnancy.
11. Eating from common plate and drinking from common glass are signs of brotherhood.

Custom

Definition

It is the transmission of a way of doing. By tradition is meant the transmission of a way of thinking or believing (Ross).
Examples:
1. Open land is meant for field defecation.
2. Latrine within the house is dirty and objectionable.
3. Apply cow dung to the floor before religious function.
4. Taking bath before food.
5. Preventing women performing religious function and forbidding entry to kitchen during menses period.
6. Walk bare foot within the house and in the temple.
7. Throwing waste outside the house through window.
8. Using pond water for human bath, animal bath, and cloth wash.
9. Holy dip in river during pilgrimage and bringing the same water as holy water to keep at home.
10 Keeping the animal within the house.
11. White washing house on all festivals.
12. Hindus are vegetarians.
13. Onion and garlic are not eaten by upper caste people.
14. Observing fasting on holy days.
15. Prolonged breastfeeding of baby by lactating mother even up to 1.5 years.
16. No colostrum is given to the newborn.
17. *Janam gutti*, honey, cows urine, and sugar water are given as first feed to the newborn baby.
18. Branding of skin, oil bath once a week, oil application to the head of the child (anterior fontanel).
19. Smoking with burning side inside the mouth.
20. Hubble bubble to all invited guests in the house.
21. Wearing *burqa* and *parda*.
22. Circumcision among muslim community.
23. Thread ceremony among Hindus.
24. *Annaprashana* at 1 year age for the child.
25. Covering their head by women when they come outside the house or when they participate in functions with men.

Habits

Definition

It is an acquired faculty to act in certain manner, without reason and deliberation or thought.
Examples:
1. Putting finger in nose, and ear.
2. Putting sticks in mouth.
3. Nail biting.
4. Eating fish, and egg as hot foods.
5. Eating curds, milk, vegetables like cucumber as cold food.
6. Alcohol consumption by higher class society
7. *Ganja, bhang, and charas* among *sadhus*.
8. Eating pan tobacco with lime and smoking.
9. Exchange of cloths in hostel life.

10. Applying *kajal* to the eyes.
11. Applying *kajal* to the cheek of kids.
12. Charcoal, *neem* twig tooth brush in the morning.
13. Hand washing after defecation and before eating food.
14. Application of turmeric powder before bath by women.
15. Walking barefoot.
16. Sleeping on the floor.

Tradition

Definition

Sets of rule associated with strict sanction that act as guide to conduct and tend to produce conformity in a community.
Examples:
1. Men eat first and women in the last.
2. Motherhood respecting religious function during first pregnancy.
3. Sending women for first delivery in their parents' house.
4. Touching the feet of elders to get their wishes.
5. Purifying bath before religious function.
6. Keeping delivered women away from *pooja* room and kitchen for 10 days and allowing entry after 11th day purifying bath.
7. Delivery by the traditional birth attendant.
8. Performing marriages within same caste and race.
9. Marriage is performed in girls' house.
10. Household articles are given at send off to husband's house after marriage.
11. Wishful gift given at housewarming ceremony.
12. Puncturing ear, and nose.
13. Offering *pan supari* after food in all social gathering.
14. Shaving is done outside house by a barber
15. Taking bath after attending funeral ceremony.
16. Performing functions such as naming ceremony, birth days, and anniversaries.
17. Child marriage as in *Rajasthanis* and tribal.
18. Polygamy, polyandry as in Himachal Pradesh *adivasis*.

Social sciences, like history and economics influence society; whereas behavioral sciences influence the human behavior which is the scientific examination of human behavior.

WEANING AND SUPPLEMENTATION (ADDITION OF SEMISOLIDS)

It is a gradual process of withdrawal of child from breastfeeding. Weaning period is a crucial period. Suitable supplementary foods such as cow's milk, fruit juice, soft cooked, rice, dhal, and vegetables are given.

Age-related Guidelines for Weaning and Supplementation

4–6 months	Start 1–2 teaspoon for each feed. Frequent feed 5–6 times a day, 4 weeks later increases to ½ cup a day No over dilution—give semisolid food Continue breastfeeding
6–9 months	Give food what family takes Mash all foods Frequent feed 5–6 times a day Continue breastfeeding
9–12 months	Can eat everything cooked at home No spices and condiments No mashing of food ½ cup 5–6 times a day Continue breastfeeding
12–18 months	Can eat all foods cooked in family, Needs ½ amount the mother eats daily Feed 4–5 times a day, and Continue breastfeeding especially at night

Desirable Qualities of Weaning Foods

High in energy, easy to digest, semisolid in consistency, low in bulk and viscosity, fresh and clean, affordable easy to prepare and culturally acceptable.

Low Birth Weight

Any infant with a birth weight 2.5 kg or less than 2.5 kg regardless of gestational age is called LBW.

Difference between Preterm Baby and Small-for-date Babies

	Preterm	Small-for-date
Birth occurring	Between 20 and 37 weeks of gestation	Preterm or at term
Intrauterine growth	Normal	Retarded
Prognosis	Easily brought back to normal	Difficult to bring back to normal
Weight	More than 10th percentile for gestational age	Less than 10th percentile for gestational age
Palmar and plantar crease	Developed	Not developed
Areola of nipple	Developed	Not developed

Indian Picture
Low birth weight (LBW) is 18.6% of live births.

Causes

Preterm babies

Acute infections, hypertension, and multiple births.

Small-for-date babies

Maternal malnutrition, anemia, toxemia, very young mother, no birth spacing, placental abnormalities, and intrauterine infections.

Prevention and Control
- Dietary improvement of pregnant women
- Control of maternal infections and diseases
- Spacing of pregnancy
- Incubatory care for LBW
- Proper feeding of LBW
- Infection control of LBW.

SOCIAL WELFARE SCHEMES FOR BETTER RCH

Programs for Mothers

There are various programs under social welfare schemes categorized under:
- Programs for the welfare of women.
- Composite programs for mother and child integrated child development (ICD) and development of women and children in rural areas (DWACRA) are examples of composite welfare scheme.
- Agencies involved are All India Women's Conference, Family Planning Association of India (FPAI). The Kasturba Memorial Fund and UNICEF.

Programs for Children

Child welfare covers physical, mental, social and economic development to the families. They give preventive, promotive, and rehabilitative services. The beneficiaries are children from below poverty line, children of working mothers, destitute and orphan and handicapped children.

Important welfare agencies are:
- Indian Council for Child Welfare
- Central Social Welfare Board
- Kasturba Gandhi Memorial Trust, and
- The Indian Red Cross.

The main activities of these agencies are:
- Day care services
- Balwadi, crèches, and nursery
- Holiday homes
- Bal Bhavans.

INTEGRATED CHILD DEVELOPMENT SERVICES (ICDS) (IMCDS)

Integrated Child Development Services (ICDS) now renamed as Integrated Mother and Child Development Services (IMCDS).

Started in 1975 with 33 experimental blocks, now there are 7,067 ICDS blocks functioning (**Fig. 12.5**).

The beneficiaries are:
- Children below 6 years
- Pregnant women
- Lactating mothers
- Women in the age group of 15–45 years.

The main objectives are:
- Improve the nutritional and health status of children in the age group of 0–6 years.
- Lay the foundation for proper psychological, physical and social development of the child.

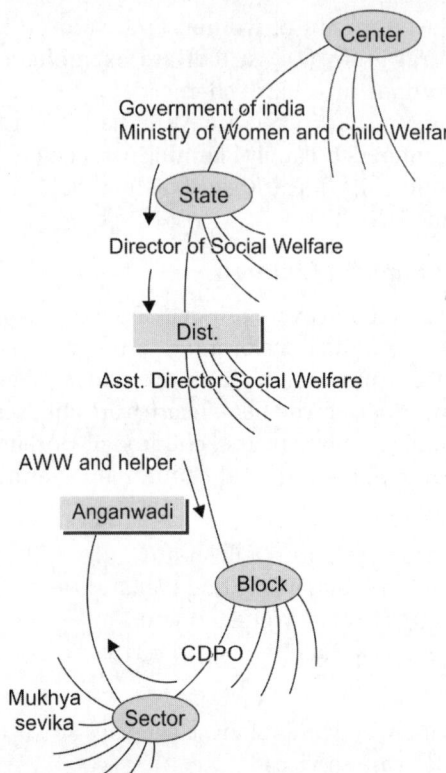

Fig. 12.5: IMCD administration.
(IMCD: Integrated Mother and Child Development Services; AWW: Anganwadi Workers; CDPO: Child Development Project Officer)

- Reduce the incidence of mortality, morbidity, malnutrition, and school dropouts.
- Achieve effective coordination of policy and implementation among the various departments to promote child development.
- Enhance the capability of the mother to look after the normal health and nutrition and needs through proper nutrition and health education.

Integrated Mother and Child Development Services (IMCD) Package of Service includes:
- Supplementary nutrition, vitamin A, IFA
- Immunization
- Health check-up
- Referral services
- Treatment of minor illnesses
- Nutritional and health education to women
- Preschool education of children 3–6 years (nonformal)
- Convergence of other supportive services like water supply and sanitation.

Integrated Mother and Child Development Services (ICDS) Blocks

Rural	Urban	Tribal
Community development block	Slums development	Tribal blocks
100,000 population	100,000 population	35,000 population
100 villages	–	50 villages

Two major evaluations conducted in 1978 and 1982. At present, 7,067 ICDS blocks are functioning adolescent girls scheme is sanctioned in all the blocks.

The following are under the proposal of Government of India:
- Universalization of IMCD
- Sanction of *Indira Mahila Yojana*
- More NGO involvement
- More coverage under World Bank assistance.

KEY INDICATORS IN REPRODUCTIVE AND CHILD HEALTH

a. Currently married women
   Percentage of married females to total females in the age
   10–14 years – 4.5%
   15–19 years – 35.3%
   20–24 years – 81.8%
   15–44 years – 79.5%
b. Mean age at marriage–22.3 years
c. No. of children per married women aged 45–49 years
   Ever born – 4.3
   Surviving – 3.7
d. Currently married women with any ANC–67.2% (any one or two of ANC check-up, TT, and IFA)
e. Currently married women with full ANC–14.8% (all had 3 ANC check-up + TT + 100 IFA/tablets)
f. Institutional delivery–35.0%
g. Safe delivery (by trained)–41.9%
h. Women with pregnancy complications–34.8%
   - Swelling hand, and feet

Chapter 12: Reproductive Maternal and Child Health

- Visual disturbance
- Bleeding
- Convulsions
- Weak or no fetal movement
- Abnormal presentation.

i. Delivery complications–36.4%
   - Premature labor
   - Obstructed labor
   - Prolonged labor

j. Postdelivery complications–42.0%
   - High fever
   - Lower abdominal pain
   - Foul smelling vaginal discharge
   - Excessive bleeding
   - Dizziness
   - Severe headache.

k. Currently married women 15–44 years of age with symptoms of RTI/STD–28.8%

l. Currently married women 15–44 years of age who are aware of acquired immunodeficiency syndrome (AIDS)–41.1%

m. Males aged 20–54 years with symptoms of RTI/STD–12.7%

n. Males aged 20–54 years who are aware of AIDS–57.4%.

SUMMARY

Briefing the elements of CSSM, emergency care is described. Growth and feeding practices are highlighted. Social welfare schemes including ICDS are described.

VIVA VOCE

1. Mention basic elements of RCH.
2. Mention services under RCH problem.
3. Stipulate five doses of vitamin A prophylaxis under RCH.
4. What is essential obstetric care?
5. Mention six services under essential newborn.
6. What is rooming in?
7. Mention child survival strategies.
8. Mention safe delivery practices.
9. What are the criteria for fast breathing in ARI.
10. Mention MCH indicators.
11. Hat is present MMR? Explain
12. What is present IMR?
13. Give present BR, DR and GR.
14. Mention functions of Under Five clinic.
15. What is exclusive breastfeeding?
16. What is Baby Friendly Hospital Initiative (BFHI)?
17. Mention social welfare schemes for better RCH.
18. Who are ICDS beneficiaries?
19. Enumerate ICDS objectives.

CHAPTER 13

School Health

Chapter Outline

- Milestone
- Health Problems
- Medical Examination
- School Health Education
- Mid-day Meal
- School Health Administration

INTRODUCTION

It is a personal health service aimed at bringing positive health of future generation, viz. school children. Special needs of school children are health guidance and education in group living. For raising health status of a nation, school age group children are to be given special care. Being future generation, school children form an economic group of the country. It is categorized under personal health services. Early days of medical examination is totally changed for a comprehensive school health services.

As per 2011 census, 18.5% of Indian population (1210.1 million) constitutes 223 million, who are of school age between 5 and 14 years of age. Therefore, health care needs and nursing care needs of 223 million school children become a stupendous task unless a formulated national guideline is prepared.

OBJECTIVES

- ❖ To promote the positive health of children
- ❖ To prevent childhood diseases
- ❖ To recognize chronic defects among children
- ❖ To create health consciousness among children
- ❖ To provide healthy school environment.

MILESTONES

1909	First school medical examination at Baroda city
1946	Bhore Committee recommends its importance.
1953	Secondary Education Committee emphasizes the need of examination and school feeding.
1960	Government of India constituted a school health committee which suggested means of improving school health.
1982	School health committee or improvement of health and nutrition
1997-2002	9th Five-Year Plan envisaged the progress of school health care.
2003-2007	Formal document has been prepared and is waiting for clearance which include widened version of school health care.

HEALTH PROBLEMS IN SCHOOL CHILDREN

Main problems noticed are malnutrition and infectious diseases. Emphasis is laid on following illness among school children.

- ❖ Skin infection including scabies and louse infestation

- Dental caries (it is a special problem)
- Measles, mumps and chickenpox
- Roundworm and hookworm infestation
- Vision alteration (it is a special problem)
- Hearing impairment (it is a special problem)
- Acute respiratory infection
- Diarrhea.

ACTIVITIES

- Medical examination
- Immunization
- Health education on personal hygiene, environmental hygiene and family life
- Mid-day school meal
- Chronic defects detection, and
- Record system.

Record System

Cumulative health record helps in giving continuing health supervision. It evaluates school health activities. It serves as a link between home and school.

Along with cumulative card, health card should also be maintained for each student. That should contain the following:
- Identification data
- Past health history
- Family history of any illness
- Findings of medical check-up
- Information on care given.

Medical Examination (Health Appraisal)

At admission and every 4 years' check-up by clinical examination and needed laboratory examination are done. The schedule of medical examination includes:
- Periodic medical examination
- Daily morning inspection
- Teachers and staff check-up
- Remedial measures, and
- Follow-up action.

Immunization

School immunization is scheduled as follows:
- 5–6 years DT
- 10 years TT, and
- 16 years TT.

School Education

Health Education

This is required for desirable change in knowledge, attitudes and practices (KAP) among children. It should include:
- Personal hygiene
- Environmental health and
- Family life.

Teacher to be educated to note and to take action on:
- Skin rash
- Respiratory symptoms
- Neck rigidity
- Eye redness
- Diarrhea
- Fever and chills
- Headache
- Vision defect
- Hearing defect
- Behaving rudely
- Flushed face
- Swollen face.

Safety Education

Safety education includes precautions to be taken to avoid accidents at school and in surrounding environment such as—(a) edge of sharp objects are kept away from the body, (b) care at walk to avoid banana peels and wet patches, (c) avoid playing with electric gadgets, (d) avoid in claiming the height, etc. Minimum training to all school children on first aid and hygiene is advocated.

Sex Education

As a component of population education, it was introduced in India through National Family Welfare Planning Programme during 1960. It includes mostly education on reproduction; however, it should also impart positive attitude to sex behavior. Sex education can motivate people to change or to modify the existing negative attitude and misbehaviors.

Main goal of sex education is to develop an ability to merge biological impulses with socially acceptable norms of sex behavior conducive to a satisfying family life as adult men and women.

It is going on as a learning process without our knowledge both in informal form (home, peer group) and formal form (School, university). Feeling of love and affection that has to be from parents in role modeling and also by siblings is not a true sex in human sexuality. It is the learning of sex attitude, sex emotion which are responsible for family relation and family responsibility that needed to be imparted in sex education.

Parents need to attempt to satisfy the natural and anxious curiosities of their child from where sex education starts. During adolescence, physiology of body, sexually transmitted diseases are to be made understandable. Sex education and counseling for adult men and women is managed by family physicians.

Mid-day School Meal and Other Nutritional Service

They include:
i. Development of school garden.
ii. Special nutrients for dental caries, endemic goiter, night blindness, PEM, anemia.
iii. Mid-day school meal.
   - It is a supplement,
   - It provides 1/3 of energy (diam or per day requirement)
   - At low cost, and
   - Simple cooking in acceptable form
   - By local foodstuff.

Menu per child per day	
Cereal and millet	75 g
Pulses	30 g
Oil	8 g
Leafy vegetable	30 g
Nonleafy vegetable	30 g

Half of pulse can be substituted by any of the following:
15 g fish,
120 g skimmed milk, and 15 g Multi Purpose Food (MPF).

iv. Balahar
70% wheat,
25% defatted groundnut meal, and 5% skimmed milk.

Menu for North Indian School Children

Menu	Program	Calorie	Protein	Cost (₹)
1. Maize Roti + rape leaves + Buttermilk	3 days a week	380	16	1.25
2. Bajra cooked + Curry		430	15	1.60
3. Tandoori roti + Aalu chole		420	16	1.80
4. Missi roti + Curd	2 days a week	560	17	1.50
5. Aalu chole + Bread		370	14	1.80
6. Marunda + Khaman Dhokla		560	27	2.40

Menu for South Indian School Children

Menu	Program	Calorie	Protein	Cost (₹)
1. Rice + Sambar + Buttermilk	3 days a week	550	15	1.80
2. Pongal + Curry + Buttermilk		500	15	1.75
3. Veg Chapaties		500	21	1.60
4. Wheat pulse porridge + Buttermilk	2 days a week	450	14	2.00
5. Sundal + Buttermilk		36	13	1.75
6. Laddu + Buttermilk		500	19	2.00

Chronic Defects Detection

This entails for the detection of impaired vision, impaired hearing (refractive error, deafness), dental health check-up, mental health check-up, and identification of handicap followed by remedial measures.

HEALTHY SCHOOL ENVIRONMENT

Location	Fair distance from busy place.
Site	On a high land.
Structure	Heat resistant and only ground floor.
Classroom	One for every 40.
Desk	Minus desk preferred (**Fig. 13.1**).
Door	Provision for cross ventilation.
Window	20% of floor area.
Paint	Only by white color.
Light	To the possible maximum extent from behind and left
Water supply	Potable water
Eating space	Separate hygienic area.
Urinals	1 per 60 students.
Latrine	1 per 100 students.

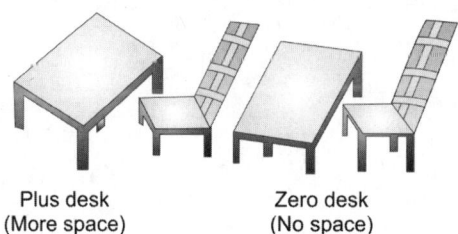

Plus desk (More space) Zero desk (No space)

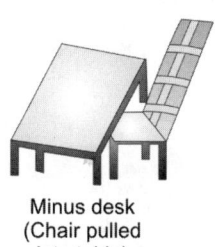

Minus desk (Chair pulled into table)

Fig. 13.1: Type of desk.

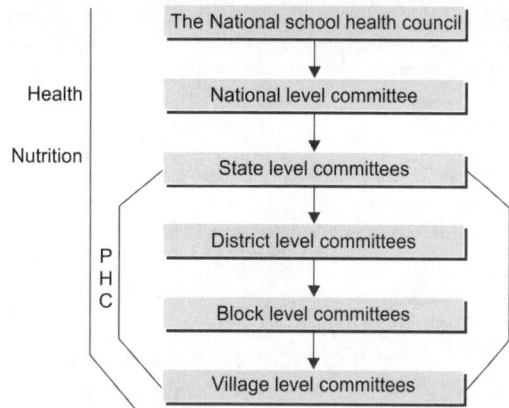

Fig. 13.2: School health administration.

School Health Administration

See Figure 13.2.

SUMMARY

Health problems of school age are described. Medical examination, scheduling health education and mid-day meal are described. Brief outline of school health administration is given.

VIVA VOCE

1. What are the objectives of school health program?
2. Schedule school immunization by DT and TT.
3. Describe Mid-day school meal.
4. What is minus desk?

SECTION 5

Section Outline

Chapter 14. Occupational Health Including Social Security
Chapter 15. Geriatrics and Health
Chapter 16. Genetics and Health
Chapter 17. Mental Health

14 CHAPTER

Occupational Health Including Social Security

Chapter Outline

- Ergonomic
- Occupational Hazards
- Pneumoconiosis
- Occupational Hazards in Agriculture
- Occupational Cancers
- Sickness Absenteeism
- Industrialization
- Occupational Risk of Health Professionals
- Prevention of Occupational Diseases
- Employees State Insurance Scheme (ESIS)

INTRODUCTION

Occupational health takes care of 2 things; the effect of work on our health, the effect of health on capacity to work. It was Bernardino Ramazzini who described the importance of occupational medicine and is called the Father of Occupational Medicine.

Earlier term *Industrial hygiene* is fully transformed to *occupational health* where application of preventive medicine is in all types of work placement. Initially with factory, now the growth of industries and varied occupation have given rise to the present concept of inclusion of all trades of services including human engineering.

DEFINITION

It is a science of labor welfare where, "Promotion of physical, mental, and social well-being of workers of all occupation, preventing disabilities out of occupations, protecting workers from occupational hazards and fitting the man to suitable job."

According to International Labor Organization (ILO), Occupational Health is defined as "The field of science which aims at promotion and maintenance of highest degree of physical, mental and social well-being of workers in all occupation, at prevention of any departure from health at work."

Occupational Environment

It is the sum total of external influences and external conditions present at the place of work that can influence the health of the worker. The interactions are:

- Different agents around man
- Machine and technology upon the healthy man
- Interhuman relationship.

ERGONOMICS (TABLE 14.1)

It is the science of norms and laws related to work or occupation.

1. *Job-fitting code:* Medical fitness as to a person's capability to work.

Table 14.1: Job fitting code.

–A	Fit for any work
+B	Got remediable diseases
++C	Not fit for employment only for limited fields of work
+++D	Unfit for any work.

2. *Job-fitting examination*:
- For the suitability of a person in specific work placement for ruling out
- Tuberculosis person in silica industry
- Anemia person in lead industry
- Skin changes and dermatosis in rubber industry.

OCCUPATIONAL HAZARDS

Occupational Hazards due to Physical Agents

Temperature

High temperature causes heat exhaustion, heat stroke, heat syncope, heat cramps, fatigue, e.g., glass industry, steel industry, foundry, jute industry, automobile industry, and mines.

Low temperature causes frostnip, frostbite, immersion foot, trench foot, e.g., ice factory. Cold shock by immersion hypothermia is also known.

Humidity

Discomfort, fatigue, throat and nose changes, e.g., textile, and jute industry.

Altitude

High altitude: Headache, insomnia, breathlessness, nausea, vomiting, anorexia, vision impairment, memory impairment, paralysis, and coma, e.g., mountaineering, and pilots.

Medical emergencies in high altitude are pulmonary edema, cerebral edema, acute mountain sickness, migraine headache, and bronchopneumonia and eardrum perforation.

Low altitude

Mental dysfunction, and unconsciousness, e.g., Caisson disease.

Radiation (Table 14.2)

Leukemia, malignant changes, genetic changes, sterility, and welder's flash (keratitis), e.g., welding, workers in X-ray unit, and workers in isotope plant.

Ionizing radiation

See **Table 14.2**.

Noise

Hearing loss, fatigue, nervousness, e.g., pneumatic drilling, and rotating tool use.

Table 14.2: Radiation by rays.

Type	In air	In tissue	Occupation	Hazard
α	Few cm	10 μ	Plutonium	Internal
β	Several meters	Few mm	Caesium	External and internal
γ	Many meters	Many cm	Cobalt therapy	External and internal
X	Many meters	Many cm	Hospital X-ray	External
Neutrons	Many meters	Many cm	Reactors	External

Log to the base of 10 of ratio of measured pressure to reference pressure are called Bels. International agreed reference levels of dB are:
- Sound pressure level (Bels) SPL
- Sound pressure level (deciBels) SPL
- Intensity (deciBels) SPL.

Lighting

Headache, corneal congestion, miner's nystagmus, e.g., TV and watch repair, mining workers.

Vibration

Physical stressors at work are seen in drills, guns, impact, grinders, sanders, buffers, saw, and vibrating pokers. Related conditions for hand arm vibration (e.g., tools) are carpal tunnel syndrome, Dupuytren's contraction. Whole body vibration is seen with use of heavy vehicles from agriculture or any work platform. If the whole body vibration is <0.315 m/s^2, person will not be uncomfortable. If it is 0.8–1.6 m/s^2, discomfort starts.

Occupational Trauma

Repeated occupational trauma affecting musculoskeletal system is known. Shoulder problems (tendinitis, capsulitis), neck problems (cervical spondylosis, thoracic outlet syndrome, and tension neck syndrome), elbow problems (lateral or medial epicondylitis), wrist and forearm (tenosynovitis, carpal tunnel syndrome).

Occupational Hazards due to Chemical Agents

Toxicokinetics

Basic knowledge of the concepts of Toxicokinetics is to understand the mechanism by which chemicals gain entry into our body. It is the study of dynamic relationship between concentration of chemical in the body fluids and tissues and biological effect on the body.

Gases

Methane, CO_2, CO, SO_2, CS_2, HCN, HCl asphyxiants, and irritants.

Dust

Organic dust
- *Bagassosis* (cane bagasse): Paper, cardboard, and rayon.
  Clinically fever, breathlessness, cough, hemoptysis, lung mottling, fibrosis, emphysema, and bronchiectasis.
  Prevention: Containment, dilution, periodic examination of workers, maintenance of 20% moisture, and use of 2% propionic acid.
- *Byssinosis* (cotton): Textile.
  Clinically fibrosis, emphysema.
  Prevention: Usual protection and exhaust ventilation.
- *Tobacosis* (Nicotine): Cigar, snuff.
  Clinically gastrointestinal—nausea, vomiting, and diarrhea.
  Cardiovascular system (CVS)—arrhythmia, myocarditis.
  Central nervous system (CNS)—neuritis, amblyopia.
  Respiratory—carcinoma lung.
- *Farmer's lung* (Hay/grain dust)
  Clinically asthma, fibrosis, cor pulmonale.

Prevention: By maintaining 20% humidity at 40°C temperature.

Inorganic dust
- *Anthracosis* (coal): Simple pneumonia to progressive massive fibrosis, disability. Anthracosis is notifiable.
- *Silicosis* (silica): Gold mine, mica mine, rock mining, and sand blasting.
  Clinically nodular fibrosis. Snowstorm appearance X-ray associated with TB.
  It is notifiable.
- *Asbestosis* (Asbestos): Roof-tile, cement, gasket silicates of Mg (chrysolate). Silicates of Fe, Ca, Na, Al (amphibole). Clinically pulmonary fibrosis, pleural thickening, emphysema.
  Sputum shows asbestos bodies.
  X-ray ground glass appearance.
  Associated with mesothelioma.
- *Iron:* Iron and steel industry.
  Clinically respiratory changes.
- *Lead* (plumbism)—battery, glass, ship building, painting, rubber, automobile.
  Inorganic lead—clinically abdominal colic, constipation, blue line in gum, stippling of red blood cell (RBC) anemia, wrist drop, foot drop.
  Organic lead—clinically insomnia, headache, mental confusion, delirium.
  Treatment: Saline purge.
  D-penicillamine 0.5–1.5 g per day for 4 weeks.
  Ethylenediaminetetraacetic acid (EDTA) 70 mg/kg/day for 5 days.
- *Manganese:* Decolorizing agent, dying, metallurgy, steel, clinically motor ataxia and pneumonia.
- *Nickel:* Electroplating (stainless steel) Clinically hemorrhagic bronchopneumonia.
- *Chromium:* Electroplating, alloys, photography, paint.
  Clinically skin lesion, perforation of nasal septum.
- *Mercury:* Vermillion, barometers avoid skin contact.
  Treatment: British antilewisite (BAL) in acute poisoning.
  First day 200 mg, later 100 mg.
- *Phosphorus* (yellow): Match industry, Rodenticide.
  Clinically phossy jaw, gastrointestinal (GI) symptom, paraplegia.
  Treatment: Tetraethyl pyrophosphate (TEPP) 10 mg oral [2.5 mg intramuscularly (IM) 6th hourly].
- *Arsenic:* Paris green, dye industry.
  Clinically skin reaction, GI manifestation, neuritis, paralysis of peripheral nerves.

Occupational Hazards due to Biological Agents

Anthrax	: Farmer, butcher, dealer in hair, wool and bone meal.
Actinomycosis	: Peasant, *dhobi*, and fisherman
Brucellosis	: Veterinary surgeons
Encephalitis	: Forest rangers, and wildlife associates
Fungal infection	: Swimmer, and animal husbandry
Hydatid cyst	: Pet dog, veterinary people, and field workers
LIH (Rat)	: Miner, sewage worker, field workers in rice, sugar, and fish workers
Psittacosis	: Birds, parrots, and pigeons
Tetanus	: Agricultural workers, and gardener.

Occupational Hazards due to Social Agents

Frustration, tension, aggressiveness, alcoholism, peptic ulcer, and hypertension.

PNEUMOCONIOSIS

Lung manifestation by inhalation of organic or inorganic dust of 0.5 micron, in the working placement causing inflammatory changes and later infective process which cause reduced pulmonary ventilatory capacity and fibrosis. This condition is called pneumoconiosis.

Example: Silicosis
Anthracosis
Byssinosis
Bagassosis
Asbestosis

OCCUPATIONAL HAZARDS IN AGRICULTURE

Disease: Tetanus, leptospirosis, anthrax.

Accidents

- Insect bite, snake bite
- Toxic effect of insecticides
- Sunstroke, radiation, burns
- Farmer's lung, asthma.

Agrochemicals

- Herbicide
- Insecticide
- Molluscicide
- Fungicide
- Rodenticide.

Occupational Hazards in Industry

Falls, fracture, loss of parts, loss of organ, loss of vision, and death.

Causes

- Human factor,
- Physical discomfort,
- Lack of experience, and
- Ignorance.

Prevention

- Job training after job fitting exam
- Safe working environment.

Occupational Dermatitis

Commonly, contact dermatitis which can be irritant contact dermatitis or allergic contact dermatitis, contact urticaria and oil folliculitis are seen.

Causes: Heat, cold, radiation, acid, dye, chemicals, fungi, and plant products.

Prevention

- Preselection examination
- Personal protective equipment
- Personal hygiene.

Occupational Hazards in "Do It Yourself Activities"

Painting, plastics, woodwork, and photography.

OCCUPATIONAL CANCER
(FIG. 14.1 AND TABLE 14.3)

Control Measure

- Detection and exclusion of carcinogen
- Personal hygiene
- Education to workers on safety.

Chapter 14: Occupational Health Including Social Security

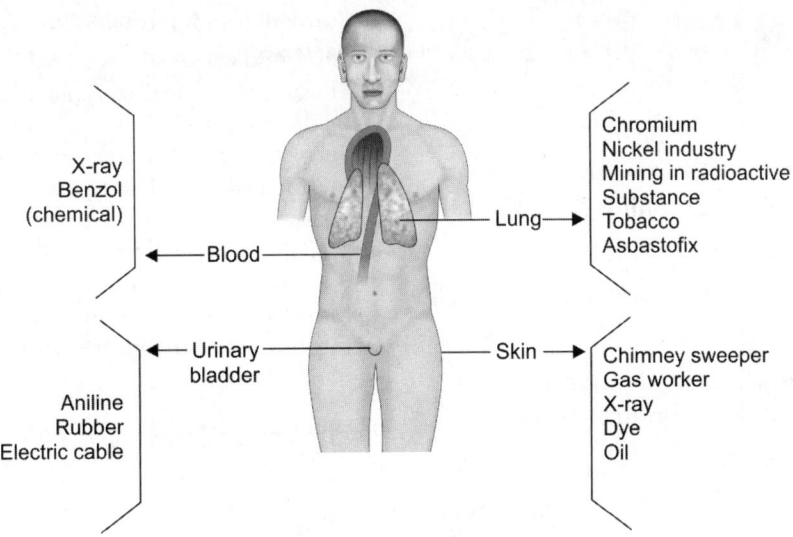

Fig. 14.1: Common occupational cancer.

Table 14.3: Occupational cancers.

Occupation	Cancer
Chromate, hardwood dust, nickel	Ca. nasal cavity
Asbestos, radon, chromate	Ca. lung
Asbestos	Ca. peritoneum Ca. pleura Ca. larynx
Benzidine (dye, rubber)	Ca. bladder
Radiation, Benzene	Ca. blood
Tar distillate	Ca. skin
Vinyl chloride monomer	Ca. liver

SICKNESS ABSENTEEISM

Worker's absence by any cause or by any means is attributed to sickness. It is around 20% as per National Productivity Council. Unauthorized absence rate of spells longer than 14 require special attention. It should be less than 5 as per standards. The rate of absence is 8–10 days per head per year. It affects both the progress and production.

Causes:
- Medical causes
- Social causes, economic causes, and
- Nonoccupational causes.

Prevention

- Use effective ergonomics
- Good human relationship, and
- Efficient management of workers in industry or factory.

INDUSTRIALIZATION

It refers to urban health, since industrialization and urbanization go hand in hand.

Health Problem

- Shortage of water, and accommodation
- Air pollution
- Sexually transmitted disease (STD), tuberculosis
- Food-borne infections
- Behavioral disorders
- Accidents
- Social problems

Work and Mental Health
- Bullying repeated negative acts in workplace
- Post-traumatic stress disorder
- Violence at work.

OCCUPATIONAL RISKS OF HEALTH PROFESSIONALS AND THEIR PREVENTION

Occupational Risks of Health Professionals by Physical Agents

Radiation: Carcinogenic
- Teratogenic
- Mutagenic
- Burns

- Cataract
- Infertility
- Anomalies

Ventilation: Nosocomial infection.

Occupational Risks of Health Professionals by Chemical Agents

- Anesthetic agents.
- Hazardous drugs (potential risks to health professionals).

Occupational Risks of Health Professionals by Biological Agents

Droplet cores: Tuberculosis and influenza.

Blood: Hepatitis B virus (HBV), hepatitis C virus (HCV), HIV.

Direct contacts: Scabies, skin parasites.

Needle stick injury.

Nursing assistant and sanitary workers at hospital are risk groups.

Occupational Risks of Health Professionals by Ergonomics

Posture: Low back pain among nurses (58%) doctors (33%)

- Repetitive strain injury
- Eye strain
- Carpel tunnel syndrome
- Depression
- Insomnia
- Headache, back pain, neck pain, shoulder pain, wrist pain, and hand pain.
- Obesity
- Hearing loss
- Urinary infection
- Digestive problems.

Occupational Risks of Health Professionals by Psychosocial Agents

- Verbal threat, and verbal abuse
- Behavioral threat at workplace
- Violence at workplace on doctors, nurses, ANM, pharmacists, radiographers, laboratory technicians.

Prevention of Occupational Risks of Health Professions

- Follow the rules of workplace, particularly by doctors, nurses and technicians
- Formation of health security council at work
- Mention source of danger at work
- Evaluate risks
- Medical examination of staff
- Give health and security education
- Make proper documentation
- Increase staff for shift or for rotation to decrease exposure to risks.

Health Protection Measures in Occupation

- Nutrition
- Disease control
- Minimum standards of physical condition (environmental sanitation)
- Mental health
- Special care for women (crèches) and child workers (above 14 years)
- Health need awareness
- Small family norm.

PREVENTION OF OCCUPATIONAL DISEASES

Medical

- Preplacement examination
- Periodic examination
- Protection of workers
- Health education.

Engineering

- Containment
- Dilution
- Substitution
- Device to protect workers.

Legislation

- Indian Factory Act (IFA)
- Employees State Insurance Scheme (ESIS).

Accident Prevention in Industry

- Preplacement examination
- Periodic examination

- Safety department with safety engineer with safety devices
- Job training to all workers
- Safe working environment
- Good reporting system, and
- Good record system.

Labor Act and Law in Occupation

To secure health and welfare of workers national policies are enacted from time to time. The mines Act for miners, the plantation Act for plantation workers, the minimum wages Act for all types of working placements are examples of welfare through legislation. Most important factory laws are:
1. Indian Factory Act (IFA)
2. Employees State Insurance Scheme (ESIS).

Indian Factory Act (IFA) (1948)

It is detailed under PH Act. The Act is applicable to any establishment where 10 or more workers are employed. Within the definition of worker, contract labor is also included. The Act details:
1. Health
2. Safety
3. Welfare
4. Prohibition of child labor
5. Hours of work
6. Privilege of leave with pay
7. Notification, enquiry on diseases and death.

Recently, employment in hazardous process and safety management therein are incorporated.

EMPLOYEES STATE INSURANCE SCHEME (ESIS) (1948) AMENDED (1975, 1984, 1989, 2010)

This covers factories, shops, hostels, cinema, transport, newspaper and almost all work placements where 10 or more employees are employed. Since 2010 even clerical, supervisory and technical workers drawing salary up to 15,000 PM are included under the provision of Act. Enhancement to ₹ 20,000 per month as limit was proposed in June 2016 by Employees State Insurance Corporation (ESIC). It is raised to ₹ 20,000 per month w.e.f. 6.9.2016.

Administration

- Labor ministry
- ESI corporation, and
- Standing committee.

Finance

- Employers contribute 4.75% of wage bill
- Employees contribute 1.75% of wage, and
- 1/8th expenditure by state, 7/8th by ESI.

Benefits

a. Medical
b. Sickness
c. Maternity
d. Disability
e. Dependent
f. Funeral.

a. *Medical benefits:* One doctor for 1,000 workers, one part-time doctor for 750 workers and insurance general practitioners take care of medical care (1:585 Doctor: Worker in ESI) (3.21 beds per 1,000 employees in ESI).

b. *Sickness benefit:* A worker is eligible for 7/12 of wage for 91 days in a year.

Extended sickness benefit (309 days):
- Bacterial—TB, leprosy
- CNS—mental, paraplegia, hemiplegia
- CVS—CCF
- Cancer
- Eye cataract 6/60 vision.

Extended sickness benefit of 124 days for:
- Respiratory—bronchitis, lung abscess
- CVS—MI, aplastic anemia, gangrene
- Bone—disk prolapse, ankylosing spondylitis, fracture of lower limb
- CNS—Parkinson's disease
- GI—cirrhosis of liver with ascites
- Eye—detachment of retina.

c. *Maternity benefit*
- 26 weeks cash benefit allowed (delivery)
- Additional maternity benefit (confinement benefit ₹ 5,000/- per confinement)
- 6 weeks of benefit in miscarriage

- 30 days of benefit in sickness of confinement

d. *Disablement benefit*
  90% of wage given for temporary and permanent disability.

e. *Dependents' benefit*
  90% to the dependents as per rule.

f. *Funeral benefit*
  Expense of ₹ not exceeding 10,000/- available.

Recently, rehabilitation allowed after retirement for medical treatment on monthly payment of ₹ 10/- by the worker.

Research Institutes of Occupational Health

- The Central Mining and Research Station, Dhanbad
- The Industrial Toxicology Research Center, Lucknow
- The Occupational Health Research Institute, Ahmedabad
- The National Environmental Engineering Research Institute at Nagpur
- The Indian Institute of Technology, Kanpur
- The All India Institute of Hygiene and Public Health, Kolkata.

SUMMARY

Briefing the ergonomics and occupational hazards are given. Pneumoconiosis is detailed. Brief outline of hazards in agriculture and occupational cancers are given. Sickness absenteeism is detailed. Prevention of occupational hazard including ESIS is detailed.

VIVA VOCE

1. Define occupational health.
2. Define ergonomics.
3. What is bagassosis?
4. Enumerate occupational hazards due to biological agents.
5. Define pneumoconiosis.
6. Give examples of occupational cancers.
7. What is sickness absenteeism?
8. Mention medical prevention of occupational diseases.
9. What are the benefits of ESIS?

CHAPTER 15: Geriatrics and Health

CHAPTER OUTLINE

- Geriatric Health Problem
- Nutritional Requirement
- Social Welfare Measures
- Elderly Citizen Facility Concept

INTRODUCTION

According to Sir James Sterling Ross, "We cannot heal old age; we can protect it, promote it and extend it."

Now that expectation of life is increased, geriatric age group is widening and we have nearly 5% of the population above 65 years of age (7.7% population is above 60 years of age). This comes to nearly 60 million people above the age of 65 years as per 2011 census.

Aging process involves changes in physiological, pathological, social and psychological conditions of a person. Changing sociocultural trend is taking elderly off from joint family system to the old age homes (those who can afford). Slowly family life by bonding is weaning off creating chaos in health status, nutrition status, metabolic status and psychological status. Sometimes the elderly are left alone to find themselves for their survival.

There are two groups of older people:
1. One is older people with healthy life.
   In them, we observe the following senescence changes:
   - ↓ Bone mineral density
   - ↓ Gastrointestinal motility
   - ↓ Glomerular filtration rate (GFR)
   - ↓ Tissue sensitivity to insulin cardiovascular system (CVS) changes
   - Respiratory changes
   - Central nervous system (CNS) changes.
2. The other is older people with frequent multiple pathology called frail older people.
   - Here, ability of man to withstand environment is reduced.
   - Geriatrics is the branch of medical science which deals with the care of the old people.
   - Old age changes are called senescence. It is a normal biological phenomenon.

Gerontology	Study of aging process
Social gerontology	Deals with old age social problems Experimental research on old age
Geriatric	Old age problem in elderly
Gynecology	Ladies

Gerontology, gereology and preventive geriatrics are areas of interest in geriatrics.

Global Proportion of Geriatric Age Group
9–10% (above 65 years).
Proportion of geriatric age group in India
5.0% (above 65 years)
7.7% (above 60 years)

Most of the geriatrics problems in India, in the order of merit, are cataract, arthritis, hypertension, neurological problems, chronic bronchitis, loss of hearing and psychiatric problems.

GERIATRIC HEALTH PROBLEMS

Social Problems of Geriatrics

* Loneliness (loss of colleagues and friends)
* Rejection (lowered status and income)

Old age problems	Chronic illness
The changes in old age is called senescence which is a natural process. Common effects of old age are: • Senile cataract • Nerve deafness • Osteoporotic changes • Bronchitis with emphysema • Changes in mental outlook and many more old age changes.	Old people are prone to a few known chronic diseases, of particular importance are: • Atherosclerosis • Heart attacks • Hypertension • Stroke • Cancer • Diabetes • Accident and fractures • Gout • Rheumatoid arthritis • Fibrocystis • Neuritis • Chronic bronchitis • Asthma • Prostate enlargement • Fibroid of uterus.
Geriatric problems	Geriatric illnesses

* Insecurity, and
* Maladjustment (boredom and generation gap).

Psychological Problems of Geriatrics

* Dementia
* Sexual problems
* Emotional disturbances, and
* Instability.

Health Problems

Special sense impairment: Visual impairment, cataract, glaucoma, auditory impairment, deafness.

Locomotor system impairment: Arthritis, osteoarthritis, spondylitis.

Pulmonary function impairment: Chronic bronchitis, asthma.

Genitourinary (GU) system malfunctions: Enlarged prostate, cervical prolapse.

CVS system malfunction:

Malignancy: Cancer prostate, cancer uterus.

Accidents: Fracture neck of femur, Colles' fracture.

Metabolic diseases: Diabetes.

Digestive diseases: Constipation, liver cirrhosis.

Economic Aspect of Geriatrics

* Dependency
* Expenditure on welfare activity of elders.

Major Health Problems of Elders

1. Vision impairment
2. Joint disorders
3. Musculoskeletal disorders
4. Neurological disorders.

NUTRITIONAL REQUIREMENT

Indian Council of Medical Research (ICMR) has worked out the nutritional requirement of old people (1990). The requirement of energy is expected to be 10% less than that of an adult.

Balanced Diet for Geriatric Age

Foodstuff	Requirement (Grams)	
	Males	Females
Cereals	350	225
Pulses	50	40
Vegetables	200	150
Leafy vegetables	50	50
Roots, tubers	100	100
Fruits	200	200
Milk and milk products	300	300
Sugar	20	20
Fats and oils	25	25

Chapter 15: Geriatrics and Health

Nutrients Required for the Old Age

Foodstuff	Requirement (Grams)	
	Male	Female
Calorie	2,200	1,700
Protein	65 g	50 g
Fat	50 g	40 g
Calcium	1 g	0.9 g
Iron	38 mg	30 mg
Vitamin A (retinol)	1,030 µg	930 µg
Thiamin	1.96 mg	1.45 mg
Riboflavin	1.78 mg	1.51 mg

Some Dietary Tips for the Elderly

The diet of the elderly may be modified according to physical activity of an individual and general health condition. The following tips are suggested for dietary management of the elderly. They are:
1. Take simple but nutritious diet.
2. Improve the quality of diet by adding liberal quantity of green leafy vegetables, fruits and whole cereals
3. Take frequent but small meals
4. Take plenty of fluids and semisolids
5. Avoid dry foods
6. Reduce total fat
7. Reduce refined carbohydrate
8. Reduce salt intake
9. Avoid fasting.

Other Indirect Nutritional Advice

1. Maintain good social and psychological environment for normal health
2. Do regular exercise like brisk walking
3. Avoid inactivity, loneliness and social isolation.

SOCIAL WELFARE MEASURES

- National assistance
- Supplementary pension
- Home service or old age homes
- Home care services or home help services
- Meals on wheels service for single-aged ones
- Sitters-up service
- Provision of health visitors service, and
- Counseling to accept old age.

Health measures to be taken for elderly people for improving quality of life of older people:
- Activities, interests, and hobbies by traditional cultural programs, old age club facilities
- Good family cordial relationship
- Good social cordial relationship, and
- Make freedom from disabilities.

ELDERLY CITIZEN FACILITY CONCEPT

- Travel concession (train, bus)
- Wheel chair facility on request
- Priority base lower birth reservation in railways
- Income tax rebate
- Accessibility of old age home
- Geriatric clinics at different level; aspirin prophylaxis in geriatric care with 150 mg per day against degenerative diseases.
- Meal on wheels (facility of hot fresh food at lunch/dinner by organization/institution to doorstep in time)
- No waiting in bank, post office, purchase and entertainment
- Free facility of hearing aids, and
- Free facility of presbyopic correction glasses.

According to German and Fried, old age preventive care can be grouped under three levels:

1. Primary Level
Good health habits like:
- Good sleep
- Good and required nutrition
- Curtailing smoking, alcohol and fatty foods
- Avoidance of overeating (obesity control).

Avoiding risk factors like:
- Care at routine to avoid accident, fracture
- Diet restrictions
- Periodic health check-up.

2. Secondary Level
- Screening for hypertension
- Early diagnosis and prompt treatment for infections.

3. Tertiary Level
- Rehabilitation for physical defects.
- Rehabilitation for cognitive defects
- Rehabilitation for functional defects
- Use of caretaker for support.

SUMMARY

Geriatric health problems are highlighted. Nutritional requirement of elderly is deduced. Available social welfare measures are highlighted. It is concluded with elderly citizen facility concept.

VIVA VOCE

1. Mention old age problems.
2. Mention chronic illness among elderly.
3. What are the health problems of elderly?
4. Give dietary tips to elderly.
5. What is elderly citizen facility?

16 | Genetics and Health

CHAPTER OUTLINE

- Genetic Disorders
- Prevention of Genetic Disorders
- Population Genetics
- Gene Therapy
- Heritability

INTRODUCTION

This discipline is the application of the principles of human genetics to medical practice. It deals with inheritance, diagnosis and treatment of diseases by gene or chromosomal factors. Genetic counseling and screening are included in the discipline.

COMMON TERMS

Mitosis:	Ordinary cell division
Meiosis:	Reproductive cell division called reduction division, diploid to haploid (46 to 23 chromosomes)
Chromosome:	Condensations of chromatin, made up of DNA, which consists genes
Genes:	Units of heredity "A length of DNA" that contains information
Genotype:	Total genetic constitution of a person
Phenotype:	Outward expression of the genetic constitution
Genome:	Genetic material made of DNA which contains information
Heterozygote:	Two genes of a pair are different from one another
Homozygote:	Identical genes
Mutation:	Process by which DNA changes
Recombination:	Crossing over gives rise to rearrangement of gene
Transgenesis:	Introduction of new gene to human cell
Transplantation:	Cell, tissue or organ is removed from one person and implanted into another person.

We have gene map which is a resource in public health. It has given us genetic screening. Man can inherit biological determinant and/or he can inherit cultural determinant. This becomes "rule of inheritance" (**Fig. 16.1**).

Genetics deals with genetic cause or inherit cause of a disease which helps us to identify predisposed individual or community.

Lifetime frequency of genetic disorders is about 7 per 1,000 which includes cardiovascular disorders. Major cause of infant deaths will be congenital malformation. Oocyte aneuploidy is about 18%, stillbirth is

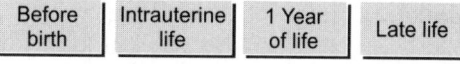

Fig. 16.1: Place of understanding endogenous genetic factors in human life.

about 5.6%, and congenital malformation is about 3.6 % in their frequencies.

Medical genetics is important on the ground that mutations are irreversible, family history of congenital defects is a risk and they have social and psychological impact. Pathfinders in the field are:

Gregor Mendel	1865 Mendelian laws
Watson and Crick	1953 Double helix DNA
Tijo and Levan	1956 Chromosomes
Victor McKusick	1994 McKusick's catalogs

GENETIC BASIS

Genes are units of heredity. They can be homozygous (alike AA) or heterozygous (not alike aA). If manifested, it is dominant, otherwise recessive. Their location is in chromosomes which are autosomes (22 pairs) and sex chromosomes (1 pair). Chromosomes are in seven groups (A to G) where X and Y sex chromosomes are in C and G groups, respectively.

Clinical Genetic Examination

Buccal smear, peripheral blood, bone marrow, skin, or testis tissues are taken. Colchicine is added to arrest metaphase (hypotonic). They swell and disperse. Later stained, fixed and studied.

Molecular Genetics

Enzymes involved in DNA and RNA synthesis are identified and made available for laboratory use.

DNA technology allows genetic diagnosis. This is useful in gene therapy.

Gene therapy allows modifying cell behavior. It is useful in prevention of genetic mutation.

Human Genome Project is a research on mapping and isolating human genes.

Human Genome Varsity Project helps in understanding human evolution.

GENETIC DISORDERS

Autosomal Dominant Genetic Disorders

- Retinoblastoma
- Marfan syndrome
- Neurofibromatosis
- Polyposis coli.

Autosomal Recessive Genetic Disorders

- Albinism
- Total color blindness
- Infantile amaurotic idiocy
- Phenylketonuria
- Fibrocystic disease of pancreas.

Common Inborn Errors of Metabolism

See **Table 16.1**.

Sex-linked Disorders

- Hemophilia (**Fig. 16.2**)
- Agammaglobulinemia
- Red green color blindness
- Neonatal jaundice
- Duchenne muscular dystrophy (**Fig. 16.3**).

Table 16.1: Common inborn errors of metabolism.

Phenylketonuria	Amino acid metabolism	AR	Deficient phenylalanine hydroxylase	Mental retardation, eczema, epilepsy
Alkaptonuria	Amino acid metabolism	AR	Deficient homogentisic acid oxidase	Dark urine, arthritis
Hyperargininemia	Urea cycle disorder	AR	Deficient arginase	Spasticity, intellectual, deterioration, ammonemia
Galactosemia	Carbohydrate metabolism	AR	Deficient galactose-1 phosphate uridyltransferase	Cataract, mental retardation, cirrhosis of liver
von Gierke's disease	Glycogen storage disease	AR	Deficient glucose-6-phosphatase	Liver enlargement, hypoglycemia
Testicular feminization	Steroid metabolism	XR	Deficient androgen receptor	External genitalia female, internal genitalia male, chromosome male

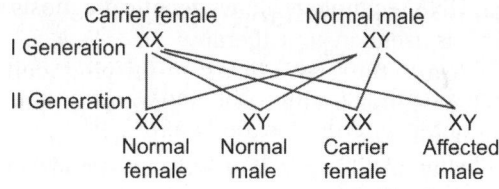

Fig. 16.2: Sex-linked genetic expressions.

Chromosomal Aberrations

- Klinefelter syndrome (abnormal male) (XXY or XXXY)
- XYY syndrome (antisocial)
- Turner syndrome (apparent female) (XO)
- Super females (XXX, XXXX).

Autosomal Aberrations

Trisomy 21: Down syndrome (Mongolism). It is associated with rising maternal age, congenital malformations, mental retardation and degenerative disorders.
Trisomy 18: Edward syndrome
Trisomy 13: Patau syndrome
Trisomy 16: First trimester fetal loss

All trisomies manifest growth retardation, mental retardation, and multiple systemic anomalies.

Diseases Associated with Genetic Predisposition

- Cancer
- Coronary heart disease
- Diabetes (insulin dependent)
- Alzheimer's disease.

PREVENTION OF GENETIC DISORDERS

Health Promotion

- *Eugenics* (improving genetic endowment)
  - Positive
  - Negative
- *Euthenics* (suitable environment for a genotype)
- *Genetic counseling*
  - Prospective
  - Retrospective
- Regulation on consanguineous and late marriage.
- a. *Specific protection from X-ray; early diagnosis* by:
  - Detection of carriers
  - Prenatal diagnostics
  - Amniocentesis and chorionic villus biopsy
  - Newborn screening
  - Preclinical case recognition.
  b. *Prompt treatment by:*
  - Available facility.

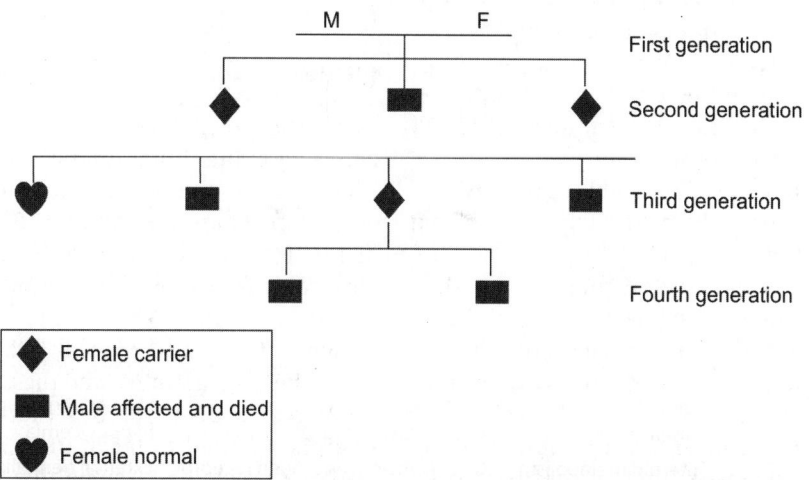

Fig. 16.3: X-linked recessive inheritance of Duchenne muscular dystrophy. Transmitted through affected females (because male do not survive).

c. *Rehabilitation*
   - Community-based rehabilitation
   - Special schools.

POPULATION GENETICS

Human being has more than 100,000 structural genes, each has two copies each. The study of precise structural genetic composition of a population constitutes population genetics.

Hardy–Weinberg equilibrium states that the relative frequencies of each gene allele tend to remain constant from generation to generation.

If the form of allele for tallness is A and for shortness a, there are three chances that a person can draw as his combination. They can be:

- AA   Tall
- Aa   Medium
- aa   Short

This follows the constancy of algebraic formula:
$a^2 + 2ab + b^2$
i.e., AA + 2Aa + aa
that is, a^2 (AA) + 2ab (Aa) + b^2 (aa)

Population genetics studies:
- Gene frequencies
- Factors influencing gene pool
- Long-term consequences.

GENE THERAPY

It is a process of introduction of gene sequence as a part of treatment in genetic disorders.

Usually, gene therapy involves introducing an adenovirus. Gene delivery to somatic cell is agreeable on ethical ground, e.g.,
- Cancer treatment (for producing cytotoxicity)
- Ischemic heart disease (IHD) (for modifying susceptibility)
- Cystic fibrosis (for correcting mutation).

Gene therapy trials are seen with brain tumor, breast cancer, malignant melanoma, myelogenous leukemia, lung cancer, and neuroblastoma.

In case of cancer therapy, gene therapy include targeted killing of diseased cells by inducing genes that encode toxins or by provoking enhanced immune response.

Human Genome Project (HGP)

This is an international research effort which analyzes the structure of human DNA and aims to determine the locations of the estimated 30,000–40,000 known and predicted genes. This was begun formally in 1990.

It is a genetic process of mapping and isolating human genes and coding them for identification. It is helpful in defining human genetic relations.

It is found very useful in:
- Genetic migration
- Genetic drift
- Genetic selection.

The procedures incorporated are:
- Molecular cloning
- DNA sequencing
- Somatic cell hybridization
- Cell sorting
- Deletion and duplication mapping
- Sequence scanning.

Methods for determining mode of inheritance:
- Multifactorial model analysis
- Segregation analysis
- Analysis of maternal effects
- Linkage analysis, and
- Sibling pair methods.

Sequencing of entire human genome was first proposed in mid-1980s by US Department of Energy. Steps are shown in **Figure 16.4**.

Cloning

Cloning is a technique for producing a genetic twin of a living thing. It entails taking DNA from an adult animal and inserting it into an egg cell from another animal. The egg then divides into an embryo. The cloned embryos have genes from only one parent. The embryo is then transferred to a surrogate mother and grown to term. The process has worked in cows, sheep, goats, mice and pigs.

A group of 40 Nobel Prize winning scientists issued a declaration supporting research on cloning, saying that a total ban "would have a chilling effect on all scientific research and that it would be unprecedented

Chapter 16: Genetics and Health

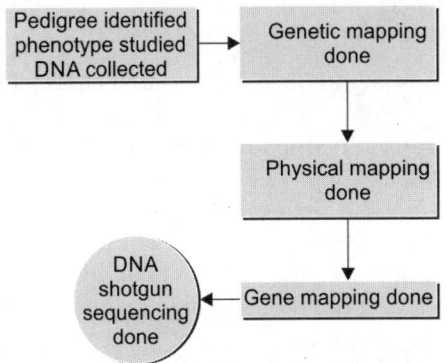

Fig. 16.4: Steps in human genome project.

and ill-conceived and would place medical R&D at a dangerous disadvantage."

HERITABILITY

It is the liability of inheritance of a given disease in the community **(Figs. 16.5 and 16.6)**.
Examples of heritability: (Proportion of the total variation of a character which can be attributed to genetic factor) **(Table 16.2)**.

Table 16.2: Heritability.

Disease	%	h^2
Asthma	4	80
Schizophrenia	1	80
Cleft lip	0.1	76
Cleft palate	0.1	76
Congenital heart disease (CHD)	3	65
Hypertension	5	62
Peptic ulcer	4	37
Congenital heart disease	0.5	35

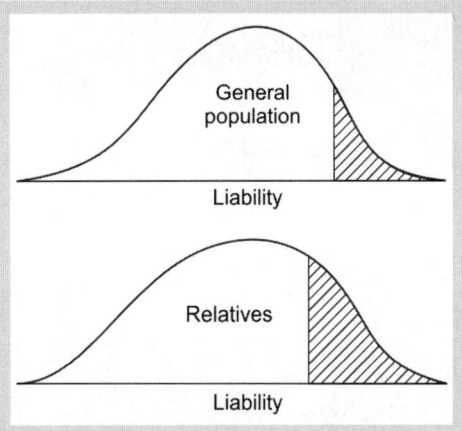

Fig. 16.5: Genetic predisposition in population.

SUMMARY

Describing genetic disorders, their prevention is detailed. Population genetics and gene therapy are given importance along with heritability.

VIVA VOCE

1. Name autosomal dominant genetic disorders.
2. Name two inborn errors of metabolism.
3. Describe hemophilia. Show how sex linked?
4. What is Trisomy 21?
5. What is genetic counseling?
6. What is human genome project?
7. Define cloning.

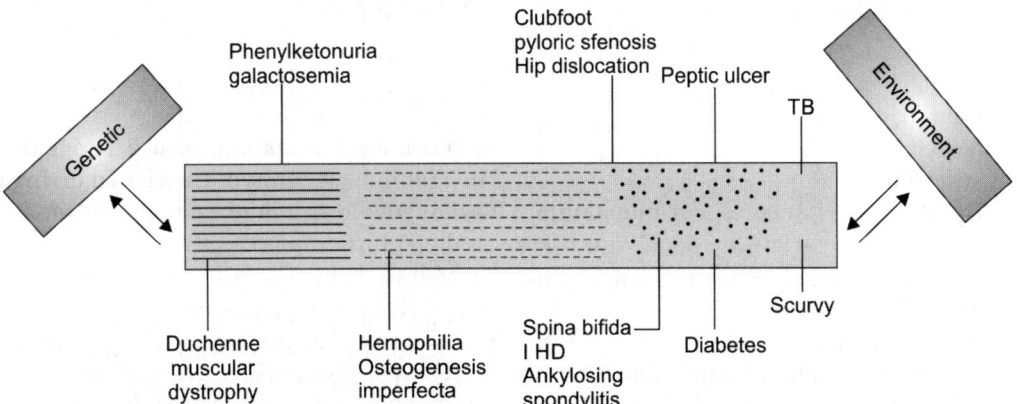

Fig. 16.6: Genetic liability in community.
(IHD: ischemic heart disease)

17 CHAPTER — Mental Health

Chapter Outline

- Current Picture
- Mental Illness
- Psychosomatic Disorders
- Alcohol and Substance Dependence
- Childhood Disorders
- Modern Therapy
- Prevention
- Community Psychiatry
- National Mental Health Programme

INTRODUCTION

Satisfaction in life and happiness are required for normal behavior of man which depends on mental health. Harmonious working of mind can lead to well-adjusted personality. Mentally ill person can disturb the family or even the community.

Personality and emotion adjusted to harmonious life for better mental health influence positive healthy life.

Until the last century, treatment to mentally sick was tedious and torturous; presently the treatment is ideally based on psychiatric treatment through drugs, counseling and community activities.

CURRENT PICTURE

- 13.7% of population has psychological stress
- Schizophrenia is 2 per 1,000 population
- Organic psychoses are 1 per 1,000 population
- Serious mental disorders are around 10–20 per 1,000 population
- Overall morbidity in India is around 18–20 per 1,000 population

COMMON DEFENSE MECHANISMS

Repression

Forgetting unacceptable idea.
For example, during fits, patient urinates which he cannot recollect a month later.

Sublimation

Diverting unacceptable feeling.
For example, unmarried is dedicated to career.

Reaction Formation

Unconscious dealing for unacceptable desire.
For example, afraid of surgery, patient cuts a joke about it.

Dissociation

Unconscious removal of painful experience.
For example, parents are charred to death in front of a child and child cannot recollect it.

Conversion

Change feelings to emotions.
For example, man who does not want to marry gets fits (Common in hysteria).

Rationalization

Give excuses (unconsciously).
For example, a girl always seen semi-nude, when asked says that she can never find anything else to wear.

Projection

Shift the blame to others.
For example, poor dancer blames uneven floor.

Regression

Childish behavior.
For example, anxious husband becomes completely dependent on wife, refusing to do even smallest thing for him.

MENTALLY ILL

Worry, no concentration, unhappy, lacking temperament, loss of sleep, depression, dislike, disturbed life, getting nervous, feeling bitter, fear, and aggressiveness.

Criteria of Abnormal Behavior

According to William C Menninger, the criteria of abnormal behavior are:
- Always worrying
- Unable to concentrate
- Unhappy without justified cause
- Very often and very easily losing temperament
- Regular insomnia
- Depression which makes incapacitated to fight
- Routine life is not normal
- Unnecessarily getting frightened
- Feeling always right or always wrong
- Somatic incurable pains and aches.

MENTALLY WELL

Secured, comfortable, feel right, group acceptance, problem-solving capacity, discharge responsibility, no fear or anger.

MENTAL ILLNESS

1. **Psychosis**
   - Schizophrenia (split personality) who are in dreamland
   - Manic depressive psychosis (vary from excitement to depression)
   - *Paranoia:* Suspicion, tendency to see world in delusion.
2. **Neurosis/psychoneurosis:** Unable to reach normality to life situation, compulsion and obsession present.
3. **Personality/character disorders:** Because of unfortunate childhood experience.

Causes

- Mental illness due to organic conditions
- Hereditary
- Economic factors like poverty, poor standard of living
- Social factors like stress, family pattern
- Environmental factors:
  - Toxic
  - Drug abuse
  - Trauma.
- Crucial points of life uncared:
  - Pregnancy
  - Under-five
  - Social age
  - Adolescence, and
  - Old age.

Need for Mental Health

- Affection
- Achievement
- Belonging
- Independence
- Self respect
- Recognition, and
- Self-realization.

PSYCHOPHYSIOLOGICAL DISORDERS (PSYCHOSOMATIC)

They are a group of disorders in which emotional factors have a demonstrable role in the etiology. They are stress-related disorders.

Common psychosomatic disorders seen in clinical practice are:
- High BP
- Asthma
- Peptic ulcer

- Ulcerative colitis
- Irritable bowel syndrome
- Arthritis
- Headache
- Eczema
- Diabetes
- Anorexia nervosa
- Obesity
- Psychogenic pain.

Common causes could be response to emotion, personality traits, family pattern and prolonged stress.

Management includes symptomatic treatment. Nursing care includes:
- Good nursing relationship
- Encourage patient to discuss his problem
- Create a feeling of acceptance
- Encourage family participation in therapy
- Teach relaxation exercises.

ALCOHOL AND SUBSTANCE DEPENDENCE

Alcohol withdrawal delirium occurs in 5% of alcoholics who stop alcohol. Corrections of dehydration, electrolyte imbalance, and control of fits are to be attended along with careful monitoring of vital signs.

Opioids, antipsychotic drugs show involuntary muscle contractions like stiff neck, stiff mouth, elevated eyeball.

Case has to be managed as inpatient along with the special nursing care of psychiatric emergencies.

CHILDHOOD DISORDERS

Proportion of childhood mental disorders can be gauged by the fact that children constitute 28–30% of our population which comes to about 363 million at present as per 2011 census.

Common causes of disorders are biological cause (heredity, illness), psychological causes (broken homes) and social causes (poverty).

Common illnesses are:
- Mental retardation
- Autism (driven to fantasy)
- Conduct disorders
- Specific development disorders
- Personality development disorders
- Hyperkinetic disorders
- Tics
- Mannerism.

MODERN THERAPY

In mentally ill person, treatment is not specific since it varies from person to person. Nurse, being closer with patient, has important role in therapy. Her action, attitude and skills to help patient to deal with his problems are themselves an essential part of his treatment.
- *Physical Therapy:* It includes drug treatment, ECT, psychosurgery.
- *Psychopharmacology:* This includes psychotherapy of individual, group, family.
- *Hypnosis:* By altered state of consciousness induced by conditioning and skilled use of suggestions.
- *Play therapy:* Very helpful for young and the old. Diversion by play can get over tension and anxiety.
- *Activity therapy:* There are specific therapies like occupational, music, dance, psychodrama, recreation and psychosocial therapies.

PREVENTION OF MENTAL ILLNESS

1. Counseling
   - Genetic counseling
   - Sex counseling
   - Marriage counseling
2. Reproductive child health (RCH)
3. School health service
4. Geriatric care.

Primary prevention	*Secondary prevention*	*Tertiary prevention*
• Personality development • Family life	• More psychiatrist in the community for treatment of mentally ill • Child guidance clinics • Health education on mental health	• Day care • Family living • Self-help in group • Industrial therapy • Home care

Substance abuse (*see* Chapter 36).

COMMUNITY PSYCHIATRY

It is a branch of psychiatry that develops and maintains organized programs for the prevention, promotion and rehabilitation of mentally ill person.

In a defined population, care given through health workers and community health guides for a continuous care and integrated with regular health service is called community mental health care.

Follow-up services are given importance. For details, *see* Chapter 33.

NATIONAL MENTAL HEALTH PROGRAMME

Government of India has launched National Mental Health Programme during Seventh Five-Year Plan with the objectives of:
- Ensuring availability of service.
- Making mental health service accessible.
- Its application in general health care.
- Promoting community participation.
- Helping for self-help.

Now, the National Mental Health Programme forms part of the comprehensive mental health program where the mentally ill is treated with common man in community.

In the year 2013, Comprehensive Mental Health Action Plan was jotted to last till 2020 to promote mental well-being, prevent mental disorders, and to provide care. This included:
- Strengthening leadership
- Integration of mental health into social care services
- Implementation of strategies laid down in the action plan
- Development of Health Information System (HIS) and research.

SUMMARY

Defining the mental health, psychosomatic diseases are enumerated. Alcohol and substance abuse is given detailing. Common childhood disorders are described. Community psychiatry is detailed. It is concluded with National Mental Health Programme.

VIVA VOCE

1. When do we call a person mentally ill?
2. What are the criteria of abnormal behavior?
3. Describe psycho-somatic disorders.
4. What is autism?
5. Describe prevention of mental illness.
6. What is community psychiatry?

SECTION 6

Section Outline

Chapter 18. Disaster Management
Chapter 19. Hospital Waste Management

18 CHAPTER

Disaster Management

Chapter Outline

- Classification
- Man-made Disasters
- Vulnerability Reduction in Disaster Management
- Emergency Preparedness
- Phases
- Common Disasters in India
- Hazards Description Scales

INTRODUCTION

Any disaster is an emergency situation and the health sector alone cannot tackle it in isolation. Local community, civil, defense, army, police, fire brigade, government organization, nongovernmental bodies and voluntary organizations should combine to reverse the effects of disaster management.

Disasters are catastrophic occurrences that invariably have profound implication on public health. It is a destructive event that results in the need for a wide range of emergency resources to assist and ensure the survival of the disease-struck population.

TERMINOLOGY

Disaster

World Health Organization's definition of disaster is "any occurrence that causes damage, economic disruption, loss of human life, deterioration in health and health services on a scale sufficient to warrant an extraordinary response from outside the affected community or area."

Hazard

WHO's definition of hazard is "any phenomenon that has the potential to cause disruption or damage to people and their environment."

Triage

Rapidly classifying the injured based on severity of injury, number of survivors. An approach for maximum benefit to all injured in a major disaster.

Tagging

Injured is identified by name, age, place of origin and triage category.

Disaster Mitigation

Designed measures in the community to reduce casualties such as building codes, land use planning, flood mitigation works.

Critical Health Supplies

Food (supply and safety), water (supply), basic sanitation, personal hygiene, vector control, and vaccination, that are also called humanitarian supplies (supply, transport, storage, distribution).

Agencies in Humanitarian Assistance

Agencies mean WHO, UNICEF, World Food Programme, FAO, CARE, Red Cross.

World Disaster Reduction Day

Celebrated on second Wednesday of October every year. Main activities are awareness on disaster, knowledge dissemination on community involvement.

CLASSIFICATION OF DISASTERS

Natural Disasters

Floods	Earthquake	Fire
Hurricane	Cyclone	Thunderstorm
Tornadoes	Snowstorms	Volcanoes
Land slides	Famine	Drought
Sea erosions	Heat waves	Epidemics of infectious diseases
Gas tragedies by chemical leakage	Multi-storey building collapse	Burst of nuclear plants
Military war	Civil war	Major accidents of ship, plane, train

Man-made Disasters

- Civil war and terrorist attacks
- Chemicals and radioactive waste disposal to sea, river
- Poisonous gas leakage in factories
- Military war and deaths of million
- Poisonous gas leakage as occurred in 1984 Bhopal Gas Tragedy at Union Carbide's company
- Blast in nuclear power plant as occurred in 1986 Chernobyl Nuclear Power Plant.

Technological Disasters

- Explosions
- Fires
- Chemical release to environment
- Radiological release to environment.

Conflict-related Disasters

Result of social, economic, political problems involving armed confrontation, e.g., Rwanda, Somalia, Bosnia.

PUBLIC HEALTH TOOLS AVAILABLE IN DISASTERS

- Information of needs
- Information of status
- Focused Health Survey reports
- Target Health Survey reports
- Focused Health Surveillance reports.

Public Health Interventions

- Environmental health control
- Communicable disease control
- Nutritional rehabilitation.

CHALLENGES IN DISASTER MANAGEMENT

- Violence in disaster area
- Early reach is impossible
- Early supply is impossible
- Women, children and elderly are vulnerable to effects of disaster very early
- Destructive technology by terrorists
- Psychological upset in families.

DOCUMENTATION AND TAGGING IN DISASTER AREAS

0—Black	Death
I—Red	Requires transport
II—Yellow	An urgent condition
III—Green	Nonurgent condition

EFFECTS OF INAPPROPRIATE HUMANITARIAN ASSISTANCE (FIG. 18.1)

Assistance appears a fairly simple solution. If it is not requested by affected community or not integrated with country's normal service and development, reduces the developmental opportunities in the areas.

VULNERABILITY REDUCTION IN DISASTER MANAGEMENT (FIGS. 18.2 AND 18.3)

Vulnerability is a function of degree of exposure to disaster hazards.

Chapter 18: Disaster Management

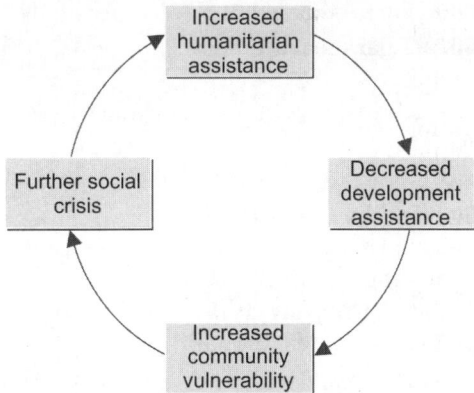

Fig. 18.1: Vulnerability by assistance.

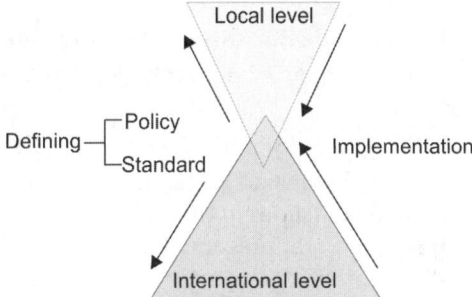

Fig. 18.2: Vertical integration of vulnerability reduction.

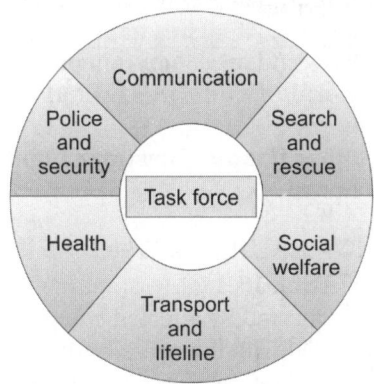

Fig. 18.3: Horizontal integration of vulnerability reduction.

Community vulnerability depends upon:
* Susceptibility (degree of exposure to hazard)
* Resilience (capacity to cope with hazard).

High or low susceptibility and resilience determine the task of disaster management.

Vertical and horizontal integration of vulnerability reduction helps to cope with disaster situations.

EMERGENCY PREPAREDNESS IN DISASTER (FIGS. 18.4 AND 18.5)

It is a long-term development activity whose goals are to strengthen the overall capacity and capability of a country to manage efficiently all types of emergency and bring about an orderly transition from relief through recovery and back to sustained development (WHO).

Prepared communities can maintain and improve their level of development.

PHASES OF DISASTERS

Natural Phases

* Pre-disaster phase
* Impact phase
* Post-disaster phase

(Rescue, relief, rehabilitation).

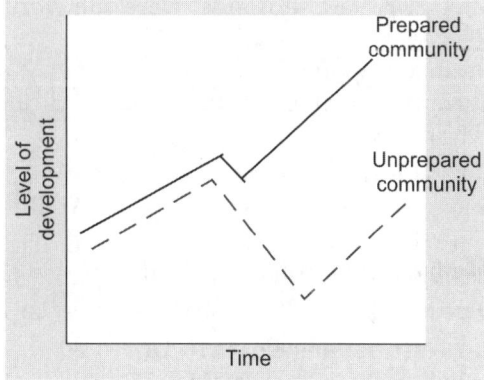

Fig. 18.4: Effect of preparedness of development.

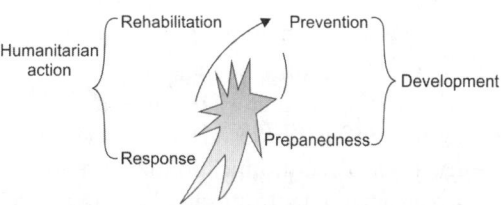

Fig. 18.5: Emergency management cycle.

Behavioral and Psychological Phases

- Impact phase (fear)
- Heroism phase (rescue)
- Honeymoon phase (shared good outcome)
- Disillusionment phase (discontentment)
- Reorganization phase.

Victim Response Phases

- Impact phase (fear, psychosis, loss)
- Interaction phase (feeling conflict)
- Acceptance phase (to survive)
- Acquiescence phase (humiliation, rage).

Important, outrageous and dangerous disasters recorded in India:

1630–Deccan famine of 1630–1632
Result of failure of three consecutive staple crops.
Death Toll: Approximately 20 lakhs.
Men began to devour each other.

1737-Calcutta cyclone
Calcutta witnessed one of the worst cyclones.
Death toll: Approximately 3 lakhs.
Destroyed nearly 20,000 ships

1770 -Bengal famine of 1770
Bihar, Orissa and Bengal were the worst affected.
Death toll: Approximately 1 crore.
Attributed in large part to rampant policies of British.

1839 - Coringa cyclone
Ancient city of Coringa in present Andhra Pradesh.
Death toll: Approximately 3 lakhs.
Destroyed 25,000 ships and vessels in its bay.

1876 - Great famine of 1876-78
Known as the Madras famine.
Death toll: Approximately 3 crores.

1899 - Third plague pandemic 1899
Death toll: Approximately 1.2 crores.
There were not enough people left alive.

1943 - Bengal famine of 1943
Death toll: Approximately 15–40 lakhs.
Series of crop failure caused localized famines.

1993 - Latur earthquake
About 52 villages were totally destroyed.
Death toll: Approximately 20,000.

2000 - Earthquakes
2001- Gujarat earthquake
Kutch district of Gujarat.
An earthquake with a magnitude of 7.7 on Richter scale.
Death toll: Approximately 20,000.

2004- Indian Ocean tsunami
Earthquake registered 9.0 on Richter scale.
Tamil Nadu was worst effected.
Death toll: Officially 10,136.

2005 - Kashmir earthquake
2006 - Earthquakes
2007- Bihar Floods
2008 – Kerala Floods
2010 - Eastern Indian Storm
2011 - Stampede Haridwar and Earthquakes
2012 – Orissa alcohol poisoning and Indian cold wave
2013- Stampede Allahabad Kumbha Mela
2013 - Temple town of Kedarnath
Floods and landslides in Uttarakhand.
5,700 people were "presumed dead".
100,000 pilgrims and tourists trapped in the valleys.

2014—Patna stampede
2015—Gujarat and Assam floods
2016—Indian heat wave and Uttarakhand forest fire
2017—Powerful monsoon rain in Mumbai
2018—Kerala floods and Kolkata bridge collapse
2019—Bihar floods, Karnataka floods and Kerala floods.

COMMON NATURAL DISASTERS IN INDIA (TABLE 18.1)

Earthquake

It may cause a large number of deaths and injuries mainly because of sudden house collapses. People residing in houses built with stones and bricks, but not conforming to the building codes are more vulnerable than those residing in houses constructed with lighter material such as wood, bamboo and mud. In the history of earthquake affected population include those residing in densely populated

Table 18.1: Effect of common disasters.

	Earthquake	Floods	Drought
Death	Many	Few	Moderate
Severe injury	Overwhelming	Few	Moderate
Food scarcity	Rare	Common	Common
Population movement	Rare	Common	Common
Undernutrition	Occasional	Moderate	Common
Communicable diseases	Risk +	Risk ++	Risk +++
Recent disasters			
	1991 Uttarkashi	1998 Kutch	
	1993 Latur	1999 Odisha	
	1999 Chamoli	2001 Bhuj	
	2001 Gujarat		

areas closer to the epicenter of the earthquake. Casualties are more during night time, when most of the people remain inside their houses. Earthquakes on ocean bed also give rise to a dangerous phenomenon called *tsunami* (Maremoto) generating a several meters high sea wave which crashes down on the coasts and engulfs people on the seashore or beach.

Floods

Among all natural disasters, flood is regarded as the most damaging in terms of human lives and property. The flood is an annual feature of major rivers and their tributaries during monsoon season. Population living on alluvial plains liable to flooding are worst affected. Mortality is high in case of sudden flooding mainly due to drowning. Besides fractures, injuries and bruises, cases of accidental hypothermia also occur during cold weather. Deaths due to bites by poisonous snakes and insects are also common.

Drought

Factors responsible for drought are low rainfall, reduction in vegetation, soil erosion and surface evaporation. In rural communities, economic factors (Agronomy) and sociocultural factors (nomads, city migration) affect the health and survival of the families. Famines and desertification are their most fearsome consequences which cause PEM, vitamin A deficiency, measles, ARI, and diarrhea with dehydration. Drought-affected population who migrate and settle down on outskirts of cities and towns face the problem of poor hygiene and sanitation. Overcrowding further exposes them to communicable diseases like diarrhea, tuberculosis, parasitic infestation and malaria.

WHAT TO DO IN AN EARTHQUAKE

* When house is built of bamboo, mud and lighter material and street is wide, one should go out and make the way along middle of the road towards a square. If the street is narrow, better to stay indoor under a doorway.
* When house is built of concrete and one stays ground floor, better to go out, walk along middle of the road towards a square. If in higher floor remain indoor near an internal pillar.
* When house is built of stones, bricks, and on above floor, one should position under a doorway in a loadbearing wall. If in ground floor, one can walk along middle of road towards a square.
* Balcony, terrace, and projections are avoided.
* Panic and confusion are avoided.

ACTION PLANS ON EARTHQUAKE BY GOVERNMENT OF INDIA

* Disaster Management Action Plan (DMAP) by a satellite network connecting all civic bodies for ensured action.

- ❖ Establishment of the National Geospatial Data Infrastructure under Department of Science and Technology is now underway.
- ❖ National Calamity Contingency Fund (NCCF) with initial corpus fund of ₹ 500 crores is set up.
- ❖ A working group of experts and professionals would be set up to advise the National Committee on Disaster Management (NCDM).

STEPS IN MANAGEMENT OF NATURAL DISASTERS

Predisaster Phase

- ❖ Training in first aid, life-saving resuscitation, victim rescue; basics of hygiene and sanitation
- ❖ Focus on environmental sanitation
- ❖ Immunization.

Disaster Phase

- ❖ Calmness
- ❖ Helping victims
- ❖ Food rehabilitation
- ❖ Dealing the dead (man, animal).

MANAGEMENT OF CYCLONIC STORM AFFECTING PHC AREA

Cyclone Disaster

- ❖ Community rescue operation
- ❖ Overcome fear, panic
- ❖ Make volunteers from PHC
- ❖ Organize for:
  a. Measures to be attended within an hour
  b. Measures which wait for few hours.

Aftermath of Cyclone

- ❖ Assess requirement
- ❖ Consider outside assistance
- ❖ Get temporary shelter sanction
- ❖ Monitor food supply
- ❖ Deal with disposal of dead
- ❖ Vaccination, nutrition, HE, sanitation and mental health.

Further Cyclone

- ❖ Disaster information
- ❖ Knowledge of risk
- ❖ Training of volunteers
- ❖ Preparedness of population.

Diseases to be Monitored

- ❖ Diarrhea
- ❖ Measles
- ❖ ARI
- ❖ Malaria
- ❖ Meningitis (Meningococcal)
- ❖ Tuberculosis
- ❖ Hookworm
- ❖ Scabies
- ❖ Xerophthalmia
- ❖ Anemia
- ❖ Tetanus.

HAZARD DESCRIPTION SCALES

They are available in standard tables prepared and set by International Emergency Management Agency.

Common scales used are:
1. Beaufort scale (storm, hurricane).
2. Hurricane disaster potential scale.
3. Frequency of tropical storms
4. Modified Mercalli scale (earthquake)
5. Landslide damage intensity scale
6. Damage probability matrix for landslides
7. Tsunami intensity scale (floods)
8. Volcanic eruption scales
9. Dangerous goods classes (explosive, inflammable, corrosive, toxic gas, etc.).

SUMMARY

Vulnerability reduction in manmade disasters is described. Emergency preparedness is detailed. A common disaster in India with their hazard description scale is described.

VIVA VOCE

1. Define disaster.
2. When is the world disaster reduction day?
3. What is tagging in disastrous areas?
4. What to do in an earthquake?
5. What is tsunami?

CHAPTER 19: Hospital Waste Management

Chapter Outline

- Classification
- Hazards
- Waste Disposal Container Code
- Treatment Option for HWM
- Important Aspects of HWM
- Major and Important Instructions in HWM through Pictures

INTRODUCTION

There has been increasing concern for effective management of hospital waste (which is clinical and hazardous waste) and infection control to reduce morbidity, mortality, improve patient satisfaction, and quality assurance and minimization of medicolegal cases. The Ministry of Environment, Government of India, has issued following notification in July 1998, "The Biomedical Waste Management Rules 1998", making it imperative to install appropriate hospital waste management system.

The treatment option for hospital waste disposal is given in **Table 19.1**.

Table 19.1: Treatment option for hospital waste disposal.

Waste class category	Waste description	Treatment method
1. Human anatomical wastes, blood, body fluids	Human tissue, organs, waste body parts, body fluids, blood and blood products; items saturated or dripping with blood body fluids contaminated with blood and body fluids removed during/after treatment, surgery or autopsy or other medical procedures	Incineration
2. Microbiological wastes	Laboratory culture stocks or specimen of microorganisms live or attenuated vaccine; human or animal cell culture used in research; infectious agents from research wastes from production of biological dishes and devices used for transfer of cultures	Incineration
3. Waste sharps	Sharps such as needles, scalpel, blades, etc., which include both used and unused	Chemical disinfection autoclaving followed by shredding
4. Discarded glassware	Wastes generated from glassware and glass equipments used	Chemical disinfection autoclaving followed by shredding

Hospital waste is divided into:
- Noninfective waste
- Infected sharp waste
- Infected waste.

Recently, while hearing a public interest litigation, the Supreme Court has directed all hospital authorities to install incinerators or/and suitable devices for safe disposal of hospital wastes.

Central Pollution Control Board and State Pollution Control Board are the regulating authorities in this aspect.

DEFINITION

Hospital waste is generated during diagnosis, treatment, immunization and research.

CLASSIFICATION

- Infectious waste
- Pathological waste
- Sharps
- Pharmaceutical waste
- Genotoxic waste
- Chemical waste
- Wastes of heavy metals
- Pressurized containers
- Radioactive waste.

HAZARDS

- Infections—HIV, Hepatitis B and C
- Chemicals—toxic, corrosive, flammable
- Genotoxic—inhalation, absorption, digestion at treatment
- Radioactive—vomiting, dizziness, headache
- Aesthetic—human organs, tissues.

WASTE DISPOSAL CONTAINER CODE AT HOSPITAL WASTE MANAGEMENT

Category	Color	Waste
1.	Yellow	Human anatomical
2.	Yellow	Animal
3.	Yellow/red	Microbiology/biotechnology
4.	Blue/white	Sharps
5.	Black	Medicine/drugs
6.	Red/yellow	Solid dressing material
7.	Red/blue/white	Solid instruments/appliances
8.	------	Liquid
9.	Black	Ash
10.	Black	Chemicals

TREATMENT OPTION FOR HOSPITAL WASTE MANAGEMENT

See **Table 19.1**.

IMPORTANT ASPECTS OF HOSPITAL WASTE MANAGEMENT

1. Never transfer sharps from person to person (**Fig. 19.1**)
2. India's vulnerability to disasters:
   - 57% land is vulnerable to earthquakes. Of these, 12% is vulnerable to severe earthquakes.
     - 68% land is vulnerable to drought.
     - 12% land is vulnerable to floods.
     - 8% land is vulnerable to cyclones.
   - Also vulnerable to chemical and industrial and manmade disasters.
3. Areas of concern:
   - How to activate an early warning system?
   - How to involve Science and Technology and Administration?
   - Communication (water, power, transport)
   - Funding
   - Weak forecasting
   - Emergency medicine and first aid.

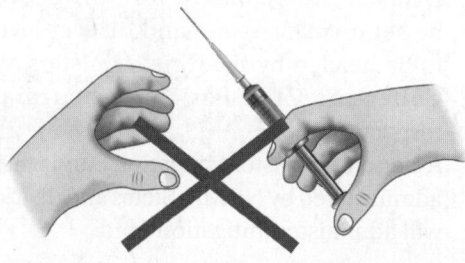

Fig. 19.1: Person to Person transferring sharps.

4. Nodal agencies for disaster management:
   - *Cyclones:* Indian Meteorological Department
   - *Earthquakes:* Indian Meteorological Department
   - *Epidemics:* Ministry of Health and Family Welfare
   - *Avian flu:* Ministry of Health, Ministry of Environment, Ministry of Agriculture and Animal Husbandry
   - *Chemical disasters:* Ministry of Environment and Forests
   - *Industrial disasters:* Ministry of Labor
   - *Rail accidents:* Ministry of Railways
   - *Air accidents:* Ministry of Civil Aviation
   - *Fire:* Ministry of Home Affairs
   - *Nuclear incidents:* Department of Atomic Energy
   - *Mine disasters:* Department of Mines
   - *Floods:* Ministry of Water Resources.
5. Dynamics of disasters:
   - High probability of a low probability event
   - Unpredictability of disaster events
   - The high-risk and vulnerability profiles make it imperative to strengthen disaster preparedness, mitigation and enforcement of guidelines, building codes and restrictions on construction of buildings in flood-prone areas and storm surge-prone coastal areas.
6. New directions for disaster management in India:
   The National Disaster Management Authority (NDMA) has been set up as the apex body for disaster management in India, with the Prime Minister as its Chairman.
   Disaster Management Authorities will be set up at the state and district levels to be headed by the Chief Ministers and Collectors/Zilla Parishad Chairman, respectively.
   A National Disaster Mitigation Fund will be administered by NDMA. States and districts will administer mitigation funds.
   - A National Disaster Response Fund will be administered by NDMA through the National Executive Committee. States and districts will administer State Disaster Response Fund and Disaster Response Fund, respectively.
   - Battalions of National Disaster Response Force (NDRF) are being trained and deployed with CSSR equipment and tools in eight strategic locations.
   - A National Disaster Management Policy and National Disaster Response Plan will also be drawn up.
7. Lessons learnt:
   - *Be prepared:* Preparedness and mitigation is bound to yield more effective returns than distributing relief after a disaster
   - Create a culture of preparedness and prevention
   - Evolve a code of conduct for all stakeholders.
8. Future directions:
   - Encourage and consolidate knowledge network
   - Mobilize and train disaster volunteers for more effective preparedness, mitigation and response (NSS, NCC, Scouts and Guides, civil defense, home guards)
   - Increased capacity building leads to faster vulnerability reduction
   - Learn from best practices in disaster preparedness, mitigation and disaster response
   - Mobilizing stakeholder participation of self-help groups, women's groups, youth groups, Panchayat Raj institutions
   - *Anticipatory governance:* Simulation exercises, mock drills and scenario analysis, indigenous knowledge systems and coping practices
   - *Living with risk:* Community-based disaster risk management

- Inclusive, participatory, gender sensitive, child friendly, eco-friendly and disabled friendly disaster management
- *Technology driven but people-owned knowledge management:* Documentation and dissemination of good practices, Public–private partnership.

MAJOR AND IMPORTANT INSTRUCTIONS IN HOSPITAL WASTE MANAGEMENT THROUGH PICTURES (FIGS. 19.2 TO 19.6)

Major and important instructions in hospital waste management are depicted in the following pictures:

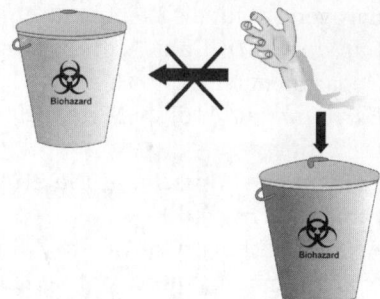

Fig. 19.4: Always incinerate human anatomical waste.

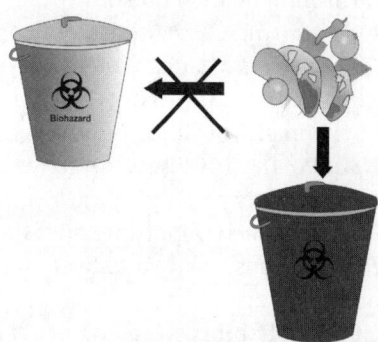

Fig. 19.5: General waste use black container.

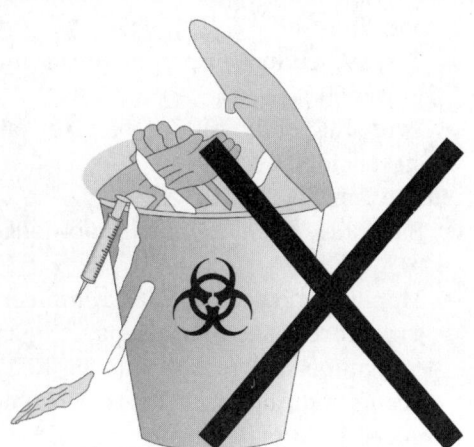

Fig. 19.2: Never overload bins.

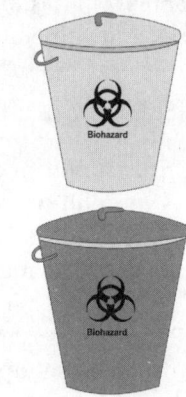

Fig. 19.6: Display biohazard waste symbol.

SUMMARY

Classification and hazards are described. The detail of waste container code is briefed. Treatment option for Health Waste Management is detailed.

VIVA VOCE

1. What are the hazards of hospital waste?
2. Describe waste disposal container code for human anatomical waste.
3. What is the color of general waste use?

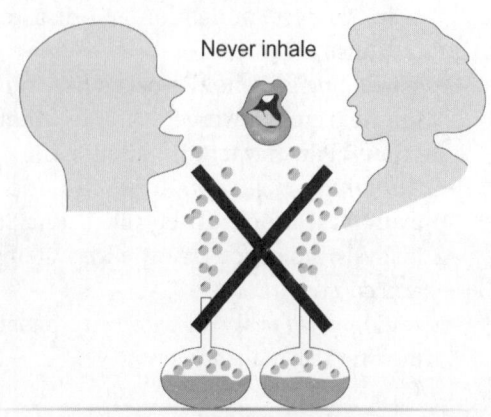

Fig. 19.3: Use mask. Never inhale.

SECTION 7

Section Outline

Chapter 20. National Health Programs
Chapter 21. Health Planning
Chapter 22. Health Management
Chapter 23. Community Healthcare

20 CHAPTER: National Health Programs

CHAPTER OUTLINE

- National Health Problems
- National Health Programs
- Major National Health Programs
  - Reproductive and Child Health (RCH)
  - National Family Planning Programme (NFPP)
  - Acute Respiratory Infection (ARI) Control Programme
  - Diarrheal Disease Control (DDC)
  - National Sexually Transmitted Disease (STD) Control Programme
  - National Acquired Immunodeficiency Syndrome (AIDS) Control Programme
  - Nation Tuberculosis (TB) Control Programme
  - National Filaria control Programme
  - National Leprosy Control Programme
  - National Malaria Eradication Programme (NMEP)
  - National Mental Health Programme
  - National Diarrhea Control Programme
  - Rural Water Supply Programme
  - National Urban Water Supply Programme
  - Basic Minimum Service Program
  - 20-Point Programme

INTRODUCTON

India being a developing country is facing various health problems which are being tackled through national health programs (NHP). They are aiming at the control or eradication of communicable diseases, for the improvement of environmental sanitation, for raising the standard of living, to give better nutrition, for stabilizing the population and to give priority to improve the rural health.

International agencies, voluntary health agencies and many foreign agencies are assisting the health programs.

NATIONAL HEALTH PROBLEMS

1. Communicable diseases
2. Population explosion
3. Nutritional health problems
4. Environmental sanitation
5. Medical care.

NATIONAL HEALTH PROGRAMS

Types of national health programs are:
1. Vertical programs implemented by central government
2. 50:50 centrally sponsored and
3. 100% sponsored by central government.

Change of Names is Observed in the following National Health Programs

1. National Family Planning Programme to National Family Welfare Programme
2. National Goiter Control Programme to National Iodine Deficiency Disorder Control Programme
3. National Leprosy Control Programme to National Leprosy Eradication Programme
4. National Tuberculosis Control Programme to Revised National Tuberculosis Control Programme
5. Expanded Programme of Immunization to Universal Immunization Programme

6. National Malaria Control Programme to National Malaria Eradication Programme and to National Antimalaria Programme
7. Maternal and Child Health to Child Survival and Safe Motherhood Programme, further to Reproductive and Child Health Programme
8. Minimum Needs Programme to Basic Minimum Services Programme.

Merged National Health Programs

1. National Cholera Control Programme now under Control of Diarrheal Diseases
2. National Trachoma Control Programme now under National Programme for the Control of Blindness
3. National Sexually Transmitted Disease (STD) Control Programme now under National Acquired Immunodeficiency Syndrome (AIDS) Control Programme.

Defunct National Health Programs

1. National Smallpox Eradication Programme of 1962 to April 1977 now is defunct
2. National Guinea Worm Eradication Programme of 1983 to Feb 2000 now is defunct
3. Applied Nutrition Programme of 1963–1980 now is defunct
1. **Disease eradication programs**
   - National Malaria Eradication Programme
   - National Leprosy Eradication Programme
   - National Yaws Eradication Programme
   - National Polio Eradication Programme
   Note: Two successful eradication programs are:
   - First eradicated disease—Smallpox.
   - Second eradicated disease—Guinea worm.
2. **Disease control programs**
   - National Filaria Control Programme
   - National Tuberculosis Control Programme
   - National AIDS Control Programme
   - National STD Control Programme
   - National Control of Diarrheal Diseases
   - National Acute Respiratory Infections (ARI) Control Programme
   - National Cholera Control Programme
   - National Trachoma Control Programme.

   Note: State Control Policy under central guidance is provided to the following which are not accorded priority under National Control Policy.
   a. Japanese encephalitis (JE)
   b. Kala-azar
   c. Dengue fever
3. **National nutritional programs**
   - Vitamin A Prophylaxis Programme
   - Nutrition Anemia Control Programme
   - Iodine Deficiency Disorder Control Programme (IDDCP)
   - Special Nutrition Programme (SNP)
   - Balwadi Nutrition Programme
   - Integrated Child Development Services Scheme (ICDS) and
   - School Mid-day Meal Programme
4. **National Water Supply and Sanitation Programme (NWS and SP)**
   - Instituted in 1954
   - In 1972, Accelerated Rural Water Supply Programme (ARWSP) was started as special program
   - In five-year plan, rural water supply included in minimum need program
5. **National Family Planning Programme (NFPP):** It was started in 1952. Separate family planning department got introduced in 1966 when small family norm and extension education approach were introduced. At primary health center (PHC) level it was integrated with maternal and child health (MCH) services in 1970. National Population Policy gave an impetus to the program in 2000. During 12th five-year plan, investment on family welfare (FW) has been ₹ 371,600 crores (2012–2017).

Now, it is on voluntary basis, adopts cafeteria approach of small family norm policy in its implementation. This got intensified through post-partum center (PPC) in 1972. Training of traditional birth attendance (TBA) is a major issue in implementation of Family Planning Programme.

Chapter 20: National Health Programs

6. **National programs to control non-communicable disease (NCD)**
   - National Programme for Control of Blindness
   - IDDCP
   - National Cancer Control Programme
   - National Mental Health Programme
   - National Diabetes Control Programme

7. **National programs for mother and child health**
   - Reproductive and Child Health (RCH)
   - Universal Immunization Programme (UIP)

Difference between Vertical Health Program and Horizontal Health Program

See **Table 20.1**.

Table 20.1: Difference between vertical health program and horizontal health program.

Vertical health program	Horizontal health program
1. Narrow base, short-term	1. Wide base, long-term
2. Special, unipurpose, expert-assisted, foreign-assisted crash program, to get quick results. When it is seen in maintenance phase it is taken to vigilance action by the states	2. Multipurpose, state health program, state budget and community development budget
3. After a pilot project, taken up at national level, tackle specific problem, unipurpose workers posted on duty. Expert training is given. Special incentive present	3. Now routine training of workers is included
4. Time bound in the beginning (normally 5–8 years) peak at the time of results, when enters maintenance it is passed on to states for taking up vigilance	4. PHC function which was following in 1952 1 MO 1 Compounder 1 Surgical attendant 2 HI 1 HV 4 Midwives (Total 10) are geared up to cope horizontal health program by present set up (2001) which include MOH 2 or 3 or 4, qualified pharmacist trained MPW's are additional staff.
5. They are at national scale and by central budget	5. Any state health program at state budget taken from time to time
6. Note unipurpose workers such as vaccinator, sanitary inspector, FP worker, malaria worker, district disease officer, state disease coordinator, etc.	6. Note multipurpose workers
7. Examples of vertical health programs: ➢ Filaria ➢ Leprosy ➢ Tuberculosis ➢ DD ➢ STD ➢ Blindness ➢ IDD ➢ UIP ➢ AIDS ➢ FP	7. Examples of horizontal health programs: ➢ Nutrition program ➢ Minimum need program ➢ Guinea worm eradication ➢ Sushruta program

Note: Programs that are both vertical and horizontal stages are (transitory):
- Malaria
- Water and water supply
- ICDS

(DD: Diarrheal disease; STD: sexually transmitted disease; AIDS: acquired immunodeficiency syndrome; UIP: Universal Immunization Programme; IDD: iodine deficiency disorders; FP: family planning; PHC: primary health center; MO: medical officer; ICDS: Integrated Child Development Services)

MAJOR NATIONAL HEALTH PROGRAMS

Reproductive and Child Health (RCH) Programme (1997)

Earlier it was called MCH and family planning (FP) and subsequently referred to as CSSM (Child Survival and Safe Motherhood Programme).

It is an integrated approach of service which provides health services to young women and young children through family welfare programs such as UIP, oral rehydration therapy (ORT), CSSM, ARI control, emergency and essential obstetric care, medical termination of pregnancy (MTP) services, reproductive tract infections (RTI) and STD control, essential newborn care and vitamin A prophylaxis.

Above components were found to overlap and cost heavily on the National Exchequer. Hence, RCH package was thought and an integrated approach was created.

Accordingly central, state and district level MCH and FP officers are redesignated under RCH scheme with specified responsibility.

Concept of Reproductive Health

- Family planning
- Mother health through antenatal care (ANC) immunization by tetanus toxoid (TT), anemia prophylaxis, referral services, care during child birth by essential obstetrics care and emergency obstetrics care, birth timing and spacing, and safe motherhood
- Child care through newborn care at home by warmth and feeding, primary immunization, vitamin A prophylaxis, ARI control, and diarrheal control including ICDS services.

Prevention of Reproductive Tract Infections

- Safe abortion services
- Effective control of STD and RTI
- Prevention and management of infertility
- Prevention, detection and treatment of reproductive tract malignancies
- Care of adolescent health.

MCH and FP services for Reproductive and Child Health Programme are being rendered through the following infrastructure in the country:

Subcenters	156231
PHC	25650
CHC	5624
RFWC	5435
HFWTC	47
PPC	1562
Health posts	871
Urban FW centers	1083

(PHC: primary health centers; CHC: community health centers; HFWTC: health and family welfare training centers; RFWC: rural family welfare center; PPC: postpartum center)

Criteria for Differential Approach in Reproductive Tract Infections

Based on birth rate and female literacy rate, 507 districts were classified into following categories:

Category	No. of districts
A	58
B	184
C	265
Total	507

Over a period of 3 years, all districts were covered in a phased manner, where weaker districts got more support.

Special Features of Reproductive Tract Infections

- Integration of fertility regulation to both men and women included
- RCH is community-based and client-oriented
- First referral units (FRU) are created at taluka level and village level and RCH facility in PHC is upgraded
- PHC will include essential obstetrics and gynecology (OBG) care viz., MTP and intrauterine device (IUD) (insertion). They are also done in subcenters
- Specialist service for STD and RTI is provided at all levels
- Outreach service to urban slum, tribal and adolescents are emphasized
- Indian system of medicine is supported by providing training in RCH
- Zilla Parishad (ZP) will have the key role in RCH scheme.

Intervention in RCH Programme include (Table 20.2)

- Essential OBG care
- Emergency OBG care
- 24-hour delivery service at PHC
- MTP
- Prevention of RTI and STD
- District surveys
- Early registration of pregnancy
- Three ANC check-up, TT (ANC).

The Package of Services

Child	Mother
• Essential newborn care • Immunization • Appropriate management of diarrhea • Vitamin A prophylaxis	• Immunization • Prevention and treatment of anemia • Antenatal care, early identification of complications • Delivery by trained person • Health promotion by trained dais • Promotion of institutional delivery • Management of obstetric emergency • Birth spacing

- Nutritional advice
- Risk identification and referral, and
- Birth spacing.

Prevention of Anemia in Pregnancy

- Increase in dietary intake of iron rich foods
- Iron folic-acid (IFA) tablets during pregnancy ensured, and
- Birth spacing for least 3 years.

Essential Obstetrical Care

- Early registration of pregnancy
- At least three antenatal check-up
- Universal coverage with TT
- Universal coverage with IFA tablet
- Advice on adequate food and rest
- Early detection and treatment of maternal complications
- Deliveries by trained personnel
- Institutional deliveries for women with maternal complications, bad obstetric history, and risk factors
- Management of obstetric emergencies
- Birth spacing.

Essential Newborn Care

- Resuscitation of newborns with asphyxia
- Prevention of hypothermia
- Prevention of infections
- Exclusive breastfeeding, and
- Referral of the sick newborn.

Five Clean Practices for Prevention of Maternal and Neonatal Sepsis

- Clear surface for delivery
- Clean hands of the attendant
- New blade for cutting cord
- Clean tie for cord, and
- No application on cord stump.

Disposable Delivery Kit (DDK) for Clean Delivery

- A piece of soap
- A new razor blade
- Two pieces of thread

Table 20.2: Intervention in RCH.

In all districts	In selected districts
• Child survival by immunization, vitamin A prophylaxis, ORT, ARI control • Safe motherhood by ANC, TT (ANC) safe delivery, anemia control • Target free approach • Training to all RCH staff • IEC activities • Urban slum, tribal included • All district hospital to have RTI/STD clinic • Equipment, staff to PHC for MTP • ZP, NGO women group involved • Adolescent health included • Reproductive hygiene included	• Intervention mentioned under is taken up in all districts • Facility to screen and treat RTI/STD at subdivision level • Drugs to FRU for emergency OBG care • Drugs + staff to PHC for essential services • Additional ANM to subcenter in weak district • Provision of equipment kit, IUD insertion ANM kit to subcenters • Facility for transport of obstetrics emergency to referral center

(RCH: reproductive and child health; ORT: oral rehydration therapy; ARI: acute respiratory infection; RTI/STD: reproductive tract infections/sexually transmitted disease; ANC: antenatal care; TT: tetanus toxoid; FRU: first referral units; OBG: obstetrics and gynecology; PHC: primary health center; IEC: information education communication; MTP: medical termination of pregnancy; ZP: Zilla Parishad; NGO: nongovernmental organization; IUD: intrauterine device; ANM: auxiliary nurse midwife)

- Two pieces of gauze, and
- Two cotton swabs.

Subcenter Drug Kits under RCH

Drug Kit A

1. IFA (Large): 15,000 tablets (100 mg)
2. IFA (Small): 13,000 tablets
3. Vitamin A: 5 bottle (100 mL each) 1 mL = 1 lakh IU
4. Cotrimoxazole: 1,000 tablets (Ped.)
5. Oral rehydration salts (ORS) Pkt: 150

Drug Kit B

1. Methylergometrine: 1,000 tablets (0.125 mg)
2. Chlorpheniramine: 400 tablets (4 mg)
3. Paracetamol: 500 tablets
4. Antispasmodic tablet: 250
5. Injection methylergometrine 5 amp (0.2 mg/mL)
6. Mebendazole: 300 tablets (100 mg)
7. Chloramphenicol (1%): 500 applicap
8. Cetrimide powder: 5 pack (125 g each)
9. Povidone ointment (5%): 5 tube (25 g each)
10. Cotton bandage: 120 roll (4 cm × 4 m)
11. Cotton absorbent: One roll (500 g).

Community Needs Assessment Approach

On the basis of community needs assessed by the health workers subcenter action plan is prepared annually.

Acute Respiratory Infections (ARI) Control

Acute respiratory infections are to be prevented to prevent deaths due to pneumonia. Training health workers on recognition and management is undertaken. Through drug kit cotrimoxazole is supplied under the scheme.

Vitamin A Prophylaxis

Five doses of vitamin A to all children below the age of 3 years, is provided each with specified dose.

9 months	–	I dose 1 lakh units
18 months	–	II dose 2 lakh units
24 months	–	III dose 2 lakh units
30 months	–	IV dose 2 lakh units
36 months	–	V dose 2 lakh units

First Referral Units in RCH (FRU)

They are responsible for essential and emergency obstetrical care at community health center and subdistrict hospitals.

Following emergency obstetrical care is expected in FRU.

A. *Surgical*
- Cesarean section
- Laparotomy and repair of ruptured uterus
- Surgical treatment of fever sepsis
- Uterine evaluation of incomplete abortion
- Repair of cervical and vaginal tear
- Amniotomy with or without oxytocin, and
- MTP.

B. *Medical*
- Management of eclampsia
- Management of hemorrhagic shock
- Management of severe anemia
- Management of septicemia, and
- Use of intravenous (IV) oxytocin for induction of labor.

C. *Manual*
- Manual removal of placenta
- Forceps delivery
- Vacuum extraction, and
- Partography.

D. *Anesthesia*
- General anesthesia (GA)
- Spinal anesthesia.

E. *Blood transfusion*
- Bleeding a donor
- Blood transfusion, and
- Performing mandatory tests.

F. *Newborn care*
- Resuscitation, and
- Management of sick newborn.

G. *Other*
- Operation theater (OT) assistance.

National Population Policy 2000 on RCH Programme

Organizing RCH camps, MCH services to remote areas, supply of equipments for newborn care, trial for home-based neonatal care, border district cluster strategy for the development of trained staff at health centers, trial for contractual appointments, development of integrated management of neonatal and childhood illness for sick infant, and introduction of hepatitis B vaccination project.

Dai Training

Involvement of districts with low safe delivery rate (below 30%) for training of dais.

Recent introduction of initiatives such as training of doctors in anesthetic skills, and delivery skills, setting up blood storage centers, training of TBAs, development of Vandemataram scheme and Janani Suraksha Yojana.

In 2001, selected states got focused attention as per the recommendations by Empowered Action Group for H and FW planning.

Reproductive and Child Health (RCH) Key Indicators

- Currently married women
  Percentage of married females to total females in the age groups of:
  10–14 years – 4.5%
  15–19 years – 35.3%
  20–24 years – 81.8%
  15–44 years – 79.5%
- Mean age at marriage–22.3 years
- Number of children per married women aged 45–49 years
  - Ever born – 4.3
  - Surviving – 3.7
- Currently married women with any ANC–67.2% (any one or two of ANC checkup, TT, IFA)
- Currently married women with full ANC–14.8% (all had three ANC checkup + TT + 100 IFA/tablets)
- Institutional delivery–35.0%
- Safe delivery (by trained)–41.9%
- Women with pregnancy complications–34.8% (swelling of hands, feet, visual disturbance, bleeding, convulsions, weak or no fetal movement, and abnormal presentation)
- Delivery complications–36.4% (premature labor, obstructed labor, and prolonged labor)
- Postdelivery complications–42.0% (high fever, lower abdominal pain, foul smelling vaginal discharge, excessive bleeding, dizziness, and severe headache)
- Currently married women 15–44 years of age with symptoms of RTI/STD–28.8%
- Currently married women 15–44 years of age who are aware of AIDS–41.1%
- Males aged 20–54 years with symptoms of RTI/STD–12.7%
- Males aged 20–54 years who are aware of AIDS–57.4%.

Universal Immunization Programme (UIP)

Universal Immunization Programme (UIP) is the name given in 1985 to existed expanded program of immunization (EPI). UIP is also called UCI (universal child immunization).

Coverage of all infants and pregnant women is primary goal of UIP. Though 80% coverage disrupts disease transmission, goal of UIP is to cover all children.

Primary immunization to infants and TT to pregnant women under UIP schedule have shown remarkable achievement, polio is being eradicated. Next priority has been given to measles and neonatal tetanus for their eradication.

This program has inclusion of the following during its implementation:

- Urban measles campaign
- Coverage of women in reproductive age group with 3 doses of TT for a goal of neonatal tetanus elimination
- A pilot project of introduction of hepatitis B vaccine.

Universal Immunization Programme (UIP) has the recommended cold chain which is a system to ensure vaccine in potent condition during transport, during storage and during handling from manufacturer to vaccination site.

1. **Walk-in Cold (WIC):** Refrigerated room at manufacture level, at state level and at regional level.
2. **Ice-lined Refrigerator (ILR):** At district level at PHC level to freeze ice pack in freezer and to store vaccine at compartment at 2–8°C. It opens at top, like freezer or cold box. If electricity fails, temperature is maintained for 10 hours.
3. **Cold box:** To transport vaccine from district to PHC. It has ice layer at 4 sides.

4. **Vaccine carrier:** To transport vaccine from PHC to subcenter or to outreach fellows or areas. The carrier contains 4 ice packs.
5. **Day carrier:** To transport vaccine from PHC to subcenter which contains 2 ice packs.
6. **Cup filled with ice:** For the use at immunization session.

National Family Welfare Programme

It was started in 1952. Separate family planning department got introduced in 1966 when small family norm and extension education approach were introduced. At PHC level it was integrated with MCH services in 1970. National Population Policy gave an impetus to the program in 2000. During 10th five-year plan, investment on FW has been ₹ 27,125 crores (2002–2007).

Now, it is on voluntary basis, adopts cafeteria approach of small family norm policy in its implementation. This got intensified through PPC in 1972.

Training of TBA is a major issue in implementation of family planning program.

Targets

Birth rate	-	21/1,000 MYP
Death rate	-	9/1,000 MYP
Couple protection rate	-	60%
NRR	-	1
Age at marriage for girls	-	20 years
MMR	-	3/1,000 LB
Growth rate	-	1.6%
Total fertility rate	-	2.9

National Family Planning Programme is backed up by comprehensive National Population Policy 2000. During 10th and 11th five-year plans expenditure were 58,920.3 crores and 136,147 crores. During the Twelfth five-year plan, the total estimated outlay is 371,600 crores.

Various national goals under 10th five-year plan are noteworthy. Among them following need to be emphasized:
- Total fertility rate (TFR) achievement by 2010 to replacement level
- Infant mortality rate (IMR) to below 30
- Maternal mortality ratio (MMR) to below 1
- Addressing the unmet need of basic reproductive need of the community
- Promoting the delayed marriages
- Universal access of information and counseling on fertility regulation and contraception
- FP as people-centered program
- Integration of Indian System of Medicine
- Differential approach for attending weaker districts.

Acute Respiratory Infections (ARI) Control Program

It was started in 1990 and is now included under RCH Programme. Health workers are trained to recognize and treat pneumonia. Through drug kit, cotrimoxazole drug is supplied under the program.

Diarrheal Disease Control (DDC) Programme

It was started in 1978, incorporated ORT in 1985. Program includes:
- Case management of diarrhea, and
- Health education on home-available fluids (HAF), ORS, feeding. Now, it is an integral part of RCH.

National Sexually Transmitted Disease (STD) Control Programme

It was started in 1949. In 1981, strategy was changed to training, teaching and research aspect. STD clinics were started for VDRL (venereal disease research laboratories) testing, health education and counseling.

Now, it is linked with human immunodeficiency virus/acquired immunodeficiency syndrome (HIV/AIDS) control because of its same behavioral component in transmission. In presence of STD, HIV transmission is more. Early diagnosis and treatment of STD form major step of control of HIV infection. There are about 510 STD clinics in the country functioning for its effective control.

Sexually transmitted disease (STD) surveillance where collection, compilation, analysis and dissemination of data for necessary action

have found utmost importance. Three types of reporting that are followed:
1. Universal reporting—every institution concerned with control is a reporting unit
2. Obligatory reporting—which is a mandatory reporting
3. Sentinel surveillance—when a few representative health care facilities are selected as reporting units.

Now, it is merged into AIDS control program which is giving services through STD reference centers, skin leprosy STD centers, and STD clinics in district hospitals.

Compilation of Data

Syndrome approach, i.e., diagnosis by signs and symptoms, genital ulcer, urethral discharge, vaginal discharge and pain in lower abdomen form the basis of syndrome approach. Further etiological approach is also included.

Sentinel surveillance is set up for reporting. Diagnosis, treatment, health education and individual counseling form the basis in control of STD.

Syndrome Approach

This is a method of management and control of STDs where diagnosis and treatment is based on a group of symptoms and signs. Treatment is targeted toward all diseases that could cause that syndrome. It allows diagnosis without extensive laboratory test and treatment with a single visit.

National Acquired Immunodeficiency Syndrome (AIDS) Control Programme

It was launched in 1987. Since 1982 National AIDS Control Organization (NACO) is coordinating control program.

Strategies

- Establishment of AIDS surveillance centers
- Identification of risk groups
- Screening for diagnosis
- Management of HIV/AIDS case
- Formulation of guidelines to blood bank and dialysis units, and
- Information education and communication (IEC) activities.

Components

- Safe blood procedures by safe blood policy
- HIV testing policy on voluntary basis with pre- and post-test counseling
- Effective STD control program, and
- Condom promotion (social marketing).

Human Immunodeficiency Virus (HIV) Surveillance is of following Types

1. HIV sentinel surveillance
2. HIV serosurveillance
3. AIDS case surveillance
4. STD surveillance
5. Sex behavior surveillance

From December 1999, National AIDS Control Programme entered a second phase with the support of World Bank.

Following are recent control measures being undertaken:
- Prevention and control of HIV/AIDS at all level
- Categorization of states according to the volume of prevalence and check interstate spread
- RTI and STD awareness in the community, and
- Awareness on RTI and STD treatment.

Since 1999, phase II of NACO Programme is effective as 100% centrally sponsored scheme in 32 states, and 3 metro cities. This has the objectives of reducing the spread of HIV/AIDS and long-term management of cases. The goal has been to maintain prevalence rate below 5% of adult population, to reduce the blood-borne transmission of HIV to below 1%, to create 90% HIV awareness among youths, condom use of more than 90% among risk groups.

In 2002, National AIDS Prevention and Control Policy was evolved for—(a) blood safety (b) counseling and testing (c) STD control (d) condom promotion (e) surveillance (f) IEC activities (g) family health awareness campaign. In 2007, NACP III launched for 5 years. In 2014, NACP IV launched for 5 years. In 2017, National Strategic Plan for HIV/AIDS and STIs for the period 2017–2014 initiated.

Goals under Tenth Five-Year Plan

- Targeted intervention for 80% coverage of risk group
- Health education in schools and colleges to cover 90% coverage for HE
- Rural population coverage for awareness to the extent of 80%
- Blood transmission control to below 1%
- District-wise establishment of voluntary counseling and testing center (VCTC)
- Mother to child transmission prevention at district level
- Achieving zero level of increase of HIV prevalence by 2007.

Since 2004, prevention among high-risk population, care at low cost and surveillance have been the priority in the control program. In this free treatment scheme for AIDS in selected states for full blown cases was introduced. World Health Organization (WHO) and UNAID sponsored *3 by 5 plan* where free treatment with 3 in 1 combination was introduced once a day with Lamivudine + Stavudine + Nevirapine.

National Tuberculosis Control Programme

This started in 1962 with following objectives:
- To make tuberculosis no more a public health problem
- Case detection to be cent per cent
- Bacille Calmette-Guérin (BCG) to newborn and infants, and
- Integration with health and family welfare services.

National Tuberculosis Control Programme (NTCP) is operated through district tuberculosis program through functioning 466 district TB centers (DTCs) covering 76% of Indian population in India.

For structure and function of DTC refer **Table 20.3**.

All tuberculosis patients receive free treatment under directly observed treatment, short course (DOTS) which is a community treatment. Under supervision MPW of PHC and local voluntary workers such as teacher, Anganwadi worker (AWW), dai, ex-patient, and social workers help in providing DOTS. Other workers are DOT agents. They receive ₹ 150/-honorarium per patient after completing treatment. The success of DOT depends on accountability, good drug supply directly observed treatment by health workers, good quality sputum microscopy, and political commitment.

The drugs are supplied in blister packs, separately for intensive phase and continuation phase. They are kept ready in boxes for supply to patients for a full course of treatment. 1 day's medication in each pack for intensive phase and 1 week's medication in each pack for continuation phase are kept in boxes.

In 1992, National TB control was revised with following strategies:
a. To achieve 85% cure rate of infectious cases by directly observed treatment.
b. To achieve 70% detection rate by quality sputum microscopy.
c. To involve NGO for IEC activities.

Activities under District Tuberculosis Center
- Case finding
- Case treatment
- BCG vaccination

Table 20.3: Structure and function of DTC.

DTC coverage (Average) 50 health institutions	
Staff	Function
1. DTO	1. Case finding
1. MO	MMR
2. Laboratory technician	Tuberculin test
2. Health visitors	Sputum exam
1 X-ray technician	2. Record maintenance
1. Team leader (Nonmedical)	3. Treatment by RNTCP (DOTS method)
1. Statistician	4. BCG vaccination
1. Pharmacist	5. Preventive treatment
	6. Rehabilitation
	7. Surveillance

(DTC: district tuberculosis center; DTO: district tuberculosis officer; MO: medical officer; MMR: maternal mortality rate; DOTS: directly observed treatment, short course; RNTCP: Revised National TB Control Program)

- Recording and reporting, and
- Supervision on supply and work.

In 1992, revised strategy of NTCP (RNTCP) was put to enforcement. Objective was to interrupt transmission, achieve 70% case detection, undertaking the diagnosis by three sputum examinations, to maintain uninterrupted drug supply.

For cure target of 80% following measures are suggested:
- Supervised short course chemotherapy in periphery should achieve 85% cure rate.
- 70% of estimated cases should be detected through quality sputum microscopy.
- IEC should involve NGOs.

Above schedule is being effected in phased manner which involves:
- Passive case finding by three acid-fast bacillus (AFB) tests of sputum
- All cases are provided with free RNTCP
- Direct observed therapy short-term (DOTS) by MPWs is incorporated
- Monitoring of disease by health service
- Health worker (HW) or nonhealth worker supervises and motivates, and
- Appropriate treatment is installed
- TB care services in the private sector and TB/HIV coordination found added the tuberculosis control.

Directly observed therapy (DOT) agent

Multipurpose worker (MPW), teacher, AWW, *Dai*, ex-patient, and social worker who give directly observed therapy for short-term is called *DOT agent*. He/she will be paid ₹ 150 per completed patient treatment.

National Filaria Control Programme

It started in 1955. In 1978, urban malaria scheme was merged with this program.

There are 206 filaria units, 199 filaria clinics and 27 survey units which are working to cover the program activities in the country.

Activities

- Survey and case detection in omitted places
- Antilarval measures, and
- Antifilaria measures.

These activities are done through filaria control units (FCU).

VHG is trained for an effective primary care in antifilaria activities.

Under revised filaria control strategy, center is providing diethylcarbamazine (DEC) tablets for mass therapy campaign and cash assistance for IEC activities.

In highly endemic areas, in order to reduce transmission, government is following WHO recommendation of annual single dose mass drug therapy with DEC as a supplement to existing National Filaria Control Program (NFCP) strategy.

Revised Strategy

In 2004, Government of India allocated funds for lymphatic filariasis elimination operations in endemic districts. It has followed WHO recommendation of annual single dose mass drug therapy with DEC with albendazole as a supplement to existing NFCP strategy in highly endemic districts.

At present, there are 210 filaria control units, 30 survey units, and 200 filaria clinics functioning.

WHO recommendation is followed in endemic areas:

"Annual single dose therapy with DEC along with NFCP strategy."

National Institute of Communicable Diseases (NICD), Delhi is conducting training and research on filaria control.

National Leprosy Eradication Programme (NLEP)

Started as control program in 1955, got changed to eradication program in 1983. The strategy of multidrug treatment (MDT) is to reduce case load to less than 1 per 10,000 population.

Leprosy control units (LCU) are situated in endemic areas with one medical officer (MO) and 20 paramedical workers (PMW) covering 4.5 lakh population. There are 778 LCU in the country.

Survey, Education and Treatment (SET) centers are situated in nonendemic areas with one nonmedical supervisor and paramedical workers. These are attached to primary health centers. There are 5,744 SET centers in the country.

Each urban leprosy center (ULC) cover 50,000 population. There are 907 ULCs in the country.

Mobile leprosy treatment units (MLTU) in nonendemic area consist of one doctor, one nonmedical supervisor, two PMWs and a driver. There are more than 350 such units working in the country.

Modified Leprosy Elimination Campaign (MLEC)

This started in 1997 with short-term training to leprosy staff. House-to-house search for new case was done throughout the country. Now, health workers are given training for subsequent rounds of MLEC. Four such campaigns were held from 1999 to 2003. Following were the year-wise targets achieved:

1999	464,000 case detection
2000	214,000 case detection
2001	165,000 case detection
2002	102,000 case detection
2016–2017	34,672 cases were detected and were put on treatment

There was an achievement of prevalence from 57.3 per 10,000 to 5.8 per 10,000 by 2002.

For early detection and proper management, SAPEL (special action project for elimination of leprosy) and LEC (leprosy elimination campaigns) for urban areas were recommended. There are about 1,500 such projects working in the country.

In 2002, leprosy elimination monitoring was initiated to cover priority endemic states.

Program implementation plan for 12th plan period 2012–2017 with the objectives of elimination of leprosy, strengthening disability prevention, and reduction of stigma.

Goals Under Ongoing 5 Year Plan are:

- Integration of horizontal and vertical programs in case of leprosy by 2007
- Redeployment of leprosy workers and laboratory technicians under integration process
- Training of existing personnel in PHC
- Provision of reconstructive surgery
- Rehabilitation and involvement of NGO.

National Malaria Eradication Programme (NMEP)

National Antimalaria Program

National Malaria Control Programme (NMCP) was started in 1953 with dichlorodiphenyl-trichloroethane (DDT) spray twice a year. By 1958, the successful result made the program to eradication called National Malaria Eradication Program (NMEP). There was reappearance (resurgence) of malaria in 1976 due to many reasons such as—(a) operational defect (b) technical defect (c) administrative defect, etc. In 1977, MPO (modified plan of operation) was launched which was mainly based on API zones (annual parasite index).

During all these period active surveillance were done, where health workers visited houses, collected blood smear of fever cases and gave treatment. In passive surveillance fewer cases come to hospitals and health centers. Health workers are given targets of smear collection in the field.

Two Main Indicators used in Malaria Effective Control are

1. Annual parasite incidence (API)

$$= \frac{\text{Confirmed cases during 1 year}}{\text{Population under surveillance}} \times 100$$

2. Annual blood examination rate (ABER)

$$= \frac{\text{No. of slides examined}}{\text{Population}} \times 100$$

In 1978, malaria control through primary health care was approved. Because of increase in malaria, malaria action program was initiated in 1994.

Later in 1997, World Bank gave support for enhanced malaria control project.

In 1998, through roll back malaria program, the health system got strengthened.

From 1999 malaria control is going on under "National Antimalaria Programme."

In 2010, new drug policy came to existence.

In 2016, malaria elimination framework launched.

In 2017, National Strategic plan for Malaria Elimination 2017–2022 launched.

Chapter 20: National Health Programs

Main activities of malaria control are as under:

In Areas with Annual Parasite Incidence (API) Above Two

- Pyrethroids spray two rounds at 6 weeks' interval
- Entomological assessment (mosquito examination)
- Active and passive surveillance
- Treatment of malaria case.

In Areas with Annual Parasite Incidence (API) Below Two

- *Spraying:* Focal sprays around severe malaria cases
- Surveillance both active and passive
- Radical treatment of detected cases
- Blood smear follow-up for 12 months (every month) from positive cases
- Epidemiological investigation.

Presumptive Treatment (PT)

All fever cases are presumed as malaria and presumptive treatment is given soon after taking blood smear (also refer page 165).

Radical Treatment (RT)

If blood smear is positive, radical treatment is given (also refer page 165).

Goals for ongoing five-year plan have been to achieve ABER of above 10%, API of less than 1.3.

Morbidity and mortality due to malaria to be brought to 25% reduction by 2007 and to 50% reduction by 2010.

Objectives of National Malaria Eradication Programme

- To prevent deaths by malaria
- To bring down malaria morbidity
- To intensify antimalaria measure for bringing back agricultural and industrial production, and
- To consolidate the gains achieved so far.

Action in Area with API more than Two

- Spraying (two rounds DDT or three rounds malathion)
- Assessment by entomologists for an effective insecticide

- Active and passive surveillance, and
- Presumptive treatment (PT) and radical treatment (RT).

Action in Area with API less than Two

- Focal spraying around *Plasmodium falciparum* cases
- Every fortnightly active and passive surveillance
- PT and RT of all cases
- MP follow-up smear on RT and later monthly for 1 year, and
- Epidemiological investigation.

Drug Distribution Center (DDC)

Drug distribution center to dispense chloroquine tablets.

Fever Treatment Depots (FTD)

Fever treatment depots to collect MP smear and to dispense chloroquine.

Urban Malaria Control Scheme

To reduce urban malaria transmission.

Containment of Severe Malaria

This is called *P. falciparum* containment program started in 1977. Sensitivity to chloroquine by *P. falciparum* is being detected in various parts of India. Health education on malaria is stressed in the program.

Presently, district malaria officer at district health and FW office is made responsible for the program implementation at the district levels.

Surveillance

It is for watch over the disease.

Active Surveillance

Multipurpose health worker (MPHW) covers a population of 10,000 collects smear from fever cases, gives PT. Later, if positive gives RT. Four MPWs are supervised by 1 HA.

Passive Surveillance

When fever case comes to health center or hospital, malaria smear is taken, presumptive treatment and radical treatment are attended. Target of 15% of OPD cases are given as target under passive surveillance.

Malaria Action Program

This is a measure for early detection and action in the area of case occurrence. Before the onset of monsoon, antimalaria month is observed in June every year to create awareness of malaria and its control.

With World Bank assistance, enhanced malaria control project is undertaken in hyper-endemic areas by intensifying antimalaria activities.

Under recent strategy all urban areas with above 50,000 population are included under malaria action program. Reporting is made compulsory if slide positive rate is 5%. Both active and passive surveillance are continued.

National Surveillance Program for Communicable Diseases

The above program was launched in 1988 for timely detection of disease outbreak, to take appropriate action and for immediate action. This included:
- Training of paramedical staff
- Provision of technical guidance
- Upgrading laboratory
- Computerization of data pertaining to diseases
- Public education.

This program is covered in three different dimensions which are:

Low priority—when there is no existing strategy.

Medium—when it is known and locally controlled.

High—when control and eradication are existing.

District epidemiological cell is established to list out institutions, general practitioners and to computerize data and weekly reporting system.

National Mental Health Programme

This was started in 1982. National Institute of Mental Health and Neurosciences (NIMHANS) is the nodal center. Training of medical officers and paramedical workers is the main activity. The objectives are to render treatment as well as care for mental and neurological disorders. The goal has been to give mental health knowledge to public for their preparations for a quality of life and to promote health. Through the program psychiatric treatment is made available to all section of the society and to promote self-help matters.

Basic Components
- Psychiatry emergencies
- Epilepsy
- Treatment at PHC
- Counseling for alcohol addiction and drug addiction
- Management of behavior problem of children.

In 1997, District Mental Programme was initiated to:
a. Educate the community on stigma
b. Collect morbidity data
c. Report to state
d. Report to center.

The mental health care bill of 2013 was passed as the Mental Health Care Act in 2017. Expert committee was formulated for action plan.

National Diabetes Control Programme

This was initiated in 1987. Main objectives of this program have been:
a. To identify high-risk people
b. To treat avoidable complications of diabetes
c. To train health personnel and paramedical staff
d. To render special care to Juvenile diabetes.

Rural Water Supply Programme

This program has the goal of providing 55 liters per head per day and 30 liters per day per cattle.

Provision of hand pump 1 per 150 persons in problem villages.

Discouraging the discrimination against caste or creed.

Rajiv Gandhi Technical Drinking Water Mission for ridding excess fluoride, arsenic, salinity and iron.

To have low cost sanitary latrine instead of dry latrine.

Urban Water Supply Programme

- This program has the main objective of 100% water supply to the community

- The scheme provides 125 liters of water per head per day through piped water supply when underground drainage is present
- The scheme provides 75 liters per head per day when no underground drainage
- Under the scheme dry latrine to be converted into low cost sanitary latrine
- Effluent to be recycled for irrigation
- Solid waste is properly disposed off.

Basic Minimum Service Programme

This was started as minimum need program in 1974 and was revised in 1980. The same was incorporated into NWS and SP in the country.

Components

A. *Expansion of health service*
   - 100% primary health care coverage
   - 1 PHC per 30,000 people (in case of tribal and hilly–1 PHC per 20,000 people)
   - 1 per 5,000 population for subcenter (in case of tribal and hilly–1 subcenter for 3,000 population)
   - 1 community health center for 100,000 population

B. *Rural water supply*
   100% water supply to problem villages
   Problems village is defined as a village, if any one of the following is prevailing:
   - Which do not have any source of water within 1.6 km of human inhabitation, water is not available within 15 meter depth from the ground
   - Water is available in 100 meter elevated place
   - If water contains saline, iron, and fluoride and if cholera is endemic.

C. *Rural housing*
   - Free house to landless farmers and for shelter less.
   - Loan is provided at the rate of 2,000/- per sq. yard to landless farmers (under this scheme 1.3 million rural houses and 0.7 million urban houses are planned).

D. *Other needs*: Rural sanitation, rural nutrition, rural road, rural electrification, rural elementary education, and rural adult education are recommended.

E. *Pubic distribution system*
   - For below poverty line—10 kg grain per month per head at 40% cost
   - For above poverty line—10 kg grain per month per head at 80% cost

F. Urban slum improvement.

20-Point Program

It was launched on 1.7.1975 but initiated on 20.8.1986.

Main components have been food, shelter, employment, and healthy environment. Other subcomponents of the program are:
- Create community asset
- Expand rural employment
- Provide agricultural seeds
- Improve the irrigation for agriculture purpose
- Surplus land to landless
- No bonded labor
- Safe water and justice to SC and ST categories
- Primary health care facility expansion
- Two children norm in the community
- Bring about gender equality
- Youth preparedness for any community health activities
- Low-cost housing
- Slum improvement
- Social forestry development
- Ecofriendly development
- Consumer protection
- Village elevation in terms of socioeconomic level
- Expansion of education.

SUMMARY

Initially national health problems are jotted down followed by major National Health Programs are described in detail.

VIVA VOCE

1. Name disease eradication programs.
2. Name disease control programs.
3. Name national nutrition programs.
4. What is the major issue in implementation of NFPP?

5. What are the differences between vertical health programs and horizontal health programs?
6. How many PHCs are in India?
7. How many sub-centres are in India?
8. What are the interventions in RCH Programme?
9. What are the interventions in essential newborn care?
10. Describe DDK.
11. Tell something about UIP.
12. Mention targets in NFPP.
13. What is syndrome approach in STD?
14. Mention staff and functions of DTC?
15. Which are the two main indicators used in malaria effective control?
16. What is presumptive treatment?
17. Define village problem.

21 CHAPTER

Health Planning

Chapter Outline

- Definitions
- Elements
- Planning Cycle
- Health Committee Reports

INTRODUCTION

When we plan for healthcare of a community, it is preceded with preplanning where idea of planning starts.

Preplanning requires the following:
- Political will of government
- Health legislation
- An organizational structure
- Administrative capacity
- Money
- Material, and
- Manpower

DEFINITIONS

Health Planning

Health planning is an orderly process of defining strategies during: (a) Formulation, (b) Execution, and (c) Evaluation. This continues in all phases of health activities. It is based on health need and health demand of the community.

Health Need

Deficiencies noted in healthcare delivery system are called health need, e.g., immunization coverage, FP coverage, etc.

Health Demand

The requirement of healthcare services as seen by the community.

Health Resources

Money, material and manpower are health resources.

Objective: Planned end of health activity.

Target

Degree of achievement of health activity.

Goal

Ultimate desired state in health activity.

Policy

Guiding principles in health activity.

Program

Sequence of action in health activity.

Schedule

Time sequence in health activity.

Procedure

Set of rules in health activity.

Budget

Financial allocation for health activity.

ELEMENTS OF HEALTH PLANNING

- Objectives
- Policies
- Programs
- Schedules, and
- Budget

PLANNING CYCLE

Steps that are followed in planning (stage by stage) involve sequence of events, which constitutes planning cycle.

The planning cycle answers queries of the healthcare delivery system.

Steps in Planning (Fig. 21.1)

1. Goals and objectives are fixed after analyzing the situation.
2. Priority is fixed after noting the resources.
3. Plan is formulated.
4. It is put to action by sequential order.
5. Implementation of the work and monitoring.
6. Impact is studied by evaluation.

Characteristics of Good Health Planning

- Health needs are properly assessed.
- Resources are made sure.
- Priorities are fixed without bias and with national commitment.
- Provision is made for additional health resources.

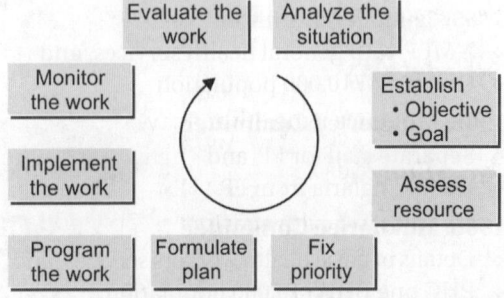

Fig. 21.1: Planning cycle.

Factors that Affect Health Planning

- Attitude of functioning government
- Legislature approval
- Parliamentary budgetary allocation
- National unexpected calamities and disasters.

Health Planning in India

Guided by various health committee reports. Government of India has set up a planning commission to draft social and economic health plans with fullest utilization of available resources.

Health planning is categorized as under:
- Central plan
- State plan, and
- District plan

The district planning by Planning Commission is new and latest decentralization activity started in 2000 AD.

Planning Commission has given due importance to health planning under five-year plans **(Tables 21.1 and 21.2)**.

In Five-Year Plan of government has given due importance to:
1. Communicable disease control
2. Strengthening health center services by expansion
3. Population control
4. Health manpower development

During 9th Five-Year Plan, district level surveillance for diseases was strengthened; appropriate systems for emergency, disaster and accidents were implemented; screening of nutritional deficiencies was implemented; growth rate reduction policy was targeted and emphasis on RTI/STD surveillance was given.

Present 12th Five-Year Plan 2012-2017

Plan commenced with annual plans in 2012.

In 10th Five-Year Plan, following areas are stressed and covered:
- Reduction of IMR to 25
- Reduction of MMR to 100
- Reduction of TFR to 2.1
- Reduction of under nutrition by 50%
- Anemia reduction to 25%
- Reduction of burden of CD

Chapter 21: Health Planning

Table 21.1: Five-year plan outlay.

First Five-Year Plan	1951-56
Second Five-Year Plan	1956-61
Third Five-Year Plan	1961-66
Annual Plan	1966-67
Annual Plan	1967-68
Annual Plan	1968-69
Fourth Five-Year Plan	1969-74
Fifth Five-Year Plan	1974-79
Annual Plan	1979-80
Sixth Five-Year Plan	1980-85
Seventh Five-Year Plan	1985-90
Annual Plan	1990-91
Annual Plan	1991-92
Eighth Five-Year Plan	1992-97
Ninth Five-Year Plan	1997-2002
Tenth Five-Year Plan	2002-2007
Eleventh Five-Year Plan	2007-2012
Twelfth Five-Year Plan	2012-17
Action Agenda of NITI Aayog	2017-2020

Table 21.2: Achievement during First Five-Year Plan to Tenth Plan (Till date).

Total plan investment (In crores)	921,291
Health sector (In crores)	339,253
FW sector (In crores)	371,600
Total PHC (No)	29,367
Total subcenter (No)	156,231
Total beds (No)	908,168
No. of medical colleges	476
No. of annual admission to medical colleges	52,646
No. of dental colleges	313
No. of allopathic doctors (registered)	1,041,395
No. of nurses	19,805,260
No. of ANM	841,276
No. of health visitors	55,625
No. of HW female	220,707
No. of HW male	71,053
No. of village health guides	613,000

* All villages to have sustained access to potable drinking water within the stipulated plan period.

Health Sector Planning

Planning Commission's implementation through five-year plans has been through health sector planning, which contains seven subsectors from the implementation point of view.
1. Water supply and sanitation
2. Control of communicable disease
3. Medical education, training and research
4. Medical care at hospitals and health centers
5. Public health services
6. FP
7. Indigenous systems of medicine.

The implemented action from village to center is monitored by Bureau of Planning (1965) under Ministry of Health, Government of India.

HEALTH COMMITTEE REPORTS

1946: Bhore Committee (Survey and Development in Four Volumes)
* Integration of curative and preventive service
* Primary health center under short-term and long-term, and
* Three months training in P and SM (Interns).

1947-48 Chopra Committee (Current Health Infrastructure)
Integration of several systems of medicine.

1962: Mudaliar Committee (Health Survey and Planning)
* Consolidation of advance made
* Strengthening of district hospital
* Assistant directors to supervise DHO
* PHC coverage of 40,000 population
* Quality, integrity: IMS in line with IAS

1963: Chadah Committee
* NMEP with general health services, and
* One BHW/10,000 population

1965: Mukherjee Committee
* Separate staff for FP, and
* Delink malaria from FP

1966: Mukherjee Committee
* Details of basic health workers services, and
* PHC one BHW/10,000 population
* Urban one BHW/15,000 population

1967: Mudhok Committee
- Small family norm, and
- Health cess on patients

1967: Jungalwalla Committee
For integration: Unified cadre, common seniority recognition of extra qualification, equal pay for equal work, special pay for special work, no private practice.

1973: Kartar Singh Committee
- Multipurpose worker scheme

1975: Shrivastava Committee
- Medical education, manpower problems, and
- Health workers from the community.

1976: Shivaraman Committee
- Basic rural doctors, and
- Emphasis on MCH, immunization, nutrition.

1977: Rural Health Scheme
- Community health workers of Shrivastava Committee, and
- ROME started

1981: Ramalingaswami Committee
- An alternate model of health organization (village to state)
- Redefine doctor, drug, and health centers under ZP.

1981: Report of Working Group on HFA by 2000
- Broad approach, and
- Targets fixed

1986: Bajaj Committee
- Policy on medical education
- ECHS (Educational Council for Health Sciences) on line with UGC, and
- Establishment of University of Health Sciences.

1991: Karunakaran Committee
- Formulation of Population Policy

1992: Krishnan Committee
- Review of progress made, and
- Urban health services

1995: Expert committee on Malaria
Malaria Action Plan

2000: National Population Policy Report
2000: UN Millennium Declaration Report
2002: National Health Policy Report

GOALS OF NATIONAL HEALTH POLICY BY 2005, 2007, 2010 AND 2015

By 2005
1. Eradicate polio
2. Eradicate yaws
3. Eliminate leprosy
4. Establish an integrated system of surveillance, National Health Accounts and Health Statistics
5. Increase state-sector health spending from 5.5 to 7% of the budget

By 2007
Achieve zero level growth of HIV/AIDS

By 2010
1. Eliminate kala-azar
2. Reduce mortality by 50% on account of tuberculosis, malaria and other vector- and water-borne diseases.
3. Reduce prevalence of blindness to 0.5%
4. Reduce IMR to 30 per 1,000 live births and MMR to 1 per 1,000 live births
5. Increase utilization of public health facilities from current level of below 20% to above 75%
6. Increase health expenditure by government as a percentage of GDP from the existing 0.9% to 2%
7. Increase share of central grants to constitute at least 25% of total health spending.
8. Increase state sector health spending from current 5.5 to 8% of the budget.

By 2015
Eliminate lymphatic filariasis

By 2015
9. National Health Policy 2017 with the objectives of (a) Strengthening of Health System, (b) Fixing performance targets, and (c) Goals for its impact.

SUMMARY

In the beginning, introduction and definition is given. Elements of Health Planning are described. Planning cycle is highlighted

VIVA VOCE

1. What are the characteristics of good health planning?
2. What is planning cycle?
3. Mention goals of health policy.

22 CHAPTER — Health Management

Chapter Outline

- Definition
- Gulick's POSDCORB
- Inventory Management
- Financial Management
- Basic Activities in Health Management
- Span of Management
- Management Methods
- Health Policies
  - NHP
  - National Education Policy
  - National Nutritional Policy
  - National Population Policy
  - National Housing Policy
  - National Blood Policy
- Health Systems in India
- Rural Development
- Evaluation of Health Services
- Milestones

INTRODUCTION

Health management is a primary force in healthcare services, where health profession does the job of getting best out of available resources. For a better and effective health care, present team approach is needed in an organizational set-up where health services are to be coordinated.

DEFINITION

Health Management

It is an art of knowing what a team leader wants to do and then to see that it is done in a coordinated effort in the best and cheapest possible way.

Health Administration

It is a process of planning to organize, command, coordinate and control to get best results.

Efficiency

In an administration or in a management, an appropriate approach is done for good outcome. A health administrator uses his managerial expertise to get optimum results in health management. Following are the main theories of management:

- Classical management theory
- Behavioral management theory
- Quantitative management theory
- Systems theory
- Contingency theory.

GULICK'S POSDCORB IN HEALTH MANAGEMENT

- Planning the things that need to be done
- Organizing the formal structure of the agency
- Staffing the organization
- Directing the work of the agency and making decisions relating thereto
- Coordinating all staff activities

- Reporting to the executive and through him to those to whom he is responsible, and
- Budgeting and all other aspects of fiscal management and control.

Staff Development

It is a requisite to see that all-round development of staff is advocated for an effective management. Since healthcare has become vast, staffs require update of knowledge and skill. If this component is ignored, the health service is downgraded and achievement of healthcare goal will be lowered. Staff development programs that are advocated from time to time for an effective use of health manpower are: (a) In-service education, (b) continued education, (c) specific orientation courses, and (d) specific skill training.

Welfare of staff: This is one of the secret areas of management which holds the crown of health management.

Working condition: It must be a friendly and homely atmosphere. Rigid actions are unwanted in genuine cases; minimum physical facilities like sitting arrangement, recreation arrangement, toilet facilities, working lunch or snack at affordable rates, etc., are expected.

Safety: Safety procedures are adopted in health care procedures. First aid and immediate healthcare provisions are made available.

Health: Free or reimbursable facility for medical care, leave allowance for the period of illness or maternity are basic health facilities that are called for.

Salaries: It is to be compensated as wage for the work. Compensation and incentive which provide basic financial need make a staff to be punctual, attentive and prompt in their discharging duties.

Benefits: Leave privilege of medical benefits, compensation, tenure and promotions are considered as the professional benefit for financial gain, power gain, prestige gain and public services.

Recreation: Holiday compensatory leave, get together, recreation facilities during off days, facility for indoor games are suggested recreation facilities under staff welfare scheme.

Medical supplies: Items used along with drugs to provide curative, preventive and rehabilitative services.

Nonmedical supplies: Nonmedical items used in providing medical care services.

Equipment: They are movable items used by medical profession which are for long-term use.

Facility: They are not movable items like dining room, latrine, dressing room, fencing for protection, etc.

INVENTORY MANAGEMENT

Right drug supply and the equipment are at the right place, at the right time, and in the right quantity in order that staff delivers quality healthcare are very crucial. Without material supply, health staff gets frustrated and patient community lacks confidence in health service.

Good material management involves the following procedures:
- Regular and systematic inventory by staff.
- Daily indenting according to actual need by sending request indent
- Indent is received and checked with request indent
- Material supplies received are stored properly and are protected from misuse.
- Procedure is followed for use for patient care.

Regular replenishment of drugs, medical supplies and nonmedical supplies are done. Regular and proper use and preventive maintenance is advocated. Preventive maintenance is checking equipment facilities regularly to keep them in good condition.

In material management, no overstocking or understocking is advised. Overstocking is not a proper material management which causes losses from pilferage and waste due to spoilage. Understocking is also poor material management because it causes shortage and hardship.

Policy and Procedure in Material Management

Within the country, many variations are seen from state to state and from hospital to hospital. In private sector, bulk purchase and a central store is maintained which supplies on daily basis. In public sector, procurement of supplies is made by central medical store on annual basis.

Material management includes proper store of drugs, medical items so as to protect them from temperature, humidity and rainfall. Facilities and equipment should be kept in good working condition.

Guidelines to staff for an effective health administration under material management are as under:

- Have an idea about past 3 years requirement sought for
- Estimate present requirement
- List the item with particulars
- Indent early allowing for appropriate time lag from the date of previous indent
- Proper bottling, accounting and labeling are necessary for good drug management
- Organize the material in the store, label them and keep an index of available items in the store. Make a tally card for up-to-date and accurate stock of material.
- Preserve rubber goods with power to avoid their deterioration
- Have weekly check of material to avoid rusting
- Accounting of stores is essential for auditing
- Train the subordinate staff for proper use and handling of supplies and equipment.
- Always keep a track on the date of expiry of medicaments
- Prompt reporting of loss, theft or damage help in replacement or condemnation
- Nonconsumable goods should have the following information:
  A. Date of purchase
  B. Source of procurement
  C. Cost at the time of purchase
  D. Cost of maintenance if under repair
  E. Reason for condemnation, if to be condemned

Intuitive method: As per requirement, commonly required are indented, stocked and followed. This is simple and appropriate method for ward management.

Perpetual inventory method: It is useful at main store level. At hospital, nursing staff must be diligent in record keeping.

ABC analysis: High priority items under A and least required under C are indented and adjusted to budgeting which help in continuous supply. This is useful at hospital level.

Example: If 12 lakhs is the budget for 1 year of hospital for drugs, then

A category—APC, aspirin, paracetamol, sulfa, piperazine, etc., are indented for ₹ 8 lakhs.

B category—dressing, antibiotics are indented for ₹ 3 lakhs

C category—fourth-generation antibiotics, such as Taxim, universal precaution gowns are indented for ₹ 1 lakh.

VED method: It is potentially appropriate at matron and hospital level. Essential, very essential categorization at indent, supply and inventory are done.

Two-bin method: This method is appropriate for ward management. Two portions, one for immediate utility and the other for next requirement are kept. When first bin completes, second bin is used. Quick provision for indent is made to see that no shortage or hardship is caused.

Health administration requires material requirement planning (MRP) which can be independent demand or dependent demand. Sometimes, just in time (JIT) planning also is suitable for unusual, rare procedures and performances.

FINANCIAL MANAGEMENT

Financial management includes law, policy, regulation, procedure and proforma related to the receipt and expense of money during patient care and patient management. Main idea is to protect misuse and waste.

Senior staff should know what a budget is. Knowledge of procedure and deadline make input possible and no lapse of allocated budget can occur. There are two types of money recognized in financial management.

Invisible Money (Budgetary Allocation)

It is for drugs, staff transport, etc., where actual money does not pass the hands, but spent through allocations. For example,

There are 20 wards in a civil hospital where 184 staff is working. These wards have a budget of ₹ 85 lakhs for drugs and medical items and ₹ 4,608,000 budget for staff salary. When the budget is released to the civil hospital, the supply is automatically done and salary is spent. In this way, the civil hospital spends ₹ 85 lakhs for drugs and ₹ 4,608,000 for salary without any money passing through the hospital.

Visible Money or Cash (Imprest Amount)

It is provided to meet unforeseen emergencies. Nursing staff is authorized to spend imprest money and then replenish the amount spent. But, imprest amount is replenished against an original receipt in order to prevent misuse of funds. Each time when imprest money is spent, it must be recorded on a cash voucher. Each cash voucher is numbered and must have a receipt attached to it from the person who has sold the goods to the hospital.

In financial management, funds allocation are done under head of account, such as:
- 213 Cabinet—nonplan
- 280 Medical—nonplan
- 281 Medical plan
- 281 Family welfare plan
- 282 Public health—plan
- 282 Public health—nonplan
- 299 Hills—nonplan
- 288 Samajik Suraksha and Kalyan (nonplan)
- 289 Relief in Natural Calamites (nonplan)

There are specified forms, vouchers, receipts, and registers that are to be used in financial management. Staff on administration should know about them which is possible by the existing compulsory departmental examination in 'accounts higher' which is the requisite qualification for an administrative post in nursing service.

BASIC ACTIVITY OF HEALTH MANAGEMENT

- Plan
- Organize
- Communicate, and
- Control

SPAN OF MANAGEMENT

The span of management is otherwise called *span of control* and sometimes it is called *span of supervision*. Under this, number of subordinates who can be controlled by a supervisor is identified; government has set up a *span of control* to a PHC to a DH and FWO, where a MOH or DH and FWO can effectively act and control. Wide span, moderate span and narrow span are usual situations a manager in health management comes across. The guidelines for span of control in health management are:
- Health situation
- Sanctioned and working staff, and
- Health administrator **(Fig. 22.1)**.

MANAGEMENT METHODS

Quantitative Methods

Cost-benefit analysis: Commonly used where cost invested and benefit obtained are compared.

Cost-effective analysis: Suitable in health field where cost invested and effect obtained are compared.

Cost accounting: Cost invested is accounted in each step and in each purpose.

Input–output analysis: Unit of input and unit of output are compared.

Health model: A base structure is prepared to limit health activities for a purpose.

Systems analysis: Whole health system is analyzed for input, activity and output.

Network analysis: Health activities are put to a cyclic form to bring out discipline. They are:

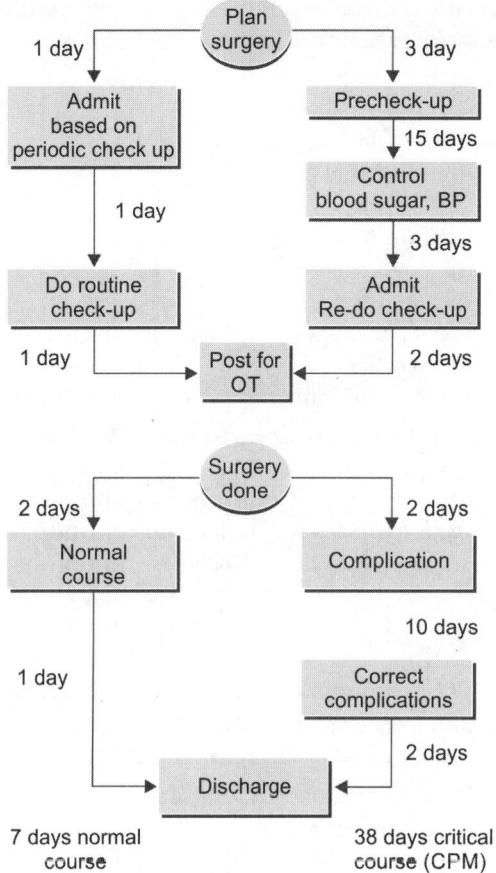

Fig. 22.1: Network analysis.

- *Program evaluation and review technique (PERT):* Logical sequence is followed with diagrammatic representations. This allows time sequence, work sequence and deviation sequence (critical sequence).
- *Critical path method (CPM):* Critical course or longest path in network **(Fig. 22.1)**.
  Plus minus and interesting analysis: Features of proposed course of action are studied and is called PMI analysis.

Force Field Analysis

Strong force and weak force are considered in understanding the betterment of operation in management. It is called FF analysis.

Strength, Weakness, Opportunities and Threats Analysis

Studies with regard to staff, fund and system is done and is also called SWOT analysis.

Planning Programming Budgeting System (PPBS)

Planning, programming, budgeting are involved, since starts with *nil* from all angle, it is called zero approach.

Work sampling: Periodic, random check in health management.

Decision making: Health management wants the flexible decision at all levels.

Qualitative Method

Organizational design: Flexible and effective organization since concepts and technology are changing.

Personal management: This is appropriate job fitting to the suitable.

Communication: Good communication brings strong health management.

Information systems: It is day-to-day information for day-to-day health activities.

Management by objectives (MBO): End point of health activities is set before health management.

Supervision and Leadership Quality

These two are main areas of effective functioning of healthcare services.

Supervision is an art or a process by which designated individuals or group of individuals oversee the work of others and establish controls to improve the work as well as the worker.

Good leadership has following characteristics:

- Coexistence with subordinates
- Assumption of responsibility
- Impartial and fair objectivity
- Capacity to understand the feelings and problems of subordinates
- Ability to take decisions and handle situations
- Willingness to make personal sacrifice to assist subordinates.

HEALTH POLICY

National Health Policy (1983)

In order to establish comprehensive health care for health development and human development, Government of India evolved a National Health Policy in 1983.

Subsectors of National Health Policy include:
- National Education Policy
- National Nutrition Policy
- National Population Policy

Elements of National Health Policy
- Health awareness and community participation
- Safe water and basic sanitation through affordable technology
- Correction of rural urban imbalance
- Giving legislative support
- Greater emphasis on correction of malnutrition
- Provision for alternative health care, and
- Emphasis on Indian system of medicine.

Components of National Health Policy
- Women welfare, child welfare
- Rural development
- Rural employment
- Reducing regional disparity.

National Health Policy Goals
- Birth rate—21/1000 MYP
- Death rate—9/1000 MYP
- IMR—60/1000 LB
- Postneonatal MR—35/1000 LB
- MMR—2/1000 LB
- 0–5 aged MR—10/1000
- Life expectancy—64 years
- Couple protection rate—60%
- NRR—1
- Growth rate—1.2%
- Family size—2.3%
- Delivery by trained TBA—100%
- ANC care—100%
- TT (Pregnant)—100%
- TT (10 years)—100%
- TT (16 years)—100%
- DPT—85%
- OPV—100%
- BCG, DT—85%
- Arrest typhoid—80%
- Arrest leprosy—80%
- Arrest tuberculosis—90%
- Blindness incidence—0.3%
- LBW—10%
- Vitamin A coverage—50%
- IFA coverage—50%
- Water supply—100%
- Night soil disposal—100%
- Malaria 0.5—API
- Goiter reduction to 95%

Specific Goals of National Health Policy

Subcenter	1/5000 population
PHC	1/30,000 population
Community	1/lakh population health center
VHG	1/1000 population
Training TBA	100%
Training of MPW	100%

The predominant areas stressed by National Health Policy are as following:
- Need to evolve 20-point Programme
- Population stabilization
- Enforcement of PFA
- List of problems that needed urgent attention like nutrition, food adulteration, water and sanitation, immunization, MCH, school health and health awareness
- Establishing health information system
- Essential drugs
- Health insurance

National Health Policy (2002 and 2017)

National Health Policy 1983 and National Health Policy 2002 gave an impetus to the National Health Policy 2017.

Main focus is to strengthen and shape health system in all its dimensions.

Expected impacts of National Health Policy 2017 are:
- Expectation of life to increase to 70 by 2025
- Decrease TFR to 2.1 by 2025
- Decrease under-five Mortality to 23 by 2025
- Decrease MMR to 100 by 2020
- Decrease IMR to 28 by 2019

Chapter 22: Health Management

- Reduction of incidence/prevalence of diseases
- Elimination of leprosy, elimination of kala-azar and elimination of lymphatic filariasis by 2018
- Reduction of TB cure rate to above 85%
- Decrease in prevalence of blindness to 0.25/1000 by 2015
- National Health Policy 2017 has given standards for health system, for health performance, for health infrastructure and for health management.

Because of significant change in many social and economic determinants, Government of India revised the National Health Policy and a new National Health Policy 2002 was evolved.

The main focus of attention was to achieve positive health of the community through decentralized public health system and could be through new establishments in infrastructure. More stress and emphasis was given on equitable distribution.

Disease burden by tuberculosis, malaria, blindness and HIV/AIDS was considered on priority in implementation of actions. Specific goals by 2005, 2007, 2010 and 2015 were established. They are enumerated and highlighted in the chapter on *Health Planning*.

National Education Policy (1974)

Article 45 conveys free and compulsory education for all children up to 14 years. It is mentioned as right of a child for right to free education.

Main social goal is basic education for all children and completion of primary education by at least 80% girls as well as boys.

National Nutrition Policy (1993)

Article 47 conveys that the state shall regard the raising of the level of nutrition and the standard of living of its people and the improvement of public health as amongst its primary duties.

Aims

- To reduce malnutrition through awareness and intersectoral coordination.
- To initiate this as part of national development policy.
- To identify short-term and long-term strategies.

Strategies

1. Communication
2. Social mobilization
3. Community participation
4. Monitoring and evaluation.

Sectoral action is being done through following sectors:
- Women and child development
- Agriculture
- Food
- Civil supplies, consumer affairs and public distribution
- Rural development
- Health and FW
- Education
- Environment.

Long-term and structural changes suggested are as given below:
- In order to achieve an annual 215 kg per capita availability of food grains, the Government recognized the need or production of 250 million tonnes and a buffer stock of 35 million tones.
- Shift from production to nutrition by cereal revolution.
- Nutritional objective is incorporated in IRDP, Jawahar Rozgar Yojana and 100 days employment of rural landless families.
- Assurance of ration of seasonally risk population.
- Accessibility to improve ANC and PNC.

Household Food Security

Access to food and purchasing power is fundamental to household food security. A household is food secure when it has access to the food needed for a healthy life for all of its members (adequate in terms of quality, quantity, safety and culturally acceptable) and when it is not at undue risk of losing such access.

National Population Policy

Basic component has been population stabilization by reducing birth rate, growth rate, infant deaths, maternal death, fertility rates and NRR.

Salient Steps

1976: NPP stressed marriageable age 18 years for female and 21 years for male.
1977: NPP stressed small family norm, on voluntary basis; family planning is family welfare.
1986: NPP stressed voluntary participation by the people for people.
2000: NPP stressed on
- Practical and effective suggestions to get best out of NPP
- 12 steps for effective use of NPP, and
- Brought out economics of NPP.

Need: For all level developments of nation.
Goal: Family size to 2.3
- Birth rate to 21
- Death rate to 09
- IMR to 60, and
- CPR to 60.

Elements

- Preferable marriageable age for girls—20 years
- Two children per family norm
- Increase female literacy rate
- Conventional contraceptive device should be extended to 42%
- Promotion of spacing
- Emphasis on UIP and ORT
- IRDP linkage
- Involvement of NGO, and
- Establishing women volunteer corps 1 per 60 families.

National Housing Policy

It was adopted in 1992.

It helps to own one's own home by the lower income group by providing land and finance.

Helps people to fetch low-cost housing technology.

Helps in getting basic amenities like water supply, sanitary latrine, drainage, smokeless chulha.

National Blood Policy

India adopted National Blood Policy (NBP) in April 2002. It aims at "Comprehensive efficient and a total quality management approach" within the country. Main objective is to ensure easy of access to adequate and safe blood supply. All blood transfusion services (BTS) are coordinated by the National Blood Transfusion Council (NBTC). Besides state blood transfusion councils, regional centers, satellite centers, Indian Red Cross and NGOs work through network. Blood banks are monitored by Drugs Controller General of India (DCGI). Technical training, provision of corpus funds for Research and Development are provided. There are well-developed 922 blood banks in the country.

Other aspects of the policy are:
- Prevention of transfusion-associated infections, viz. HIV/AIDS, hepatitis B, syphilis and malaria
- Blood donation shall be voluntary and nonremunerative
- Quality assurance
- Administrative commitment for blood in hospitals
- Human resources and financial resources
- Donor's record
- Rational use of blood.

HEALTH SYSTEM IN INDIA (TABLE 22.1)

Structure, functioning and essentiality of health system in India is unique. Center makes health policy and states run healthcare independent of center.

2011 first stage census drafted 24.9 (249,501,663) million households, 6.5 lakh villages (649,481), 7,935 towns and cities which function on three-tier system of healthcare.

National Health Policy is backing up three-tier health system.

Three-Tier System In Health

District is main unit for health system in India with an average of 3 million population.

Types of Four-3 Tier Systems

Type I

Central health and FW service, state health and FW service and district health and FW service

Chapter 22: Health Management

Table 22.1: Health system in India.

District (763)		
DH and FWO and ZP	District surgeon	Corporation health Authorities
PHC (25,650) Subcenter (156,231)	District hospital (763)	
States and Union Territories (29+7)		
State ministry	Directorate	
Center (Government of India)		
Union Ministry	DGHS	CCH (Chairman and members)
Union function	International Health Regulations Drug standard	Policy of health legislation
Concurrent function	Medical store PG training ME/Med research CGHS Central Health Education Bureau (CHEB) Medical Library	Grant-in-aid cooperation with state

Type II
State health and FW service, district health and FW service, and village health and FW service.

Type III
- Zila parishad
- Mandal panchayat
- Village panchayat

Type IV
- Primary health center
- Subcenter
- Village health guide

Historical Perspectives

1946:	Bhore Committee recommended primary, secondary and tertiary unit in health care
1952:	Later, we see establishment of block development
1977:	Rural Health Scheme.
1981:	Health for All
2000:	National Strategy for Health for All
2000:	The Millennium Development Goals

Healthcare Facilities under 3-tier System

1. *Tertiary:* Teaching hospitals (medical college hospital)
   Super-specialty hospitals (cancer, neuro-surgery, trauma, cardiology)
   Regional hospitals (railway hospital).
2. *Secondary:* District hospitals, community health centers
   Where surgeon and specialists are available with qualification Diploma Public Health (DPH), medicine, pediatrics, surgery, OBG and Bachelor of Shuddha Ayurvedic Medicine (BSAM).
3. *Primary:* PHC for 30,000 population, subcenter for 5,000 population, and VHG/TBA/AWW for 1,000 population.

	Present position
Medical colleges	476 Annual admission is 52,646
Doctors allopathic	1,041,395
Nurses	1,980,526
Hospitals + dispensaries	43,322
Total beds	908,168
Subcenters	156,231
PHC	25,650
Community health centers	5,624
Anganwadies	1,363,000
Integrated Child Development Services (ICDS) blocks	5,320
Dental colleges	313
ANM	841,276
HV	55,675
HW female	220,707
HW male	50,163
BEE	3,512
Health assistant male	12,288
Health assistant female	14,267

Drawback in 3-tier System Noticed

- Bed population ratio is less
- No MPW or VHG in some villages
- No doctors in some PHC
- Infrastructure inadequate.

Village level worker cover 10 villages (5–6 thousand population)		
IRDP*	IRDP*	IRDP*
Communication education	Community development block	
Sanitation housing social welfare	Covers 100 villages (1 lakh population)	

*IRDP = Integrated rural development program

Fig. 22.2: Scheme of rural development.

RURAL DEVELOPMENT (FIG. 22.2)

Since 1952, all-round development of rural community is taken up.

The scheme of rural development is given above.

EVALUATION OF HEALTH SERVICES

Correction and improvement of health service is possible by periodic check which is through evaluation process.

Types of Evaluation

1. Structure evaluation
2. Function evaluation
3. Outcome evaluation

Successful evaluation depends upon following elements:
- Adequacy
- Accessibility
- Acceptability
- Efficiency
- Effectiveness
- Impact, and
- Relevance

Medical Audit

Systematic examination of accounts of medical system for finding out mistakes. Audit helps to correct mistakes and help in improving efficiency. This also evaluates professional work of doctors. It can be internal audit or an external audit.

Components are qualifications of staff, quality of medical services, time spent, fee charged and the outcome.

MILESTONES IN PUBLIC HEALTH IN INDIA

Before Independence

1859: Royal Commission was appointed for health and sanitary condition investigation.
1946: Bhore Committee report.

After Independence

1948: India joined WHO
1950: India became republic
1952: Community Development Programme started
1973: Minimum Needs Programme incorporated
1977: Rural Health Scheme launched
1981: Strategy for HFA, and
1987: New 20-point programme launched
1995 to
2001: Pulse Polio Initiative (PPI) or Intensified Pulse Polio Immunization Programme (IPPI)
1997: Reproductive and Child Health (RCH) Programme
1999: Towards certification of Guinea worm eradication
2000: National Population Policy announced.
2002: National Health Policy
2002: National AIDS Prevention and Control Policy
2002: National Blood Policy
2003: Umbrella Programme for Vector-borne diseases
2004: Integrated Disease Surveillance Project
2005: Janani Suraksha Yojana, National Rural Health Mission launched
2006: IMNCI launched (Integrated Management of Neonatal and Childhood Illness)
2007: Senior Citizen Bill passed
2008: NCD (Noncommunicable Disease) Programme launched
2009: New Mother Child Protection Card came to use; guidelines for Human Stem Cell research by NIH

2010: ICMR standards for Indians for Nutrition
2011: Decennial census; Patient Protection and Affordable Care Act
2013: National Health Mission launched
2014: Declared polio free
2015: NITI Aayog replaced Yojana Aayog; IPV use in immunization; Swachh Bharat Abhiyan launched
2016: Malaria Eradication Plan 2016–2030 launched: Polio tOPV to bOPV changed
2017: NHP 2017
2018: National Health Protection Scheme
2019: World Health Summit in Berlin

VIVA VOCE

1. What is inventory management?
2. Mention four basic activities of health management
3. What is cost benefit analysis?
4. Describe PERT
5. What is critical path method?
6. Describe national population policy
7. Describe three-tier systems
8. What is present doctor population ratio?
9. Which are the types of health evaluation?

SUMMARY

With definition, Planning, Organizing, Staffing, Directing, Coordinating, Reporting and Budgeting (POSDCORB) is described. Inventory and Financial Management are described. Span of management is detailed. Different managerial methods are described. Major National Health Policies are described. Health systems in India are detailed.

Community Healthcare

CHAPTER OUTLINE

- Concept of Healthcare
- Primary Healthcare
- Community Development Program (CDP)
- Essential Healthcare
- Health for All (HFA)
- Millennium Development Goals (MDG)
- Health Programs
- Levels of Healthcare
- Healthcare Delivery System

INTRODUCTION

As the very name implies, healthcare services should reach entire country with more focus on rural areas. Apart from medical care (curative) it should include healthcare (basic sanitation, housing, prevention of diseases, etc.). To render acceptable level of health for all, the country has to see that both urban orientated and rural oriented healthcare is considered, both curative and preventive care is considered and it is made accessible to all section of the society. Medical care is a component of healthcare.

Community healthcare should be:
- According to health needs of community
- Reached out-reach people also
- Participated by community

CONCEPTS OF HEALTHCARE

1. **Comprehensive healthcare (1946)**
   Way back in 1946, Bhore Committee has defined comprehensive healthcare as "integrated promotive, curative and preventive health services from womb to tomb." Certain criteria are fixed for comprehensive healthcare. They are:
   - Service given at the doorstep of the community
   - There shall be community participation
   - Must be available to one and all without considering their ability to pay
   - Vulnerable and weaker sections are given preference
   - At family and at working place creation of healthy environment.

   Preventive + curative + promotive health care through National 5-year plans have given good experience for the past 55 years.

2. **Basic healthcare (1965)**
   This is the network of coordinated peripheral and intermediate health units capable of performing effectively a selected group of functions essential to the health of a geographic area by competent professional and auxiliary personnel.
   A selected function by health units by competent auxiliary is also found and shared by comprehensive healthcare services.

3. Total health care (all required health care)
4. Integrated healthcare (curative + preventive)
5. Primary healthcare (first contact care)

PRIMARY HEALTHCARE

The Alma Ata Declaration in 1978 has defined Primary Healthcare (PHC) as under: "Primary healthcare is essential healthcare made universally accessible to individuals and acceptable to them, through their full participation and at a cost the community and country can afford."

Elements of Primary Healthcare

- Health education on health problems and their control
- Promotion of food supply and proper nutrition
- Safe and wholesome water and basic sanitation
- Maternal and child health (MCH) and family planning (FP) [reproductive and child health (RCH)]
- Immunization against vaccine preventable diseases [universal immunization program (UIP)]
- Prevention and control of locally endemic diseases
- Appropriate treatment of common diseases and injuries
- Provision of essential drugs

Principles of Primary Healthcare

- *Equitable distribution:* Health services must be shared equally by all people irrespective of their ability to pay. Rural or urban, rich or poor all must have access to health services.
- *Community participation:* Involvement of individuals, families and communities in promotion of their own health and family welfare.
- *Intersectoral coordination:* In addition to health sector, coordination with related sectors such as agriculture, animal husbandry, food, industry, education, housing, public works, communication, and transport.
- *Appropriate technology:* Technology that is scientifically sound, adaptable to local needs, and acceptable to those who apply it and those for whom it is used at an affordable price.

Community Health Center
First Referral Unit

Each community health center (CHC) covers 100,000 population (80,000 in hilly/tribal) in a community development block. It has 30 beds having specialists in medicine, surgery, obstetrics and gynecology (OBG) and pediatrics. It will have X-ray and laboratory facilities. There are about 5,510 community health centers in the country.

It covers about 3–4 PHCs.

Staff Pattern

- 1 Community health officer (medical or nonmedical)
- 4 Medical officers (MO)
- 7 Nurse midwifes
- 1 Dresser
- 1 Pharmacist
- Laboratory technician
- X-ray technician
- Ward boys
- 1 Dhobi
- Sweepers
- 1 Mali
- 1 Chowkidar
- 1 Aya
- 1 Peon

Community health center (CHC) refers cases to district level hospitals or medical college hospitals (teaching hospitals).

Primary Health Center

It is an outcome of Bhore Committee Report. PHC provides integrated health services. We have about 25,650 PHCs in the country. It covers about 5 subcenters (SC).

Staff: [at PHC level which cover 30,000 (20,000 in hilly/tribal) population]

- 1 MO
- 1 Pharmacist
- 1 Nurse midwife
- 1 Health worker (HW) (Female)
- 1 Health educator
- 1 Health assistant (HA) (Male)
- 1 HA (Female)
- 1 Upper division clerk (UDC)
- 1 Lower division clerk (LDC)

- 1 Laboratory technician
- 1 Driver (subject to availability of vehicle)
- 3 Class IV employees

Functions

- Medical care
- Reproductive and child healthcare
- Family welfare planning
- Water supply and sanitation
- Control of communicable diseases
- Collection of vital statistics
- Health education
- Carry out National Health Programs
- Referral services
- Training of auxiliary staff such as health assistants, health workers, health guides, and local dais
- Basic laboratory services
- Provision of essential drugs for primary healthcare

Primary health center (PHC) is equipped with the following procedures:

- Tubectomy
- Vasectomy
- Medical termination of pregnancy (MTP)
- Minor operation theater (OT) procedures.

Government has proposed and brought to the action that each medical college should adopt three primary health centers for reorientation of medical education.

Subcenter

It is an outpost attached to a PHC covering a population of 5,000. One multipurpose worker (MPW) (M) and one MPW (F) are posted to work under a subcenter. Mainly RCH, immunization and FP are emphasized. Government is trying to give facility for intrauterine device (IUD) insertion and urine examination for albumin and sugar. Health assistant female supervises the activity of MPW (F).

It covers a population of 5,000 (3,000 in hilly/tribal) areas and has following staff:

- MPW (M)–1
- MPW (F)–1
- Voluntary health guide–1

The functions are the same as PHC with limited services; but restricted to the population it covers viz., 5,000 population. There are about 156,231 subcenters in the country.

a. Community Health Guide (Village Level)

He is a literate volunteer who can secure people's participation. Scheme of Village Health Guide (VHG) came in 1977.

They are chosen from the community. They act as a link between PHC and public. Criteria in their selection are:

- Local residents
- Able to read and write (6th std)
- Acceptable to community
- Should spare 2–3 hours per day for community work.

They undergo training for 3 months (with stipend) of 200.00 per month. After training they receive a working manual and a medicine kit. They spare 2–3 hours a day, get 50.00 stipend per month and drugs worth ₹ 600.00 per year.

As on today there are about 324,000 CHGs working in the country.

b. Dais

They are called TBA (traditional birth attendants). They are given 1 month training with 300.00 stipend. After training, they are provided with a delivery kit. She gets 10.00 for every registered case of pregnancy and 3.00 for every registered infant. Total trained *Dais* are about 700,000 in India. Each trained TBA covers 1,000 population.

c. Anganwadi Worker

Under integrated child development services (ICDS) an AWW is selected from the community. She undergoes training for 4 months. She is paid ₹ 1,000.00 per month honorarium for her service (When State Government Assistance is present). She helps in health checkup, immunization, supplementary nutrition, health education, nonformal education, and referral services. Each AWW covers a population of 1,000.

Panchayat Raj System

Zilla Parishad

President (political) Secretary (executive) District Health and FW Officer (Technical advisor).

Mandal Panchayat

Mandal Pradhan (Political)

Village Panchayat

Panchayat Chairman (Political)

Corporation (in Urban areas)

Mayor (political) Commissioner (executive) City health Officer (Technical advisor).

Panchayat Raj System has three-tier system which are:

1. Village Panchayat at village level (5,000 population)
2. Mandal Panchayat or Mandal Samiti at Block level (100,000 population)
3. Zilla Parishad at district level (1–2 million population).

Panchayat at Village Level

Gram panchayat is an executive organ responsible for village development. It has a president (*Sarpanch*), vice-president and a secretary. Administration, sanitation, public health, socioeconomic development are discussed by them. When they give legal verdict it is called *Nyaya Panchayat*.

Panchayat Samiti at Block Level

About 100 villages of 100,000 population has a *samiti* consisting of *sarpanchs* of the block. Block Development Officer (BDO) acts as secretary of *samiti*. It is responsible for community development program of the block.

Zilla Parishad at District Level

It is a rural local self-government of the district. All heads of panchayat samiti are members. Deputy Commissioner (Collector) is a nonvoting member. It will have above 60 members. Health services including family planning services of the district come under *Zilla Parishad*.

Rural Health Services

It comprises three levels cadre of health centers namely community health center, primary health center, and subcenter.

COMMUNITY DEVELOPMENT PROGRAM (CDP)

Community development is a process designed to create conditions of economic and social progress for the whole community with its active participation and the fullest possible reliance upon the community's initiative. Here people are united for their development.

CDP was launched in 1952 for the all round development of rural areas. It is an organized program by community development blocks, each covering 120,000 population. There are about 6,100 community development blocks in the country.

It envisages following programs:
- Improvement of agriculture
- Improvement of communication
- Education
- Health
- Water and sanitation
- Housing.

The community development block will work for intensive development for 5 years followed by continued work in second phase of 5 years. It is mainly a Centrally Sponsored Program. By this program, it is tackling rural poverty and unemployment.

ESSENTIAL HEALTHCARE

- **Essential obstetrical care:** This aims at providing basic maternity services to all pregnant women and brings down maternal mortality ratio (MMR). The components include early registration of pregnancy within 16 weeks of last menstrual period (LMP), 2 doses of tetanus toxoid (TT), 100 iron–folic acid (IFA) tablets, 3 antenatal care (ANC) checkups, safe delivery either at home or at hospital, 3 postnatal care (PNC) checkups.
- **Essential newborn care:** Main goal of essential newborn care is to bring down perinatal and neonatal mortality. They include resuscitation of newborn, management of asphyxia, prevention of hypothermia, prevention of infections, exclusive breastfeeding, and referral of sick newborn.

HEALTH FOR ALL (HFA)

Member countries of World Health Organization (WHO) have defined HFA as under: "Attainment of a level of health that will enable every individual to lead to socially and economically productive life."

It is to fill the gap between service givers and consumers in healthcare services. It serves to achieve social goals. Simple, acceptable, cheap, and accessible health to all form the scheme of health for all. The HFA does not mean treatment of sick component to make everybody healthy. But it touches the component of availability of healthcare services.

India developed its policies, strategies and plan of action to launch HFA under its own norms and indicators. WHO has established 12 global indicators as the basic point of reference to assess the progress toward HFA. Two major goals that all member countries have adopted are: (a) Life expectancy of 60 years and (b) Infant mortality rate (IMR) below 50 per 1,000 live births (LB).

In India, the laid down goals for HFA are:
1. Attaining IMR below 60 per 1,000 LB
2. Rise in expectation of life to 64 years
3. To reduce crude death rate (CDR) to 9 per 1,000 MYP
4. To reduce crude birth rate (CBR) to 21 per 1,000 MYP
5. To achieve net reproduction rate (NRR) of 1
6. To provide potable water to the entire population.

Basic Principles of HFA

- Intersectoral coordination
- Community participation
- Integrated approach, and
- Creating health awareness.

Plan of Action

- Policy
- Strategy
- Political commitment
- Worked out cost
- Who and when is decided, and
- Training to personnel.

Working Group

Indian Council of Medical Research (ICMR) and Indian Council of Social Science Research (ICSSR) issues are basis of national health policy which was formed in 1982 and got approved in 1983.

In HFA, essential healthcare strategies are developed for regional and global action.

Health concepts included in HFA are:

- Income
- Nutrition
- Education
- Sanitation
- Water, and
- Healthcare availability.

HFA services are given through district health administration (593 revenue districts) from following established network:

- 5,624 community health centers
- 25,650 PHC, and
- 156,231 subcenters.

Targets of HFA

- Birth rate 21/1,000 MYP
- Death rate 9/1,000 MYP
- Annual growth rate 1.2%
- IMR 60/1,000 LB
- Postneonatal mortality rate 35/1,000 LB
- 0–5 mortality rate 10/1,000 0–5 age group
- MMR 2/1,000 LB
- Life expectancy 64 years
- NRR 1.0
- Couple protection rate above 60%
- Family size 2.3, and
- Potable water to all.

Special area emphasized in HFA

- Socioeconomic strategy in national planning
- Development of health management information system (HMIS)
- **Primary healthcare by:**
  - Water
  - Sanitation
  - Immunization, and
  - Essential drug at 1 hour walking distance.

Healthcare by health organization through health programs for existing health problems.

MILLENNIUM DEVELOPMENT GOALS (MDG) SET BY UNITED NATIONS IN 2000

Main aims of MDG are: Poverty reduction, hunger reduction, tackling ill health, tackling gender inequality, tackling illiteracy, and access to clean water.

Indicators of millennium development goals are:
- Prevalence of underweight children
- Proportion of population below minimum level of dietary energy consumption
- Under five mortality rate
- IMR
- Proportion of 1 year children immunized for measles MMR
- Proportion of births attended by skilled health persons
- Human immunodeficiency virus (HIV) prevalence among young people
- Condom use in high risk population
- Ratio of children orphaned.

Malaria death rate, malaria prevalence rate, proportion of population under age 5 in malaria risk areas using insecticide treated bed nets, proportion of population under age 5 with fever being treated with antimalarial drugs, tuberculosis (TB) death rate, TB prevalence rate, proportion of acid fast bacilli (AFB) positive cases, proportion of smear positive pulmonary TB cases detected cured under directly observed treatment short-course (DOTS).

Proportion of population using biomass fuel.

Proportion of population with sustainable. Access to an improved water source (rural and urban areas).

Proportion of urban population with access to improved sanitation.

Proportion of population with access to affordable essential drugs on a sustainable basis.

Health Problems

- Communicable diseases
- Malnutrition
- Poor sanitation
- Healthcare problem
- Population problem
- Emerging health problem

HEALTH PROGRAMS

See **Table 23.1**.

Health Resources

Enough resources are needed to meet the needs of healthcare in the country. For efficient healthcare basic resources are:
- Manpower development
- Money or financial resources
- Material resources and
- Time management

Table 23.1: National health programs.

CD	NCD	Reproductive health	Population	Others
Malaria eradication	Blindness control			
Filaria control	Iodine deficiency disorder control program	UIP	FP program	NWS and SP
Leprosy eradication	Cancer control Mental health program	RCH		Minimum need program 20-Point Program
TB control AIDS control	Diabetes control			

(AIDS: acquired immunodeficiency syndrome; CD: communicable disease; NCD: noncommunicable disease; UIP: Universal Immunization Program; RCH: reproductive and child health; FP: family planning; NWS and SP: National Water Supply and Sanitation Programme; TB: tuberculosis)

LEVELS OF HEALTHCARE

- **Primary level (First level care) (First contact care), by:** VHG/TBA/AWW (village) MPW (SC) PHC staff (PHC)
  An essential healthcare given very close to the people and health problems are solved at community level. This is found very effective since it looks into the needs and limitations. This binds the human culture and human communication system.
- **Secondary level:** District level hospitals and community health centers.
  Little more complex health problems are tackled at this level.
- **Tertiary level:** Specialty hospitals. This level requires superspecialty services. Sound referral system develops continuity of care and gives confidence to the community.

HEALTHCARE DELIVERY SYSTEMS

For the effective healthcare, system adopted and existed in our country is multifaceted and they are working within the framework of national socioeconomic and political systems. They are:

1. **Government Sector (Public Health)**

Health centers
- Subcenters
- PHC
- Community health center.

Hospitals
- Taluk hospitals
- District hospital
- Regional hospital
- Specialty hospital
- Teaching hospitals (medical colleges)

Health Insurance
- Employment State Insurance Scheme (ESIS)
- Central Government Health Scheme (CGHS).

Others
- Defense healthcare services
- Railway healthcare services

2. **Private Sector (Profit or not for Profit- NGO or Charitable)**
- Private clinics
- Private nursing homes
- Private hospitals

3. **Indian Systems of Medicine (AYUSH)**
- Ayurveda
- Sidda
- Unani
- Tibbi
- Homeopathy
- Other traditional healers

4. **Voluntary Health Agencies**
   Nonprofit and nonpolitical private group for (a) Disease control, (b) RCH (c) Rescue and relief, (d) Family welfare, (e) Community development, (f) Professional activities.

Job Responsibilities of Staff of PHC and SC

- **Medical Officer of Health**
  - Team leader
  - Curative, preventive and rehabilitative care
  - Supervision
  - Training
- **Health Assistant (Table 23.2)**
- **Health Worker (Table 23.3)**

Table 23.2: Duties of male and female health assistants.

Common	Male	Female
Supervision	Malaria	RCH
Guidance	Leprosy	Training
Meeting	Tuberculosis	UIP
Camps, campaigns	• Environmental sanitation • UIP • FP (Vasectomy and condom) • Nutrition • Blindness control • Registration of vital events • Epidemic control measure	FP (Tubectomy, OC, IUD)

(UIP: Universal Immunization Program; RCH: reproductive and child health; FP: family planning; OC: oral contraceptives; IUD: intrauterine device)

Chapter 23: Community Healthcare

Table 23.3: Duties of male and female health workers'.

Common	Male	Female
Multipurpose	Records maintenance	Registration
Work	Malaria	Care at home
	Leprosy	Care at clinic
	TB	Care at community
	Environmental	Dai training
	Sanitation	FP (IUD, OCP, tubectomy)
	UIP	
	FP (Condom, vasectomy)	
	Epidemic control measure	

SUMMARY

Primary Healthcare and Essential Healthcare are discussed. Health Programs are described including levels of Healthcare. Healthcare delivery system is detailed.

VIVA VOCE

1. What is primary healthcare?
2. Name staff and functions of PHC
3. What is essential healthcare?
4. Tell something about HFA
5. Which are the levels of healthcare?

SECTION 8

Section Outline

Chapter 24. International Health Organizations

Chapter 25. Voluntary Health Organizations

Chapter 26. Nongovernmental Health Organizations

CHAPTER 24: International Health Organizations

CHAPTER OUTLINE

- History in the Development of International Health
- Organizations
  - WHO
  - UNICEF
  - FAO
  - ILO
  - UNDP
  - UNFPA
  - UNESCO
  - UNIDO
  - UNAIDS

INTRODUCTION

Quarantine, which started in days of plague and detaining travelers and crew members whenever there was a doubt about their health, hallmark the international health consciousness. Since, there was no specific knowledge at that time, it was a failure on the part of organizations.

HISTORY IN DEVELOPMENT OF INTERNATIONAL HEALTH

- 150 years ago—First International Sanitary Conference to tackle cholera, plague, and yellow fever.
- 100 years back—Establishment of Pan American Sanitary Bureau developed PAS codes. Now, it is WHO's regional office.
- In 1907, Paris office called "Office International d'Hygiene Publique" was established. Supervision of quarantine and information on diseases was intended by the office.
- In 1923, the Health Organization of League of Nations was established. Apart from CCD and quarantine, it looked into nutrition, housing and rural hygiene.
- In 1943, the United Nations Relief and Rehabilitation Administration was set up. Malaria and typhus were the main focus.
- On 7-4-1948, WHO under UN got ratification on WHO.

ORGANIZATIONS

- WHO
- UNICEF
- FAO
- ILO
- UNDP
- UNFPA
- World Bank
- UNESCO
- UNIDO
- UNAIDS

World Health Organization

World Health Organization (WHO) is a nonpolitical world health agency of United Nations, WHO recently made a tremendous impact by developing a major health policy through (a) Alma-Ata Conference, and (b) Global strategy for health for all.

Membership—194 countries (2016)

Functions

Following are the major functions of World Health Organization:
- Directing, coordinating healthcare.
- Helping and strengthening health services.
- Gives central technical service for:
  - Warning on health
  - International health regulation
  - International statistics of health
  - International standardizations
  - Medical and health publications
  - Research activities

Structure: World Health Assembly
- Executive Board (gives effects to decision and policies of Assembly)
- Secretariat headed by DG of WHO with 14 secretariat divisions.

Regions
- South-east Asia—Delhi (India)
- Africa—Harare (Zimbabwe)
- America—Washington DC (USA)
- Europe—Copenhagen (Denmark)
- Eastern—Alexandria (Egypt) Mediterranean
- Western Pacific — Manila (Philippines)

South-East Asia Region has 11 Member Countries

They are:
1. India
2. Myanmar
3. Sri Lanka
4. Thailand
5. Indonesia
6. Nepal
7. Maldives
8. Mongolia
9. Bangladesh
10. Korea
11. Bhutan

WHO Day Theme of the Century

2000	Safe blood starts with me—blood saves lives
2001	Stop exclusion—dare to care
2002	Move for health.
2003	Shape the future of life—healthy environment for children
2004	Road safety is no accident
2005	Make every mother and child count
2006	Working together for health
2007	International health security
2008	Protecting health from climate change
2009	Save lives. Make hospitals safe in emergencies
2010	World Health Day 2010 will focus on urbanization and health.
2011	Antimicrobial resistance: no action today, no cure tomorrow.
2012	Good health adds life to years
2013	Healthy heartbeat, healthy blood pressure
2014	Vector-borne diseases
2015	Food safety (with 5 keys; Key 1: Keep clean, Key 2: Separate raw and cooked food, Key 3: Cook food thoroughly, Key 4: Keep food at safe temperatures, Key 5: Use safe water and raw materials).
2016	Diabetes: Scale up prevention, strengthen care, and enhance surveillance
2017	Depression: Let's talk
2018	Universal health coverage: everyone, everywhere
2019	Health for all—everyone, everywhere

United Nations International Children's Emergency Fund (UNICEF)

- It was established in 1946.
- It has a 36-member national executive board
  - Africa — 8
  - Asia Pacific — 7
  - Eastern European — 4
  - Latin America and Caribbean — 5
  - Western Europe and Others — 12
- It collaborates with WHO and FAO.

Headquarters: New York.

Regional headquarters of UNICEF are situated in Columbia (America and Caribbean), Geneva (Europe), Bangkok (East Africa and Pacific), Kathmandu (South Asia), Nairobi (East and South Africa), Jordan (Middle East and North Africa), and Abidjan (West and Central Africa). *South Central Asian Region:* New Delhi.

Functions

The principal functions and objectives of United Nations International Children's Emergency Fund are as given below:
- Child health and welfare
- Mother health and welfare
- Mother and child nutrition
- Family welfare
- Education

Present Strategy
- GOBI (Growth monitoring, oral rehydration, breastfeeding, immunization). In addition, it involves infertility control, female adult literacy and iron (Ferrum) supplementation.
- UBS (Urban basic services)
- IPPI (Intensive Pulse Polio Immunization).

Food and Agricultural Organization (FAO)

It was founded in 1945 and its headquarters is in Rome.

The major functions of FAO are the following:
- Helping nations to raise standards
- Improvement of nutrition
- Development of farming, forestry and fisheries.

Recent Campaign
Freedom from hunger campaign (1960).

Coordination
- Nutritional surveys
- Nutritional training
- Nutritional research

International Labor Organization (ILO)

It was established in 1979 for a coordinated effort toward improving working condition and living condition of workers in their occupation.

Headquarters is in Geneva.

Functions
The main functions of ILO are as following:
- Development of policies, justice and codes of labor
- Promotion of social justice, and
- Improvement of occupational health through health and welfare of workers.

The United Nations Development Programme

- It was set up in 1966.
- Member countries (There are 51 countries in UN) (2019) take its help for their national development.

The principal functions of the United Nations Development Programme (UNDP) are:
- Funding to poor countries
- Giving technical assistance
- Helping agriculture development
- Helping industry development
- Helping education development
- Helping health development
- Helping for social welfare

UNDP

It works in collaboration with
- WHO
- UNICEF
- World Food Programme
- ILO
- FAO
- UNESCO (United Nations Educational Scientific and Cultural Organization)
- UNIDO (United Nations Industrial Development Organization)

The United Nations Fund for Population Activities (UNFPA)

It helps in development of family welfare infrastructure and availability of family welfare services.

Functions
The major functions are the following:
- Development of contraceptive manufacture
- Development of education program
- Introducing innovative approach of FW

World Bank

It is a specialized agency of United Nations; popularly called IBRD (International Bank for

Reconstruction and Development), which was established in 1944. World Bank has billions of dollars of capital which is managed by a Board of Governors and Executive Directors.

India took help in Family Planning Programme, tuberculosis control, cataract surgery and malaria control. Other programs and projects helped by World Bank are RCH, AIDS control, Rural Water Supply and Sanitation Program, Chennai Water Scheme, and Mumbai Sewage Disposal Project. State governments have taken World Bank's loan for slum improvement and hospital strengthening.

Functions

It provides loans for projects on:
- Economic growth
- Agriculture, water supply, education
- Road, railway, electricity, family planning
- Health and environment
- World Bank assistance to hospital care.

UNESCO

Founded in 1945 and has 188 member countries. Collaborates and promotes education, science, culture and communication for world's peace and security.

UNIDO

Founded in 1966 under United Nations. Helps in industrial development and industrial consultancy.

UNAIDS

Under United Nations, it targets expanded response to HIV epidemic and AIDS.

SUMMARY

With history of International Health Organization, major International Health organization are detailed. WHO and UNICEF are emphasized.

VIVA VOCE

1. What is WHO theme of 2020?
2. Tell about Intensive Pulse Polio in India.

25 CHAPTER: Voluntary Health Organizations

CHAPTER OUTLINE

- Role of Voluntary Organization
- Functions of Voluntary Health Organizations
- Organizations
  - For Communicable Diseases
    - Tuberculosis Association of India (TAI)
    - Hind Kusht Nivaran Sangh (HKNS)
  - For Noncommunicable Diseases
    - All India Blind Relief Society
  - For RCH
    - Indian Council for Child Welfare
    - Central Social Welfare Board
    - The Kasturba Memorial Fund
    - All India Women's Conference
    - Child Relief and You (CRY)
  - For Rescue and Relief
    - India Red Cross Society
  - For Family Welfare Planning
    - Family Planning Association of India
  - For Rural Health
    - Bharat Sevak Samaj
  - For Community Development
    - Voluntary Health Association of India
  - For Professional Activities
    - Indian Medical Association
    - Indian Dental Association
    - The Trained Nurses Association of India
    - Associations of Community Health

INTRODUCTION

Community health activities of the past, the present and the future are relied upon voluntary health organization, which have explored new ways and means and thus pioneering in research and development of health sciences. They are social service organizations and social developmental institutions motivated to meet the needs of disadvantaged in a society.

They are non-profit and non-political private group of individuals set up with the intention of relief, welfare, as professional body and for providing health services.

Voluntary health organizations have certain characteristics. They are enumerated as under:
- They are organized
- Have an autonomous board
- Hold meeting
- Collect fund
- Conduct public health program
- Create health awareness
- Help in policy making
- They are small enough to reach any place

ROLE OF VOLUNTARY HEALTH ORGANIZATION

- They stimulate government activities.
- Take care of community at no cost.
- Have patented many healthcare services, and
- They are real coordinators of health and welfare services.

Role in Social Reforms

- Education
- Old age care
- Child care
- War victim care
- Aid at natural calamities
- Insure the community

Recent Areas of Involvement

- Home makers
- Shopping
- Meals on wheels
- Transportation of sick
- Hospital care

Basic Inception Ideology

- Mostly autonomous
- Conduct board meetings
- Raise fund
- Involve education and research

FUNCTIONS OF VOLUNTARY HEALTH ORGANIZATIONS

- Stimulate and supplement government in healthcare service
- Provide new concepts and pioneer the research activities
- Experiment and demonstrate many health and welfare activities
- Guide in implementation of healthcare activities
- Set up regulation criteria, and
- Help in public health legislation.

ORGANIZATIONS

For Communicable Diseases

Tuberculosis Association of India

It started in 1939 and has many branches in India. It mobilizes Fund through "TB seal campaign", trains medical and paramedical in chemotherapy. There are many leading Tuberculosis Institutions in India which are run by Tuberculosis Association of India (TAI). Main activities are control, prevention, training and research on tuberculosis.

Hind Kusht Nivaran Sangh

Hind Kusht Nivaran Sangh (HKNS) started in 1950 with its headquarters in Delhi. Financial assistance to leprosy homes, health education by posters and training of physiotherapists are main activities of HKNS. Main activities are eradication, training and research on leprosy.

For Noncommunicable Diseases

All India Blind Relief Society

Started in 1946, is associated with eye camps for identification of preventable blindness and conducting cataract surgery camps with postoperative follow-ups and free spectacles for refractory corrections. Recently, All India Blind Relief Society has introduced cataract surgery with IOL implantation which otherwise is not affordable by a common man. Main activities are eye camps and eye relief measures.

For Reproductive and Child Health

Indian Council for Child Welfare

It started in 1952. It has network of state councils in India. Its main objectives are to provide social and economic security to child by legislative means through right of the child.

Central Social Welfare Board

This was started in 1953. Under Ministry of Education, this board is formed as an autonomous organization. It is identifying voluntary welfare organizations and rendering financial aid to them for welfare activities. Running balwadies, mother crafts, play centers and women self-employment assistance are its other added popular schemes. Main activities are family service and child service.

The Kasturba Memorial Fund

It started in 1944. It aims at helping rural women through gram sevikas. Main activity is woman improvement.

Chapter 25: Voluntary Health Organizations

All India Women's Conference

Started in 1926, is running antenatal and postnatal care clinic, child guidance clinics, adult education centers, milk distribution centers and family planning clinics. Main activities are women health and welfare.

Child Relief and You

Child Relief and You (CRY) was founded in 1981 by Rippan Kapur in order to take care of street children, bonded children, children of prostitutes, and children of remand homes. It helps in schooling as well as sports. CRY supports other agencies and has instituted Rippan Kapur Fellowship. It raises fund through greeting cards.

For Rescue and Relief

Indian Red Cross Society

Indian Red Cross Society founded in 1920. Junior Red Cross is an active section. There are many branches across the country executing relief work during earthquake, floods, drought and disease epidemics. It is providing assistance to fetch milk and medical supplies to many hospitals, RCH centers and orphanages. The primary obligation of the Red Cross is to take care of wounded, sick or injured armed forces. For permanently disabled ex-servicemen, Red Cross has initiated "Red Cross Homes".

Recently, great attention of Indian Red Cross has fallen on first aid, voluntary blood donation and family planning clinic which can bring medical relief and social relief to the society. Red Cross day is detailed in Chapter 36.

For Family Welfare Planning

Family Planning Association of India

Founded in 1949. Main activities are training, service and research on family planning.

For Rural Health

Bharat Sevak Samaj

Founded in 1952. Village sanitation and guide self sufficiency. It is helping people to achieve health by their own effort and actions.

For Community Development

Voluntary Health Association of India

It is a federation of organizations for health development. This develops health education material, helps in popularization of well-baby clinic and imparts training to health workers.

For Professional Activities

Indian Medical Association

It is a professional body which is guiding Medical Council of India. Indian Medical Association (IMA) is helping in setting up quality standards in professional education in medical profession and health science profession. It is also involved in organizing relief camps and medical relief during natural calamities. It coordinates with Indian Red Cross Society.

Over hundreds of health check-up camps, health awareness camps, blood donation camps, screening camps are conducted every year thus providing access to health and welfare to common man.

Indian Dental Association

It is a professional body which is guiding Dental Council of India. Indian Dental Association is helping in setting up quality standards in professional education in dental profession.

Over hundreds of dental check-up camps, dental health awareness camps and screening camps are conducted every year, thus providing access to health and welfare to common man.

The Trained Nurses Association of India

By 1952, we could see an organized effort of grouping among trained nurses but without any registered body. Of late, various specialized courses are being made available such as community health nursing, midwifery, operating assistant and rehabilitation nursing. In 1960s, an organized group called Trained Nurses Association was formed with the objective of involvement into community welfare activities, such as:

- Nursing care of children
- Nursing care of elderly

- Blood donation campaign and camps
- First-aid facility
- Vocational rehabilitation
- Relief work with Red Cross, IMA and general practitioners.

Associations of Community Health

They involve in professional standardization, academic activities, healthcare camps and health research.

SUMMARY

Role and Functions of Voluntary Health Organization are described. Voluntary Health Organizations are described as per their activities in India.

VIVA VOCE

1. Tell about IMA.
2. Tell about Indian Red Cross Society.
3. What are the functions of Indian council of child welfare?

CHAPTER 26: Nongovernmental Health Organizations

Chapter Outline

- Organization List
- Organizations
  - International Red Cross
  - Rockefeller Foundation
  - Ford Foundation
  - CARE
  - Oxfam
  - Save the Child Fund
  - Aga Khan Foundation
  - Freedom from Hunger

ORGANIZATION LIST

Nongovernmental health organizations are major and important promoters of healthcare. They are independent nonprofit organizations working for the development, research and relief operations in the world.

Following are the major internationally renowned health organizations:

- International Red Cross
- International Planned Parenthood Federation
- International Agency for the Prevention of Blindness
- World Federation of the Deaf
- International Leprosy Association
- Rockefeller Foundation
- Ford Foundation
- CARE
- World Federation of Medical Education
- International Union against Cancer
- The Population Council
- Oxfam
- Save the Children Fund
- Agha Khan Foundation
- Freedom from Hunger.

ORGANIZATIONS

International Red Cross

- It was founded by Henry Dunant in 1859.
- It serves for international peace.
- It readily comes to the rescue and relief operations during war and natural calamities.
- This organization symbolizes universal brotherhood.

Major role: War, peace, natural disasters.

Other role: First aid, nursing education, RCH welfare.

Red Cross Day is detailed in Chapter 36.

Rockefeller Foundation

It was founded by John D Rockefeller in 1913. Since 1920, it is associated with public health programs in India. It covers the areas of:

- Public Health
- Advancement of Life Sciences
- Advancement of Social Sciences
- Advancement of Agricultural Sciences
- Advancement of Medical Education.

All India Institute of Hygiene and Public Health at Kolkata was established by Rockefeller Foundation.

Fellowship and travel grants in Medical Education are awarded by this foundation.

Rockefeller Foundation is supporting the following at present:
- Rural training
- Family welfare planning
- Agricultural development.

Ford Foundation

Ford foundation has been working for better administrative schemes for developing countries.

In India, it has established National Institute of Health Administration and Education at Delhi.

Ford Foundation is supporting at present the following projects:
- Research in reproductive biology
- Solutions to basic problems of environmental sanitation
- Training courses to health personnel, medical personnel and paramedical personnel. (Through orientation training centers)
- Support research in Reproductive Biology.

Cooperative for Assistance and Relief Everywhere (CARE)

It is popularly known as CARE, which was started in 1945. It is operative since 1950 in India providing food support to children in the age group of 6–11 years. Many health and nutrition projects are ongoing that are mainly concerned with women and children through CARE.

CARE started as a program in Europe; got extended to everywhere. CARE has its head office in Belgium. It has 11 regional headquarters based in Atlanta (USA), London (UK), Canberra (Australia), Ottawa (Canada), Paris (France), Bonn (Germany), Oslo (Norway), Tokyo (Japan), Wien (Austria), Copenhagen (Denmark), and Ea Den Haag (Netherlands).

It is one of the biggest developmental and international relief organizations.

CARE is supporting at present:
- Food support to vulnerable age groups
- Health of adolescent girls, and
- RCH development.

OXFAM

An autonomous NGO committed to fight poverty and injustice. This is helping in many developmental activities in India.

Save the Children Fund

Founded in 1919 in UK. It provides emergency relief to malnourished children around the world.

AGA KHAN Foundation

Founded in 1967. It helps in rural development and health systems. Child care and child development are given importance.

Freedom From Hunger

Founded in 1946. It provides self-help to hunger and poverty.

SUMMARY

In the beginning, organizations list is provided. Important Nongovernmental Health Organizations such as International Red Cross, Rockefeller Foundation, Ford Foundation, CARE etc., are described.

VIVA VOCE

1. What is the major role of International Red Cross?
2. What is CARE?

SECTION 9

Section Outline

Chapter 27. Urban Health
Chapter 28. Medical Ethics
Chapter 29. Public Health Law

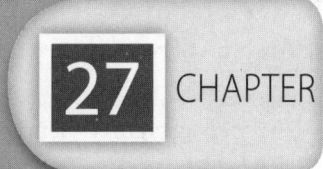

27 CHAPTER

Urban Health

CHAPTER OUTLINE

- Urban Health Problems
- Process of Urban Life
- Suggested Education Activity
- Service on Urban Slum Areas and Services on Urban Area
- Agenda for Sustainable Ecological Balance
- Krishnan Committee Report (1982) on Urban Health

INTRODUCTION

Cities have been growing dramatically since 1900. In 1900, 1 in 10 (1:10) lived in city. By 1948, it came to 3 in 10 (3:10) urbanized. According to UN, about 47% population are living in urban world.

The extent of urbanization in three major cities of India (2000) is indicated below:

Mumbai 18.1 million
Kolkata 12.9 million
Delhi 11.7 million

According to WHO SEARO, New Delhi, trends expected in these cities by 2015 are:

Mumbai 26.1 million
Kolkata 17.3 million
Delhi 16.8 million

The proportion of urban slum and shanty town is highest in Mumbai which is around 48.9% and lowest in Patna which is 0.25%.

Highest urban population is recorded in Tamil Nadu as 43.9% and lowest in Bihar at 10.5%.

According to United Nations' definition, if a city has the population of more than 10 million, it is considered as a mega city. At present, there are 47 mega cities in the world.

There are 35 urban cities with more than one million population in the world. Mega cities of Delhi, Kolkata and Mumbai are in India with above 1 million population.

India has 7,935 towns and 475 urban conglomerations.

A direct consequence of population explosion is referred to as "urban crisis" and urban explosion. As a consequence numerous problems are becoming more and more difficult to tackle with existing resources. Slums and shanty town are increasing; migrant population has temporary shelters using roadside, pavement and footpaths.

INDIA: TREND IN GROWTH OF URBAN POPULATION

In 1960, urban population stood at 1 billion and rural stood at 2 billion population.

1961	80,000,000
1981	160,000,000 Doubling in 20 years
1971	109 million
1991	217 million (25.72% increase). There were 4,615 cities and towns. (doubling in 20 years)

Contd...

Contd...	
2001	285 million (27.8% increase). There are 5,161 cities and towns.
2007	3.3 billion urban population and 3.4 billion rural population; an equal status noticed.
2011	377.1 million. There are 3 mega cities; 7,935 towns; 475 urban conglomerations
2016	4 billion urban population and 3.4 billion rural population is observed
2050	68% of urban population is expected in the world

Annual exponential urban growth = 3.09% (Rural 1.8%).

In India, there were 751 million urban population in 1950. This has been exponentially increased to 4.2 billion in 2018. Annual urbanization increase is 2.8%.

URBAN HEALTH PROBLEMS

Common urban health problems are:
- Cholera
- Malnutrition
- Mental illness
- Chronic respiratory infection.

Since 5 years, healthy city vision and healthy cities for better life has started (1996). It has identified five types of urban health problems. They are:

Medical

Typhoid, hepatitis, skin infection, STD, CVS, diarrhea, cancer, degenerative disease.

Social

Alcohol, drug abuse, prostitution.

Environmental

Traffic accidents, air pollution, river pollution.

Economic Problem (Poverty)

Diarrhea, ARI, TB, effect of inflation resulting in rise in population following below poverty line (BPL).

Psychological

Mental illness, street violence, suicide.

HISTORY OF URBAN HEALTH

- 19th century Industrial Revolution.
- Land of farm to smoking factory (Dark Satanic mills)
- 20th century social aspect of environment.
- Housing Finance Agency Act, 1981.
- Employees' State Insurance Amendment Act, 1989
- Panchayat Raj Act, 1994
- National Family Health Survey, 1999
- National Commission on Population, 2000
- Maintenance of Parents and Senior Citizen Bill, 2007
- National Health Mission, 2013
- Swachh Bharat Abhiyan, 2015
- National Health Protection Scheme, 2018.

PROCESS OF URBAN LIFE (FIG. 27.1)

Process of Urban Health

- Rural poverty induced urbanization, e.g., Uttar Pradesh,, Bihar.
- Rural prosperity-induced urbanization, e.g., Punjab, Haryana.

According to National Institute of Urban Association (NIUA):
- About 41% by natural growth.
- About 40% migration.
- About 19% reclassified settlement.

In mega cities, 50% of population is in slums.

Urban Problems Related to Poverty

Diarrhea, ARI, TB, typhoid, hepatitis, malaria, skin infection, malnutrition and STD.

Urban Problems Related to Affluent

CVS, cancer, mental illness, degenerative diseases.

Urban Problems Related to Ecology

Traffic accidents, air pollution, river pollution, alcoholism, drug abuse.

Problems of Cities

The major problems facing the Indian cities are:

Chapter 27: Urban Health

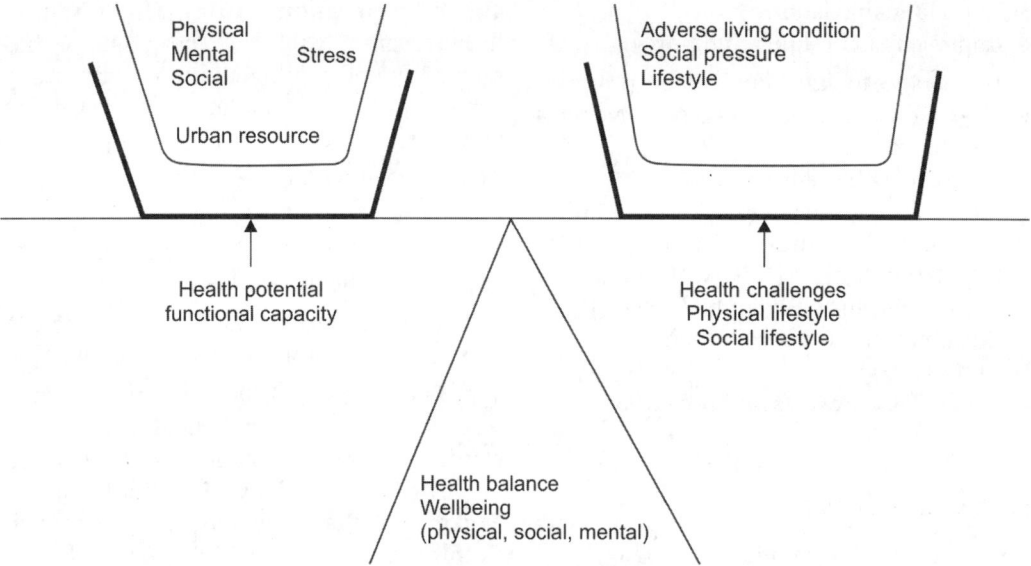

Fig. 27.1: Process of urban life.

- Lack of food, clean water, shelter
- Overcrowding
- No facility for waste disposal
- Hazard working condition
- Atmospheric pollution, and
- Accident, street violence, suicide, juvenile delinquency.

Healthy city movement is an interaction of economic, cultural, social activity within cities, its resource and environment for:
- Small family norm
- Quality and quantity of food
- Healthy physical environment
- Specific preventive measures
- Therapeutic measures.

Slum improvement movement is an initiative for better city life.

Strategies to convert city to health cities (ABC strategy).
- Setting up task forces.
- Formation of local committee to implement decisions taken by task force.
- Action at community level.
  - Health awareness on habit and lifestyle
  - Community participation
  - Urban law implementation
  - Seminar and conference to share each others' experience
  - Healthy management of urban wastes.

SUGGESTED EDUCATION ACTIVITY

Following educational activities are suggested for urban society:
- Theme broadcast on AIR/TV
- Future articles for good message
- Good publicity material
- Exhibitions and display on urban problem
- Use of folk media for awareness
- Cultural programs imbibing urban message
- Competitions on city improvement activities.

SERVICE ON URBAN SLUM AREAS AND SERVICES ON URBAN AREA

Following are the welfare actions suggested for Indians' urban society:
- Encourage local agricultural-based industry
- Rural shifting of hazardous industry
- Planning of road, office, residence to reduce traffic
- Development of green belt, park, trees
- Public transport and pooling vehicle to reduce traffic
- Building plans for reduced noise pollution
- Encourage use of biodegradable material for package
- Library and recreation centers in residential areas

- Good human relations
- Improvement of slum condition

Slum clearance to slum improvement program.
- Slum improvement projects as overseas development. Agency—(ODA) assisted effort and UCD efforts.
- World Bank assisted Indian population projects [Mumbai, Chennai, India Population Project (IPP)-V, Kolkata, New Delhi, Bengaluru, Hyderabad, IPP-VIII].
- Environmental improvement of urban slums (EIUS).
- Urban Basic Services for Poor (UBSP).

AGENDA FOR SUSTAINABLE ECOLOGICAL BALANCE

- Garbage recycling policy
- Excreta disposal policy
- Safe drinking water in cities
- Dangerous industries
- Ozone depletion
- Global warming and greenhouse effect
- Air pollution in cities

KRISHNAN COMMITTEE REPORT (1982) ON URBAN HEALTH

The committee has recommended primary healthcare for urban slum where more than 40% of population is poor. This is called urban revamping scheme. The committee has recommended health manpower for primary urban care as per population congregations which are as under:

Type A—below 5,000 population (1 nurse midwife)

Type B—5,000 to 10,000 population (1 male and 1 female health worker)

Type C—10,000 to 25,000 population (2 male and 2 female health workers)

Type D—25,000 to 50,000 population (1 LMO, 3 nurse midwives, 3 male health workers, 1 class IV, 1 clerk and 1 voluntary health worker).

At present, we have 871 health posts working after the recommendation of Krishnan Committee Report and 1,083 urban family welfare centers.

SUMMARY

In the beginning, Urban Health Problems are described. Process of urban life is detailed. Services on urban slum areas are described. Krishna Committee report on Urban Health is highlighted.

VIVA VOCE

1. Mention urban health problems.
2. Mention problems of cities.

28 CHAPTER

Medical Ethics

CHAPTER OUTLINE

- Indian legislations related to medical ethics
- Heteronomous and autonomous ethics
- Major principles of medical/bioethics
- Perspectives of medical ethics
- Ethics of the individuals
- Organ donation
- The ethics of human life
- Cloning
- Recent approaches in gene therapy
- Prolongation of life
- Advanced life directives
- Death and dying
- Professional ethics
- Research ethics
- Area of ethical interest in present day practice
  - Ethical issue of symbols
  - Ethical issue of pushing for cheaper drugs
  - More controversy in euthanasia
  - Components of an ethically valid informed consent for research
  - Ethical issues with alternative medicine

INTRODUCTION

Teaching of human values to health professionals constitutes the curriculum of medical ethics. It deals with how we conduct ourselves in medical profession. It is formed with beliefs and practices. It differentiates acceptable (right) and unacceptable (wrong in hospital practice and in community health practice).

DEFINITIONS

Medical Ethics

It is of concern for a patient who is suffering from illness and his relatives. Next it is for the doctor who is treating. This medical ethics has principles governing moral behavior.

Box 28.1 enumerates the merits and demerits of medical ethics.

Meta-ethics

This concerns the essential and basic concept.

Box 28.1: Merits and demerits of medical ethics.

- Merits of medical ethics
- Sets responsibilities on doctor
- Regulates doctor
- Improves professional image
- Guides the conduct of a doctor with his patient
- Creates awareness
- Improves medical care
- Demerits of medical ethics
- Not normally put to practice
- Heterogeneous nature of medical profession do not help everyone each time
- No uniformity

Normative Ethics

It concerns setting standards.

Applied Ethics

This concerns patient examination and specific ethical issues.

INDIAN LEGISLATIONS RELATED TO MEDICAL ETHICS

- 1940–The Drugs and Cosmetics Act
- 1948–The Pharmacy Act
- 1954–The Drugs and Magic Remedies Act
- 1971–Medical Termination of Pregnancy Act
- 1986–Juvenile Justice Act
- 1989–Blood Safety Program
- 1995–Legislation on Transplantation of Human Organ
- 1996–Prenatal Diagnostic Techniques (PNDT)
- 1998–Management and handling of Biomedical waste rules
- 2013–National Mental Health Mission

HETERONOMOUS AND AUTONOMOUS ETHICS

Heteronomous ethics deals with desirability of a thing particularly useful in health practice which is subject to external law.

Example: Defective newborn cannot be allowed to die.

Autonomous ethics deals with desirability of a thing particularly usefulness in health practice which is independent of others or in other words under one's own law.

Example: Sin to get abortion done by religious norm.

Bioethics deals with problems that have arisen out of recent developments in science and technology.

Example: Cloning, surrogate mother.

MAJOR PRINCIPLES OF MEDICAL/BIOETHICS

- Principle of doing good which is called beneficence in ethics.
- Social and distributive justice to one and all with a view to serve the ill with fairness, equity and impartiality, this is called justice in ethics.
- Full freedom, right of individual to make choice, right to make decision for themselves. This is called the respect for autonomy. Self-determination and liberty are other names for autonomy.
- Principles of not harming patients. It is called nonmaleficence.

PERSPECTIVES OF MEDICAL ETHICS

- Babylonian code
- Egyptian code
- Ancient Indian codes of Atreya, Anushasana, Charaka Samhita and Sushruta Samhita
- Hippocrates oath
- Nuremberg code
- The declaration of Helsinki
- World Health Organization (WHO) declaration of Geneva
- International code of medical ethics
- Indian Medical Council (IMC) Act (1956)
- Medical Council of India (MCI) code of ethics (1980), and
- The Patient Self-Determination Act

ETHICS OF THE INDIVIDUALS

- The patient as a person
- The right to be respected

Each person has right to call for assistance and help from his fellowmen at an emergency and illness. A doctor has his role play to treat the sick. There is a social obligation for a doctor to treat the sick and for a patient to seek medical help. In this interaction all individuals have the right to be respected.

- Truth and confidentiality.

An individual often has many roles and many events in his or her life time. Illness is one such event. If a person is suffering from tuberculosis or leprosy or psychological disturbances, the situation is true. There lies the truth in his/her illness. The truth is that he or she is a patient of a given disease which makes him/her a social outcaste. The information on this will be with the doctor or the profession which is connected largely with the patient's privacy.

An individual has every right to privacy over the issue of truth. This aspect of professional secrecy is called confidentiality.

Chapter 28: Medical Ethics

Medical oath and medical declaration make a doctor obliged to maintain confidentiality.

Examples of Truth in Medical Profession

- Homicide
- Fitness for service
- Insurance coverage and claim
- Accident (Hit and run)

Examples of Confidentiality in Medical Profession

- Hospital or survey record of health of an individual.
- Confidential information collected by the doctor for the purpose of treatment.
- Scientific publication of a case study when a pseudonym is used.
- No gossip done by the profession on information about the patient's sexual habit.

Troubling Problems in Truth and Confidentiality (Dilemmas)

- A patient is diagnosed to suffer from sexually transmitted disease.
- A patient who is human immunodeficiency virus (HIV) positive is on operation table for an emergency operation.
- When an insurance company compels for personal information.
- A patient has a highly infectious communicable disease which is notified by the Municipality Act.
- A person selected in Railways and Communication as a railway driver is found to have color blindness. (*Note*: Truth takes off the job and confidentiality can kill thousands of innocents!).

ORGAN DONATION

Treatment involving use of organ to the sick. It is not possible without formal procedure. Values and norms are drawn and ethical issue is a big-scale phenomenon.

Common organs used are kidney, cornea, blood, liver, fetal brain tissue, bone marrow and heart.

The Anatomical Gift Act of United States of America (USA), Human Organ Transplant Act of United Kingdom (UK) and World Health Assembly Proclamation are controlling the unethical practice of commercialization.

Organ replacement is imminent treatment for damaged organ among suffering patients to save their lives. Present set of line of treatment in them is involving use of organ to the sick. It is not possible without formal procedures. Values and norms are drawn and ethical issue has a great significance in organ transplantation. Since, organs are not available and that the demand is very high, they have created many ethical issues. Common ethical problems are:

- Very expensive
- Force for an organ for life
- Compulsion for an organ for life
- Loss of lives for want of organs occurring
- Unethical practice of commercialization (money, agency and commission raise their ugly head in the issue)

Administrative problem, such as too long a waiting time and a scientific factor, such as donors' compatibility can create ethical problem.

Common organs used in organ donation are:

- Kidney
- Cornea
- Blood
- Liver
- Fetal brain tissue
- Bone marrow
- Heart

Requirements in Organ Donation

- Compatibility in live donors
- Close relatives for good take
- Will, consent and declaration are required
- Age of the donor must be above 3 years
- Brain death proof is required on many occasions.

Anatomical Gift Act

Any person above 18 years of age can donate his/her organ or part. This Gift takes effect upon his/her death. India is following the Model Act of United States of America.

Court has no powers to allow certain procedures under the Gift Act by the donor. An illustration is available from Australia Court, which denied a bereaved woman the chance of becoming pregnant by her dead fiancée (2003).

Human Organ Transplant Act

This has come up as an ethical issue in many countries because of the demand for kidney transplantation to save lives. The first Act was at United Kingdom in 1989. Model Acts are seen in Turkey and in India. Organ donations do not include any reproductive organs.

World Health Assembly Proclamation 1991 on Organ Donation

The Proclamation 1991 includes the following:
- Donation by the deceased
- Donation by the living
- Consent is a must
- Recipient care must be undertaken
- Should be genetically related
- Risk, benefit and consequences of the consent should be known
- Should be an adult above 18 years
- No commercial transaction
- Should not be on financial need
- Only on a medical indication done
- Only on life saving need

Organ Donation for Life after Death

Nine out of 10 enquiries would say that they have thought about organ donation for life after death. But given a chance the proportion may go up. In case of critical injury to the brain due to accident or stroke, patient succumbs to brain death. In such cases 9 out of 10 have no ventilator support to protect organs for donation for life after death.

Medical ethics and bioethics allow living person to get a chance to voice his or her decision with regard to the donation of organs after his or her death.

Views of major religions on the subject of organ donation for life after death was brought out by The New York Regional Transplant Program.

THE ETHICS OF HUMAN LIFE

Ethics of conception is related to:
- Inheritance of property
- Adoption
- Divorce
- Polygamy

Ethics of Human Life includes

- Medical termination of pregnancy (MTP)
- Prenatal sex determination
- In vitro fertilization
- Artificial insemination husband
- Artificial insemination donor
- Surrogate motherhood
- Gamete intrafallopian tube transfer
- Semen intrafallopian tube transfer, and
- Zygote intrafallopian tube technique

The technology covers the following procedures under the ethics of human life:
- IVF-ET: In vitro fertilization and embryo transfer
- GIFT: Gamete intrafallopian transfer
- ZIFT: Zygote intrafallopian transfer
- PROST: Pronuclear stage embryo transfer
- Transfer of gamete
- Transfer of embryo
- Surrogate motherhood
- Micromanipulation of gametes
- Intrauterine insemination
- Sperm intrafallopian transfer
- Sperm intraovarian transfer
- Intraperitoneal sperm transfer

CLONING

Gene cloning requires a host cell and uses a vector which should have marker. When inserted to a host cell by microinjection, develops a replica (without a natural biological process).

Cloning is a technique for producing a genetic twin of a living thing. It entails taking deoxyribonucleic acid (DNA) from an adult animal and inserting it into an egg cell from another animal. The egg then divides into an embryo. The cloned embryos have genes from only one parent. The embryo is then transferred to a surrogate mother and grown to term. The process has worked in cows, sheep, goats, mice and pigs, while attempts have failed with rabbit, rat, cat, dog, monkey and horse. Barely 10% or fewer of cloning attempts succeed. Many cloned animals have subtle brain defects or other problems that could be devastating in human. Yet another cloning technique called germ line genetic engineering alters eggs and sperm in what could lead to a total reconfiguration of the human species. A British Columbia based company has announced a new technique for using artificial human chromosomes to alter children's health, appearance, personality and lifespan. Another company that offers cloning services for $200,000 has received many inquiries. The demand is there, and the patients are willing to accept these risks for a fancy come true.

According to scientists, cloning per se is not bad. Cloning a whole animal or a human-being, however, is a much more difficult proposition, even without considering moral implications. The basic method sounds deceptively simple: scientists allow an egg to mature in a culture dish. They strip out the genetic material from this egg. Then they insert the genetic material of a separate cell, an adult cell. Next, using a chemical mixture or electrical stimulation, researchers trick the egg into thinking that it has been fertilized by sperm. This will activate the cell to start dividing. Essentially, scientists are trying to reprogram the egg to create a new organism. The concept of using stem cells to create embryos called as "Therapeutic cloning" still has a long way to go before a cure to Parkinson's and related disorders is available.

RECENT APPROACHES IN GENE THERAPY

Transfer of genes into the brain by liposome coated in a PEG (polyethylene glycol). This has a potential to treat Parkinson's disease.

Short interfering ribonucleic acids (siRNAs) are detected to be found helpful to silence Huntington's chorea.

Thalassemia, cystic fibrosis and some cancers are found to be benefited by new gene therapy approach which repairs errors in messenger RNA derived from defective genes.

Tiny liposome (25 nanometers) called DNA nanoballs are discovered which can boost gene therapy.

Sickle cell is successfully treated in mice and has given some hope among scientists.

PROLONGATION OF LIFE

Following biotechnologies have put forth an effort to prolong human life when illness or disability occurred.
- Immunization
- Advanced life support techniques
- Advanced life saving procedures
- Organ transplantation
- Intensive care unit (ICU)
- Intensive critical care unit (ICCU)
- Respirators
- Cardiac pacemakers
- Surgical removal of diseased organ, and
- Dialysis

Components of Prolongation of Life
- Enhancing life expectation in years with interventions
- Keeping more person years in good health with interventions
- Enhancing validity years with intervention.

Ethical Issues Related to Prolongation of Life
- Right to die with dignity
- Huge unbearable expenditure to the family no hope of benefit by prolongation
- Person remains unconscious for over 3 months even with life supporting systems
- Profession has no obligation to use extraordinary means of prolongation of life
- Lack of relatives and no care takers due to unexpected inability of near relatives
- Person who is physically and mentally handicapped and disabled.

ADVANCED LIFE DIRECTIVES

- *The living will*
  Declaration by a person giving future course of action. It is different from dying declaration.

❖ *Euthanasia*
Euthanasia is the act of deliberately ending the life of a patient which can be active or passive. By no means, it is looked upon as ethical. In another definition, euthanasia is "unethical procedure of taking life of a patient, with/without consent of the patient in irreversible or terminally-ill patients". The deliberate taking away of human life is a crime.

Euthanasia is of four types:

1. Active euthanasia	It is an act of commission to kill the suffering by a merciful act, e.g., poison injection
2. Passive euthanasia	Life sustaining measures are not allowed or terminated to kill the suffering by a merciful act
3. Voluntary euthanasia	Act done with the consent of the dying person
4. Nonvoluntary euthanasia	Act done without the consent of the dying person who is in coma

Mercy killing is not permitted by any law to cruelty of allowing suffering and slow death. No one can take off a human life under any circumstance, excepting war field situations. Taking life of a patient with/without consent of patient always amounts to unethical procedure.

❖ *Cancer and terminal care:* These are conditions which do not have reversal to normalcy at any professional cost.

DEATH AND DYING

Brainstem death is legal death and is consistent with ethics in unplugging of life supporting system and organ donation.

Modern medicine including intensive care does not accept the definition of death given by layman. By artificially maintaining a patient's vital function, such as respiration and heartbeat, it may be difficult to pronounce a patient really dead. There is certain ambivalence about death, such as pulling out the plug, spare parts surgery. The treating team mediates between death and life.

Use of life supporting systems, such as invasive hemodynamic monitoring image technology assessment, mechanical ventilators, renal support, and intensive care units involves bioethics under the law of fundamental right to refuse life supporting systems.

The right to die with dignity: Medical and bioethical code has always been for:
❖ Preservation of life
❖ No action in taking away life by any means
❖ No international uniform direction for termination of life of patient

Contrary to this, patient's bill of right justifies the right to die with dignity. He can refuse treatment, can refuse emergency surgery and can refuse life supporting systems.

The problems of right to die with dignity arise in cancer and terminal care of patient. He expects mercy killing which by no means is available legally.

PROFESSIONAL ETHICS

Professional ethics has moral principles which are guiding the professionals in their dealing with each other, with their patient, with their society and the government. Following are areas that are looked into by the professional ethics.
❖ Contract
❖ Confidentiality
❖ No fee splitting
❖ Rational use of drugs, and
❖ No over-investigating the patient

A code of conduct is made by norms and values from tradition and convention. This is to be followed by any profession, lest it may feel inadequate in discharging its duties and responsibilities. A code of conduct is a crossway of social regulation and is not equivalent to legislation. Code of conduct is a time honored social legislation in civil life.
❖ Atreya Anushasana
❖ Charaka Samhita
❖ Sushruta Samhita
❖ The Hippocratic Oath

Chapter 28: Medical Ethics

- The Indian Medical Degree Act 1916, as a regulatory body
- The IMC Act 1933 for safeguarding the status of medical education
- The Nuremberg code 1947
- The Dentist Act 1948
- The IMC Act 1956
- The MCI code of ethics 1980
- The WHO declaration of Geneva 1982
- International Code of Medical Ethics 1983
- The patient self-determination Act 1990
- The International Guidelines for ethical review of epidemic states
- The International Guidelines for ethical review of research involving human subjects.

RESEARCH ETHICS

This is the area which faithfully differentiates what is right or wrong in animal experiment and human experiment.

In animal experiment humaneness and other procedures are strictly followed. Early permission as per international committee on laboratory animals is required if they are to be sacrificed. Animal experiment with only tissues and organs is more advanced ethical issue.

Human experimentation should follow modified Helsinki declaration and should follow human experimentation protocol. Human volunteer research should be with informed consent. Drug trial has special ethical issue involved.

Research is an essential tool needed if at all there is progress anticipated in medical world. Medical research is carried out on animals and human beings apart from laboratory procedures in the laboratory. Thus, research ethics decide what is right and what is wrong in our doing in the name of research.

Human experiment is required to know physiological and pathological changes in health and disease. It also can show the impact of an intervention. In the present situation, all community measures are time tested as harmless procedures before they are taken on to community health services.

Research ethics denotes an area of delineating of doing right or wrong in professional activities.

Clinical case review, change of drug or therapy, allowing for additional investigations, selection of patients or volunteers for future observations, retrospective record review, experiments on animals followed by human experiments are the committed fields in research ethics.

Human Voluntary Research

This involves stringent rules which are regulated by national and international codes of conduct. In human voluntary research, we seek the benefit to the human subjects; we intend to have potential benefit to a group of patients and a long-term benefit to humanity; apart from getting a gain in human knowledge in the management of diseases and disabilities.

Human volunteer research is guided by the following ethical principles:
- Ethical consideration of research on the patient
- Medical confidentiality
- Informed consent
- Doctor and volunteer relationship
- Profession not doing anything for the sake of money.

Ethics Related to Human Immunodeficiency Virus/Acquired Immunodeficiency Syndrome (HIV/AIDS)

There is increase in seropositivity of HIV and acquired immunodeficiency syndrome (AIDS) cases which has made tremendous impact on ethical issues related to HIV/AIDS.

From 1980 to 2000, the development and progress in the field of HIV/AIDS is no doubt more than 100-fold. From 2000 to 2005, it further has developed another 100-fold. Enigma behind this disease being behavioral in nature has claimed top seat under communicable diseases of public health importance. There is an increase in the seropositive feature of HIV cases and AIDS cases, which has made a tremendous impact on ethical issues related to HIV/AIDS.

Major principles that guide the profession are:
- Compassion
- Confidentiality
- Element of informed consent
- Information
- Obligation to treat
- Respect for persons
- Solidarity, and
- Wellbeing or beneficence

Our working criteria toward decision relies upon gathering all scientific factors, all human factors, and all value factors. Decision shall be at alleviating pain and suffering and toward cure, in good faith and to the best of our ability.

Ethics Related with Cadaver for Dissection in Health Science Colleges

Ethical issue is associated with selling the dead body from graveyard, from medical college, transport or illegal commercial transaction of cadaver. News media is highlighting this unethical transaction from medical institutions. Police are intercepting vehicles carrying dead bodies sold for dissection in institutions.

In modern days, medical education is fast growing and request for dead body for dissection is there in all systems of medicine. There are about 5,924 health institutions which include more than 207 medical colleges and 163 dental colleges in the country. Most of the health science institutions require cadaver for learning activities. This need is increasing because of upcoming new medical and dental colleges. It is estimated that about 10–12 bodies per year are required for a medical college for dissection purpose.

Body may be donated if the person, at any time before his death, had expressed an intention in writing, in the presence of two or more witnesses, that his body or any part of it be given to an approved institution after his death for the purpose of conducting anatomical examination and dissection or other similar purpose.

AREAS OF ETHICAL INTEREST IN PRESENT DAY PRACTICE

- Ethical issue of symbols.
- Ethical issue of egg donation.
- Ethical issues of quality of syringes and needles.
- Ethical issue of pushing for cheaper drugs.
- Ethical issue in intracytoplasmic sperm injection technique.
- The emerging focus on the quality of end-of-life care and how to improve it.
- More controversy in euthanasia.
- Computer ethics
- Ethical issue of cyber crimes.
- Ethical standards for e-research
- Ethical issue of cross-cultural medical ethics.
- National security system and ethics.
- Ethical conduct of clinical research involving children.
- Ethics in digital dilemma.
- Ethics teaching: contempt of content.
- Components of an ethically valid informed consent for research.
- Ethically, it is not "nothing is lost" but it is "everything is lost" as far as stem cell research is concerned.
- Ethical issues with alternative medicine.

Five main areas are discussed below:

Ethical Issue of Symbols

A red cross on a white background is the most common symbol associated with medical profession. Anybody and everybody in the medical field–be it a hospital, an ambulance, a doctor are found proudly flaunting the sign. But the original holder of the symbol. The Indian Red Cross Society has now objected to the abundant use of the symbol.

The symbol is for the International Red Cross Society only. For doctors, for hospitals, and for an ambulance there are internationally acknowledged distinctive signs. Hence, ethically Red Cross has to be used only by the Red Cross Societies and by Army Medical Corps. This has been directed by Secretary General of Indian Red Cross Society (IRCS) also.

Indian Red Cross Society (IRCS) has already taken up the matter with the center following which the drug controller of India has issued a circular to pharmacies to use their own symbol which is a green cross.

Misuse of the emblem has many times put IRCS in an awkward position particularly when it served people in conflict zones of Jammu and Kashmir, and the North East. Even during the riots, people have used the symbol in a manner and spirit which is not in conformity with the Red Cross Motto of absolute neutrality.

The Geneva Conventions make misuse of the Red Cross emblem a punishable offense. The punishment includes a fine of Rs. 500 and forfeiture of the goods or vehicles on which the emblem has been used.

The correct use of symbol for Red Cross, for a doctor, for a hospital, for an ambulance, and for pharmacy is shown in **Figure 28.1**.

Ethical Issue of Pushing for Cheaper Drugs

Protecting public health is the key priority and the World Trade Organization rules on intellectual property must not be allowed to endanger that.

There is a need for some measures on compulsory licensing, parallel imports, to locally produce medicine, to locally import medicine in spite of their patented nature. The TRIPS, The trade related intellectual property rights could not do its best in spite of good effort in the control of pushing for cheaper drugs.

Ethics lies in the fact that prices are hiked on drugs due to patents. Demands from developing countries are growing concern on how medicine prices are shooting up because of patents. The concern turned to outrage when drug companies and the USA government took action against developing countries that were trying to make medicines more affordable. The European Union appears to be more amenable to the developing countries' position.

Can governments override full patient rights by taking measures such as compulsory licenses and parallel imports to provide cheaper medicines to the public? This is debated hotly under the ethical issue of pushing for cheaper drugs.

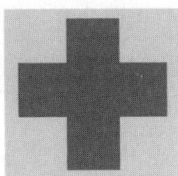
Red Cross symbol; this can be used only by Red Cross Movement members and Army Medical Corps

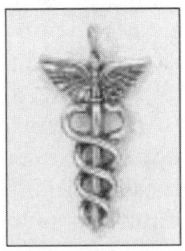
This symbol can be used by the doctor

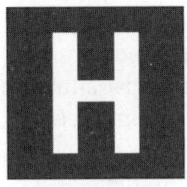
This symbol can be used by a hospital

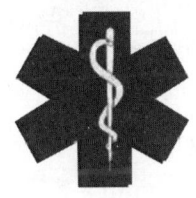
This symbol can be used by an ambulance

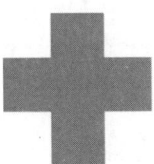
This symbol can be used by pharmacy

Fig. 28.1: Can use and cannot use about symbol by doctor.

More Controversy in Euthanasia

Doctors are sedating many terminally-ill patients until death. In some cases without artificial feeding or without hydration.

However, these do not come under mercy killing. Researchers estimate that terminal sedation occurred in about 10% of the total deaths in a given year.

As sedation is considered normal medical treatment, doctors are not legally obliged to report their actions as they must in euthanasia. But terminal sedation is now seen as an alternative to euthanasia for many Dutch patients.

First intension must be to alleviate symptoms. But how to exclude the explicit intension to hasten death? Ethically, terminal sedation is defined as "the administration of drugs to keep the patient in deep sedation or coma until death without giving artificial nutrition or hydration".

Doctors almost always discussed treatment with relatives, but not always with patients who were often no longer able to communicate.

According to Professor Van der Maas, ensuring that a dying patient remains asleep until death—mostly by giving benzodiazepines or combining these with morphine—had more or less become established medical practice. According to them, it is relevant alternative to euthanasia for suffering unbearably. But, all emphasize that the primary intension in most cases was alleviating symptoms not shortening life.

All are requesting for clear professional guidelines to define terminal sedation. Involving of the legal profession in a normal medical practice is a frightening prospect according to them!

Components of an Ethically Valid Informed Consent for Research

For an informed consent to be ethically valid, the following components must be present.

Informed consent is required by law. "no investigator may involve a human being as a subject in research covered by these regulations unless the investigator has obtained the legally effective informed consent of the subject or the subjects legally authorized representative".

The potential participants must be given the opportunity to give full consideration regarding the decision whether or not to participate in the research study without undue influence from his/her physician, family or the scientific investigator. No informed consent may contain any exculpatory language by which the participant waives any legal rights or releases the investigator or sponsor from liability for negligence.

As a general rule, deception is not acceptable when doing research with humans. This deception jeopardizes the integrity of the informed consent process and can potentially harm participants.

Routine educational experience constitutes simple study and is eligible for exempt status from obtaining approval.

Disclosure: The potential participant must be informed as fully as possible of the nature and purpose of the research, the procedures to be used, and the expected benefits to the participant and/or society, the potential of reasonably foreseeable risks, stresses, and discomforts and alternatives to participating in the research. There should also be a statement that describes procedures in place to ensure the confidentiality or anonymity of the participant. The informed consent document must also disclose what compensation and medical treatment are available in the case of a research-related injury. The document should make it clear whom to contact with questions about the research study, research subjects' rights and in case of injury.

Understanding: The participant must understand what has been explained and must be given the opportunity to ask questions and have them answered by one of the investigators. The informed consent document must be written in lay language, avoiding any technical jargon.

Voluntariness: The participant' consent to participate in the research must be voluntary, free of any coercion or promises of benefits unlikely to result from participation.

Competence: The participant must be competent to give consent. If the participant is not competent due to mental status, disease, or emergency, a designated surrogate may provide consent if it is in the participant's best interest to participate. In certain emergency cases, consent may be waived due to the lack of a competent participant and a surrogate.

Consent: The potential human subject must authorize his/her participation in the research study, preferably in writing, although at times an oral consent or assent may be more appropriate.

Ethical Issues with Alternative Medicine

Following alternate medicines have found their place that are totally accepted by the community and praised by the ancestors for their accessibility, affordability and simplicity, and naturality.

- Ayurveda
- Unani
- Siddha
- Homeopathy
- Naturopathy
- Herbal medicine
- Yoga
- Massage
- Acupuncture
- Magnetotherapy

Allopathic or modern medicine has become expensive, not natural and cannot give relief in many illness; has runs into dissatisfaction with the people. Both trained and untrained persons are trying the alternate medicine and thus are attached with quackery.

Value assessment is required in alternative therapies. Can this be done in a healthy attitude? Ethically, standards and qualifications of doctors in alternate medicine are to be insisted. If inappropriate preparations are used to treat, what could be the ethical value of alternate medicine?

Allopathic practitioner practicing with alternative medicine and vice versa is unethical. Indiscriminate use of modern medicine and allopathic medicine are producing adverse results.

Ethical correction was sought by the integrated medicine training and practice but has not been successful.

On one side Government of India is promoting Indian system of medicine. On the other side knowledge and ethics of its practitioners is ethically questionable. Ethical problem also exists with the poor inter-professional relationship.

With high acceptance and respect of Indian people, Indian system of medicine should be streamlined with good ethical, moral, social aspect through Central Council of Indian Medicines and Central Council of Homeopathy which can regulate the practitioners.

SUMMARY

Heterogeneous and Autonomous Ethics are described. Ethics of individual, Organ donation, Ethic of human life description is followed. Cloning and gene therapy are highlighted. A note on Death and Dying is also given. Areas of ethical Interest in Present Day Practice are highlighted.

VIVA VOCE

1. What are the merits of medical ethics?
2. What are the major principles of medical ethics?
3. Specify requirements in organ donation.
4. What is cloning?
5. Define professional ethic.
6. What is euthanasia?

Public Health Law

CHAPTER 29

CHAPTER OUTLINE

- Troubling Problems in Medical Ethics
- Legal Rights and Responsibilities in Modern Medicine
- Health Law in India
- Major Acts
  - IFA 1948 (Act LXIII of 1948)
  - The Food Act 1954 (Amended 1986)
  - The Drug Act 1940
  - State Public Health Act
  - Karnataka Private Nursing Home (Regulation) Act 1976
  - Municipal Act (1964)
  - Population Law (1974)
  - The MTP Act 1971 (Medical Termination of Pregnancy)
  - The Environmental Law

INTRODUCTION

Legislation in health field is mainly to execute health services and family welfare services through an established and recognized organization.

Planning, execution and evaluation depends upon health law existing in the area.

Public health law depends on:
- Social values
- Social standards
- Interprofessional relationship
- Local government.

Public health law comprises of:
- **Health law**
  - Dealing rights and duties
  - Legal Acts
  - Legal procedures
  - Jurisprudence
- **Health ethics**
  - Social and individual values
  - Religion
  - Health philosophy
- **Doctor and patients**
  - Performance of medical Act
  - Privacy
  - Confidentiality
  - Right to refuse
  - Social regulations
  - Malpractice

Legal Aspect in Public Health

- **In curative care:**
  - Efficiency
  - Emergency
  - Infectious case
  - Organ transplant
  - Blood transfusion
  - Surgery and anesthesia
  - Psychiatric management
  - Autopsy
  - Drug reaction, shock, sudden death
- **Professional duties in social work:**
  - Fitness in occupation
  - Medical certification
  - Court witness
  - Blood test
  - Treatment of prisoners, hunger strikers.
- **In preventive activities:**
  - Immunization

- Mass screening
- Hotel closure, cinema house inspection, market inspection, slaughter house sanitation.
- Limiting commercial activity
- Limiting religious activity.
- **In coverage of risk, benefit, injury.**

TROUBLING PROBLEMS IN MEDICAL ETHICS

- Affirmative action in medical school admission.
- Drug testing in prison (sociological, penological and constitutional characteristics).
- Treating children without parental consent.
- Right to refuse treatment.
- Right to privacy when lives are at stake, e.g., organ donation.

LEGAL RIGHTS AND RESPONSIBILITIES IN MODERN MEDICINE

- Defective newborn to die
- Paternalism
- Animal experiment
- Religion and family planning
- Great suffering to die
- Artificial insemination by husband (AIH) and artificial insemination by donor (AID).

HEALTH LAW IN INDIA

- **Before Independence:**
  1825: The Quarantine Act promulgated
  1973: The Birth and Death Registration Act promulgated
  1880: The Vaccination Act passed
  1881: The Indian Factory Act passed
  1897: The Epidemic Disease Act promulgated
  1920: Municipal Act passed
  1930: Sharada Act came into effect
  1940: The Drug Act passed.
- **After Independence:**
  1954: PFA Act passed
  1956: SITA Act passed [Now, Immoral Traffic (Prevention) Act, 1986]
  1969: The Central Births and Deaths Registration Act promulgated
  1970: The Drugs (Price Control) Order promulgated.
  1971: MTP Act passed
  1975: ESI Act amended
  1976: IFA amended, PFA amended
  1981: Air Prevention and Control of Pollution Act was enacted
  1984: The ESI Bill approved; the Workmen Compensation Act came into force; the Juvenile Act came into force
  1985: The Lepers Act repealed
  1986: The Environment (Protection) Act promulgated and the Juvenile Justice Act, 1986, came into force
  1987: The Factory Act, 1987 operated
  1989: The ESI Act, 1989 operated
  1992: The infant milk substitute, feeding bottle and infant foods (Regulation of Production Supply and Distribution) Act, 1992, came into force
  1994: The Panchayat Raj Act came into force
  1995: The Organ Donation Act enacted
  1996: The Prenatal Diagnostic Technique Act came into force.
  2003: The Preconception and Prenatal Diagnostic Technique (Prohibition of Sex Selection) (PC-PNDT) Act, 2003.

MAJOR ACTS

- **Central Act:**
  - IFA
  - The Food Act, and
  - The Drug Act
- **State Act:**
  - PH Act and
  - Nursing Home Act.
- **Local Self-government Act:** Municipal Act.

The Factory Act, 1948 (Act LXIII of 1948) (Amended 1987)

This Act is applicable to any establishment with 10 or more workers employed where power is used. It details health, safety and welfare in III, IV and V chapters; working hours of adults are given in chapter VI; prohibition of child employment below 14 years and related to employment of young persons is dealt in chapter VII. This Act also deals with:

(a) power to require medical examination, and (b) power to make rules. There are 17 main lists of notifiable diseases which include lead poisoning, mercury poisoning and silicosis.

The Food Act, 1954 (Amended 1986)

"The Prevention of Food Adulteration Act" to make provision for prevention of adulteration of food was enacted by the Indian Parliament in 1954. This Act makes provisions uniform, broad-based and more deterrent to some of the lacunae in existing food laws of states and municipalities.

The consumer and voluntary organizations have been empowered under the Act to have sample of food analyzed by giving notice to the vendor.

For a case of proven order, a fine of ₹1,000 and 6 months' imprisonment is allowed for adulteration.

With Amendment (1986), the consumer and voluntary organization have been empowered to take samples of food.

The Drug Act, 1940

This Act envisages the regulation of import, manufacture, distribution and sale of drugs.

State Public Health Act

Based on legal provisions of Municipalities and Local Boards Act of 1920, Government of India made a draft model of PH Act for the country. This was adopted in the states of Chennai, Mumbai, Mysuru and Hyderabad in the year 1920, 1921, 1933 and 1956, respectively.

Main areas under Public Health Act are:
- Water supply
- Sewage board
- City improvement board
- Town planning
- Dangerous diseases
- Notifiable diseases
- Food establishments
- Entertainment taxation
- Swimming pools
- Central Acts through state from time to time.

Karnataka Private Nursing Home (Regulation) Act, 1976

This came into force with effect from 1-1-1977. Main idea was to bring uniformity in the fee charging and accessibility of service to all.

The Act makes the following mandatory:

Accommodation
- Waiting room 100 sq ft
- Examination room 15 sq ft
- OT 250 sq ft
- Wards 20 sq ft per person
- Labor room 150 sq ft

Staff
- 25 beds/doctor
- 50 beds/2 doctors
- 20 beds/doctor (for the remaining)
- 1 pharmacist
- 1 laboratory technician
- 1 X-ray technician
- 1 assistant/nurse for 20 beds

Facility
- For outpatient departments (OPD) and inpatient departments (IPD)., for examination, linen, bed sheet, bed pan, etc.

Fee
- Consultation fee per visit ₹30
- Later visit ₹10
- General duty doctor fee ₹5 per visit.

Procedure
- There are 438 procedures under medicine, surgery, obstetrics and gynecology with stipulated fees.

Some of the examples are:

Tumor removal skin	75.00
Minor OT	75.00
Thyroidectomy	300.00
Piles injection	75.00
Hemorrhoidectomy	400.00
Breast removal	500.00
Hip replacement	3,300.00
Mandibulectomy	600.00

Chapter 29: Public Health Law

Laboratory Investigations

All blood tests	40.00
Urine test	3.00
Stool test	3.00

Inspection fee for 20 beds and above is ₹100.00.

Inspection fee for no bed hospital and clinic is ₹10.00.

Inspection done for sanitation, staff, facilities, and accommodation.

License is to be obtained in January every year in prescribed form.

Penalty of ₹1000, 3–6 months imprisonment, for hospitals above 20 beds not fulfilling requirement, and ₹250 penalty to clinic (with no beds) for not fulfilling the mentioned requirements.

Municipal Act (1964)

Karnataka Municipality Act (1964) similar to other State Municipal Acts was amended from time to time.

This contains the following:
- Water supply
- Building sites, building works
- Drains, privies, other receptacles for filth
- Restrain of infection
- Registration of births, deaths, disposal of dead, and
- Removal of sewage, rubbish and offensive matters.

Karnataka Municipal Act of 1976 under chapter 18 and section 401 to 420 details the procedure of prevention of diseases.

Population Law (1974)

Based on human right law, it covers privacy, family, home, correspondences and health.

Abortion surveillance and policy liberalization is:
- Not permitted in civil law, e.g., Ireland, Philippines, Francophone and Africa.
- Permitted on medical ground: Saudi Arabia, Somalia and Spain.
- Permitted on medicosocial and ethical grounds
  - Common law countries.
  - Commonwealth countries.
- Permitted on social and economic grounds: Finland, India, USA.
- At the request of pregnant mother: Hungry, erstwhile Zeck, Japan.

Following global indicators are used in abortion surveillance:
- Rate of legal abortion in female of 15–45 years of age.
- Rate of legal abortions in relation to normal deliveries.

The MTP Act, 1971 (Medical Termination of Pregnancy)

This lays down the conditions, persons to perform and place to perform for MTP.

Indications

Medical	–	When pregnancy causes injury or death to mother
Eugenic	–	When abnormal growth is established
Humanitarian	–	When rape has caused pregnancy
Socioeconomic	–	When socioeconomic cause can lead to death or injury to mother
Failure of contraceptive	–	Failed FP methods causing pregnancy

Written consent of guardian when pregnant woman is lunatic or minor is a requirement.

Person to Perform MTP

By Registered Medical Practitioner (RMP), if below 12 weeks, who has an experience in Obstetrics and Gynecology (OB/GYN).

By 2 RMPs' opinion, if above 12 weeks, who have an experience in OB/GYN.

Place to Perform MTP

It must be in a hospital, health center or any approved place.

Following amendments are done in 1975 in MTP:

- DH and FWO can certify a doctor to conduct MTP.
- An RMP who conducts 25 MTPs in a hospital is permitted to conduct MTP.
- Experience in OB/GYN means:
  - 6 months' house surgency in OB/GYN.
  - PG in OB/GYN.
  - RMP of before 1971 needs 3 year OB/GYN practice.
  - RMP of after 1971 needs 1 year OB/GYN practice.
- DH and FWO can certify place of conducting MTP.

Thus, MTP is a safe, legal abortion made universally available for family planning in the country.

The Environmental Law

This covers nuclear installation, marine pollution, statutory nuisance of noise and air pollution, water supply, waste disposal, housing, food safety.

Public health law has the following major tasks in the coming centuries:
- Interrelationship of poverty and disease.
- Sanitation as a part of legal program.
- The program of technical assistance.

SUMMARY

In the beginning, Troubling Problems in Medial Ethic are given. Legal rights and responsibilities in Modern Medicine are described. Health Law in India is described. Major Acts in Vogue are described.

VIVA VOCE

1. Tell about IFA.
2. What is nursing home Act?
3. Mention amendments in MTP.

SECTION 10

Section Outline

Chapter 30. Essential Medicine
Chapter 31. Rational Drug Management
Chapter 32. Health Information System

Essential Medicine

CHAPTER OUTLINE

- Criteria for Inclusion of a Medicine in National List of Essential Medicine
- Criteria for Deletion of a Medicine from NLEM
- History
- Uses of Essential Medicine
- National List of Essential Medicines (NLEM) 2015

DEFINITION

As per the WHO, essential medicines are those that satisfy the priority healthcare needs of the population. The list is made with consideration to disease prevalence, efficacy, safety and comparative cost-effectiveness of the medicines. Such medicines are intended to be available in adequate amounts, in appropriate dosage forms and strengths with assured quality. They should be available in such a way that an individual or community can afford.

Examples

Following are recommended essential drugs:
- Oxygen—medicinal gas
- Phenobarbitone tablet—anticonvulsant
- Mebendazole tablet—anthelmintic
- Trimethoprim tablet—antibacterial
- Metronidazole tablet—antiamebic
- Chloroquine tablet—antimalarial
- Digoxin tablet—cardiac glycoside
- Norethisterone tablet—hormone
- Chlorpromazine tablet— psychotic drug.

Ministry of Health and Family Welfare, Department of Health Research, ICMR, AIIMS jointly prepared National list of essential medicine in 2015.

CRITERIA FOR INCLUSION OF A MEDICINE IN NATIONAL LIST OF ESSENTIAL MEDICINE

- The medicine should be approved/licensed in India.
- The medicine should be useful in disease which is a public health problem in India.
- The medicine should have proven efficacy and safety profile based on valid scientific evidence.
- The medicine should be cost-effective.
- The medicine should be aligned with the current treatment guidelines for the disease.
- The medicine should be stable under the storage conditions in India.
- When more than one medicine are available from the same therapeutic class, preferably one prototype/medically best suited medicine of that class to be included after due deliberation and careful evaluation of their relative safety, efficacy, cost-effectiveness.
- Price of total treatment to be considered and not the unit price of a medicine.

- Fixed dose combinations (FDCs) are generally not included unless the combination has unequivocally proven advantage over individual ingredients administered separately, in terms of increasing efficacy, reducing adverse effects and/or improving compliance.
- The listing of medicine in NLEM is based according to the level of health care, i.e., Primary (P), Secondary (S) and Tertiary (T) because the treatment facilities, training, experience and availability of healthcare personnel differ at these levels.

CRITERIA FOR DELETION OF A MEDICINE FROM NLEM

- The medicine has been banned in India.
- There are reports of concerns on the safety profile of a medicine.
- A medicine with better efficacy or favorable safety profiles and better cost-effectiveness is now available.
- The disease burden for which a medicine is indicated is no longer a national health concern in India.
- In case of antimicrobials, if the resistance pattern has rendered a medicine ineffective in Indian context.
- There were 348 medicines listed in NLEM 2011. A total of 106 medicines have been added, and 70 medicines have been deleted to prepare NLEM 2015 which now contains a total of 376 medicines.

HISTORY

1970	Tanzania listed essential drugs
1975	WHO prepared preliminary list
1977	WHO listed 186 essential medicines
1985	Guided procurement, distribution, rational use and quality assurance
1996	Total 279 medicine listed
2015	Total 376 medicine listed

USES OF ESSENTIAL MEDICINE

- Guide safe and effective treatment of priority disease conditions of a population
- Promote the rational use of medicines
- Optimize the available health resources of a country. It can also be a guiding document for: State governments to prepare their list of essential medicines
- Procurement and supply of medicines in the public sector
- Reimbursement of cost of medicines by organizations to its employees
- Reimbursement by insurance companies
- Identifying the 'MUST KNOW' domain for the teaching and training of healthcare professionals.

NATIONAL LIST OF ESSENTIAL MEDICINES (NLEM) 2015

Section 1: Anesthetic agents.

Section 2: Analgesics, antipyretics, nonsteroidal anti-inflammatory medicines, medicines used to treat gout and disease modifying agents used in rheumatoid disorders.

Section 3: Antiallergics and medicines used in anaphylaxis.

Section 4: Antidotes and other substances used in poisoning.

Section 5: Anticonvulsants/Antiepileptics.

Section 6: Anti-infective medicines.

Section 7: Antimigraine medicines.

Section 8: Antineoplastic/immunosuppressives and medicines used in palliative care.

Section 9: Antiparkinsonism medicines.

Section 10: Medicines affecting blood.

Section 11: Blood products and Plasma substitutes.

Section 12: Cardiovascular medicines.

Section 13: Medicines used in dementia.

Section 14: Dermatological medicines (Topical).

Section 15: Diagnostic agents.

Section 16: Dialysis solutions.

Section 17: Disinfectants and antiseptics.

Section 18: Diuretics.

Chapter 30: Essential Medicine

Section 19: Ear, nose and throat medicines.
Section 20: Gastrointestinal medicines.
Section 21: Hormones, other endocrine medicines and contraceptives.
Section 22: Immunologicals.
Section 23: Muscle relaxants and cholinesterase inhibitors.
Section 24: Medicines for neonatal care.
Section 25: Ophthalmological medicines.
Section 26: Oxytocics and antioxytocics.
Section 27: Psychotherapeutic medicines.
Section 28: Medicines acting on the respiratory tract.
Section 29: Solutions correcting water, electrolyte disturbances and acid-base disturbances.
Section 30: Vitamins and minerals.

SUMMARY

Essential Medicine is defined. Criteria for inclusion of Medicine National List are described. Use of Essential Medicine is highlighted. National List of Essential Medicine is given.

VIVA VOCE

1. Define essential medicine.
2. What are the uses of essential medicine?

CHAPTER 31

Rational Drug Management

CHAPTER OUTLINE

- Types of Irrational Drug Use
- Drugs
  - Traditional Drugs
  - Modern Drugs
  - Complementary Drugs
- Prescription
- Compliance
  - Doctor Compliance
  - Patient's Compliance
  - Placebo
- Self-Medication
- Irrational Use of Drugs
- National Drug Policy
- Drug Economics

INTRODUCTION

Use of drugs has been for treatment of illness, relief of suffering and psychosociological satisfaction. Rational therapy depends on clinical trials, patient satisfaction, physician factors and evidence-based medicine and cost.

Rationale of Rational Treatment

❖ Meet real *medical need*, i.e., their use is likely to improve a particular health problem
❖ Be effective therapeutically, i.e., they must do what is claimed of them
❖ Be acceptably safe, i.e., their likely benefits should be outweighing their risks
❖ Offer good value for money, i.e., those that cost less and work as well as other drugs
❖ Be provided with adequate and clear information for optimal and safe use
❖ Be available and
❖ Be affordable.

Above demands are reasonable. They need radical changes in medical practice. Existing policy or actions are piecemeal. For example, essential drug program has however been instituted but unable to provide regular access to essential drugs to all **(Fig. 31.1)**.

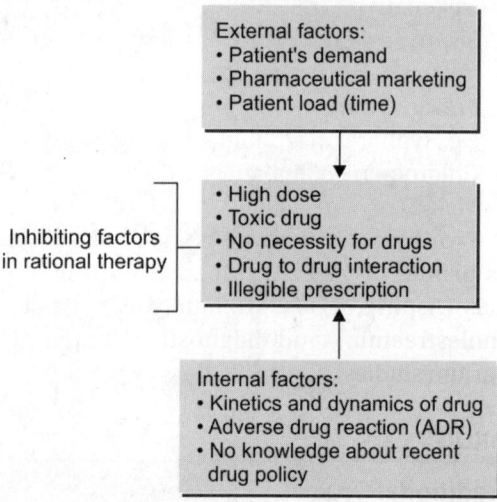

Fig. 31.1: Inhibition factors leading to rational drug management.

Chapter 31: Rational Drug Management

Present requirement for rational drug use are:
- Improvement in prescribing practice
- Educational reforms in health and pharmacy
- Balance between technology and humanity
- Reinforcement of social, cultural, economic and political dimensions
- Right dose of drug at right time, at right place, right duration and proper route
- Benefit versus risk
- Efficacy versus safety.

TYPES OF IRRATIONAL DRUG USE

1. Incorrect prescription
2. Overprescription
3. Multiple prescription
4. Underprescription
5. Improper combinations

Principle Ways to Drug Use

a. Primary therapy for cure
   e.g., Chloramphenicol in typhoid curative (present trend)
   e.g., Ciprofloxacin in typhoid
b. Secondary therapy for auxiliary treatment (palliative)
   e.g., General anesthesia (GA) for surgery, oxytocin in OB/GYN.
c. Suppressive therapy for maintenance treatment, e.g., metoprolol in hypertension.
d. Preventive therapy for protective treatment
   e.g., typhoral in typhoid endemic area
   Chloroquine in malaria area
   Mala D in married life.

Prophylactic therapy is also classified as primary (Oral contraceptives), secondary (Aspirin in post MI, Lipolytic in hypercholestraemia), and diagnostic (Barium in Barium studies).

DRUGS

Traditional Drugs

They are medicaments being used since olden times. It varies from no use to effective remedy. In all, they are cost-effective and are distributed in many systems called traditional medicine. They include Ayurveda, Unani, Siddha, Homeopathy, Anthroposophical medicine, Applied Kinesiology, Kirlian photography, Reflexology, Osteopathy, Chloropractice, Impact therapy, Rolfing, Breathing, Cymatics, Psionics, Radiesthesia, Radionics, Orgone therapy, Pyramid therapy, Naturopathy, Dianetics, Interferential therapy, Aromatherapy, Flower therapy, Biochemics, Orthomolecular medicine, Bioenergetics, Enlightenment Intensive, Magnetotherapy, Gem therapy, Acupuncture, Hydrotherapy, etc.

Metallic powder (churna) in jaundice is not only harmful to liver but also useless; on the other hand, Foxglove preparation (Digitalis) in heart disease: Cinchona bark extract (Quinine) in malaria: *Rauvolfia serpentina* (*sarpagandha*) extract (Reserpine) in hypertension even today are effective remedies. England venture on digitalis, South American venture on quinine and Indian venture in reserpine are gems in therapy.

Thus, task of science is to find out gems in traditional medicine and to discard the dross.

Modern Drugs

General tendency is to explain harmful effects of modern drugs rather than their beneficial effects. We should agree that modern drug cures disease, but not the life expectation or death. Conspiracy between medical profession and pharmaceutical industry should be stopped and drug effects are not to be ignored or concealed. Low standard of prescribing should be changed to prescribing better. Modern drugs have become customary, used for maintenance (prolonged therapy) in the middle of their definite cure in known areas of therapy.

Complementary Drugs

Drugs are given on complementary basis which is a close attention to patient's personal feeling. Here, following cults exist.
- Very low scientific way of thinking
- Naive acceptance of anybody's said hypothesis
- Uncritical acceptance of causation.

The term complementary drug is used with an ambitious claim and preference given continuously. We see in homeopathy the revival of traditional drugs to adaptation of more modern cults. Homeopathic drugs are complementary medicine.

For economic reason, if scientific medicine is not accepted and if traditional drugs are removed, we can do nothing to certain sectors of population. Hence, government is supporting evaluation and encouragement to complementary drugs.

PRESCRIPTION

Time-tested scientific method of drug prescription is taught in pharmacology. But irrational drug management is upsetting correct way of drug prescription. Accurate diagnosis is a prerequisite for rational therapy, even though it has to be made with limited locally available resources. Rational drug prescription precedes good clinical history, skillful clinical examination, problem-oriented case records and judicious use of laboratory tests.

Following factors determine drug prescription.
- Choice of drugs
- Cost and range
- Trial and satisfaction can lead to habit
- Pharmaceutical marketing.

COMPLIANCE

Doctor Compliance

Compliance is not a concept for patients alone but doctors also have the duty to comply.
a. Not to be ignorant
b. Inform patients what they need to know
c. To warn hazards, and
d. Clear, legible and unambiguous prescription.
e. Update latest trend in therapy.

At any cost, it should not be for an effective marketing of drugs.

The interactions between doctor and patient should be used for a benefit. The empathy created could be used to enhance compliance with prescription, advice, reduce wastage, needless self-medication, education on drug role.

Other important ideas like prevention of disease, the self-limiting nature of common diseases and the value of simple home remedies (ORS, nutrition in diarrhea) could be given when interacting with patients.

Doctors' compliance also lies in drug history taking to overcome reactions, adverse effects, false results and residual effects.

Patient's Compliance

Getting nontherapeutic prescription for a benefit or advantage by a patient is disregarded. Because of noncomprehension of instructions, patient's compliance may be affected. Level of education and intelligence are not factors in patient's compliance. Undiscovered noncompliance can invalidate therapeutic trials.

Placebo

It is a vehicle for cure by suggestion and surprisingly found successful. All treatments carry placebo including surgery, psychotherapy, and physiotherapy. All treatments have psychological component whether to please (true placebo effect) or to vex (negative placebo effect). They are used for two purposes.
- Therapeutic trial (drug evaluation)
- Psychological therapy.

SELF-MEDICATION

For the people started caring for themselves because they do not want to feel unwell, pain, indigestion, nervousness, sleeplessness, cough, depression are common symptoms where "do-it yourself" (self medication) is practiced. Self- medication is blamed for drug abuse, drug resistance and drug-tolerance. Rational drug management does not advocate self- medication.

Prescribing, dispensing or verbally recommended drug by not authorized persons also constitute self-medication.

Recommendations by relatives or friends contribute to self-medication. Drugs may also be given by traditional practitioners, quacks or doled out by medical detail men as gifts or samples.

This area is treated as "inappropriate use of drugs in the community".

IRRATIONAL USE OF DRUGS

Risk in Irrational Use of Drugs

a. Adverse side reactions
   - Allergy
   - No pharmacological response
   - Side effects, and
   - Carcinogenicity.
b. Iatrogenic disorders (long-term NSAID in peptic ulcer, phenothiazine in Parkinsonism)
c. Drug reactions which can be unintentional or life threatening (β-blockers + calcium channel blockers)
d. Cost of treatment will increase
e. Treatment failure.

Risks to Irrational Drug Use can be Prevented

- Informed careful prescription
- Responsible prescription
- Better knowledge of disease
- Topical or local use when needed.
- Short list safe drugs
- Improve clinical skill
- CME on drug information
- Active involvement of pharmacist in health care system
- Banning unsafe and irrational combination through policy.

Injury in Irrational Use of Drugs

Injury by a drug is possible and the irrational use of drug precedes compensation for injured person. Following are the examples of injury in irrational use of drugs:
- Optic neuropathy by clioquinol,
- Oculomucocutaneous syndrome by practolol
- Phocomelia (seal-like extremities) by thalidomide
- Care in new drugs after trial and drug standardization procedure will take care of injuries in irrational use of drugs.

Hazards in Irrational Use of Drugs

- Long-term therapy called chronic pharmacology (renal damage, cancer growth in prolonged administration of drug).
- Resurgence of chronic disease (IHD, autoimmune disease)
- Metabolic change (Development of diabetes)
- Specific cell injury (retinal damage in phenothiazine).

Prevention of these hazards is possible by the following ways:
- Correct information to patients
- Understanding of drug (Pharmacology)
- Risk–benefit weighment.

Adverse Medical Cascade

Adverse medical cascade is a process in rational drug management. In rational therapeutics, there are a few positive processes that are dominated as negative reflections. They can be small errors in communication process between patient and doctors. On many occasions, this medical cascade becomes frustrating and uncontrollable situations. Progressive riskier course can lead on to unnecessary costlier interventions.

NATIONAL DRUG POLICY (FIG. 31.2)

The evolution of a national drug policy is the outcome or the identification of following areas:
- Essential drug listing
- Use of generic and not brand name
- Advertising and drug promotion
- Procurement, self-sufficiency
- Self-medication
- Basis for registration of pharmaceuticals
- Pricing

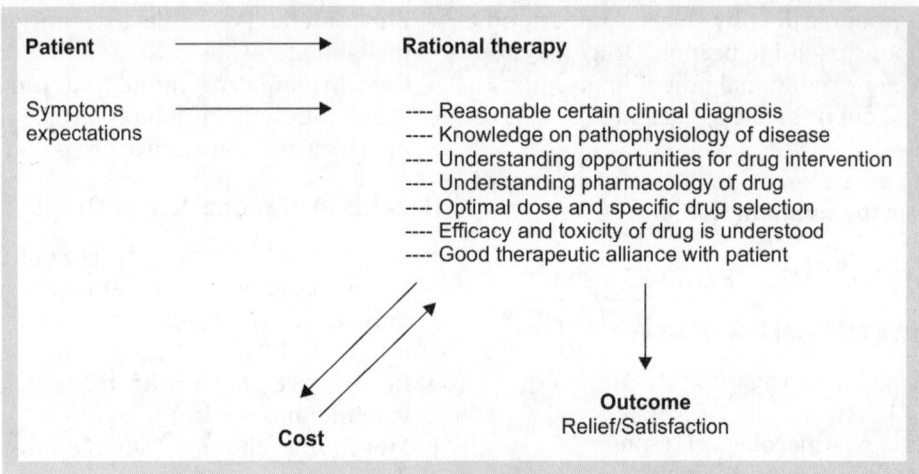

Fig. 31.2: Process of rational drug management.

- P drugs (personal drug or selected physician list).

Cardinal principles of rational drug policy are as given below:
- Tolerance
- Efficacy
- Safety
- Economy (cost)
- Accessibility.

These measures attempt to include concepts of rational drugs use, stop irrational drug prescription and will stop the doctors who have a tendency to prescribe one or more drugs that were rejected or withdrawn from the essential list.

National drug policy should have the priorities for: (a) Regulatory mechanism, (b) Manufacture of drugs, (c) Procurement of drugs.

DRUG ECONOMICS

Increasing attention is given to individual and community. Economy in drug management is individual sick role and community health service.

Wasteful prescribing is not advocated, prescription is an opportunity cost (cost spent not available again).

Cost effectiveness and cost benefit are looked in rational drug management.

Needs are defined and resources are deployed for a better person year in good health.

SUMMARY

Introduction to Rational Drug Management is given. A note on Prescription is detailed. Self-medication is highlighted. National Drug Policy is highlighted. A description of Drug Economics is given.

VIVA VOCE

1. What is irrational drug use?
2. Mention factors which determine drug prescription.
3. What is placebo?
4. Describe National Drug Policy.

32 CHAPTER — Health Information System

CHAPTER OUTLINE

- Qualities of Good Health Information System
- Components of Health Information System
- Uses of Health Information System
- Sources of Health Information System
- Recent Approach in Medical Informatics and Public Health Informatics

INTRODUCTION

Health statistics was given social and political value to be called *health intelligence*. But consolidated data is popularly known as *health information*. Health information of hospitals and institutions are referred to as *medical informatics*. But population-based data is becoming increasingly popular and is called *public health informatics*.

DEFINITION

Health Information

It is a mechanism for the collection, processing, analysis and transmission of information required for organizing and operating health services and also for research and training.

Public Health Informatics

It is the application of information on science and technology to public health practice and research.

Data

Attributes, variables, events or discrete observations.

Information

Reduced, tabulated and summarized data.

Intelligence

Information of social and political value.

QUALITIES OF GOOD HEALTH INFORMATION SYSTEM

- It should be population-based data
- The data should have a sensible correlation
- It should use operational terms and functional terms
- This should be along with data presentations by diagrams, figures and charts
- Data feedback should be possible.

COMPONENTS OF HEALTH INFORMATION SYSTEM

With the following components recommended by WHO, the health information system (HIS) becomes a comprehensive health information system.

- Vital events
- Demographic characteristics
- Health data like morbidity, mortality, disability, and quality of life
- Health resources like money, material and manpower
- Health service utilization, e.g., bed occupancy
- All health service outcomes, e.g., polio prevented, cure rate, etc.

USES OF HIS

- Health status of community is measured
- Healthcare need is assessed
- Health problems are identified
- Health status comparison is possible
- Planning, organizing, executing and evaluation are possible
- Impact of health services is assessed, and
- A tool for research activity.

SOURCES OF HEALTH INFORMATION SYSTEM

- Registration of vital events like live births, fetal deaths, marriages, divorces, adoptions, legitimating, annulments, recognitions and legal separations.
  1873 – Births, Deaths and Marriages Registration Act
  1969 – The Central Birth and Death Registration Act
  Of late – Lay reporting by Voluntary Health Guides
- *Notification of diseases*
  1897 – Epidemic Disease Act
  1930 – Madras Public Health Act
  International health regulations – cholera, plague, yellow fever.
  International surveillance – louse-borne typhus, relapsing fever, polio, influenza, malaria, rabies, salmonellosis.
  Notification of cancer, mental illness, congenital malformation, stroke, and handicap are extensions.
- *Census*
  Process of collecting, compiling, publishing demographic, economic and social data at a specified time covering all persons in a country.
  Started in 1881. Census is done once in 10 years. Latest was in the year 2001.
  1948 – Census Act was passed.
- *Sample registration system*
  1965 – Initiated. Dual record system by enumeration of births and deaths + half yearly survey as a check.
- *Hospital records*
  It forms an integral part of National Statistical Programme: but is not representative of Population. MRD in hospital is emphasized.
- *National Registry of Diseases*
  Established permanent record. Useful to know natural history of diseases. National registries for stroke, MI, cancer, blindness, congenital defects, congenital rubella, tuberculosis, leprosy are available.
- *Survey report*
  Survey of evaluation, investigation and administration. In survey, interview, health examination, record survey, mailed questionnaire are followed. Household survey, school children survey and occupational groups' survey are common sampling units.
- *Screening report*
  Screening is detailed in chapter 15.
- *Surveillance report.*
  Surveillance systems are set up for many diseases control program such as tuberculosis, leprosy, malaria, filaria, etc.
- *Statistics related to health*
  Demographic, economic, social security, etc.

RECENT APPROACH IN MEDICAL INFORMATICS AND PUBLIC HEALTH INFORMATICS

- Local area network (LAN)
- World wide web (www)
- National Library of Medicine (Medline)
- Environment and sick build (CDC and EPA)
- Morbidity and mortality (CDC Wonder). Successfully used and popular among systems are Epi Info, CDC Wonder and AIDS reporting system from CDC computer system.

SUMMARY

Quality and Components of Health Information System (HIS) is described. Use of HIS is highlighted. Sources of Health Information System are enumerated. Medical Informatics is described.

VIVA VOCE

1. What are the uses of Health Information system?
2. Which are the sources of Health Information System?

SECTION 11

Section Outline

Chapter 33. Recent Area of Interest in Community Medicine

CHAPTER 33: Recent Area of Interest in Community Medicine

Chapter Outline

- Acute Flaccid Paralysis (AFP) Surveillance
- Adverse Events Following Immunization (AEFI)
- Acquired Immunodeficiency Syndrome (AIDS) Day
- Acquired Immunodeficiency Syndrome (AIDS) Surveillance
- Anthrax–Bioterrorism
- Avian Influenza (Birds Flu, Avian Flu, or Fowl Plague)
- Ayushman Bharat Program
- Baby-Friendly Hospital Initiative (BFHI)
- Chikungunya Fever Epidemic
- Community Dentistry
- Community Ophthalmology
- Community Psychiatry
- Consumer Protection Act (COPRA)
- Dengue Burden in India: Recent Trends and Importance of Climatic Parameters
- Coronavirus Epidemic 2019–2020
- Desmotology
- Early Childhood Development (ECD)
- Emporiatrics
- Essential Drugs
- Family Medicine
- Genetic Engineering
- Global Warming
- Guinea Worm Disease Eradication: Indian Scenario
- Handigodu Syndrome (Endemic Familial Arthritis)
- Hospital Waste Management
- Hypothermia
- Intensive Pulse Polio Immunization (IPPI)
- Janani Suraksha Yojana
- Kangaroo Mother Care
- Leptospirosis: An Emerging Public Health Problem
- Medical Informatics
- Meta-analysis
- Millennium Developmental Goals
- National Days
- National Health Goals by 2015
- National Rural Health Mission (NRHM)
- National Sociodemographic Goals by 2010
- National Urban Health Mission (NUHM)
- National Health Policy (NHP) 2017
- Nipah Viral Infection
- National Institution for Transforming India (NITI) Aayog 2015
- Poison Control Information
- Portograph
- Postpartum Program
- Recent Global Tuberculosis (TB) Strategy
- Red Cross Day
- Rights of Persons with Disability Bill 2016
- Rome
- Sanitation at Fair, Festival, Pilgrimage
- Severe Malaria
- Social Accountability of Hospitals and Medical Colleges
- Social Marketing
- Sociometric Analysis
- Substance Abuse
- Sulabha Shauchalaya
- The Preconception and Prenatal Diagnostic Techniques (PC and PNDT)
- Trends in Recent Immunization
- Tribal Health
- Universal Declaration of Human Rights
- World Health Organization (WHO) Day
- Women's Hygiene Kit (WHK)
- Zika Viral Infection

ACUTE FLACCID PARALYSIS (AFP) SURVEILLANCE

The eradication of polio is based on our knowledge about polio, good effective vaccine and effective methods for the control. The surveillance is "Collection and analysis of data for action". We have passive surveillance and active surveillance carried by institutional and community-based surveillance. Acute flaccid paralysis (AFP) is defined as sudden onset of weakness and floppiness in any part of the body in a child before 15 years of age or paralysis in a person of any age in whom polio is suspected.

We have achieved highest vaccination coverage. We have successfully implemented nationwide mass immunization. Now, we have to strengthen the surveillance of acute flaccid paralysis so that all cases are detected, investigated and controlled.

AFP surveillance is carried out for all cases of AFP and not just for poliomyelitis (**Fig. 33.1**).

Acute Flaccid Paralysis (AFP) Case is Reported Positively

Institutional surveillance (hospital): By touring hospital, meeting with hospital staff, weekly hospital report is collected, verification of reporting is done, and feedback is provided.

Field and health centers [primary health center (PHC)]: DIO initiates the investigation of reporting, does 60 days follow-up and monthly reporting continued. Isolation of wild poliovirus from stool is the best way to confirm the diagnosis of paralytic poliomyelitis. For all AFP cases, two specimen should be collected within 2 weeks after the onset of paralysis, 24–48 hours apart (8 g of specimen is suggested), each specimen is given an EPID number and sent to laboratory for test. It takes 28 days to isolate and identify poliovirus.

Following program surveillance indicators help the ongoing AFP surveillance.
1. Rates of AFP.
2. Monthly negative reporting.
3. Percentage of AFP cases with two stools taken within 2 weeks after paralysis onset.

In India, AFP surveillance is practiced for detection of poliovirus transmission based on case reporting, investigation, stool collection and laboratory investigation at local, district, state, and national levels.

ADVERSE EVENTS FOLLOWING IMMUNIZATION (AEFI)

Vaccines used in National Immunization Program are made 100% proof for safety, efficiency and clarity. Even worldwide experience is

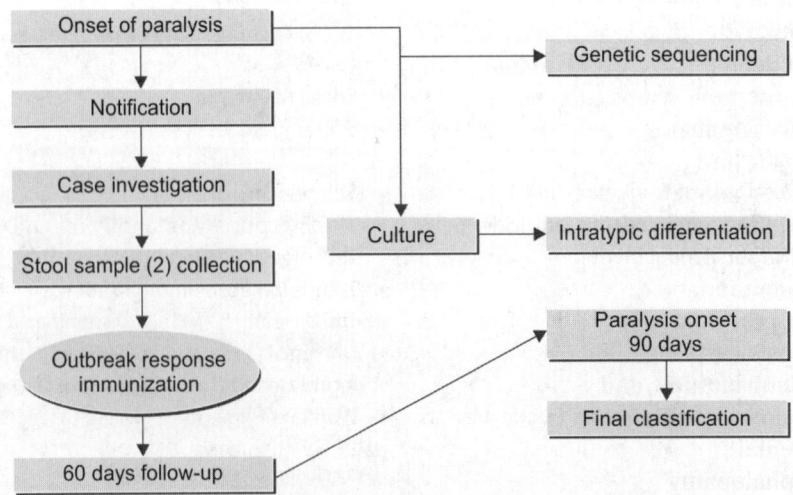

Fig. 33.1: Surveillance flowchart.

Chapter 33: Recent Area of Interest in Community Medicine

documented in this regard. In India, annual turnover of vaccine is 650 million doses and 500 million injections to women and children. Although, adverse events are rare, none is entirely without risk and occurrence of some severe adverse events. But the adverse events are minute in comparison with benefits of prevented illness, complication and deaths. They can be: (a) Vaccine reaction (b) Program error (c) Coincidental (d) Injection reaction or (e) Unknown.

India started monitoring of AEFI in 1985 with the following objectives:
a. To identify any programmatic error
b. To allay public fear
c. To provide moral support to health workers
d. To pool information on AEFI

Government has constituted experts from pediatrics, microbiology and community medicine for investigation of severe adverse events. Deaths following immunization, especially those that occur in clusters are expected to be investigated within 48 hours. State reproductive and child health (RCH) officer and minister of health and family welfare (FW) are required to be notified immediately in case of death following immunization.

Adverse Events Following Immunization (AEFI)

I. Inherent vaccine induced
   * Mild and common
     - Local reactions, fever and irritability
     - Moderately severe and uncommon
     - Suppurative lymphadenitis
     - Shock/collapse
     - Severe and rare
     - Encephalopathy
     - Hypersensitive reactions, and
     - Paralytic polio
     - Programmatic
     - Abscess
     - Sepsis
   * Drug substitution, and
   * Traumatic neuritis
II. Coincidental
   * Encephalopathy
   * Sudden infant death syndrome (SIDS)
   * Aspiration, and
   * Infections/antecedent illness

Measures to prevent AEFI due to programmatic errors:
1. Immunization session on scheduled day and no door to door vaccination.
2. Steam sterilization preferred over boiling for syringe and needle.
3. One syringe and one needle for one injection.
4. Measles vaccine should be used within 4 hours of reconstitution.
5. An opened vial of measles vaccine should never be reused.
6. Vaccine and drug must be separately kept.
7. Reporting of programmatic error like abscess should be compulsory by health worker.
8. Training for high quality of service.
9. Field monitoring and correction of deficiency should be in a timely manner.
10. Community pressure and demand for quality services should be promoted.

Events to be reported and investigated immediately	Events which are to be reported in the monthly reporting forms
Any death, hospitalization, disability or other serious illnesses	Persistent inconsolable screaming of more than 3 hours
And unusual events that are thought by health workers	Hypotonic hyporesponsive episode
Or, the public to be related to immunization	Severe local reaction
Anaphylaxis	Injection site abscess
Toxic shock syndrome	Seizures including febrile seizures
Anaphylactoid reaction	Brachial neuritis
Acute flaccid paralysis	Thrombocytopenia
Encephalopathy	Lymphadenitis
Sepsis	Disseminated BCG infection
Any event where vaccine quality is suspected	Osteitis/osteomyelitis
Any cluster of events	

(BCG: bacillus Calmette-Guérin)

ACQUIRED IMMUNODEFICIENCY SYNDROME (AIDS) DAY

Themes of World AIDS Day Celebrated on Every 1st December

Year	Theme
1988	Communication: Global mobilization against AIDS
1989	AIDS and youth
1990	Women and AIDS
1991	Sharing the challenge
1992	AIDS—a community commitment
1993	Time to act
1994	AIDS and the family
1995	Shared rights, and shared responsibilities
1996	One world, and one hope
1997	Children living in a world with AIDS
1998	Force for change—world AIDS campaign with young people
1999	Listen, Learn, Live—world AIDS campaign with children and young people
2000	AIDS—men make a difference
2001	I care, do you?
2002	Stigma discrimination and human immunodeficiency virus (HIV)/AIDS
2003	Stigma and discrimination: Live and let live
2004	Women, girls, and HIV
2005	Stop AIDS: Keep the promise—make the promise
2006	Stop AIDS: Keep the promise—accountability
2007	Leadership (stop AIDS. Keep the promise)
2008	Leadership (follow promises to stop the epidemic)
2009	Universal access and human rights
2010	Universal access to human rights
2011	Getting to zero
2012	Together we will end AIDS
2013	Zero discrimination
2014	Close the gap
2015	On the fast track to end AIDS
2016	Hands up for HIV prevention
2017	My health my right
2018	Know your status
2019	Communities make the difference

Red Ribbon of AIDS

This is an international symbol of AIDS awareness that is worn by people all year round and particularly around World AIDS Day to demonstrate care and concern about HIV/AIDS/and to remind others of the need for their support and commitment.

It is grass root effect. Any red ribbon and a safety pin will do the job.

AIDS Day Theme 2000
AIDS—men make a difference (2000)

The campaign aims at increasing the role that the men play in prevention of HIV/AIDS. Over 80% of HIV occurs through sexual relationship. Men have a larger influence in sexual relationships which make women particularly vulnerable. Experience in world has shown that when men are actively engaged in fighting HIV/AIDS they are able to change the course of epidemic. Concerted efforts can change men's behavior and change in behavior can contain the spread of the infection. Involving men more fully in efforts against HIV/AIDS therefore, can and will make a difference.

AIDS Day Theme 2001
"I Care, Do You?"

Awareness on determinants and distribution of HIV/AIDS is prime requisite in its control and prevention. Community should know about it, society should have awareness and thereby each unit of society shall have knowledge which influences our attitude and practice. The theme advocates to break silence to talk about it, it helps to keep HIV/AIDS at distance and not the patient, the reminiscence of the role of monogamy and safe sex.

It is caused by human immunodeficiency virus causing serious disorder of immunosystem causing life-threatening infections, including unusual malignancies. Sources are:
a. Heterosexual 74.2%
b. Not specified 10.1%

Chapter 33: Recent Area of Interest in Community Medicine

c. Intravenous (IV) drug users 7.1%
d. Blood 8.1%
e. Homosexual 0.5%

The agent lentivirus (subfamily retrovirus) with reverse transcriptase enzyme which copies ribonucleic acid (RNA) to deoxyribonucleic acid (DNA) which integrate to cell chromosome. Reservoir are patient and healthy carriers. Latent period 5-10 years. Definite sources are blood, semen, vaginal fluid; probable source is breast milk but saliva and tears are not a source.

Among patient, factors are: (i) age 15-24 years, (ii) 70% men, (iii) drug user and sexually transmitted diseases (STD) case are risk group, white cells below 500 per cubic mm and hyper-T cells (CD) do not assist B cells and antibody to fight infection are major pathologies.

Social factors are—acceptability of certain indigenous sex practices, war, civil disturbance, nonavailablility of interventions, social acceptance of condoms, status of women in society, ethnic practice such as circumcision, tattooing, sacrification, illiteracy, high mobility, migration, alcohol use, drug use, and development of high-risk behavior by urbanization.

Transmission occurs by sexual intercourse, blood transfusion, transplantation, IV drug use, mother to child transmission.

In man, stages such as primary, early immune, middle immune and late immune deficiency are seen.

Start taking care when:
a. Weight loss (below 10% without valid reason).
b. Fever over 4 weeks not responding to treatment.
c. Diarrhea over 4 weeks not responding to treatment.

AIDS Day Theme 2002
Stigma Discrimination and HIV/AIDS

Major obstacles to effective HIV/AIDS prevention and care are stigma and discrimination. Fear of discrimination prevents people from seeking treatment. They cannot acknowledge their HIV status publicly. HIV suspect will be turned away from health care services, he is denied housing and employment, they are shunned by their friends and colleagues, they are turned down for insurance coverage, and they are refused entry into foreign countries.

Eviction from homes, divorce from their spouses, suffer physical violence and even murder. Stigma and discrimination attached can extend into next generation and place emotional burden on children who are trying to cope with death of their parents.

AIDS Day can help in this issue of dimension of a difficult social issue. It is a unique challenge.

AIDS Day Theme 2003
Live and Let Live

HIV/AIDS pandemic presents area of the greatest medical and social challenges. AIDS has claimed 20 million. About 40 million are living with HIV.

About 2.3 million children are affected and 4.1 million are newly infected. Nearly, 50% of them die before they are 35 years of age.

AIDS Day focus to eliminate stigma and discrimination by helping to fight fear, ignorance and injustice in the world.

AIDS Day Theme 2004
Women, Girls, HIV and AIDS

About half of people living with HIV are female. Globally, women and girls are becoming infected with HIV at a faster rate than men and boys. Despite this alarming trend, women know less than men about how HIV/AIDS is transmitted and how to prevent infection and what little they do know is often rendered useless by the discrimination and violence they face.

Today there are 41 million living with HIV/AIDS. Theme focuses on Women, Girls HIV/AIDS. Empowering women in this struggle must be our strategy for the future. Our job is to furnish women and girls with hope.

AIDS Day Theme 2005
Stop AIDS (Keep the Promise: Make the Promise)

Goals and plans will be developed for progress toward acting universal access to treatment, care and prevention. Promises made for progress will be kept up and answered.

Slogan relating to accountability will be generated according to settings.

Encouragement for organizational and individual campaign promoting public awareness activities through local government.

Action on promise are done through coordinated approaches.

Promote and improve work role that local government can do to prevent and fight HIV/AIDS.

World leaders have promised to reduce number of young people with AIDS by 25% globally before 2010, in most affected countries by 2005, increase number of young people with access to information and education, to fight stigma and discrimination and to provide treatment to all needed.

AIDS Day Theme 2006

Stop AIDS: Keep the Promise–accountability

2006 theme focuses on accountability to keep up our promise of earlier years. This is based on all ongoing HIV/AIDS work around the world. We will account the inputs till date for overall civil society development.

The theme focuses on universal access to treatment, care of HIV/AIDS, prevention of HIV/AIDS and to set goals toward these objectives.

Red color is used in all promotional objects. The theme reinforces the notion of leader responsibility. Political leaders shall abide by enhanced accountability on their promises on AIDS. Creating awareness and engaging with AIDS problem go side by side. Local adaptation is done in accountability on HIV/AIDS.

The year is targeted for development of media on health education.

AIDS Day Theme 2007

Leadership (Stop AIDS. Keep the Promise)

Leaders are distinguished by their action, innovation and vision.

Leadership must be demonstrated at every level to get ahead of the disease—in families, in communities, in countries and internationally. Much of the best leadership on AIDS has been demonstrated within civil society organizations challenging the status quo. Making leadership as the theme of World AIDS Days will help encourage leadership on AIDS within all levels and sectors of society. We hope it will inspire and foster champions within a range of different groups and networks at local and international levels.

AIDS Day Theme 2008

Leadership (Follow Promises to Stop the Epidemic)

2008 World AIDS Day puts leadership in the spotlight; allowing everyone to follow through with their promises to stop the epidemic.

AIDS Day 2008 marks the 20th anniversary of World AIDS Day. Since 1988, efforts made to respond to the epidemic have produced positive results, however, the latest United Nations Program on HIV/AIDS (UNAIDS) report on the global AIDS epidemic indicates that the epidemic is not yet over in any part of the world.

Together with its partners, the World AIDS Campaign set this year's theme for World AIDS Day as "Lead-Empower --Deliver", building on last year's theme of "Take the Lead". Designating leadership as the World AIDS Day theme for 2007–2008 provides an opportunity to highlight both the political leadership needed to fulfill commitments that have been made in the response to AIDS—particularly the promise of universal access to HIV prevention, treatment, care and support by 2010 and celebrating the leadership that has been witnessed at all levels of society.

AIDS Day Theme 2009

Universal Access and Human Rights

World AIDS Day is important in reminding people that HIV has not gone away, and that there are many things still to be done.

According to UN AIDS estimates, there are now 33.4 million people living with HIV, including 2.1 million children. During 2008 some 2.7 million people became newly infected with the virus and an estimated 2 million people died from AIDS. Around half of all people who become infected with HIV do so before they are 25 and are killed by AIDS before they are 35.

The vast majority of people with HIV and AIDS live in lower- and middle-income countries. But HIV today is a threat to men, women, and children. Global leaders have pledged to work toward universal access to HIV and AIDS treatment, prevention and care, recognizing these as fundamental human rights. Valuable progress has been made in increasing access to HIV and AIDS services, yet greater commitment is needed around the world if the goal of universal access is to be achieved. Millions of people continue to be infected with HIV every year. In low- and middle-income countries, less than half of those in need of antiretroviral therapy are receiving it, and too many do not have access to adequate care services.

The protection of human rights is fundamental to combating the global HIV and AIDS epidemic. Violations against human rights fuel the spread of HIV, putting marginalized groups, such as injecting drug users and sex workers, at a higher risk of HIV infection. By promoting individual human rights, new infections can be prevented and people who have HIV can live free from discrimination.

AIDS Day Theme 2010

Universal Access and Human Rights

Understanding HIV and AIDS from a human rights perspective can be difficult. Human rights are often misunderstood With "Universal Access and Human Rights" being the theme of this year's World AIDS Day, the key slogans are:
   I am accepted.
   I am safe.
   I am getting treatment.
   I am well.
   I am living my rights.
   Everyone deserves to live their rights.
   Right to Live.
   Right to Health.

Access for all to HIV prevention, treatment, care and support is a critical part of human rights.

The 2010 World AIDS Day theme, "Universal Access and Human Rights," is highlighted in events around the globe For Rights campaign.

On World AIDS Day 2010, the events encourage 100 cities to dim the lights on public landmarks to remember the devastating affect AIDS has had, and then to turn the lights back on to illuminate the fundamental human rights shared by all.

AIDS Day Theme 2011

Getting to Zero

"Getting to Zero" is the theme selected by the World AIDS Campaign to commemorate this year's World AIDS Day on 1st December. The new theme, that will be used until 2015, echoes the UNAIDS vision of achieving "Zero new HIV infections. Zero discrimination. Zero AIDS-related deaths."

The decision to choose "Getting to Zero" as the theme came after extensive consultations among people living with HIV, health activists and civil society organizations.

It will focus on zero AIDS related deaths, but it is time to use our imaginations and let everyone know that getting to zero is a must.

AIDS Day Theme 2012

Together we will end AIDS

Getting to Zero: Zero new HIV infections. Zero deaths from AIDS-related illness. Together we will end AIDS is the theme of World AIDS Day 2012. Given the spread of the epidemic today, getting to zero may sound difficult but significant progress is underway. In 2011, 2.5 million people were newly infected with HIV. An estimated 1.7 million people died. That is 700 000 fewer new infections worldwide than 10 years ago, and 600 000 fewer deaths than in 2005. This burden require to put the efforts of all individuals together and work for getting zero discrimination.

AIDS Day Theme 2013

Zero Discrimination

Between 2011 and 2015, World AIDS Day has the theme: "Getting to zero: Zero new HIV infections. Zero discrimination. Zero AIDS-related deaths". The WHO's focus for the 2013 campaign is improving access to prevention, treatment and care services for adolescents (10–19 years). It is continued effort for zero discrimination.

AIDS Day Theme 2014
Close the Gap

On World AIDS Day 2014 WHO released new guidelines on providing antiretrovirals (ARVs) as an emergency prevention following HIV exposure, and on the use of the antibiotic co-trimoxazole to prevent HIV-related infections.

The guidelines provided advice on providing ARVs as postexposure prophylaxis ("PEP") for people who have been exposed to HIV—such as health workers, sex workers, and survivors of rape. In 2013, a record 13 million people were able to access life-saving ARVs.

But too many people still lack access to comprehensive HIV treatment and prevention services. The 1st December supplement to the WHO consolidated guidelines on the use of antiretroviral drugs for treating and preventing HIV infection, released in June 2013, aims to help bridge that gap.

AIDS Day Theme 2015
On the Fast Track to end AIDS

The world has come a long way since 2000, achieving the global target of halting and reversing the spread of HIV. New infections have fallen by 35% since 2000 and AIDS-related deaths by 24%. Some 16 million people are now receiving antiretroviral treatment.

But now it is time to act even more boldly, to take innovative steps so the world can meet the sustainable development goal target of ending the epidemic by 2030. This September, world leaders agreed ambitious interim targets to fast track efforts to end AIDS.

To help achieve these targets.

AIDS Day Theme 2016
Hands up for #HIV Prevention

Like every year, World AIDS Day 2016 will give an opportunity to speak out about AIDS, educate people about the condition, increase awareness, raise money for the cause and fight prejudice. Since the first HIV cases, 35 million people have died due to conditions related to AIDS and 78 million have been tested positive for HIV infection. So, although science has progressed and today we have a life-saving HIV treatment, AIDS is still winning. Thousands of people get infected with HIV each year, and there is no decline in the number of new HIV infection among adult. The risk of contracting HIV infection is high among young women and few communities like the gay community as there is a poor rate of testing for HIV, high-risk of HIV infection and adherence to the treatment is poor. So, for World AIDS Day 2016 the theme is Hands up for HIV prevention.

AIDS Day Theme 2017
My Health, My Right

The campaign, *My Health, My Right*, focuses on the right to health and explores the challenges of people around the world face in exercising their rights. "All people, regardless of their age, gender, where they live or who they love, have the right to health," No matter what their health needs are, everyone requires health solutions that are available and accessible, free from discrimination and of good quality."

The campaign reminds people that the right to health is much more than access to quality health services and medicines, that it also depends on a range of important assurances including, adequate sanitation and housing, healthy working conditions, a clean environment and access to justice.

Most of the sustainable development goals are linked in some way to health. To achieve the sustainable development goals, including ending the AIDS epidemic as a public health threat by 2030, will depend heavily on ensuring the right to health for all.

My Health, My Right encourages people to share their views and concerns around ensuring their own right to health and to create a movement highlighting the importance of erasing health inequalities. Campaign materials include suggested tweets, downloadable posters and postcards and an information brochure that includes key messages about the right to health.

Chapter 33: Recent Area of Interest in Community Medicine

AIDS Day Theme 2018
Know your Status

World AIDS Day 2018 theme encourages everyone to know their HIV status. This year's theme is "Know your status". Significant progress has been made in the AIDS response since 1988, and today three in four people living with HIV know their status. But, we still have miles to go, as the latest UN AIDS report shows, and that includes reaching people living with HIV who do not know their status and ensuring that they are linked to quality care and prevention services.

Unfortunately, many barriers to HIV testing remain. Stigma and discrimination still deter people from taking an HIV test. Access to confidential HIV testing is still an issue of concern. Many people still only get tested after becoming ill and symptomatic.

The good news is that there are many new ways of expanding access to HIV testing. Self-testing, community-based testing and multidisease testing are all helping people to know their HIV status.

AIDS Day Theme 2019
Communities make the Difference

It is an important opportunity to recognize the essential role that communities which play and continue to play in the AIDS response at the international, national, and local levels.

Communities contribute to the AIDS response in many different ways. Their leadership and advocacy ensure that the response remains relevant and grounded, keeping people at the center and leaving no one behind. Communities include peer educators, networks of people living with or affected by HIV, such as gay men and other men who have sex with men, people who inject drugs and sex workers, women and young people, counselors, community health workers, door-to-door service providers, civil society organizations, and grass-roots activists.

The theme highlight the role of communities at a time when reduced funding and a shrinking space for civil society are putting the sustainability of services and advocacy efforts in jeopardy. Greater mobilization of communities is urgently required to address the barriers that stop communities delivering services, including restrictions on registration and an absence of social contracting modalities. The strong advocacy role played by communities is needed more than ever to ensure that AIDS remains on the political agenda that human rights are respected and that decision-makers and implementers are held accountable.

AIDS SURVEILLANCE

Surveillance is the continuous scrutiny of factors involved in the distribution and trends of incidence of a disease through the systematic collection, consolidation and evaluation of mortality and morbidity and other relevant data. It must be linked with the system of feedback and action.

AIDS surveillance is collection of information on AIDS and STD for action on control of and prevention of AIDS infection in the community.

The surveillance of AIDS is mingled with STD by their nature of being transmitted by sexual route. It involves:
- The collection of data on the various types of STD
- The compilation of data collected
- The analysis of data
- Feedback and taking action based on surveillance data.

Etiological diagnosis is done at STD clinic and sentinel centers.

Syndrome approach: It is a method of management of STD patients where patient categorized to anyone of the following four syndromes on the basis of symptom or signs. They are:
  i. Genital ulcer
  ii. Urethral discharge
  iii. Vaginal discharge
  iv. Pain in lower abdomen

Following STD are kept in mind in etiological diagnosis:
- Syphilis
- Gonorrhea

- Chancroid
- Lymphogranuloma venereum (LGV)
- Herpes
- Pelvic inflammatory disease (PID)
- Chlamydia
- Candidiasis
- Tuberculosis (TB) infection, and
- Bacterial vaginosis.

Facility survey of STD clinics is done by covering the following areas:
- Practice of healthcare providers in STD clinics
- Interaction with healthcare providers
- Interview with patients
- Infrastructure and manpower.

ANTHRAX—BIOTERRORISM

By creating a dark sore on skin, it is named anthrax from Greek meaning coal. Bacteria called *Bacillus anthracis* causes anthrax which is carried by cow, sheep, goat, horse, and pig. Since centuries it is known in man and animal.

By nature of acquiring it can be: (a) cutaneous, (b) inhalational and (c) intestinal. A bacterium becomes tough coated spore when it comes in contact with air which can stay in soil for years.

Through liquids or powders it can be delivered as biological warfare agent. Hence, letter or pocket found doubtful in terms of—(a) title, (b) address, (c) unusual features such as discolored, unusual smell, unusual pack, protruded foil are to be identified as suspicious.

Table 33.1 gives the ways of handling suspicious packages.

Management of person who handled suspicious package include the following:
- No medication is needed
- No chemoprophylaxis till laboratory report is obtained
- If treatment started and laboratory test of package is negative, drug should be discontinued
- In case of laboratory test positive a course of drug is recommended.

Table 33.1: Showing how to handle intact and non-intact packages, which are suspicious.

In the case of intact package	In the case of nonintact package
• Not to get panic	• Do not clean the leak
• Should not open	• Switch off fans
• Should not smell	• Take bath with soap and water
• To be kept in another container	• List people in room plus
• Wash hands with soap and water in intact package	• Other precautions
• Inform police	
• Send sample to designated laboratory	

Drug Treatment

Ciprofloxacin, amoxicillin, and doxycycline are drugs of choice. Based on sensitivity, second line of treatment could be with chloramphenicol, erythromycin or aminoglycosides.

Treatment if Anthrax is inhaled

Adult including pregnant

Ciprofloxacin 400 mg IV every 12 hour for 60 days

Alternative
- Penicillin G 4 million units IV every 4 hours
- Streptomycin 1 g daily intramuscularly (IM) for 60 days.

Children

Ciprofloxacin 20–30 mg/kg/day in 2 hours (maximum dose 1.0 g).

Alternative
- Below 12 years—penicillin G 50,000 units/kg IV 6 hourly
- Above 12 years—penicillin G 4 million units IV 4 hourly

Note: Oral drug is substituted when clinical condition is improved.

In case of exposure to contaminated, proved positive in laboratory test, then a course of treatment is recommended which shall be as follows (all oral):

Adults including pregnant

Ciprofloxacin 500 mg orally 12 hourly for 60 days.

Children

Ciprofloxacin 20–30 mg/kg/day in 2 doses (max g) for 60 days.

Alternative
Amoxicillin 500 mg 8 hourly.
Or
Doxycycline 100 mg 12 hourly.
    Amoxicillin 500 mg 8 hourly for child above 20 kg.
    Amoxicillin 40 mg/kg in 3 doses 8 hourly for child below 20 kg.
    Amoxicillin 500 mg 8 hourly for pregnant women.

Vaccine Treatment

There is no human tested vaccine available at present. Hence, it is of no value as on today.

Confirmation of Anthrax

This can be done by laboratory test in teaching hospitals (medical colleges). Usually, 48 hours are required for confirmation by:
i. Direct examination under microscope
ii. Culture
iii. Polymerase chain reaction (PCR)
    In the absence of evidence of exposure, there is no need for investigation of persons. All suspected waste should be disinfected as under:
i. Autoclave
ii. Incineration
iii. 0.5% hypochlorite disinfection

Environmental Decontamination

This is done by 0.5% hypochlorite solution (one part bleaching powder to nine part of water).

Transport

Suspected samples should be transported as under:
- Labeling high risk
- Keep in screw tight container
- Separate bag for each sample
- Externally disinfected secondary container is used
- Later a sturdy tertiary container is used
- Labeled as:
  - Biohazard
  - Not to be opened
  - Reference laboratory address

Bioterrorism differ from natural outbreak as under:
- Occur in a discrete population with many diseases and death
- Unusual route of exposure present in unusual place by unusual vector
- Potential agents used will be:
  a. *Aerosol-spread:* Anthrax, plague, tularemia, smallpox, and ebola
  b. *Water-spread:* Enteric infection
  c. *Vector-spread:* Dengue, yellow fever

Counter Measure for Bioterrorism

Following counter measures are suggested:
- Early detection by epidemiological investigation
- Information and communication for preparedness and response capability
- Specified intelligence to prevent recurrence
- Punishment to terrorist to deter the Act of Bioterrorism.

AVIAN INFLUENZA (BIRDS FLU, AVIAN FLU, OR FOWL PLAGUE)

Avian influenza is a public health problem in Asia particularly in South East Asian countries. Hong Kong, China, Netherlands, Vietnam and Thailand have witnessed outbreaks of human diseases due to avian influenza viruses. These epidemics are seen associated with outbreaks of avian influenza in poultry caused by the same virus subtype.

Outbreaks of avian influenza in poultry coinciding with outbreaks of human disease due to avian influenza virus are also recorded in Hong Kong, Netherlands, Vietnam and Thailand. Primarily chickens are affected and mortality is recorded in terms of deaths of millions of chickens. Ducks, Geese, and Turkeys are also known birds to cause avian influenza.

The virus nomenclature is based on hemagglutinin "H"; Neuraminidase "N" and subtypes "B and "C" viruses.

Hemagglutinin protein	Neuraminidase protein	Subtypes
H1, H2, H3, H4, H5, H6, H7, H8, H9, H10, H11, H12, H13, H14, and H15	N1, N2, N3, N4, N5, N6, N7, N8, and N9	Influenza B Influenza C

Global epidemiology has shown that highly pathogenic avian influenza (HPAI) is caused by H5N1 avian influenza virus which was first detected in December 2003 in the republic of Korea. The migratory birds have spread the virus to other places. H1N1, H2N2, and H3N3 are human influenza A viruses whereas, H5N1 is avian influenza virus A which has single strand of RNA with 8 segments.

Great influenza pandemic of 1918 caused havoc killing 50 million population. H2N2 strain genetic reassortment caused 1957 pandemic killing of more than 1 million population. H3N3 strain caused 1968 pandemic killing of another million population.

Since March 2009, pandemic influenza A (H1N1) 2009 spread rapidly throughout the world. In India, there were many outbreaks. During 2014, 937 cases 218 deaths reported giving 23.2% case mortality rate.

In 2011, WHO adopted new name influenza A (H1N1) Pdm09. This is susceptible to oseltamivir and zanamivir drugs.

Under prophylaxis, chemoprophylaxis is available since oseltamivir is the drug of choice to health workers and all contacts.

Pandemic periods are classified into four periods with specific descriptions. They are: Concern that warrant careful monitoring. The concern is that Indians have no immunity and there are no vaccines available; the new virus not only replicates in humans and cause disease, but also efficiently transmitted from human to human.

Period	Description
Inter-pandemic period	First phase: Low risk period. No infections in man. Animal infection may be present. Second phase: Animal influenza is present. There is risk seen.
Pandemic alert period	Third phase: New subtype is detected. Very rare human spread by contact is observed. Fourth phase: Localized spread in man is seen. Virus adaptation is not seen. Fifth phase: Virus adaptation is seen. Pandemic risk starts appearing.
Pandemic period	Sixth phase: Increased transmission of cases in the population is seen.
Postpandemic phase	Seventh phase: The situation returns to interpandemic period phase.

Workers handling poultry in farms, markets involved in culling activity, veterinary workers, and health workers are at higher risk of acquiring the infection. Even the family members of these workers are at higher risk. Any type of influenza tends to be more serious in children, elderly persons above the age of 65 years and the chronically sick persons.

Migratory birds are reservoirs. Birds that survive infection excrete virus for at least 10 days orally and in feces thus, facilitating further spread. It spreads from birds to man through close contact with live infected poultry through inhalation. The mode of transmission from man to man is yet to be established. H5N1 virus can survive for 3 months at cool temperature. 1 g of contaminated manure contains enough viruses to infect more than 1 million birds. Droplet nuclei and dust are possible air-borne transmission.

Case Definition (H5N1 influenza A)

Suspect case of	Probable case	Confirmed case
Contact history with case	Suspect case with antibodies	Viral culture positive
Visit to a poultry farm within a week where outbreaks are there		PCR positive
Handling samples		Rise in specific antibody titer

Systems

Symptoms in birds	Symptoms in man
• Ruffled feathers • Soft shelled eggs • Depression • Droopiness • Loss of appetite • Cyanosis • Diarrhea • Edema • Swelling of head and eyelids • Bleeding nostrils • Cannot walk • Respiratory distress	• Fever • Cough • Sore throat • Muscle aches • Eye infection • Pneumonia • Acute respiratory distress

Laboratory Diagnosis

- Antigen in nasal secretions by immunofluorescence test, antigen capture enzyme-linked immunosorbent assay (ELISA) with monoclonal antibody to the nucleoprotein, and PCR
- Virus isolation in cell line Madin-Darby canine kidney cells (MDCK) and egg inoculation
- Serological test for paired samples [done in National Institute of Naturopathy (NIN) Pune and National Institute of Communicable Diseases (NICD), Delhi]
- Diagnosis in animals is done in high security animal disease laboratory at Bhopal
- If rapid test is done, it has to be confirmed by specific test.

Clinical Samples for Laboratory Diagnosis

They are to be collected within 72 hours of illness and sent to laboratory within 24 hours of collection:
- Nasopharyngeal wash
- Nasopharyngeal swab
- Oropharyngeal swab
- Paired samples of serum, one in acute phase and another at 15th day.

International Surveillance

Confirmed cases of influenza A/H5 should be reported.

National Surveillance

Indian Council of Medical Research (ICMR) has identified the following institutions; for national surveillance purpose.
a. AIIMS New Delhi
b. Enteroviral unit, Kolkata
c. Regional Medical Research Center (RMRC), Dibrugarh
d. King Institute, Chennai
e. National Institute of Virology (NIV), Pune

Treatment

Admission to hospital, intensive care, antibiotic therapy to prevent secondary infection, and ventilator for breathing support.

Oseltamivir

Therapeutic	Prophylactic
Adult 75 mg twice daily for 5 days Infant 15 mg/kg Children 15–23 mg/kg	Adult 75 mg/day for 7 days once a day

Vaccine

Influenza vaccination is not a part of routine immunization. Available to only rich countries; not available for global prevention.

Other Relevant Useful Information

They include virus isolation, PCR and immunofluorescence to demonstrate the presence of the virus, exchanging information, organizing regular consultations and advising the national governments. The concern of environmentalists about the wanton killing of birds and animals is normally justified. Birds' flu is not a new disease. The concern is that number of cases in birds and in human is increasing. Within the country it spreads from farm to farm. Outside the country it is by trade in birds and migratory birds infected with virus. There is no specific vaccine at present. However, targeted high risk group can help in averting pandemic. Common drugs used are: (a) M2 inhibitors (amantadine and rimantadine) and the neuraminidase inhibitors (oseltamivir and zanamivir).

We need to develop national pandemic influenza preparedness, since it involves animal health and man's health.

Prevention

Preventive measures include aggressive outbreak containment in poultry, enhancing animal and human surveillance, sharing information and laboratory materials, strategic stockpiling of antiviral and personnel protective equipment (PPE), building partnerships with national and international partners and strengthening health system and human resource capacity.

H5N1 influenza has never occurred in India earlier. There is geographical proximity to the affected countries. There is risk of getting disease by faster modes of travel. Surveillance of the disease through identification of strains of virus in India is a requisite.

Use of N95 masks, use of disposable latex gloves, disposable apron, head cover to cover hair, use of goggles, proper waste management are additional preventive steps.

Hospital waste in bird's flu is infectious in nature and classified under infectious waste. Swabs and gauges are put in yellow bags and the contents are incinerated. Gloves, face masks, disposable syringes are put in blue or white autoclavable biosafety bags which are autoclaved before disposal. Staff should follow biomedical waste management and handling rules, 1998, for waste management.

Suspected and confirmed poultry carcasses can be incinerated or buried deep using lime and soil in the ratio of 1:3. The site of bird's death is disinfected with 5% formaldehyde (even 2% glutaraldehyde can also be used).

Covering nose and mouth while sneezing or coughing, washing hands after touching respiratory secretions and selective isolation of patients from children, elderly are additional advocated precautionary measures.

AYUSHMAN BHARAT PROGRAM

This is one of the major National Initiative in Health Care System in India. It was announced in the year 2018.

Under this program, 1.5 lakh health and welfare centers do work for domiciliary care. Free drug distribution and free diagnostic services are provided. Under this Program, PRADHAN MANTRI JAN AROGYA YOJNA (PM-JAY) help in free in patient care and free day care services.

It provides cashless and paperless medical access to public coverage; which include 1,350 procedures. This service is made available anywhere in the county. It covers targeted poor and deprived rural families.

Ayushman Bharat Program follows listed deprivation criteria. It covers household without shelter, destitute, manual scavengers, primitive tribal, bonded laborers, rig pickers, beggars, construction workers and any type of coolies.

Preventive care and health care services are covered at primary, secondary and tertiary levels. This is popular as ***National Health Protection Scheme*** through Health and Wellness Centers.

The Physiology, Clinical Management and Principles of Adolescent Health Including Adolescent Reproductive Sexual Health (ARSH) Clinics

Adolescent girls care and their health started as part of integrated child development scheme (ICDS) beneficiary which included girls 11–18 years of age. Their health check-up, nutrition and health education including supplementary nutrition was covered under objectives of ICDS.

With ICDS infrastructure, Kishori Shakti Yojana implemented for 11–18 years girls. Self-development was stressed in the program. Literacy was major component to develop skills.

Nutrition program for adolescent girls is implemented in ICD scheme area.

This approach was initiated in 2006 under RCH II in the form of adolescent reproductive sexual health (ARSH) clinic to provide counseling on sexual and reproductive health issues.

The Government of India has a comprehensive package for meeting health needs of the adolescent and offers a roadmap for programs and priorities that aim to address adolescent health. Promotive, curative counseling services to strengthen adolescent friendly clinics and further outreach programs.

Focuses on reorganizing the existing public health system in order to meet the service needs of adolescents. Under this program counseling services, routine check-ups at primary, secondary and tertiary levels of care is provided on fixed days and fixed time to adolescents, married and unmarried, girls and boys during the clinic sessions.

To make the clinics adolescent friendly, states have branded the clinics in the name of "Maitry in Maharashtra, UDDAN in Uttarakhand, and Sneha in Karnataka" and so on. The objective of it being addressing the stigma behind accessing the adolescent services. This has a systematic training of 5 days for auxiliary nurse-midwife (ANM), 3 days to MOs are incorporated. ANM and ASHA are the key in the success of adolescent health in the country.

Adolescent make up 22% of our population and are a heterogeneous group of people. They vary in age, marital status, economic status, cultural background, religious beliefs, etc. This calls for health interventions that are flexible and responsive to their needs. The ARSH program has evolved keeping these needs in mind. It plans to increase the health seeking behavior in the adolescent age group and provide them with the right knowledge about various aspects of their growing life.

BABY-FRIENDLY HOSPITAL INITIATIVE (BFHI)

Exclusive breastfeeding provides best nutrition and protects the child from infections, hypothermia and malnutrition. This initiative is created by WHO and UNICEF; supported by professional bodies in India and abroad.

Exclusive breastfeeding means that except for breast milk no other food or fluids, including prelacteal feeds and water should be given to a child from birth till 4 months of age. Prelacteal feeds and water reduce milk intake and increase risk of infection. Breastfeeding should be initiated within the first hour of birth, should be frequent and on demand, to ensure adequate milk flow. After cesarean baby should be allowed to suck the breast as soon as mother comes to stable which is usually 6 hours after the operation.

All hospitals and health facilities providing maternity services are expected to actively promote exclusive breastfeeding as part of essential newborn care practices. Hospitals where exclusive breastfeeding is the norm are called "Baby-Friendly" hospitals. Medical colleges, district hospitals and postpartum centers must take measures to see that a child delivered in hospital is not denied of benefits of exclusive breastfeeding. Other supportive activities for child survival are adopted by these Baby-Friendly Hospitals.

Ten steps are given that all "BF" hospitals are expected to follow:
1. Policy of BFHI is communicated to staff
2. Maternal and child health (MCH) staff trained to help breastfeeding
3. Benefits are explained to pregnant mother
4. Help mother to breastfeed within an hour of normal delivery or with 4 hours after cesarean
5. Encourage breastfeeding on demand
6. Rooming-in of mother child allowed
7. Exclusive breastfeeding till 4–6 months
8. No teats, no advertisement near hospital
9. Maintenance of lactation shown to mother
10. Mother to mother help and family counseling is encouraged

CHIKUNGUNYA FEVER EPIDEMIC

Epidemic Polyarthritis and Rash

The causative agent called Buggy Creek Virus belongs to family Togaviridae and Genus *Alphavirus*. It is a positive sense, single stranded RNA virus. Vector which transmits chikungunya is culicine mosquitoes *(Ae. aegypti, Ae. africanus, culex and mansonia)*. It is not related to eating chicken or bird flu. It is different from dengue, malaria, yellow fever or JE.

After an incubation period of 3–12 days, sudden flu-like symptoms including headache, chills, fever, joint pain, nausea, and vomiting appear. Joints of extremities get swollen and painful to touch. Recovery is common in 3–5 days. Some suffer joint pain for months. Neurological symptoms are present in pediatric age group.

Chikungunya is a self-limiting febrile viral disease with a host range of mammals, primates, birds and man. Common geographic distribution has been Africa, India, South East Asia and Philippines.

Past Epidemics

- Kolkata epidemic 1963–1964
- Chennai epidemic 1965

- Found rudimentary and not significant till 2005.

Recent Epidemics

- February 2005 Fresh island of Reunion in Indian Ocean where 258,000 cases and 219 deaths are recorded.
- 2005 epidemic of Mauritius where 3,500 cases are recorded.
- 2005 epidemic of Odisha where 5,000 cases are recorded.
- March 2006 epidemic in Maharashtra, Malegaon of Nasik where 2,000 cases are recorded.
- 2006 epidemic in Andhra Pradesh where 200,000 cases are recorded in Prakasam district and Nellore district. Kurnool has the record of 139 positive cases.
- December 2005 to May 2005 epidemic in Karnataka has shown more than 80,000 cases in the area of Gulbarga, Tumkur, Bidar, Raichur, Bellary, Chitradurga, Davanagere, Kolar, Bijapur.
- May 2006 epidemic at Bangalore manifested with arthritis and rashes. During the same period other areas such as Gulbarga, Koppal, Gadag and Dharwad have recorded cases.
- In total there were 1.5 lakh reported cases of chikungunya in Karnataka till the end of May 2006. Cases reported in May 2006 is 78,175 cases in 61 talukas of 15 districts of Karnataka. Following is the reported cases district-wise in Karnataka state:

After 2016 disease declined till 2014. Again from 2015 cases emerged more than expectations.

- 2016 cases 64,100 from 28 states.
- 2017 cases 28,800 from 25 states.

From Karnataka alone 18,100 cases reported in 2017.

Bengaluru rural	2,631
Bengaluru urban	219
Bidar	22,659
Kolar	3,886
Gadag	1,362
Bagalkot	1,815
Shimoga	1,322
Davanagere	1,500
Bijapur	3,764
Chitradurga	12,064
Raichur	18,022
Bellary	3,749
Tumkur	25,673
Gulbarga	52,353
Haveri	737
Belgaum	178
Dharwad	889
Hassan	119
Chikmagalur	1,037
Koppal	2,433

In all above cited places, stagnation of water which provides fertile breeding grounds for vector seem to be culprit, which if avoided can control chikungunya fever.

Increased severity of rashes and arthritis can be due to genetic sequence, altering the virus' coat protein which potentially allows it to multiply more easily in mosquito cells.

Laboratory test suggested are blood test and X-ray of affected joints (erosions or bone appositions).

Screening tests suggested in clinical practice are total white cell count, electrolytes, renal functions, liver enzyme, calcium level, phosphate level, protein electrophoresis, C-reactive protein, erythrocyte sedimentation rate (ESR), rheumatoid factor, antinuclear factor, extractable nuclear antigen. Confirmation is by blood test with identification of virus.

In all triad of symptoms being fever, joint pains and rash; need supportive treatment with paracetamol, nonsteroidal anti-inflammatory drugs (NSAIDs), rest, avoiding rubbing or avoiding massaging joints. Apart from pain management, physical therapy and occupational therapy are also required.

Handling of spills includes covering with absorbent paper, application of 1% sodium hypochlorite and wash after 30 minutes of contact period.

Counter measures include control of mosquito bite by the use of mosquito repellents (suitable ones suggested are DEET, DEPA, DIMP, citronella oil, lemon, eucalyptus oil) apart from dimethyl phthalate and dibutyl phthalate. Mosquito mesh and mosquito netting are advocated. The larvae settled in water stored for over 4 days should be destroyed using temephos, an organophosphorous compound using 1 mL for 10 liters of water at 1:49 dilution.

Immunization and prophylaxis none available.

COMMUNITY DENTISTRY

Dominant dental health problem in society such as caries, periodontal diseases drew attention in mid-twenties. Historically, sticky heavy sugar in dental ill-health dates back to 1873 and dental fluorosis in 1930.

Loss of teeth (Edentulism) of 45% is among below 60 years which is influenced by education, occupation and income highlights the relative importance in our society.

Care of teeth in pregnant women, in infancy, in old (Gerodontics) are area of interest in community dentistry. Filling, onlay, crowns, dentine cement have become artificial prosthesis in management.

Caries: Among 10% of children and up to 35 years loss of tooth is only by caries. Pulp chamber involvement produces pain, which becomes excruciating by involvement of ligament and bone.

Below given are the measures to control the dental loss due to caries:
* Oral hygiene to start at birth
* Water fluoridation (school water supply)
* Topical application 2% fluorine
* Pits and fissures by plastic sealants
* Refined carbohydrate reduced in eatables, and
* Weekly mouth rinsing 0.2% sodium fluoride.

Periodontal Disease

Gingivitis in child is reversible. In adults this leads to damages. It becomes irreversible damage if:
* Periodontal ligament is involved.
* Bone destroyed.

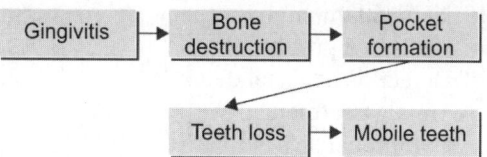

Fig. 33.2: Mechanism of edentulism.

The mechanism of edentulism is depicted in **Figure 33.2**.

Following are the measures to control edentulism:
* Oral hygiene
* Prophylaxis by scaling curettage
* Proper use of floss, tape, brush, and
* Role of traditional herbs like neem.

Malocclusion

Tooth loss, thumb sucking, other habits and sometimes genetic are attributed to malocclusion.
* 29% warrant therapy
* 5% warrant psychic counseling
* Space maintenance with wiring and orthodontic management.

Oral Cancer

* Males are more prone to oral cancer.
* Smoking, alcohol and nicotine consumption influence dental disease, oral hygiene and in turn malignancy.

Special Patients

Mentally retarded and those who are on an immunosuppressive therapy need special attention in community dentistry.

Other Descriptive

Oropharyngeal and tonsillar pathology influence good dental care.

Age Specific Recommendations

* Infant teeth are being cleaned by cloth wash
* Elderly teeth clean by finger wash.

COMMUNITY OPHTHALMOLOGY

Following are the major tasks ahead for community ophthalmology:

- National trachoma control
- Vitamin A prophylaxis
- Detection of visual defects
- Timely treatment
- Comprehensive eye care
- Primary eye health care
- Occupational hazard prevention
- Toxic amblyopia prevention
- Diabetic retinopathy prevention
- Hypertensive retinopathy prevention
- School camps for visual defect and eye disease, and
- Industry camps for visual defects and eye disease

Through the health awareness programs and camp approach the above said tasks can be achieved.

Content of health education are as following:
- Problem of blindness
- Cataract elimination
- Adventure of adolescent (Ramabana, Patakshi)
- Role of nongovernmental organization (NGO), and
- Eye banks and eye donation
- Cultural behavior (kajal application, watching TV, indoor smoking)
- Unhygienic practice (common handkerchief)
- Belief (which prevents seeking treatment)
- Nutritional blindness
- School eye health education
- Industry eye health education.

Common community eye health problems are as following:
- Cataract
- Refractive error
- Squint
- Injuries
- Eye infection
- Corneal ulcer
- Trachoma
- Xerophthalmia
- Glaucoma
- Drooping of lids
- Corneal opacities, and
- Eye in hypertension.

Current Status

- Mobile ophthalmic units during survey and camps for cataract surgeries in rural area.
- Eye banks in cities conducting corneal grafts to selected cases.

COMMUNITY PSYCHIATRY

Setback

There are 430 million mentally ill in the world, about 140 million mentally ill in India, 20 million epileptic, and 200 million mentally incapacitated. Among general public 20% are mentally sick.

Figure 33.3 depicts community psychiatry approach.

Following are the measures required to take the mental health to the needy people:
- Data collection
- Population survey
- Record system, and
- Mental health training.

Thailand was the first to take mental health to village followed by Chile, China and India.

Nonspecialist in primary mental health care levels:
a. Chandigarh study showed that LHW can initiate and supervise treatment of mentally sick (Ambala).
b. Bangalore study showed that PHC physician and ANM can treat and follow-up mentally ill in rural areas (Anekal).

Following diseases are given more priorities generally:
- Acute psychosis
- Chronic psychosis
- Depressive disorders
- Epilepsy
- Mental retardation.

Minimum essential drugs needed are:
- Chlorpromazine tablet and injection
- Phenobarbitone tablets
- Imipramine tablets.

Goals of Community Psychiatry

The major goals of community psychiatry are as following:

- Country to have a mental health policy
- Improvement of mental health of the community
- Cheap essential drugs to community health worker (CHW) at PHC level
- Development of information and technique in mental health, and
- Periodic evaluation of mental health status.

CONSUMER PROTECTION ACT (COPRA)

One who purchases health services for his use is a consumer. The user of health service with permission is also a consumer.

Service given should be free from defects, deficiencies and unfair trade practices. Receipt, bill, cash memo against all services are compulsory. Consumer can demand good service in exchange of money. Consumer Protection Act (1986) ensures rights covering all health services in government hospitals, private hospitals, nursing homes, private clinics, cooperative clinics and consultation centers. Consumer court set up under COPRA, 1986 at national state and district level provide simple, inexpensive and speedy redressal of consumer disputes including excess price charged. Complaint can be made for compensation on plain paper without court fee and without a lawyer.

District forum can be approached for compensation up to 5 lakhs; the state commission should be approached if it is between 5 and 20 lakhs and the national commission, if it exceeds 20 lakhs. The department of consumer affairs under the central ministry of Government of India is in charge of the above.

Factors taken note in the Act:
- Consumer health awareness
- Existing constraints in the infrastructure
- Misuse by the consumer, and
- Safeguard of health service providers.

Counterfeit Medicine and its Prevention

Drugs, medicamentation or pharmaceutical preparation which do not have original ingredient, which do not have authenticity and which do not have effectiveness are called counterfeit medicine. Sometimes active ingredients will be in inappropriate quantity. On occasion drug may not be there which are on the label. Fake package or fake labels also constitute counterfeit medicine.

Counterfeit medicine is seen from time immemorial has constituted drug scam or drug fraud.

Drug resistance is common impact of counterfeit drugs.

Generic drug which are low cost has become consumer friendly. This cannot be called as counterfeit drug. Generic drug has normal regulations of a country.

Hazardous, adulterated, substituted misrepresented old under false name may cause several dangerous health complications, side effects, or allergic reaction.

According to WHO, annual earnings from substandard drugs is overwhelming.

Development of drug resistance and life threatening are reported.

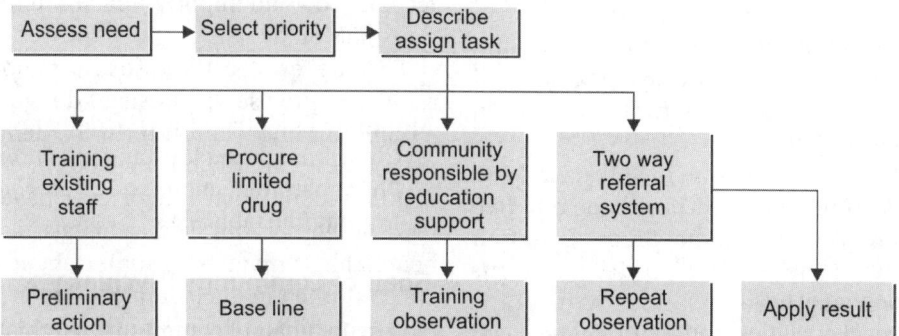

Fig. 33.3: Community psychiatry approach.

Radio frequency identification still not satisfactory in identifying counterfeit drugs. Advanced Raman Spectroscopy and EDXRD (energy dispersive X-ray differentiation) are tried to identify counterfeit drugs in the packages.

National survey by Central Drug Standards Control Organization of India in 2009 has found out 0.046% were spurious. Similarly, study in 2017 showed 3.16% of drugs were substandard. Commonly prescribed drugs are commonly counterfeited.

Free to access anticounterfeit platform is being tried all over the world.

Illegal and recreational drugs such as lysergic acid diethylamide (LSD), cannabis, methamphetamine, cocaine are another mode of counterfeit drugs.

Selective ultraviolet (UV) wavelength, custom package seal, authentication labels, holograms security printing are valued as part and parcel of security system.

DENGUE BURDEN IN INDIA: RECENT TRENDS AND IMPORTANCE OF CLIMATIC PARAMETERS

India has confirmed dengue cases with cases reported from across the country. Dengue is endemic in India. Transmission occurs year-round in southern areas and from April through November in northern states.

Dengue is a vector-borne disease. It is a major public health threat globally. It is caused by the dengue virus (DENV, 1–4 serotypes), which is one of the most important arboviruses in tropical and subtropical regions. Since the mid-1990s, epidemics of dengue in India have become more frequent, especially in urban zones, and have quickly spread to new regions, where dengue was historically nonexistent.

Dengue in India was first reported in Chennai in 1780.

First outbreak occurred in Kolkata in 1963.

Subsequent outbreaks have been reported in different parts of India. Since 1956, four serotypes (one to four) of dengue virus have been reported in various parts of the country. The total number of dengue cases has significantly increased in India since 2001.

Inadequate vector control measures have created favorable conditions for dengue virus transmission and its mosquito vectors. Both *Aedes aegypti* and *Aedes albopictus* are the main competent vectors for dengue virus in India. Infected with dengue exhibit a wide spectrum of clinical symptoms ranging from asymptomatic to severe clinical manifestations, such as dengue shock syndrome. A dengue vaccine, Dengvaxia˙, has been registered in several countries. Dengvaxia˙ is a live attenuated tetravalent vaccine that is currently under evaluation in phase 3 clinical trials in Asia (Indonesia, Malaysia, Philippines, Thailand and Vietnam) and Latin America (Brazil, Colombia, Honduras, Mexico and Puerto Rico). Dengvaxia˙ has not yet been approved by the Ministry of Health and Family Welfare, Government of India, because more clinical trials are thought to be necessary in India.

Many studies have reported changing spatial patterns in dengue transmission. The reasons for such changes are related to several factors, ranging from the globalization of travel and trade, which favors the propagation of pathogens and vectors, to climatic changes or modified human behavior.

Indian monsoon rainfall provides ample breeding habitats for *Ae. aegypti*, thus leading to high vector densities.

The extrinsic incubation period (EIP) is the viral incubation period between the time when a mosquito draws a viremic blood meal and the time when that mosquito becomes infectious. Since the 1900s, the EIP has been recognized as an important factor in dengue transmission dynamics.

For the effective control of disease outbreaks, rapid and precise diagnosis of dengue is of paramount importance. In India, dengue is diagnosed primarily on the basis of clinical manifestations (such as high fever, headache, retro-orbital pain, myalgia, arthralgia, rash and hemorrhagic manifestations). Dengue cases are confirmed in the laboratory by the MAC-ELISA method on the basis of the detection of IgM antibodies.

Chapter 33: Recent Area of Interest in Community Medicine

From 1998 to 2018, the highest dengue incidence was reported in Pondicherry, Dadra Nagar Haveli and Delhi. Similarly, high dengue incidence, ranging between 31 and 50 per million, was reported for the states of Punjab, Gujarat, Karnataka, Kerala, Tamil Nadu, and Odisha.

Dengue syndrome constitutes:
* Undifferentiated dengue fever
* Actual dengue fever
* Dengue hemorrhagic fever (DHF) without shock
* DHF with shock.

In India, epidemics are occurring and creating public health problem. Major epidemic is recorded in 1996. Another epidemic is recorded in 1998 when pandemic of dengue syndrome was seen across the countries. In India every year, on an average 12,000 cases are occurring and about 200 deaths are occurring. Classical dengue known as *breakbone fever* is caused by four serotypes. *Aedes aegypti* mosquito is the main vector. DHF is clinically differentiated into four grades depending upon bleeding and shock. Hemoconcentration and thrombocytopenia help in diagnosis.

Common breeding places of vectors are found to be discarded tin, broken bottle, fire bucket, flower pot, earthen pot, tree hole, tier, overhead tank, water cooler, flower vase, and defreeze container of fridge.

Diagnosis is done by clinical examination for fever, hemorrhage, positive tourniquet test (above 20 petechiae per square inch). Incubation period is commonly 5–6 days.

CORONAVIRUS EPIDEMIC 2019–2020

Introduction

Corona in Latin is "Crown". Its surface has series of spikes like crowns, that is where it has got the name "Corona".

The coronavirus was first identified in China on December 31, 2019. Within few days of identification, it caused panic in China and within few weeks, it became serious threat to the world. During the period of December 31, 2019 to February 29, 2020, total number of cases has been 85,206 and total deaths have been 2,923.

During the above period, global distribution of cases and deaths country-wise is as under:

Country/Area/Pocket	No. of cases	No. of deaths
China	79,252	2,835
South Korea	2,931	16
Italy	889	21
Iran	388	34
Japan	234	5
Diamond Princess Cruise ship	705	6
Other Countries*	620	6
	85,206	2,923

*Singapore, Hong Kong, USA, Germany, France, Kuwait, Thailand, Bahrain, Taiwan, Spain, Australia, Malaysia, UK, Vietnam, Canada, Switzerland, Sweden, Macao, Iraq, Israel, Austria, Norway, Oman, Croatia, Greece, Lebanon, Philippines, Finland, India, Romania, Denmark, Georgia, Mexico, Netherland, Pakistan, Russia, Afghanistan, Algeria, Azerbaijan, Belarus, Belgium, Brazil, Cambodia, Egypt, Estonia, Iceland, Lithuania, North Macedonia, Monaco, Nepal, New Zealand, Nigeria, San Marino, Sri Lanka.

Case fatality ratio (CFR) = 2.0%, incubation period = 2–14 days, among old age above 80 years + CFR= 14.8%, more seen among men = 2.8%, very common comorbidity = CVS.

In the beginning, the virus was called by temporary names like:
* 2019-nCoV acute respiratory disease
* Novel coronavirus pneumonia.

On February 11, 2020, WHO named the virus CoViD-19 (Co = Corona, Vi = Virus, D = disease)

Still there lies no confirmed epidemiological connections. Disease has spread to 60 countries.

COVID-19 epidemic has caused communist China's biggest health emergency, viz. fast transmission, wide range of infection and most difficult to prevent or control.

After new deaths and infections in Europe, West Asia, and Asia, WHO has warned "PREPARE FOR VIRUS PANDEMIC."

Common signs and symptoms shown are cough, cold, severe bodyache, high temperature, breathlessness and GI symptoms. Severe forms manifest pneumonia, respiratory distress, GI problem and kidney failure.

Vaccine Ventures (All are Early Stages)

- December 31, 2019, China alerts WHO about pneumonia-like cases in Wuhan
- January 10, 2020, China shares genetic code of nCoV-2019
- January 23, 2020, CEPI announces 3 programmes to develop vaccines with a goal of clinical testing in 4 months
- University of Queensland, Australia, DNA technique targets viral surface proteins to improve identification by the immune system
- Curevac and Moderna Therapeutics, US, is developing vaccine based on messenger RNA that tells body to produce proteins to fight disease
- Inovio US iscusing DNA-based technology human trial of vaccines for MERS coronavirus
- Pasteur Institute, France, is modifying measles vaccine to work against the coronavirus
- Center for Diseases Control and Prevention, China, started plans to develop vaccine and started developing vaccine.

VACCINE DEVELOPMENT CYCLE

- Identification of pathogen
- Clinical development in three phases [produce antigen, preclinical study (below 100, above 100 and above 1000 human trial)]
- Regulatory application
- Regulatory approval and surveillance.

DRASTIC PREVENTIVE MEASURES

- 56 million in Hubei and Wuhan under quarantine
- Bank notes disinfection with UV light or high temperature, stored for 14 days and put to circulation

- TCM (Traditional Chinese Medicine for cases' trial.
- Avoid mass gathering, cancel public event, no emperor birthday celebration and cancellation of marathon
- All arrival—self quarantine for 14 days
- Postponement of annual Parliament session
- Spray disinfectants at market places
- Tourists confined to their rooms for easy monitoring
- Strict quarantine of public in their houses
- UN Health Agency warns of very grave global threat
- WHO declares PREPARE FOR VIRAL PANDEMIC
- Saudi halts Mecca and Medina
- No passengers taking from China, Japan, Italy, Iran, India and Pakistan.

DESMOTOLOGY

The word is derived from Greek word "Desmoterion meaning Prison". This deals with the concept of Prison Health.

The discipline desmotology deals with health of inmates in jails, prisons and juvenile detention facilities. It is estimated that about 12 percent of inmates seek services (**Fig. 33.4**).

The complex problems associated with this discipline are:
- AIDS
- Multidrug resistant TB
- Hepatitis
- Neuropsychiatric illness

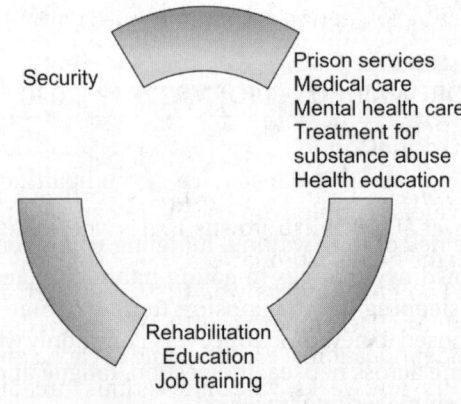

Fig. 33.4: Priorities in desmotology.

- Suicide
- Trauma
- Violence
- Substance abuse
- Epilepsy.

EARLY CHILDHOOD DEVELOPMENT (ECD)

The acronym ECD refers to a comprehensive approach to policies and programs for children from birth to 8 years of age, their parents and caregivers. Its purpose is to protect the child's rights to develop his or her full cognitive, emotional, social and physical potential.

Community-based services that meet the needs of infants and young children are vital to ECD and they should include attention to health, nutrition, education, water and sanitation in homes and communities.

The approach promotes and protects the right of the young child to survival, growth and development.

In the year 2001, UNICEF has chosen to focus on the earliest years of child viz., 0–3 years for attending to the neglected policies, programs and budgets.

The nourishment and the care that 0–3 years of age children receive during this earliest period influences their developments in later life, both in terms of their intellectual and physical growth.

Other synonyms used for ECD (World Bank Title) are:
- Early childhood care and (initial) education (UNESCO)
- Early childhood education and care (OECD).

EMPORIATRICS

This deals with the science of the health of travelers. People who travel are exposed to the risk of long waiting, mingling with overcrowding, changes in eating habit, changes in sleeping habit, exposure to new climate, exposed to new time zone. Very commonly we come across nausea, indigestion, fatigue and insomnia among travelers.

They are exposed to infectious and communicable diseases (CD) in developing countries. Travelers are away from their hometown and are devoid of readily accessible medical care.

"International Travel and Health, Vaccination requirements and Health advice" from WHO gives guidance to travelers.

It is advisable to carry medical kit for travelers that should contain minimum of following contents:
- Sun cream
- Mosquito repellent
- ORS
- Medication for diabetes, hypertension, etc.
- Dressing material
- Disinfectant.

In Emporiatrics, it is mandatory to a traveler to keep a record of his drug sensitivity, his chronic health disorders, blood group, etc.

Preventive Emporiatrics include the following:
- Food hygiene in travel
- Safe inactivated hepatitis A (HAV) vaccine administration
- No bath in polluted water
- Protect from excessive heat and humidity
- Chemoprophylaxis for malaria
- Hepatitis B vaccination
- Awareness of STD and their prevention
- Use of disposable needle and syringe in case of requirement
- Yellow fever vaccine if traveling to South America and Africa
- Booster tetanus if not taken.

ESSENTIAL DRUGS

Essential drugs are those that satisfy the health care needs of the majority of the population, they should therefore be available at all time in adequate amounts and in the appropriate dosage forms (WHO). Refer chapter 30 for detail.

Selection criteria of a drug as essential are:
- Disease prevalence
- National resources
- Efficacy of drug is known
- Safety of drug is known

- Bioavailability is assured
- Cost benefit ratio
- Formulated as single compound.

Examples

Following are recommended essential drugs:
- Oxygen—medicinal gas
- Phenobarbitone tablet—anticonvulsant
- Mebendazole tablet—anthelmintic
- Trimethoprim tablet—antibacterial
- Metronidazole tablet—antiamebic
- Chloroquine tablet—antimalarial
- Digoxin tablet—cardiac glycoside
- Norethisterone tablet—hormone
- Chlorpromazine tablet—psychotic drug.

FAMILY MEDICINE

Definitions

This is an academic and scientific discipline with its own educational content research, evidence base and clinical activity and a clinical specialty orientated to first contact care or primary care (European definition of Family Medicine, 2002).

General Practitioner

A licensed medical graduate, who gives personal primary and continuing care to a family, practicing in clinic, practicing through home visits, takes initial diagnosis, undertakes the management of chronic, recurrent illnesses, develops trust by repeated contact, and gives his professional responsibilities to the community (Leeuwenhorst 1974).

Family Practice

A discipline that trains and sustains medical doctor to practice arts and sciences of family medicine.

Family Physician

Doctor trained in family practice, has attitude, skill and knowledge to provide comprehensive health care and does the job within available resources. He seeks community participation in all matters of health.

Clinical Audit

Procedure followed to review clinical performance and help to avoid departure from best practices.

Principles

1. It offers holistic approach toward a patient and not as a specific illness.
2. Context of illness is taken note of
3. Adheres to health education and first level prevention with contact of the patient.
4. Patient is considered as a risk case in the population.
5. Doctor will be part of the community.
6. Doctor shares the platform of patients.
7. Home visits are commonly undertaken.
8. Importance is given to subjective aspect of manifestations.
9. Management will be within available resources.

Scope

Expanding and dynamic in providing vital event family care with the understanding patient's culture, tradition and behavior.
- It has better communication and better patient-doctor relationship in the practice of medicine.
- Can take care of adolescent health, geriatric health and palliation including bereavement in a family.
- It is evidence-based practice of medicine.

Philosophy

Patient is to be viewed from his family background, his community background and his social background at examination and at treatment. Emotional care, psychological care, behavioral counseling and management considering socioeconomic aspect of patient are major philosophy of family medicine.

Role of Doctor

- Survey, screening and surveillance of infectious diseases
- Routine immunization to infants, pregnant and children
- Creating awareness on cause and prevention of diseases
- Counseling of the needy

Chapter 33: Recent Area of Interest in Community Medicine

- Friend, philosopher and guide to a patient whom he is treating.

Family Crisis

Incurable disease in a family, trauma and accident, criminal acts in family, terminal illness, death and bereavement, separation or divorce etc., constitute crisis.
- Confidence, communication, unity, supportive friends, and friendly relatives can help in such crisis.
- Crisis is determined by challenges, problems, assets, liabilities, strength and weaknesses of family.
- Short-term therapy to assist individual and family by doctor who is practicing family medicine is of utmost help.

GENETIC ENGINEERING

Genetic engineering is known popularly as "gene cloning". Gene manipulation, recombinant DNA technology are procedures to isolate a specific DNA fragment from a genome of an organism to determine its base sequence and assessing its function.
It covers the following areas:
a. Gene research
b. Useful protein production
c. Transgenic plant generation
d. Transgenic animal generation

Genetic fingerprinting is used in forensic science and paternity testing.

Gene cloning which is a genetic process will help in developing a replica without a natural biological process.

Following are public health importance of genetic engineering:
a. Diagnosis of genetic disease
b. Vaccine development
c. Production of insulin, interferon and growth hormone
d. Gene therapy

GLOBAL WARMING

The emission of greenhouse gases (GHG) called "The greenhouse effect" has a threat to forest, agriculture and life in general. GHGs and CO_2, methane, nitrous oxide, though they are essential for life, their excessive concentration makes the earth warmer leading to climatic changes.

Following are available observations:
a. Biomass burning has an impact on global warming (Indian Council of Forestry, Research and Education).
b. Atmospheric changes and rise in sea level occurs (Indian Meteorological Department and National Institute of Oceanography).
c. Level of methane emission from paddy field is increased [Council of Scientific and Industrial Research (CSIR and IARC)].

The data indicates that the earth's temperature has risen by 5°C since 1860. Emission of GHG depends on human activity. CO_2 and CFC (Chlorofluorocarbon) depends on fossil fuel burning.

By current predicted model, the global temperature raises another 1°C above the present value by 2025 and 3°C by the year 2100. Global mean sea level is expected to rise 20 cm by 2030 and 65 cm by 2100.

Global warming affects the availability of water resources and biomass. Precipitation and temperature changes the disease pattern.

Sustainable Measures

- There is a need to promote multidisciplinary scientific studies.
- Development of viable energy resources including renewable resources and sustainable agricultural practices.

GUINEA WORM ERADICATION: INDIAN SCENARIO

It is a second disease to be eradicated in India after smallpox, which is caused by *Dracunculus medinensis*.

Transmission

Through drinking water from unsafe sources such as step well, ponds containing water fleas (cyclops).

Result

Pain, swelling, ulceration, discomfort, incapacitation and economic loss.

Disease Load: India

1947	25 million
1957	5 million
1967	89,000
1996	09

Risk Load

1980–1981—60 lakhs in India.

Public health experts identified guinea worm disease as potentially eradicable disease on the following grounds:
Simple life cycle
- Vector is confined to water source, and
- Tool for control is available.

The disease was exclusively of rural poor and the maximum incidence was seen during the summer months which also are the main season of intensive agricultural activity. Thus, there is a link between ill-health due to guinea worm and impaired agricultural activity.

NGWEP (GWEP): The National Guinea Worm Eradication Program was launched in 1983–1984 as a centrally sponsored scheme. Ministry of Rural Development Government of India, and State Public Health Engineering Department (Rural Water Supply) assisted the program through:
a. Provision and maintenance of safe drinking water source
b. Conversion of unsafe drinking water source.

Defined Strategies

- Case detection
- Surveillance through search operation
- Regular monthly reporting
- Case management
- Vector control by Abate (OMS-786) at the concentration of 1 mg per liter
- Vector control by temefos in unsafe water source, 8 times a year
- Use of nylon cloth strainers to filter cyclops
- Health education.

Impact of Guinea Worm (GW) Eradication

1984	39,792 cases
1996	Only 9 cases
1998	Till date zero cases

Last Case Reported

July 1996 in Aau village in Peelwa PHC area, Jodhpur district of Rajasthan.

Zero Guinea Worm

Seventh independent evaluation of GWEP in 1999 validated the zero GW disease status in India. In July 1999, India showed 3 years of zero incidences.

Free of Guinea Worm

WHO team visited our country in November 1999 to validate the zero GW disease status for certification of GWE in India. It is a major achievement in disease control of India. Following activities continued till date:
- Health education of school children and women
- Rumor investigation
- It is a notifiable disease
- Guinea worm surveillance continued
- Supervised action for safety of hand pumps.

Gender Issues and Women Empowerment

Millennium development goal has target for achieving gender equality and empowering woman. United Nations Organization (UNO) declared 2012 as the International day for girl child.

Opportunity to be borne, opportunity to grow in safe environment and opportunity to develop are issues in women empowerment.

Strong culture to have son, dowry practice, girl child is *paraya dhan*, girl child is not useful to get *moksha* are existing customs that influence gender issue and women empowerment.

Education for the elimination of gender equality and empowering women is a known arrow to de-root gender issues. School dropout are influenced by—(a) child marriage, (b) household work, (c) assisting family members, (d) looking after the siblings, and (e) distant school, lack of female teachers and lack of toilet facilities.

Neglect and discrimination against girl child delays them basic human rights.

Violence such as rape, trafficking, child labor, beggary, and son preference and daughter discrimination determine women empowerment.

Human trafficking for sexual exploitation and for cheap labor are other social stigma. India has much legislation such as:
- The Child Marriage Restraint Act 1929
- Immoral Traffic (Prevention) Act 1951
- Child Labor Act 1986
- Juvenile Justice Act 2000
- Preconception and Prenatal Diagnostic Techniques (PC PNDT) 2003
- Free and compulsory education 2010
- Female Infanticide Act

HANDIGODU SYNDROME (ENDEMIC FAMILIAL ARTHRITIS)

It was first noticed in Handigodu village of Sagar taluk in Shimoga district of Karnataka and hence, the name Handigodu syndrome. Later it was also detected in Balehonnur of Chikmagalur district of Karnataka.

No animal cases are seen. Among men, gradual onset, punctuated by pain of moderate degree in lower limbs, lumbosacral region, hips and knee joints, sometimes leading to immobilization by crippling flexon deformities of knee and hip joints. Radiologically, destruction of articular surfaces of femur, tibia and osteophytic lipping of several bones were seen—rarefaction of bones around destruction, varying degree of osteoarthritic changes are common features.

Survey has indicated following associations:
a. Familial character of the disease
b. Relation of achondroplasia dwarfism
c. Osteomalacia
d. Rickets-like manifestations

Attributable causes by field studies are:
a. Habit of eating dead crabs.
b. Consuming fish found in ponds paddy field of Malnad [(Swampy districts like Shimoga, Chikmagalur in Karnataka state are called "Malnad" (rain forest area)] imperiled by residue of endrin and pathion (insecticides).
c. Farm laborers not served food from land owners went for searching crabs around.
d. Green revolution by high-yielding paddy which required synthetic chemicals.
e. Under nutrition prevailed among villagers.
f. Consumption of illicit liquor.
g. Tradition of consanguineous marriage in village.

Control Measures

- Not specific
- But attending to attributable causes is advocated.

HOSPITAL WASTE MANAGEMENT

There has been increasing concern for effective management of hospital waste (which is clinical and hazardous waste) and infection control to reduce morbidity, mortality, improve patient satisfaction and quality assurance and minimization of medicolegal cases. The Ministry of Environment, Government of India has issued following notification in July 1998, "The biomedical waste management rules 1998" making it imperative to install appropriate hospital waste management system. Refer Chapter 19 for detail.

The treatment option for hospital waste disposal are given in **Table 33.2**.

Hospital waste is divided into:
1. Noninfective waste
2. Infected sharp waste
3. Infected waste

Recently, while hearing a public interest litigation, the Supreme Court has directed all hospital authorities to install incinerators or/and suitable devices for safe disposal of hospital wastes.

Central Pollution Control Board and State Pollution Control Board are the regulating authorities in this aspect.

HYPOTHERMIA

Hypothermia is a major cause of death in early neonatal period. All newborns are at risk of fall in body temperature since the ambient

Table 33.2: Treatment option for hospital waste disposal.

Waste class category	Waste description	Treatment method
1. Human anatomical wastes, blood, body fluids	Human tissue, organs, waste body parts, body fluids, blood and blood products; items saturated or dripping with blood body fluids contaminated with blood and body fluids removed during/after treatment, surgery or autopsy or other medical procedures	Incineration
2. Microbiological wastes	Laboratory culture stocks or specimen of microorganisms live or attenuated vaccine; Human or animal cell culture used in research; infectious agents from research wastes from production of biological dishes and devices used for transfer of cultures	Incineration
3. Waste sharps	Sharps such as needles, scalpel, blades, etc., which include both used and unused	Chemical disinfection autoclaving followed by shredding
4. Discarded glassware	Wastes generated from glassware and glass equipment used	Chemical disinfection autoclaving followed by shredding

temperature to which they are born is always by several degrees cooler than the temperature in the womb and their body temperature.

The delivery room and postnatal ward should be warm (temperature at which adult feels comfortable is cold for the newborn).

Newborn body temperature is 99.5°F and hypothermia occurs if room temperature is below 97.5°F. After birth heat-loss occurs by evaporation of amniotic fluids from the body of wet newborn.

Prevention

1. After birth, baby is quickly dried with clean cloth and wrapped with cotton clothing (turkey towel—two-towel method).
2. Skin to skin contact with mother at breast-feeding is allowed.

Risk to hypothermia is more among low-birth weight, premature, asphyxiated newborns. Radiant warmer in hospital is helpful.

Seventy-five percent are home deliveries. Hence, traditional birth attendant (TBA) and mother's awareness about steps to prevent hypothermia reduces child mortality considerably.

INTENSIVE PULSE POLIO IMMUNIZATION (IPPI)

Between 1995 and 1999 the program of polio eradication was called PPI (pulse polio immunization). It is defined as sudden, simultaneous, mass administration of extra two doses of oral polio vaccine (OPV) on a single day before the transmission season to children below 5 years of age.

Pulse polio immunization days in India during 1996–1998:

I round	II round
9th December 1995	20th January 1996
7th December 1996	18th January 1997
7th December 1997	18th January 1998
6th December 1998	17th January 1999

Despite this, due to noncoverage of certain percentage of eligible children complete eradication has not been possible. Therefore, it was decided to intensify this operation in four rounds (Based on Brazil experience) through booth based on first day and house to house visit on second to third days. This intensified program is called "IPPI".

Chapter 33: Recent Area of Interest in Community Medicine

National Immunization Days in India since 1999 till date are as under:

Year	Days
1999	October 13th, 14th, and 15th
1999	November 21st, 22nd, and 23rd
1999	December 19th, 20th, and 21st
2000	January 23rd, 24th, and 25th
2000	December 10th, 11th and 12th
2001	January 21st, 22nd, and 23rd
2001	December 2nd, 3rd, and 4th
2002	January 20th, 21st, and 22nd
2003	January 5th, 6th, and 7th
2003	February 9th, 10th, and 11th
2004	January 4th, 5th, 6th, and 7th
2004	February 22nd, 23rd, 24th, and 25th
2004	April 4th, 5th, 6th, and 7th
2004	October 10th, 11th, 12th, and 13th
2004	November 9th, 10th, 11th, and 12th
2004	November 21st, 22nd, 23rd, and 24th
2005	April 10th, 11th, 12th, and 13th
2005	May 15th, 16th, 17th, and 18th
2006	April 9th, 10th, 11th, and 12th
2006	May 21st, 22nd, 23rd, and 24th
2007	February 11th, 12th, 13th, and 14th
2007	August 20th, 21st, 22nd, and 23rd
2008	January 7th, 8th, 9th, and 10th
2008	October 2nd, 3rd, 4th, and 5th
2009	February 22nd, 23rd, 24th, and 25th
2009	August 20th, 21st, 22nd, and 23rd
2010	Scheduled 10.01.2010, 07.02.2010, February 5th, 6th, 7th, and 8th
2011	January 13
2012	May 25
2013	October 31
2014	January 19
2015	January 18
2016	January 17, 18, 19
2017	January 29 and April 2
2018	January 28 and March 11
2019	June 20 to June 24

Following Mop up operations are observed in India:

Year	Days
2000	June 18th, 19th, and 20th
2000	July 16th, 17th, and 18th
2003	(Nanded) June 29th, 30th, and July 1st
2003	(Nanded) August 10th, 11th, and 12th
2003	(Bellary) July 27th, 28th, and 29th
2003	(Bellary) September 7th, 8th, and 9th
2003	November 9th, 10th, and 11th

Following Special National Immunization Days have also been observed in India:

Year	Days
2001	March 12th, 13th, 14th, 15th, and 16th
2001	October 14th, 15th, and 16th
2004	May 9th, 10th, 11th, and 12th

Why PPI is Changed to IPPI?

- Pulse polio immunization (PPI) two rounds reduced polio cases not sufficient to reach eradication target may be due to low routine coverage.
- Persistent wild virus circulation needs additional rounds.
- 11 months between two usual PPI large birth cohort and missed children, which is a large susceptible group.
- More PPI rounds by IPPI will result in fewer chances for wild virus establishment.
- IPPI is needed to flush out wild polio virus from the community and environment.

Micro planning for social mobilization, information education and communication (IEC) activities and coordination, has helped IPPI a success. Already existed PPI infrastructure and machinery, mobilized the resources for better IPPI.

2016 is marked with SWITCH where trivalent oral polio vaccine (tOPV) replace bivalent oral polio vaccine (bOPV).

2013–2018 polio eradication and endgame strategy plan has substantial impact in polio eradication. Polio surveillance continued with following actions:

- AFP case finding
- Early stage stool sample transport for examination

- Polio virus isolation
- Mapping virus if found.

JANANI SURAKSHA YOJANA

This was earlier known as National Maternal Benefit Scheme. In 2005, it is renamed as Janani Suraksha Yojana. It is centrally sponsored scheme. It integrates with National Rural Health Mission.

Cash assistance is 1,400/- in low performing areas.

Cash assistance is 1,000/- in high performing areas.

During 2016, 104.16 lakh pregnant women received benefit under this scheme.

In 2011, Government of India introduced Janani Shishu Suraksha Karyakaram along with Janani Suraksha Yojana. This envisages 24 hours care for severe malnourished, help in therapeutic feeding. It also provides micronutrient supplementation.

Further, Government of India introduced Navjaat Shishu Suraksha Karyakram to train health workers in newborn care and in resuscitation.

All these are integrated under "INTEGRATED MANAGEMENT OF NEONATAL AND CHILDHOOD ILLNESS"

One more project "Rashtriya Bal Swasthya Karyakram of 2013 envisage early intervention services.

KANGAROO MOTHER CARE

This method of care of the newborn was developed by Rey and Martinez of Colombia for the purpose of effective way to meet low birth weight baby's need for warmth, breastfeeding, and protection from infection, stimulation, safety and love.

Basis of Kangaroo Mother Care is to provide continuous prolonged skin to skin contact. To provide needed exclusive breastfeeding at hospital and continuation at home, to enable low birth weight babies be discharged early.

Kangaroo Mother Care is a gentle and effective method of newborn care.

Kangaroo Position

Baby is placed between mother's breasts in an uplift position, maintaining chest to chest contact.

This position gives care for changing diaper, haggis and cord care.

Length and duration of Kangaroo Mother Care position is 40 weeks.

Mother can feed in Kangaroo position.

Mother should be watchful on the following Baby's breathing difficulties:
- Spells of apnea
- Body temperature rise
- Convulsion
- Diarrhea
- Yellow skin

Advantages

Exclusive breastfeed at discharge increases from 6% to 37% (Hurst et al. 1997).

Daily breast milk volume increases from 400 mL to 640 mL and daily feed increases from 9 to 12 (Schmidt et al. 1986).

Exclusive breastfeeding at 6th month increases from 23% to 70% (Charpak et al. 1994).

Support binders (Carrying pouches) are of three types (**Fig. 33.5A to C**). They are:
(1) Carrying Pouch Type I; (2) Carrying Pouch Type II; and (3) Carrying Pouch Type III

Kangaroo Mother Care is useful to save 20 million low birth weights occurring in the world.

In developing countries it is better for economic condition, better for lifestyle and better for nutrition. In developed countries it is a boon to preterm births and for impaired intrauterine growth.

LEPTOSPIROSIS: AN EMERGING PUBLIC HEALTH PROBLEM

For the first time in 1886, Weil described clinical description of leptospirosis (**Fig. 33.6**).

In 1915, leptospirae were recovered from infected cases. It is known by various names such as mud fever, trench fever, rice field fever,

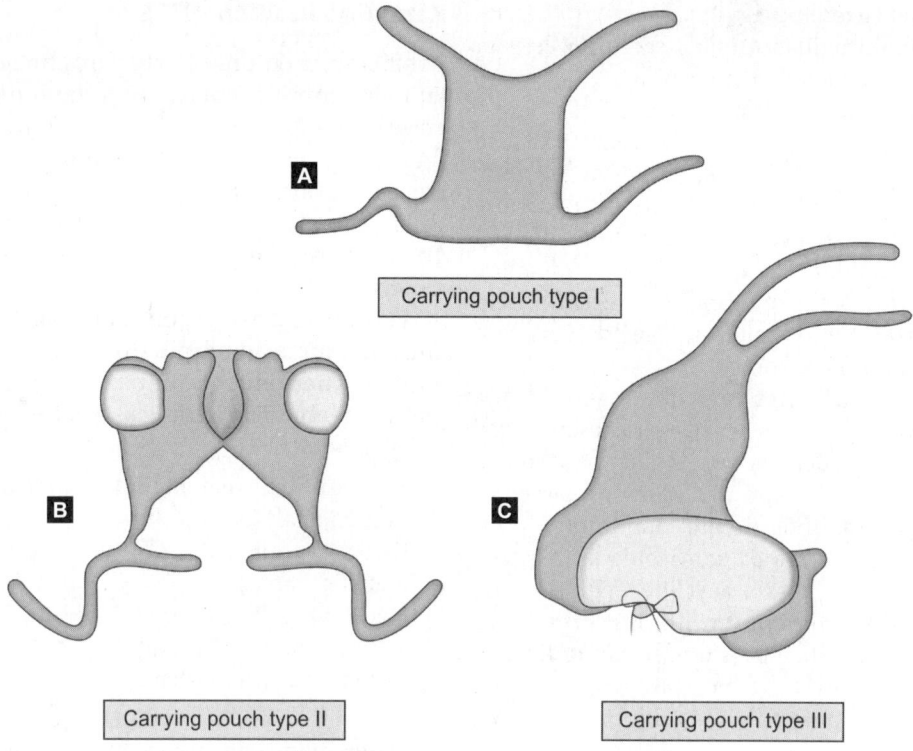

Figs. 33.5A to C: Support binders for baby care.

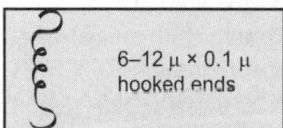

Fig. 33.6: Leptospira.

cane cutters fever, swamp fever, flood fever, 7 days fever, etc. At present, 18 serogroups having 180 serofars are identified. Common serogroups are *icterohemorrhagica, canicola, pyrogenes, autumnalis, australia, pomane, hebdomadis, grippotyphosa, andamana*. Common serotars are *icterohemorrhagiae, copenhagen, smithi, budapest*.

They are visualized by dark ground microscope and electron microscope. Normal staining is by silver impregnation method. Enriched rabbit serum is used in culture (Korthof's, Stuart's, and Fletcher's). Intraperitoneal inoculation to guinea pig is laboratory procedure. Man gets infected through water contaminated by urine of carrier animal, or entry through cuts, abrasion, or through intact mucosa of mouth, nose and conjunctiva.

Clinically mild pyrexia to severe hepatorenal damage is seen. Involvement of different systems or organs produce the manifestations such as vomiting, headache, ocular pain, fever, jaundice, rigors, purpura hemorrhagica, albuminuria, aseptic meningitis, and abdominal symptoms.

Laboratory diagnosis is possible by:
a. Leptospira demonstration by dark ground microscopy or electron microscopy or immunofluorescence.
b. Isolation in culture (enriched rabbit serum media) in chorioallantoin membrane (egg), in animal (intraperitoneal inoculation and heart blood collection).
c. Serological tests (genus specific or type specific tests) complement fixation test, ELISA, agglutination absorption test (reference laboratory for India is in Andaman and Nicobar).

d. Blood examination in early stage (I week), urine examination in late stage (II week) for demonstration of leptospira.
e. Guinea pig inoculation tests.

Domestic animals and rats excrete leptospira as carriers. Infected animals contaminate water, paddy field, sugarcane field which act as sources apart from infected pig and poultry. Floods help in dissemination. It is also an occupational infection for field workers, miners, soldiers, veterinarians, and slaughterhouse workers.

In cities, water tank or water storage damaged by rodents easily get contaminated with urine of infected rats. Studies have shown 4.4% of serum samples show presence of leptospira antibody in the community.

Treatment can be completed by selected antibiotic such as tetracycline, erythromycin, penicillin or streptomycin. But preventive measures directed as under can definitely reduce the prevalence:
a. Identification of potentially contaminated water.
b. Protection of occupationally exposed population by providing protective clothing (gum boots, gloves, aprons).
c. Prevention of environment (water, food) contaminated by animal excreta by their effective disposal.
d. Rodent control in rural, urban and recreational areas of human habitations, sugarcane field, rice field, etc.
e. Health awareness particularly to occupationally exposed population about modes of transmission, avoidance of use of contaminated sources of water and need for use of protective clothing.
f. Immunization of pet animals, particularly dogs with prevalent dominant local strains to prevent clinical illness.
g. Mechanization in agricultural operation.
h. Disinfection of water and bathing pools with chlorine, barns and pigsties with cresol; field area with copper sulfate.
i. Burning of dry leaves and bushes in sugarcane filed particularly before harvest.

MEDICAL INFORMATICS

Medicine is enlarging with minute details of pain, cornea, lipids, etc., which further have hair-splitting details. These details are stored, processed and retrieved by numeric, images and sound in high capacity computers. Similar to our brain neural network, this is the emerging modern science of medical informatics.

Fertility, morbidity, mortality, social and mental component, environmental component and demographic component are put to comprehensive quick data in medical informatics.

Following are the major medical informatics:
❖ System analysis
❖ Design technique
❖ Statistical analysis
❖ Decision system
❖ Networking
❖ Communication system
❖ Expert system.

Activities of medical informatics are such as:
❖ Patient care
❖ Health management
❖ Community health measures
❖ Medical education
❖ Medical research.

The available medical informatics now are:
❖ Bibliographic service
❖ Text-based service
❖ Internet
❖ Health management information system
❖ Distant expert consultation.

Organization attached is:
❖ NIC (National information center, GOI)
  Systems available:
❖ Medlars
❖ Medline
❖ Cancerlit
❖ Health Plan
❖ Toxline

Network available:
❖ National Informatics Center Network (NICNET)

Chapter 33: Recent Area of Interest in Community Medicine

META-ANALYSIS (TABLE 33.3)

It is a technique for the aggregation and synthesis of prior research. Meta-analysis has become an important part of scientific methods.

Epi statistical software is used to calculate individual study odds ratio by Mantel-Haenszel method. The combined risk ratios and 95% confidence interval are calculated as per Piegorsch method. In meta-analysis, the homogenicity of odds ratio between different studies are based on Chi Square Statistics; with degree of freedom n – 1.

Examples
Following studies depict respiratory diseases by dust exposures:
1. Cross-section study of carpentry (Denmark) by Sabroe et al. 1979
2. Cohort study of styrene industry (USA) by Losimer et al. 1976
3. Cohort study of woodworkers (Sweden) by Alexandersson et al. 1989
4. Cross-section study of paint and soldering (India) by Gupta et al. 1993

Gupta et al. study (n = 208) with control (n = 411) showed some odds ratio by calculation. It is grouped as under:

Thus, all the findings of a study can be tabulated. Even lung function tests like forced vital capacity (FVC), forced expiratory volume (FEV1), FVC/FEV1% are considered.

Suppose such many studies are pooled to compare odds ratios, the observation can look like as given:

Table 33.3: Pooling studies to compare odds ratio.

Pooled symptoms	Pooled odds	Ratio 95% LCL	Confidence limit UCL
Cough	2.14	2.08	2.21
Expectoration	2.37	2.29	2.46
Breathlessness	2.90	2.74	3.08
Chest pain	2.77	2.66	2.88
Wheezing	1.85	1.70	2.01
Chronic bronchitis	1.19	1.15	1.23
Irritation of nose and throat	5.04	4.64	5.48

(LCL: lower confidence limit; UCL: upper confidence limit)

Cough			Expectoration			Short of breath			Chest pain		
E	C	OR	E	C	OR	E	C	OR	E	C	OR
41	44	2.05	41	44	2.05	24	14	3.69	53	45	2.78

Note: E = Exposed = 208, C = Control = 411 OR = Odds Ratio

Thus, inference from meta-analysis can be:
1. Frequency of lung obstruction
2. Association between symptoms and lung functions, etc.

THE MILLENNIUM DEVELOPMENT GOALS

United Nations (UN) General Assembly adopted the Millennium Development goals in 2000. Targets were fixed for the development by the year 2015.

This is popularly called HEALTH RELATED MILLENNIUM DEVELOPMENT GOALS IN INDIA.

Goals:
1. Eradicate extreme poverty and hunger
2. Reduce child mortality
3. Improve maternal health
4. Combat HIV/AIDS
5. Combat malaria
6. Combat tuberculosis
7. Ensure environmental sustainability which include biomass fuel, safe drinking water, and improved sanitation
8. Develop global partnership for development with emphasis on essential medicine

In 2015, Government of India launched 17 sustainable developmental goals to be achieved by 2030.

NATIONAL DAYS

January 1	New Year Day
January 12	International Youth Day
January 15	Army Day
January 26	Republic Day/International Customs Day
January 30	Sarvodaya Day/Martyr's Day/Antileprosy Day
February 1	Deaf and Dumb Day

February 4	World Cancer Day
February 14	Valentine Day
February 16	Tuberculosis Day
February 22	Scout Day
February 24	Central Excise Day
February 28	National Science Day
March 3	World Science Day
March 8	International Women's Day
March 9	Anganwadi Workers Day
March 15	World Consumer Rights Day/World Disabled Day
March 16	Measles Day
March 21	World Forestry Day/International Day for the elimination of racial discrimination
March 23	World Meteorological Day
April 5	National Martian Day
April 7	World Health Organization Day
April 12	National Fire Fighters Day
April 17	Hemophilia Day
April 18	World Heritage Day
April 22	Earth Day
April 30	Child Labor Day
May 1	May Day (World Labor Day)
May 3	Press Freedom Day
May 8	Ascension Day/World Red Cross Day
May 11	National Technology Day
May second Sunday	Mother's Day
May 15	International Day of the Family
May 17	World Telecom Day
May 21	Antiterrorist Day
May 24	Common Wealth Day
May 25	Milk Day
May 31	World No Smoke Day
June 4	International Day of Innocent children victims of aggression
June third Sunday	Father's Day
June 5	World Environment Day
June 6	World Children's Day
June 21	International Day of Yoga
June 26	International Day of Drugs and Illicit Trafficking
June 27	World Diabetes Day
July 1	Doctors' Day
July 6	World Zoonoses Day
July 8	World Zoonotic Day
July 11	World Population Day
August 1 first Sunday	World Breastfeeding Day
August 2	Sanskrit Day
August 3	International Friendship Day
August 5	World Breastfeeding Practice Day
August 6	Hiroshima Day
August 8	Senior Citizen's Day
August 9	Nagasaki Day/Quit India Day
August 15	Independence Day
August 19	Photography Day
August 29	National Sports Day
September 5	Teachers' Day
September 8	World Literacy Day
September 10	All India Flag Day for Blind
September 14	Hindi Day
September 15	Engineers' Day
September 16	World Ozone Day
September 21	Alzheimer's Day
September 24	National Service Scheme (NSS) Day
September 26	Day of the Deaf
September 27	World Tourism Day
October 1	International Day of the Elderly
October 2	Gandhi Jayanti
October 3	World Habitat Day
October 4	World Animal Welfare Day
October 6	World Senior Citizens' Day
October 8	Indian Air Force Day
October 9	World Post Office Day
October 10	World Mental Health Day/National Post Day
October 13	UN International Day for Natural Disaster Reduction
October 14	World Standards Day
October 15	World White Cane Day (Guiding the Blind)
October 16	World Food Day/World Anesthesia Day
October 24	UN Day/World Development Information Day

Chapter 33: Recent Area of Interest in Community Medicine

October 30	World Thrift Day
November 1	Red Cross Flag Day
November 8	World Radiology Day
November 10	World Science Day
November 14	Children's Day in India
November 15	World Diabetes Day
November 18	World Epilepsy Day
November 19	National Integration Day
November 20	Africa Industrialization Day
November 24	National Cadet Corps (NCC) Day
November 29	International Day of Solidarity with Palestinian People
December 1	AIDS Day
December 2	National Pollution Prevention Day
December 3	World Day of the Handicapped
December 4	Navy Day
December 7	Flag Day (Armed Force)
December 8	National Day for the Mentally Retarded
December 9	Home Guards Day
December 10	World Human Rights Day (UN)
December 11	UNICEF Day
December 23	Kisan's Day
December 25	Christmas Day

NATIONAL HEALTH GOALS BY 2015

Eliminate lymphatic filariasis	2015
Elimination of Kala-azar	By 2010
Achieve zero level growth of HIV/AIDS	By 2007
Reduce mortality by 50% on account of tuberculosis, malaria and other vector-borne and water-borne diseases	By 2010
Reduce prevalence of blindness to 0.5%	By 2010
Reduce IMR to 30 per 1,000 and MMR to 1 per 1,000 live births	By 2010
Improve nutrition and reduce proportion of LBW from 30% to 10%	By 2010
Increase utilization of public health facilities from current level of below 20–75%	By 2010
Increase health expenditure by Government with respect to GDP from existing 0.9–2.0%	By 2010
2% of budget for medical research	By 2010
Allocation of health resources–55% for primary health sector, 35% for secondary health sector and 10% for tertiary sector	By 2010

(IMR: infant mortality rate; MMR: maternal mortality ratio; HIV/AIDS: human immunodeficiency virus/acquired immunodeficiency syndrome; LBW: low birth weight; GDP: gross domestic product)

NATIONAL RURAL HEALTH MISSION (NRHM) (TABLE 33.4)

Health is determined by the economic development and social development. Any nation should improve the quality of life of its citizen. In order to improve the basic healthcare delivery system in the country, NRHM was launched by Government of India, on 12th April 2005. This has the budget outlay of Rs. 6,500 crores for 2005–2006 and a commitment of the Government to raise public health expenditure from 0.9% to 2.3% of gross domestic product. The goal of the mission is to improve the availability of and access to quality healthcare by people in rural areas, the poor, women, and children.

The aim of NRHM is to improve the acceptability of healthcare by strengthening healthcare systems for efficient service delivery through accountability, decentralization and equity.

The expected outcomes related to health by NRHM are:
- Good sanitation
- Personal and environmental hygiene
- Better nutrition
- Safe drinking water provision
- Allowing more expenditure on health
- Utilization of Indian systems of medicine
- Removing health infrastructure imbalance
- Pooling available resources
- Emphasizing integration of health services
- Optimizing health manpower
- Strengthening district health administration
- Allowing community participation
- Upgrading community health centers to function as hospital, meeting public health standards in each community developing country (IPHS)

The NRHM is made to play key role in the following National Health Programs:
- RCH project II (Reproductive and Child Health)
- NDCP (National Disease control Programs)
- IDSP (Integrated Disease Surveillance Project)
- AYUSH (Ayurvedic, Yoga, Unani, Siddha and Homeopathy Systems)

Initial focus of NRHM is on 18 "High focus" states which are:
- Uttar Pradesh (UP)
- Uttarakhand
- Madhya Pradesh (MP)
- Chhattisgarh
- Bihar
- Jharkhand
- Odisha
- Rajasthan
- Himachal Pradesh (HP)
- Jammu and Kashmir
- Assam
- Arunachal Pradesh
- Manipur
- Meghalaya
- Nagaland
- Mizoram
- Sikkim
- Tripura.

Strategies

See **Table 33.4**.

Ongoing Activities

- State and district health mission constitution
- Health and FW societies merging
- Identification of sectoral needs
- Shaping benchmarks for performance
- District action plans
- Community health center upgrading for AYUSH inclusion
- Rogi Kalyan Samitis formation
- Strengthening immunization in rural and outreach areas by alternate vaccine delivery system
- Arrangement of mobile medical services camp for women and children household toilets provision
- Subsidized hospital service for below poverty women under JSY and ASHA
- Training and drug kit to ASHA health education
- Norm development for infrastructure, equipment, laboratory, blood storage facilities, and drugs

Network in National Rural Health Mission (NRHM)

- Subcenters 156,231 (Cover 5,000 population in rural and 3,000 population in tribal/desert areas)
- Primary health center (PHC) 25,650 (Cover 30,000 population in rural and 20,000 population in tribal/desert areas)
- Community health center 5,624 (Cover 100,000 population in rural and 80,000 population in tribal/desert areas)
- NRHM is a statement of hope and conviction. It envisages a key role of Panchayati Raj Institutions in the implementation of health programs in India. There is a need for political leadership, administrative

Table 33.4: Strategies under NRHM.

Main strategies	Other strategies
1. Planning and management of district health administration 2. Appointing village women residents in age group of 25–45 years with formal education up to 8th standard as accredited social health activist (ASHA) for services under Janani Suraksha Yojana (JSY), directly observed treatment short (DOTS) course chemotherapy, Revised National Tuberculosis Control Program (RNTCP), district health mission (DHM) promoting household toilets under total sanitation campaign 3. Strengthening health service infrastructure 4. Promoting social participation of nonprofit sector	1. Private sector regulation in health care 2. Provide public private partnerships 3. Reorientation of medical education 4. Social insurance to raise health security

(NRHM: National Rural Health Mission)

commitment and buoyant community participation to fulfill the ambitious agenda of the National Rural health Mission.

NATIONAL SOCIODEMOGRAPHIC GOALS BY 2010

- Address the unmet needs for basic reproductive and child health services, supplies and infrastructure
- Make school education up to age 14 free and compulsory and reduce dropouts at primary and secondary school levels to below 20% for both boys and girls
- Reduce IMR to below 30 per 1,000 live births Reduce MMR to below 100 per 100,000 live births
- Achieve universal immunization of children against all vaccine preventable diseases
- Promote delayed marriage for girls, not earlier than age 18 and preferably after 20 years of age
- Achieve 80% institutional deliveries and 100 percent deliveries conducted by trained persons
- Achieve universal access to information/counseling and services for fertility regulation and contraception with a wide basket of choices
- Achieve 100% registration of births, deaths, marriage, and pregnancy
- Prevent and control communicable diseases
- Integrate Indian system of medicines in the provision of RCH services
- Promote vigorously the small family norm to achieve replacement levels of total fertility rate (TFR) 2.1
- Contain the spread of AIDS, and promote greater integration between management of reproductive tract infections (RTI) and sexually transmitted infections (STI) and National AIDS Control Organization (NACO)
- Bring about convergence in implementation of related social sector programs so that family welfare becomes a people centered program

NATIONAL URBAN HEALTH MISSION (NUHM)

- In 2013, health mission by Government of India incorporated and brought many programs together under rural mission and urban mission.
- Urban mission is called NUHM (National Urban Health Mission) to cater RCH and Adolescent Health Reproductive, Maternal, Newborn, Child and Adolescent Health (RMCCH+A), control of communicable diseases and noncommunicable diseases
- Access to urban slum, shanty town and urban poor, covering all towns with a population of above 50,000. All district headquarters are covered.

Following achievements are seen:
- IMR has come down to 34
- MMR has come down to 1.3 TFR has been 2.3
- TB incidence 204 per lakh population
- TB mortality 31 per lakh population
- Leprosy prevalence came to below 1 per 10,000 population
- Annual malaria incidence to less than 1/1,000 population
- Development of urban PHC to cater 50,000 population with OPD consultation, basic laboratory tests, free drug distribution, and contraceptive distribution
- Staff under urban PHC:
  - 1 Medical officer (MO) full time
  - 2 MO part time
  - 3 Nurse
  - 1 Lady health visitor (LHV)
  - 1 Pharmacist
  - 5 Auxiliary nurse midwife (ANM)
  - 1 Manager
  - 3 Support staff +community health volunteers
- Functions being carried out are:
  - Mahila Arogya Samiti formation
  - ASHA training
  - Delivery in public health facility.

RCH services which include registration, antenatal care (ANC), tetanus toxoid (TT), immunization, referring maternal and child problem, control of communicable diseases (malaria and tuberculosis), and control of noncommunicable diseases (diabetes, cancer, and hypertension)

NATIONAL HEALTH POLICY 2017

National Health Policy 1983 and National Health Policy 2002 gave an impetus to the National Health Policy 2017. Main focus is to strengthen and shape health system in all its dimensions.

Expected impacts of National Health Policy 2017 are:
- Expectation of life to increase to 70 by 2025
- Decrease TFR to 2.1 by 2025
- Decrease under five mortality to 23 by 2025
- Decrease MMR to 100 by 2020
- Decrease IMR to 28 by 2019
- Reduction of incidence/prevalence of diseases
- Elimination of leprosy, elimination of kala-azar and elimination of lymphatic filariasis by 2018
- Reduction of TB cure rate to above 85%
- Decrease in prevalence of blindness to 0.25/1,000 by 2015.

National Health Policy 2017 has given standards for health system, for health performance, for health infrastructure, and for health management.

NIPAH VIRAL INFECTION

- Nipah viral infection is a zoonotic disease and is an emerging infectious disease.
- Nipah is a village in Malaysia. This was first identified in 1999. Kerala state in India has shown an epidemic outbreak in 2018 (19 cases and 17 deaths).
- Infected bats, infected pigs, infected people are source of infection. Incubation period range is from 4 to 14 days.
- ARI and encephalitis are common clinical manifestations.
- ELISA test is a diagnostic test for Nipah viral infection.

- No drugs are available for the case management. No vaccine is available for its prevention.
- Creating awareness and giving health education are available preventive steps in epidemic areas.

NATIONAL INSTITUTION FOR TRANSFORMING INDIA (NITI) AAYOG 2015

- NITI stands for National Institute for Transforming India. NITI has replaced planning commission.
- It is a thinktank to Central Government and State Governments. NITI guides through technical advice.
- Main functions of NITI are:
  - Monitoring health programs
  - Evaluation of health programs
  - Helping in technology upgradation
  - Helping in capacity building.

POISON CONTROL INFORMATION

Poisoning due to chemicals, pharmaceuticals, plants and animals toxins are occurring more and more.

The poisoning depends on various reasons. These are:
- Intentional
- Accidental
- Occupational
- Acute
- Chronic.

Acute poisoning presents medical emergencies.

Mass poisoning has occurred due to accidental contamination of food and medicine. Industrial disasters have occurred during manufacture and transport (Bhopal tragedy where methyl isocyanate from Union Carbide Plant resulted in 2,500 deaths and 150,000 disabilities).

Most common cause of poisoning in India is by pesticides, reasons being agriculture-based economics, poverty, easy availability of toxic pesticides.

Poison control information can contribute to the prevention of poisoning by:

- Alerting responsible authorities to act
- Encouraging manufacturers to employ less toxic formulations
- Informing general public on how to avoid poisoning
- Give special warning to professional health care worker.

PARTOGRAM

Prolonged labor or obstructed labor due to poor uterine contractions is a common obstetrical emergency and could be a cause of maternal death. Poor uterine contraction is guided by the criteria that cervix dilates slowly and incompletely. This becomes indication for cesarean section.

If the clinical conditions of mother are favorable, for a case of prolonged labor, vaginal delivery may be considered in a hospital under medical supervision. However, a cesarean section is indicated if there is fetal distress. Prolonged or obstructed labor can lead to rupture of uterus and fetal death. Slow progress of labor can cause postpartum hemorrhage (PPH), infection and obstetric fistulae.

When there are no facilities for emergency obstetric care (e.g., health center) it is important that signs of obstructed or prolonged labor are identified early so that pregnant woman is transferred to a hospital in time.

A partogram is a tool to help in the management of labor for the identification of women who are not likely to have a normal delivery and who need medical assistance.

The progress of labor is monitored by:
a. Cervical dilatation
b. Descent of head (by abdominal palpation of the head)
c. Uterine contraction (Frequency per minute and duration).

Fetal rate and maternal condition are additional monitors.

Partogram should be started after checking that there are no complications of pregnancy which require immediate action.

If progress is satisfactory, the plotting of cervical dilatation will remain on or to the left of the alert line in active phase of partogram.

POSTPARTUM PROGRAM (PPP) (PPC) (PPPC)

This program provides family planning (FP) information and services to urban women of low socioeconomic status in settings where delivery is institutional.

The 3 months following delivery or abortion (postpartum period) constitutes a significant period of high motivation during which women can be approached concerning future child-bearing. Antenatal, natal and postnatal period seem to offer unique opportunity to reach women in a systematic manner.

Teaching hospitals are preferred since it includes the aspect of training undergraduate (UG), postgraduate (PG) and paramedical.

Postpartum program was launched in India in 1969, and now it has wide establishment in different hospitals and upgraded centers.

Following infrastructure of Government of India is used for services:

Infrastructure	Number (2018)
Subcenter	156,231
Primary health center	25,650
Community health center	5,624
Rural family welfare clinic	5,435
Health and family welfare training center	47
Postpartum program center	1,562
Health posts	871
Urban family welfare center	1,083

Program Operation

- Informing all delivery and abortions about FP methods available.
- Set up informal network of "word of mouth" through friends, relatives and neighbors.

Program Implementation

A. ***Information education and communication (IEC)***
   - At antenatal clinic, antenatal ward, postnatal ward, and obstetric ward
   - Husband/visitor waiting room
   - Pediatric wards. Content of IEC
     - Conception
     - Child birth

- Feeding and care of newborn
- Hazard by repeated child birth
- Importance of spacing, and
- FP methods available

B. **Service**
C. **Training**
D. **Coordination:** Evaluation is done by the acceptance of FP by women after delivery or abortion and by calculating birth aversion rates.

A. ***Direct Acceptance (Acceptance within 3 months)***

Immediate direct acceptance (Before leaving hospital)	Other direct acceptance (After leaving hospital but before 3 months)

B. ***Indirect Acceptance (Later acceptance)***
- Not obstetrical case
- Not abortion case but accepted FP
- All vasectomy included.

RECENT GLOBAL TUBERCULOSIS (TB) STRATEGIES

- About 3 million cases are missed and are called "missed Millions" which contribute public health failure.
- Drug resistance continue to thrive
- TB is leading cause of death
- United Nations Sustainable Developmental Goal evolved TB Strategies and DOTS Strategy, STOP Strategy and END strategy.
- 1994 DOTS strategy
- 2006 Stop Strategy
- 2015 End strategy
- Main Target has been:
  - 75% reduction of TB deaths by 2025
  - 50% reduction of TB incidence by 2025
  - End of TB by 2035
  - Reduce TB affected family from catastrophe to zero
- Advocated 90-90-90 target is as under:
  A. Reach 90% of all TB cases
  B. Approach 90% of key population
  C. Achieve 90% success in treatment.

RED CROSS DAY

May 8th of every year is celebrated as Red Cross Day throughout the world which happens to be the birth anniversary of Henry Dunant. His passion to serve the humanity was extraordinary and unique which no other person could show. Henry Dunant sowed the seeds of Red Cross which is a unique organization. Actually, he was an outstanding businessman who worked for the improvement of his business. In the year 1859, as usual he intended to visit French emperor on business campaign. In his visit he saw the battle of Soldering, which was the battle between France and Austria. He was shocked to see thousands of dead and thousands wounded. Happening was the same what we saw with Emperor Ashoka in the battle of Kalinga. Without his knowledge he set aside his business visit and involved in the war relief work. His friends from Solferino also joined hands with him in relief work.

Henry Dunant wrote his experience in Solferino with the title "A Memory of Solferino."

He emphasized the need for international cooperation and trained volunteers. This was the theme in first international conference in Geneva in 1863. The groundwork of this conference created the renowned Geneva Convention.

In 1867, he was found totally bankrupt after spending all his wealth to the suffering humanity. He spent some time in asylum in Heiden at Switzerland. In 1901, he got First Nobel Peace Prize and he bequeathed the money to his dreamt charitable cause. He died in 1910 leaving the Red Cross. Now, every person on the earth knows what could be the ubiquitous vehicle bearing the emblem of the Red Cross and that is how we remember the Red Cross Day.

THE RIGHTS OF PERSONS WITH DISABILITY BILL 2016

The main idea behind this act has been care, protection, maintenance and welfare of disabled person.

Further to strengthen the training, education and rehabilitation of socially handicapped children or handicapped person.

Government of India has jotted down 21 disabilities under this Act. Further combinations such as deaf and blind are laid down for the purpose of Act.
They are:
01 Blindness
02 Low vision
03 Cured leprosy
04 Hard of hearing
05 Locomotor disability
06 Dwarf
07 Hard of hearing
08 Very low intelligence quotient (IQ)
09 Mentally ill
10 Autism
11 Cerebral palsy
12 Muscular dystrophy
13 Chronic neurological conditions
14 Disabled for learning
15 Multiple sclerosis
16 Speech disability
17 Thalassemia
18 Hemophilia
19 Sickle cell disorder
20 Acid attack victim
21 Parkinson's disease

The Rights of Persons with Disabilities Bill 2016 looks to strengthen the family, helps to make disabled to live happy and useful in life.

RE-ORIENTATION OF MEDICAL EDUCATION (ROME)

It was launched in 1977.
Main objectives: Involvement of medical colleges in community health problems and in direct delivery of healthcare services to the rural population.

Specific Objectives

- Exposing medical students to rural environment
- Exposing faculty of medical college to rural environment
- Upgrading quality of health service through specialized service such as laboratory service and X-ray service, and
- Phased transfer of total healthcare to the district.

Guidelines for Activities

- Each medical college is to adopt three PHC if possible. Affiliated Universities are suggesting to adopt one PHC in the beginning and to go for others later
- Involvement at all levels of health care system
- Suitable time-table for posting Bachelor of Medicine and Bachelor of Surgery (MBBS) students
- All faculties of medical college involvement
- Research to be rural-oriented.

For example, PG dissertation work (community medicine, OBG, pediatrics) at PHC field practice area.

- Baseline data information collection
- Various level coordination committee formation, and
- Mobile clinics are provided which serve the rural areas for the specialists' visit and service.

Teaching and Training

i. Family side teaching instead of bedside teaching by all the faculties is insisted.
ii. Community health posting of UG insisted.
iii. Compulsory interns posting at PHC, their stay in dormitory hostel, attending to healthcare service, supervisory service is insisted.

Rain Water Harvesting

This is one of the oldest and simplest method of self-supply of water for households. Larger systems are generally costlier.

Collection and storage of rain water rather than allowing it to drain off from roof and is redirected to tank, pit, borehole or regular sumps.

In urban areas, rain water collection can be used for urban agriculture, which has many facet of agro economics.

In India, all states have made legal implications in urban development, regular housing construction; to have rain water harvesting made compulsory.

Instead of using roof for catchment area, new approach for rain saucer which looks like an upside down umbrella which collects rain water directly from sky. The purity is unquestionable.

Recently, rain water harvesting by solar power panels is gaining importance in the world.

Advantages are:
- Provides independent water supply
- Supplements the main water supply
- Avoids flooding of low lying areas
- Helps in the availability of potable water.

For rain water harvesting system building, use of digital tools is useful for finding out rainwater harvesting potential, community need. This helps to save money and time for project to set up during house construction.

SANITATION AT FAIR, FESTIVAL, PILGRIMAGE

Human congregation for fair, festival and pilgrimage has attained importance for its causing:
- Epidemics
- Accidents.

Management

1. Planning of arrangements: First aid, road, layout, information to public.
2. Accommodation.
3. Medical relief arrangement for illness, epidemics and accidents.
4. Sanitary arrangement protected water supply superficial trench latrine
    - [Two seats per 1,000 people (1 day fair).]
    - Deep trench latrine
    - [One seat for 100 people (1 week fair)] Adequate urinals
    - One sanitary worker for 2,000 pilgrims: Adequate waste bins for waste storage.
5. Food supply—strict supervision.
6. Cholera inoculation in endemic areas.
7. International certificate of vaccination applicable to specified noted areas.
8. Arrangement of health inspection check post.
9. Handling of problems of prostitutes through public education by social workers.

SEVERE MALARIA

Severe malaria is caused by *Plasmodium falciparum* infection. The risk of population exposed to severe malaria is 40 percent of world's population.

Two global epidemiological factors are identified in severe malaria transmission. They are:
1. Modern rapid means of travel makes rapid transmission of malaria.
2. People from nonmalarious area getting exposed to infection, started showing serious effect after their return home.

Main public health importance of severe malaria is that malaria parasites (MP) smear examination and immediate treatment if not done, mortality by multiorgan involvement even within few hours is expected. Prompt action is especially important for high-risk groups such as young children and pregnant women.

Uncomplicated Severe Malaria

The fever is persistent rather than tertian (spikes of fever on alternate days). One of the epidemiological observation is that the expectation that *P. falciparum* malaria should have a tertian fever (alternate day fever) may lead to the diagnosis of malaria being missed.

Fever, headache, aches, pains over body, abdominal pain, and diarrhea are common in uncomplicated malaria. In children irritability, refusal to eat, and vomiting are special features.

Following presentations are always of severe malaria when a patient with severe malaria shows MP +ve, confusion or drowsiness with extreme weakness (prostration):
- Cerebral malaria defined as unarousable coma
- Generalized convulsions
- Severe normocytic anemia
- Hypoglycemia

- Metabolic acidosis with respiratory distress
- Fluid and electrolyte disturbances
- Acute renal failure
- Acute pulmonary edema and adult respiratory distress syndrome (ARDS)
- Circulatory collapse, shock septicemia (Algid malaria)
- Abnormal bleeding
- Jaundice
- Hemoglobinuria
- High fever
- Hyperparasitemia.

Management of Severe Malaria

Following are the ways to manage severe malaria:
- General management
- Nursing care, and
- Specific antimalarial chemotherapy

Antimalarial Drugs in Severe Malaria

1. Quinine by rate controlled infusion 20 mg/kg in dextrose in 4 hours
   - 10 mg/kg in later dose 8 hours after repeated till patient swallows
   - (Diluted to 60 mg/mL can be used for IM) Then 10 mg/kg—8 hourly × 7 days
2. *Artemisinin:* 10-40 mg/kg (Intrarectal suppository formulations).
3. *Artesunate*
   - 2.4 mg/kg 1 hour
   - 1.2 mg/kg 12-24 hours, later 1.2 mg/kg × 6 days (Oral, IM, IV and rectocap preparation).
4. *Artemether*
   - 3.2 mg/kg IV
   - 1.6 mg/kg × 6 days
5. *Sulfadoxine—pyrimethamine*
   - 500 mg + 25 mg
   - Contraindicated in early pregnancy and neonate.
6. *Chloroquine:* 10 mg in isotonic IV infusion 8 hours 15 mg/kg over next 24 hours.
7. *Mefloquine:* Available only in tablet form used to complement parenteral therapy with artesunate/artemether.

SOCIAL ACCOUNTABILITY OF HOSPITALS AND MEDICAL COLLEGES

In British India, limited number of hospitals and limited number of medical colleges were there to cater to patient care and medical education in the country. Later in independent India, during the period 1947-2006, many hospitals and many medical colleges have come up in the country. Hospitals come under the directive of Central and State Medical Directorate whereas medical colleges are regulated by Medical Council of India.

Primary care, secondary care, and tertiary care by various hospitals in the country, both government and private, need to take up responsibilities in its activities of health care that they should be acceptable and accessible for the common man. Thus, social accountability of hospital is a responsibility to society that should guide the hospital's scope of medical care, investigations, surgical interventions and service cum research.

Similarly, both government and private medical colleges in the country have the obligation to direct education, research and public service activities toward addressing the priority health concerns of the village, taluka, district, state, and the country. Social accountability is thus a responsibility to society that should guide the college's entire scope of activities in medical education, medical service, and medical research.

Thus, new paradigms of healthcare and medical colleges have social accountability as a direct obligation to direct their activities so that it can be a mandate to serve the community.

Social accountability counts on the social justice focusing on the poor and the marginalized, i.e., needs of the disadvantaged. There will be a mechanism of involvement of the community with additional values such as integrity, justice, empathy or concern, competence, self-reliance, self-learning, and continuing education.

Vision, objectives and recommendations on hospital services and medical colleges are already met with by quality standards enforced by the regulatory bodies, viz., of Directorate General of Health Services (DGHS) and Medical Council of India (MCI) on Medical Education Institutions and Hospitals.

Survey by various government and private organizations on hospital services has emphasized the need for social accountability. Interviews and case studies such as the one conducted by Rajiv Gandhi University of Health Sciences have made it clear about approaches both qualitative and quantitative as far as community development and nation's needs are concerned. Vision, mission, values, beliefs and goals have been the specific areas of focus and that focus have been on relevance, quality, equity, cost-effectiveness, perceived priorities, leadership roles of both hospitals and medical colleges.

With the emphasis on social accountability 25,650 primary health centers, 156,231 subcenters, 5,624 community health centers, and 460 medical colleges and innumerable number of nursing homes and clinics in the country need to have their priorities realized to meet their social responsibilities to the society. Karnataka also show a greater number in the field. There are total 59 medical colleges (29 Government and 30 private) and 11 Deemed University Medical colleges in Karnataka and accountability initiated by Rajiv Gandhi University of Medical Sciences of Karnataka (RGUHS) for the first time in the country.

SOCIAL MARKETING

In health science, community acceptability is achieved to meet the social purpose. This process involves proper planning, price fixing, communication and market distribution, e.g., Social marketing of Condom, Social marketing of Mala-N.

Social Marketing Involve Two Stages

1. Advertisement giving public an idea about a health product.
2. Actual release of the health product.

Process of Social Marketing

With example of "Women's hygiene kits" (WHK) a recent approach of social marketing of women's hygiene kit (sanitary pad) is being taken up.

Phase I: Collection of Basic Data: Personal hygiene of adolescent girls and women particularly during menstrual cycle has been of very low standards, reflecting in higher prevalence of RTI, which will result in various gynecological problems. This component of RCH is tackled by necessary intervention with "women's hygiene kit".

Phase II: IEC activities: Availability of suitable communication material flipbook, single sheeted are produced and distributed through teachers, AWW, ANM.

Phase III: Training: Training of ANM, teachers and AWW before distribution of WHK.

Phase IV: Pilot survey: Pilot survey of a sample of population is done to have baseline data.

Phase V: Actual distribution: Actual distribution of sanitary pad through public distribution system (PDS) at subsidized rate (A pack containing 10 pieces of sanitary pad of about Rs. 20-25 will be supplied through PDS, AWW and ANM at a cost of Rs. 5.00).

Phase VI: Evaluation: Evaluation of impact and utilization done by resurvey.

Difference between Social and Commercial Products

Social product		Commercial product
Controversial idea	More	Less
Complexity of product	More	Less
Consumers	Low socioeconomic	High socioeconomic
Literacy	Low	High
Utilization rate expected	Very high	Low
Consumer satisfaction	Less	More

Contd...

Contd...

Social product		Commercial product
Examples	Nirodh	Amul icecream
	Mala D	Gutka
	Women's Hygiene kit	Thums up

Advantages of Social Marketing

Following are the main advantages of social marketing:
- Government takes care of production and hence available almost at cheaper rate
- Accessibility is made
- Takes away inhibitions gradually and improve acceptability
- Underprivileged/target group gets free of cost.

SOCIOMETRIC ANALYSIS

It is a method of discovering, describing and evaluating social status, structure and development through the extent of acceptance or rejection between individuals in groups. It is a measure of attraction and repulsion between individuals in a group.

Uses

- Helps to configurate group relation
- Social position is identified, and
- Influencing factors are identified.

Outcome

- Choice
- Rejection, and
- Ignoring.

Methods

- Graphic analysis
- Index analysis
- Statistical analysis, and
- Matrix analysis.

SUBSTANCE ABUSE

Earlier terminology "drug abuse" is replaced by "Substance abuse", since definition of drug confuses the issue of addiction, when a substance is taken is not for therapeutic purpose.

Habit forming substances which are consumed repeatedly is detrimental to the health of an individual and society. Substance consumption such as drug, alcohol, plant extract taken produces toxic intoxication, which gradually makes a person dependent on it physically and psychologically.

Chronic substance abuse produces high tolerance level.

Substance abuse is one of the major social problems of the society.

WHO has recommended using the word drug dependence for drug abuse and substance abuse for nondrug addiction conditions.

Causes of Substance Abuse

- Change in socioeconomic condition
- Urban rural drift
- Loosening of informal means of social control
- Increasing stress and strain in modern society.

Following are the preventive and controlling measures:
- Medical treatment
- Change in environment
- Psychotherapy
- Education of target group
- Support of parent, teacher community leader
- Control of supply and demand of substance.

SULABH SHAUCHALAYA

Sulabh shauchalaya is a simple latrine model devised by the organization called Sulabh. The founder of this Sulabh organization is Dr Bindeshwar Pathak. The main objective of sulabh shauchalaya is to provide clean toilet facilities to public on a small payment. The amount collected is utilized for the maintenance of latrine.

The latrine is low cost latrine designed with pan and water seal. It is connected to a pit of the size 3 cubic feet volume, digestion is by anaerobic digestion. Small quantity of water is used by pouring which flush the night soil. In some of the areas a lavatory block with several seats is constructed. It employs an attendant who collects Rs. 0.50 or Rs. 1.00 and looks after the maintenance of latrine.

THE PRENATAL DIAGNOSTIC TECHNIQUES (PNDT) AND PRECONCEPTION (PC)

(Prenatal diagnostic techniques (Regulation and Prevention of Misuse) Act No. 57, 1994. (20th Sept 1994)

PC and PNDT Act 1994 and Amendments No. 14 of 2003 [The Preconception and Prenatal Diagnostic Techniques (Prohibition of Sex Selection) Act] [14th Feb 2003].

Prenatal Diagnostic Techniques (PNDT)

The Act Prenatal Diagnostic Technique, Prevention of misuse and Regulation Act came into being in 1994 only to check female feticide following steady decline in female ratio across the country.

Efforts are being made since then for strict implementation of the Act by preparing agenda for its implementation in the future.

Doctor or a person if performs female feticide without valid reasons is liable for punishment. Central Government, State Governments, Indian Medical Association and Federation of Obstetrician and Gynecologists are involved in the implementation of the Act.

Main focus of attention has been:
- PNDT should be implemented strictly to check female feticide
- It shall help in creating awareness in medical fraternity
- It shall coax them to participate in the battle against female feticide
- Shall help in strict implementation of the Act in the letter and spirit and series of interactions with medical bodies.

The Act provides, in 8 chapters, the regulation of the use of prenatal diagnostic techniques for the purpose of detecting genetic or metabolic disorders or chromosomal abnormalities or certain congenital malformations of sex linked disorders and for the prevention of the misuse of such techniques for the purpose of prenatal sex determination leading to female feticide; and, for matters connected therewith or incidental thereto.

- Chapter 1 deals with title and definitions of appropriate authority, board, genetic counseling, genetic clinic, genetic laboratory, gynecologist, medical geneticist, pediatrician, prenatal diagnostic procedures, prenatal diagnostic techniques, prenatal diagnostic tests, prescribed, rural medical practitioners (RMP) and regulations.
- Chapter 2 deals with regulation of genetic counseling centers, genetic laboratories and genetic clinics.
- Chapter 3 deals with regulation of prenatal diagnostic techniques for chromosomal abnormalities, genetic metabolic diseases, hemoglobinopathies, and sex-linked genetic diseases, congenital anomalies and any other abnormalities or diseases as may be specified by the central supervisory board. Following criteria should be satisfied:
  - Pregnant woman is above 35 years
  - If there is 2 or 3 spontaneous abortions or fetal loss
  - Exposed to radiation, infection, chemicals and teratogenic drugs
  - Mental retardation, spastic or genetic disease and any other condition specified by CSB (Central supervisory body)
- Chapter 3 also specifies that determination of sex is prohibited
- Chapter 4 deals with central supervisory board (CSB)
- Chapter 5 deals with appropriate authority and advisory committee
- Chapter 6 deals with registration of genetic counseling centers, genetic laboratories and genetic clinics
- Chapter 7 deals with offences and penalties. Provision of this Act shall be punishable with imprisonment for a term which may extend to 3 years and with fine which may extend

to Rs. 10,000/- and on any subsequent conviction, with imprisonment which may extend to 5 years and with fine which may extend to Rs. 50,000/- rupees.
* Chapter 8 deals with miscellaneous items like maintenance of records, power to search and seizure records, protection of action taken in good faith.

Preconception (PC) Prenatal Diagnostic Techniques (PNDT)

During the course of the implementation of PNDT Act, certain inadequacies and practical difficulties in the administration came to the notice of Government. Techniques have been developed to select the sex of the child before conception that was taken note of by the Supreme Court in its various orders and the Court had also observed that amendments to the PNDT Act are necessary. The purpose is to ban the use of sex selection techniques before or after conception as well as the misuse of prenatal diagnostic techniques for sex selective abortions and to regulate such techniques. To make this clear, the long title of the Act has been suitably amended to read as under:

"An Act to provide for the prohibition of sex selection, before or after conception, and for regulation of prenatal diagnostic techniques for the purposes of detecting abnormalities or metabolic disorders or chromosomal abnormalities or certain congenital malformations or sex-linked disorders and for the prevention of their misuse for sex determination leading to female feticide and for matters connected therewith or incidental thereto."

The Title of the Act is amended as *"The Preconception and Prenatal Diagnostic Techniques (Prohibition of Sex Selection) Act."*
The contents of the amendment of act are as follows:
* Chapter 1 Introduction
* Chapter 2 Definitions
* Chapter 3 Registration
* Chapter 4 Prohibitions
* Chapter 5 Instrumentalities for Implementing the Act
* Chapter 6 Maintenance and Preservation of Records
* Chapter 7 Search and Seizure

Followed by Annexure 1–8 and Appendix 1–4.

The Implementation of the Act is being monitored by Supreme Court.

The Supreme Court has defined the terms cognizable offense, complaint, nonbailable offense and noncompoundable offense.

Cognizable Offense

An offense for which the police may arrest without a warrant, the offender, or a person who is suspected of committing the offense on account of reasonable belief.

Complaint

Any allegation made orally or in writing to a Magistrate with the intension of requiring him to take action under the Criminal Procedure Code against a person who has allegedly committed an offense.

Nonbailable Offense

Offenses for which getting bail is not the right of the accused. Bail may be granted or refused based on the discretionary power of the Court.

Noncompoundable Offense

Those offenses on the commission of which no prosecution can be withdrawn or in simple terms where no settlement between the parties is possible to drop the criminal proceedings.

The registration fee is Rs. 3,000 for centers and Rs. 4,000 for hospitals.

The qualified people include gynecologist, medical geneticist, pediatrician, RMP, radiologist, sonologist and imaging specialist.

Penalties include

Imprisonment up to 3 years and fine up to Rs. 10,000 for person who acts contrary to the prohibitions.

Imprisonment up to 5 years and fine up to Rs. 50,000 for subsequent conviction.

Imprisonment of 3 years and fine of Rs. 50,000 for a person seeking the aid of the bodies for sex selection.

Imprisonment of 5 years and fine of Rs. 100,000 for subsequent conviction.

Suspension of registration for RMP.

Imprisonment of 3 months and fine of Rs. 1,000 or both for a person who contravenes the provision of the Act.

Additional fine of Rs. 500 per day for subsequent contravention if continues.

The offense under the Act shall be tried only in a court of the Metropolitan Magistrate or a Judicial Magistrate of the First Class.

Gynecologist

Having experience of performing at least 20 procedures in chorionic villi aspirations per vagina or per abdomen, chorionic villi biopsy, amniocentesis, cordocentesis fetoscope, fetal skin or organ biopsy or fetal blood sampling, etc., under supervision of an experienced gynecologist in these fields.

Sonologist, Imaging Specialist, Radiologist or RMP

Having postgraduate degree or diploma or 6 months training or 1 year experience in sonography or image scanning.

Sale of Ultrasound (USG) Machine

No organization including a commercial organization or a person, including manufacturer, importer, dealer or supplier of ultrasound machines/imaging machines or any other equipment, capable of detecting sex of fetus, shall sell, distribute, supply, rent, allow or authorize the use of any such machine or equipment in any manner, whether on payment or otherwise, to any genetic counseling center, genetic laboratory, genetic clinic, ultrasound clinic, imaging center or any other body or person unless such center, laboratory, clinic, body or person is registered under the Act.

Others

The Supreme Court of India on 11.12.2001 has directed 9 companies to supply the information as to how many machines they have sold to various clinics within last 5 years including their names and addresses and also service contract to those clinics or individuals.

About the use of ultrasound machines/scanners: The Supreme Court of India has asked to take the help of following Associations (a) Indian Medical Association (IMA) (b) Indian Radiologist Association (IRA) and (c) The Federation of Obstetric and Gynecological Societies of India (FOGSI).

TRENDS IN RECENT IMMUNIZATION

Indian Academy of Pediatrics (IAP) recommended immunization schedule for children aged 0 through 18 years–India, 2014 and updates on immunization

There is a need to review/revise recommendations about existing vaccines in light of recent developments in the field of vaccinology. Following an IAP Advisory Committee on Vaccines and Immunization Practices (ACVIP) meeting on April 19 and 20 2014, a draft of revised recommendations for the year 2014 and updates on certain vaccine formulations was prepared and circulated among the meeting participants to arrive at a consensus.

The major changes in the 2014 immunization time-table include:

Two doses of MMR vaccine at 9 and 15 months of age.

Single dose recommendation for administration of live attenuated H2 strain hepatitis A vaccine.

Inclusion of two new situations in "high-risk category of children" in context with "pre-exposure prophylaxis" of rabies.

Creation of a new slot at 9–12 months of age for typhoid conjugate vaccine for primary immunization.

Recommendation of two doses of human papillomavirus vaccines with a minimum interval of 6 months between doses for primary schedule of adolescent/preadolescent girls aged 9–14 years.

There would not be any change to the committee's last year's (2013) recommendations on pertussis vaccination and administration schedule of monovalent human rotavirus vaccine.

Table 33.5: IAP recommended vaccines for routine use.

Age (completed weeks/months/years)	Vaccines	Comments
Birth	BCG OPV 0 Hep-B 1	Administer these vaccines to all newborns before hospital discharge
6 weeks	DTwP 1 IPV 1 Hep-B 2 Hib 1 Rotavirus 1 PCV 1	**DTP:** DTaP vaccine/combinations should preferably be avoided for the primary series DTaP vaccine/combinations should be preferred in certain specific circumstances/conditions only No need of repeating/giving additional doses of whole-cell pertussis (wP) vaccine to a child who has earlier completed their primary schedule with acellular pertussis (aP) vaccine-containing products **Polio:** • All doses of IPV may be replaced with OPV if administration of the former is not feasible • Additional doses of OPV on all supplementary immunization activities (SIAs) • Two doses of IPV instead of three for primary series if started at 8 weeks, and 8 weeks interval between the doses • No child should leave the facility without polio immunization (IPV or OPV), if indicated by the schedule **Rotavirus:** • 2 doses of RV1 and 3 doses of RV5 • RV1 should be employed in 10 and 14 weeks schedule, instead of 6 and 10 weeks • 10 and 14 weeks schedule of RV1 is found to be far more immunogenic than existing 6 and 10 weeks schedule
10 weeks	DTwP 2 IPV 2 Hib 2 Rotavirus 2 PCV 2	**Rotavirus:** If RV1 is chosen, the first dose should be given at 10 weeks
14 weeks	DTwP 3 IPV 3 Hib 3 Rotavirus 3 PCV 3	**Rotavirus:** Only 2 doses of RV1 are recommended at present If RV1 is chosen, the 2nd dose should be given at 14 weeks
6 months	OPV 1 Hep-B 3	**Hepatitis-B:** The final (third or fourth) dose in the Hep B vaccine series should be administered no earlier than age 24 weeks and at least 16 weeks after the first dose
9 months	OPV 2 MMR-1	**MMR:** • Measles-containing vaccine ideally should not be administered before completing 270 days or 9 months of life • The 2nd dose must follow in 2nd year of life • No need to give stand-alone measles vaccine

Contd...

Contd...

Age (completed weeks/months/years)	Vaccines	Comments
		Typhoid:
9–12 months	Typhoid Conjugate Vaccine	• Currently, two typhoid conjugate vaccines, Typbar-TCV and PedaTyph available in Indian market • PedaTyph is not yet approved; the recommendation is applicable to Typbar-TCV only • An interval of at least 4 weeks with the MMR vaccine should be maintained while administering this vaccine • Should follow a booster at 2 years of age
12 months	Hep-A 1	**Hepatitis A:** • Single dose for live attenuated H2-strain Hep-A vaccine • Two doses for all killed Hep-A vaccines are recommended now
15 months	MMR 2	**MMR:**
	Varicella 1	The 2nd dose must follow in 2nd year of life
	PCV booster	However, it can be given at any time 4–8 weeks after the 1st dose during 2nd year
16–18 months	DTwP B1/ DTaP B1	**Varicella:**
	IPV B1, Hib B1	• The risk of breakthrough varicella is lower if given 15 months onward • The first booster (4th dose) may be administered as early as age 12 months, provided at least 6 months have elapsed since the third dose.
18 months	Hep-A 2	**DTP:** • First and second boosters should preferably be of DTwP • Considering a higher reactogenicity of DTwP, DTaP can be considered for the boosters
		2nd dose for killed vaccines; only single dose for live attenuated H2- strain vaccine
2 years	Typhoid booster	• Either Typbar-TCV® or Vi-polysaccharide (Vi-PS) can be employed as booster • Typhoid revaccination every 3 years, if Vi-polysaccharide vaccine is used • Need of revaccination following a booster of Typbar-TCV® not yet determined
4–6 years	DTwP B2/ DTaP B2	**Varicella:**
	OPV 3 Varicella 2	2nd dose can be given at any time 3 months after the 1st dose
	Typhoid booster	
10–12 years	Tdap/Td HPV	**Tdap:**
		Tdap is preferred to Td followed by Td every 10 years
		HPV: • Only 2 doses of either of the two HPV vaccines for adolescent/ preadolescent girls aged 9–14 years • For girls 15 years and older, and immunocompromised individuals 3 doses are recommended • For two-dose schedule, the minimum interval between doses should be 6 months. • For 3 dose schedule, the doses can be administered at 0, 1–2 (depending on brands) and 6 months

Chapter 33: Recent Area of Interest in Community Medicine

Indian Academy of Paediatrics (IAP) recommended vaccines for High-risk* children (Vaccines under special circumstances)
1. Influenza vaccine
2. Meningococcal vaccine
3. Japanese encephalitis vaccine
4. Cholera vaccine
5. Rabies vaccine
6. Yellow fever vaccine
7. Pneumococcal polysaccharide vaccine (PPSV 23)

*__High-risk category of children:__ *Congenital or acquired immunodeficiency (including HIV infection); Chronic cardiac, pulmonary (including asthma if treated with prolonged high-dose oral corticosteroids), hematologic, renal (including nephrotic syndrome) and liver disease; Children on long-term steroids, salicylates, immunosuppressive or radiation therapy; Diabetes mellitus, Cerebrospinal fluid leak, Cochlear implant, Malignancies; Children with functional/anatomic asplenia/hyposplenia; During disease outbreaks; Laboratory personnel and healthcare workers; Travelers; Children having pets in home; Children perceived with higher threat of being bitten by dogs such as hostellers, risk of stray dog menace while going outdoor.*

(BCG: bacille Calmette-Guerin; DTaP: diphtheria, tetanus, and acellular pertussis vaccine; Hep: hepatitis; IPV: inactivated poliovirus vaccine; OPV: oral polio vaccine; Tap: tetanus, and pertussis; DTP: diphtheria, tetanus and pertussis; PCV: porcine circovirus type 1; TCV: typhoid conjugate vaccine; MMR: measles, mumps, and rubella; IAP: Indian Academy of Pediatrics)

There is no need of providing additional doses of whole-cell pertussis vaccine to children who have earlier completed their primary schedule with acellular pertussis vaccine-containing products.

A brief update on the new Indian Rotavirus vaccine, 116E is also provided. The committee has reviewed and offered its recommendations on the currently available pentavalent vaccine (DTwP+Hib+Hepatitis-B) combinations in Indian market.

Measles and Measles, Mumps, and Rubella (MMR) Vaccination

The new schedule will have a dose of MMR at 9 months instead of measles, and another dose (2nd) at 15 months of age. The earlier recommendation of 2nd dose of MMR at 4–6 years of age has been removed.

Live Attenuated Hepatitis A Vaccine

Now, a single dose of this vaccine is recommended at 12 months of age over-riding the previous recommendation of two doses of the same vaccine.

Rotavirus Vaccines

Monovalent Rotavirus Vaccine, RV1

The available results do not warrant any change in the existing schedule of RV1 vaccine that includes the first dose at 10 weeks of age instead of 6 weeks in order to achieve better immune response, and the second dose at 14 weeks to fit with existing National immunization schedule.

Indian Rotavirus Vaccine, 116 E

This vaccine developed by Bharat Biotech (Rotavac) is a live, naturally attenuated vaccine containing monovalent, bovine human reassortant strain characterized as G9 P [11], with the VP4 of bovine rotavirus origin, and all other segments of human rotavirus origin.

Six cases of intussusceptions (all occurring after administration of 3rd dose) were recorded in the vaccines and two in the control group. This vaccine has already been licensed in India and would soon be available for use in Indian market. It is a moderately effective vaccine against rotavirus diarrhea in India.

Pre-exposure Prophylaxis for Rabies

Recommended that practically all children need vaccination against rabies and following two situations to be included in high-risk category of children for rabies vaccination:
  i. Children having pets at home; and
  ii. Children perceived with higher threat of being bitten by dogs such as hostellers, and those with risk of stray dog bite while going outdoor. These children should be offered pre-exposure prophylaxis (Pre-EP) against rabies. This must be preceded by a one-to-one discussion with the parents. The Pre-EP is not included in the IAP immunization schedule for all children. Three doses are recommended to be given intramuscularly on days 0, 7 and 28 (day 21 may be used if time is limited, as with imminent travel, but day 28 is preferred). The intradermal schedule has been shown to be effective, but is not approved for this purpose in office practice.

Typhoid Conjugate Vaccines

A new slot for typhoid conjugate vaccine for primary immunization at 9–12 months of age in the IAP Immunization schedule. There are currently two typhoid conjugate vaccines (Typbar-TCV and PedaTyph), available and licensed in the country. However, this recommendation would be applicable only to the former as the committee is awaiting more data on the latter. Only a single dose of the vaccine is recommended for primary series. An interval of at least 4 weeks with the measles/MMR vaccine should be maintained since the data on interference with the measles/MMR vaccine are not yet available.

Those who received a dose of conjugate vaccine at 9–12 months can be prescribed booster of either Vi-polysaccharide (Vi-PS) or the conjugate vaccine at 2 years of age.

Catch-up schedule: Catch-up vaccination is recommended throughout the adolescent period, i.e., up to 18 years of age.

Recommendations for Public use

Typhoid vaccine (Vi Polysacharide vaccine) given once in 3 years for the Public.

Human Papillomavirus (HPV) Vaccination Schedule

Recommendations: Two doses of HPV vaccine are advised for adolescent/preadolescent girls aged 9–14 years; for girls 15 years and older, current 3 dose schedule will continue.

Update on Pertussis Immunization

There is no need of repeating or giving additional doses of whole-cell pertussis (wP) vaccine in order to boost immunity in children who have earlier completed their primary schedule with acellular pertussis (aP) vaccine-containing products. However, it should be ensured that all the remaining doses are wP vaccine-containing products. This is to be reiterated here that wP vaccine is permitted till 7 years of age.

Pentavalent (DTwP + Hib + Hepatitis-B) Vaccine

There are concerns among pediatricians related to the quality, suitability and preference of available different wP-vaccine containing pentavalent vaccines in the market since the publication of IAP recommendations on pertussis immunization.

Cost: All the currently available liquid pentavalent combinations cost around INR 600, except Quinvaxem which is around 2.5 times more expensive. The committee thinks the price of the product cannot be justified considering all the attributes and performance.

Major Changes in Recommendations for IAP Immunization Time-table, 2014

Measles and MMR immunization
- Two doses of MMR at 9 and 15 months
- No standalone measles dose at 9 months
- No MMR at 4–6 years of age

Typhoid immunization
- Slot for "typhoid conjugate vaccine" for primary immunization at 9–12 months of age
- Recommendation applicable only for Typbar-TCV
- Booster of either Typbar-TCV or Vi-polysaccharide (Vi-PS) vaccine at 2 years of age
- Typhoid revaccination every 3 years, if Vi-polysaccharide vaccine is used
- Need of revaccination following a booster of Typbar-TCV not yet determined

Contd...

Chapter 33: Recent Area of Interest in Community Medicine

Contd...

Hepatitis-A immunization
- Single dose administration of live attenuated H2 strain hepatitis A vaccine at 12 months
- Previous recommendations of two-dose is now scrapped
- Two doses for inactivated (killed) hepatitis-A vaccine

Human Papillomavirus (HPV) vaccination
- Two doses of HPV vaccine for adolescent/preadolescent girls aged 9–14 years
- For two-dose schedule, the minimum interval between doses should be 6 months
- Three dose schedule for adolescent girls aged 15 years and older to continue

Rabies immunization
- Two new situations, children having pets in home and children perceived with higher threat of being bitten by dogs to be included in "high-risk category of children" for rabies vaccination
- These groups of children should now be offered "pre-exposure prophylaxis" against rabies

Pertussis immunization
- No change in pertussis immunization recommendations of 2013
- No need of repeating/giving additional doses of wP vaccine to children who had earlier completed their primary schedule with aP vaccine-containing products
- Review and recommendations on the currently available wP vaccine containing pentavalent (DTwP + Hib + Hepatitis-B) products in Indian market

Other changes
- A brief update and recommendation on use of new Indian Rotavirus vaccine, 116E
- The comments and footnotes for several vaccines are also updated and revised

Conclusion: All the available liquid pentavalent combinations satisfy the licensing criteria set by the Indian National Regulatory Authority (NRA) and fulfills the requirement of WHO prequalification, except Comvac-5.

TRIBAL HEALTH

Tribal population constitutes 8.6 percent of population covering 104 million populations. All scheduled tribes come under tribal health.

Literacy rate is less (59%), life expectancy is less (63.9 years), immunization in tribal children is also less (estimated 55%). Hence, tribal health got greater importance.

Malnutrition, communicable diseases and addictions are major burdens in tribal population. Animal attack and violence are additional burdens.

One primary health center for 20,000 population; one subcenter for 3,000 population cater health services under tribal health.

Since October 2013, Ministry of Health and Family Welfare and Ministry of Tribal Affairs jointly work for the cause of tribal health.

ASHA (Accredited Social Health Activist) and Doctors are motivated with increased salary and increased facility to cater tribal community.

UNIVERSAL DECLARATION OF HUMAN RIGHTS

This was adopted and proclaimed by General Assembly resolution 217 A (III) of 10 December 1948 by United Nations.
- UN High Commissioner for Human Rights ... www.unhchr.ch
- National Human Rights Commission, New Delhi ... www.nhrc.nic.in
- World Human Rights Day is celebrated on every 10th December

1. All human beings are born free and equal in dignity and rights. They are endowed with reason and conscience and should act toward one another in a spirit of brotherhood.
2. Everyone is entitled to all the rights and freedoms set forth in this declaration, without distinction of any kind, such as race, color, sex, language, religion, political or other opinion, national or social origin, property, birth or other status. Furthermore, no distinction shall be made on the basis of political, jurisdictional or international status of the country or territory to which a person belongs, whether it be independent, trust, non-self-Governing or under any other limitation of sovereignty.
3. Everyone has the right to life, liberty and security of person.
4. No one shall be held in slavery or servitude; slavery and the slave trade shall be prohibited in all their forms.

5. No one shall be subjected to torture or to cruel, inhuman or degrading treatment or punishment.
6. Everyone has the right to recognition everywhere as a person before the law.
7. All are equal before the law and are entitled without any discrimination to equal protection of the law. All are entitled to equal protection against any discrimination in violation of this declaration and against any incitement to such discrimination.
8. Everyone has the right to an effective remedy by the competent national tribunals for acts violating the fundamental rights granted to him by the constitution or by law.
9. No one shall be subjected to arbitrary arrest, detention or exile.
10. Everyone is entitled in full equality to a fair and public hearing by an independent and impartial tribunal, in the determination of his rights and obligations and of any criminal charges against him.
11. a. Everyone charged with a penal offense has the right to be presumed innocent until proved guilty according to law in a public trial at which he has had all the guarantees necessary for his defense.
    b. No one shall be held guilty of any penal offense on account of any act or omission which did not constitute a penal offense, under national or international law, at the time when it was committed. Nor shall a heavier penalty be imposed than the one that was applicable at the time the penal offense was committed.
12. No one shall be subjected to arbitrary interference with his privacy, family, home or correspondence, nor to attacks upon his honor and reputation. Everyone has the right to the protection of the law against such interference or attacks.
13. a. Everyone has the right to freedom of movement and residence within the borders of each state.
    b. Everyone has the right to leave any country, including his own, and to return to his country.
14. a. Everyone has the right to seek and to enjoy in other countries asylum from persecution.
    b. This right may not be invoked in the case of prosecutions genuinely arising from nonpolitical crimes or from acts contrary to the purposes and principles of the United Nations.
15. a. Everyone has the right to a nationality.
    b. No one shall be arbitrarily deprived of his nationality nor denied the right to change his nationality.
16. a. Men and women of full age, without any limitation due to race, nationality or religion, have the right to marry and to find a family. They are entitled to equal rights to marriage, during marriage and at its dissolution.
    b. Marriage shall be entered into only with the free and full consent of the intending spouses.
    c. The family is the natural and fundamental group unit of society and is entitled to protection by society and the state.
17. a. Everyone has the right to own property alone as well as in association with others.
    b. No one shall be arbitrarily deprived of his property.
18. Everyone has the right to freedom of thought, conscience and religion; this right includes freedom to change his religion or belief, and freedom, either alone or in community with others and in public or private, to manifest his religion or belief in teaching, practice, worship and observance.
19. Everyone has the right to freedom of opinion and expression: this right includes freedom to hold opinions without interference and to seek, receive and impart information and ideas through any media and regardless of frontiers.

20. a. Everyone has the right to freedom of peaceful assembly and association.
    b. No one may be compelled to belong to an association.
21. a. Everyone has the right to take part in the government of his country, directly or through freely chosen representatives.
    b. Everyone has the right of equal access to public service in his country.
    c. The will of the people shall be the basis of the authority of government; this will shall be expressed in periodic and genuine elections which shall be by universal and equal suffrage and shall be held by secret vote or by equivalent free voting procedures.
22. Everyone, as a member of society, has the right to social security and is entitled to realization, through national effort and international cooperation and in accordance with the organization and resources of each state, of the economic, social and cultural rights indispensable for his dignity and the free development of his personality.
23. a. Everyone has the right to work, to free choice of employment, to just and favorable conditions of work and to protection against unemployment.
    b. Everyone, without any discrimination, has the right to equal pay for equal work.
    c. Everyone who works has the right to just and favorable remuneration ensuring for himself and his family an existence worthy of human dignity, and supplemented, if necessary, by other means of social protection.
24. Everyone has the right to rest and leisure, including reasonable limitation of working hours and periodic holidays with pay.
25. a. Everyone has the right to a standard of living adequate for the health and well-being of himself and of his family, including food, clothing, housing and medical care and necessary social services, and the right to security in the event of unemployment, sickness, disability, widowhood, old age or other lack of livelihood in circumstances beyond his control.
    b. Motherhood and childhood are entitled to special care and assistance. All children, whether born in or out of wedlock, shall enjoy the same social protection.
26. a. Everyone has the right to education. Education shall be free, at least in the elementary and fundamental stages. Elementary education shall be compulsory. Technical and professional education shall be made generally available and high education shall be equally accessible to all on the basis of merit.
    b. Education shall be directed to the full development of the human personality and to the strengthening of respect for human rights and fundamental freedom. It shall promote understanding, tolerance and friendship among all nations, racial or religious groups, and shall further the activities of the United Nations for the maintenance of peace.
    c. Parents have a prior right to choose the kind of education that shall be given to their children.
27. a. Everyone has the right freely to participate in the cultural life of the community, to enjoy the arts and to share in scientific advancement and its benefits.
    b. Everyone has the right to the protection of the moral and material interests resulting from any scientific, literary or artistic production of which he is the author.
28. Everyone is entitled to a social and international order in which the rights and freedoms set forth in this declaration can be fully realized.
29. a. Everyone has duties to the community in which alone the free and full development of his personality is possible.

b. In the exercise of his rights and freedoms, everyone shall be subject only to such limitations as are determined by law solely for the purpose of securing due to recognition and respect for the rights and freedoms of others and of meeting the must requirements of morality, public order and the general welfare in a democratic society.
c. These rights and freedoms may in no case be exercised contrary to the purposes and principles of the United Nations.
30. Nothing in this declaration may be interpreted as implying for any state, group or person any right to engage in any activity or to perform any act aimed at the destruction of any of the rights and freedoms set forth herein.

WORLD HEALTH ORGANIZATION (WHO) DAY

The World Health Day will be commemorated on 7th April of every year and is dedicated to the theme of human well-being. It aims to draw global attention to the mankind about health and disease, how to have positive health and how to prevent or control disease.

The World Health Organization (WHO) under United Nations is the lead agency for the successful organizing and planning of global, regional and national events to mark World Health Day. At global level, the WHO will launch The World Health Reports and organizes a high-level meeting in conjunction with the launch of WHO Day Theme. It plans a number of activities for World Health Day to stress our commitment to protecting our greatest assets: the health and the environment.

Themes of World Health Day Celebrated on Every 7th April since 1950

Year	Theme
1950	Know your own health services
1951	Health for your child and the world children
1952	Healthy surroundings make healthy people
1953	Health is wealth
1954	The nurse, pioneer of health
1955	Clean water means better health
1956	Destroy disease carrying insects
1957	Food for health
1958	10 years of health progress
1959	Mental illness and mental health in the world today
1960	Malaria eradication—a world challenge
1961	Accidents need not happen
1962	Preserve sight—prevent blindness
1963	Hunger, diseases of millions
1964	No truce for tuberculosis
1965	Smallpox—constant alert
1966	Men and his cities
1967	Partners in health
1968	Health in the world of tomorrow
1969	Health, labor and productivity
1970	Early detection of cancer saves lives
1971	A full life despite diabetes
1972	Your heart is your health
1973	Health begins at home
1974	Better food for a healthier world
1975	Smallpox—point of no return
1976	Foresight prevents blindness
1977	Immunize and protect your child
1978	Down with high blood pressure
1979	A healthy child, a sure future
1980	Smoking or health—the choice is yours
1981	Health For All (HFA) by 2000 AD
1982	Add life to years
1983	HFA by 2000 AD—the countdown has begun
1984	Children's health, tomorrow's wealth
1985	Healthy youth—our best resource
1986	Healthy living—everyone a winner
1987	Immunization—a chance for every child
1988	Health for all—all for health
1989	Let's talk health
1990	Our planet—our health think globally, act locally
1991	Should disaster strike be prepared
1992	Heart beat—the rhythm of health
1993	Handle life with care—prevent violence and negligence
1994	Oral health for a healthy life

Year	Theme
1995	Target 2000—a world without polio
1996	Healthy cities for better life
1997	Emerging diseases—global alert, and global response
1998	Safe motherhood—pregnancy is a special event, let us make it safe
1999	Active aging—makes the difference
2000	Safe blood starts with me—blood saves lives
2001	Stop exclusion—dare to care
2002	Move for health
2003	Shape the future of life—healthy environment for children
2004	Road safety is no accident
2005	Make every mother and child count
2006	Working together for health
2007	International health security
2008	Protecting health from climate change
2009	Save lives. Make hospitals safe in emergencies
2010	World Health Day 2010 will focus on urbanization and health. Make cities healthier
2011	Antimicrobial resistance: No action today, no cure tomorrow
2012	Good health adds life to years
2013	Healthy heart beat, healthy blood pressure
2014	Vector-borne diseases
2015	"Food safety" (with 5 keys; Key 1: Keep clean, Key 2: Separate raw and cooked food, Key 3: Cook food thoroughly, Key 4: Keep food at safe temperatures, Key 5: Use safe water and raw materials).
2016	Diabetes: Scale up prevention, strengthen care, and enhance surveillance
2017	Depression: Let's talk
2018	Universal health coverage: Everyone, everywhere
2019	Health for All: Everyone, Everywhere

WHO Day Theme 2000

Safe Blood Starts with me—blood saves lives

Health awareness on blood groups, blood donation and voluntary blood donation is requisite of the day, since everyday this has been a life saving measure.

Blood testing against STD, AIDS, and hepatitis B make the blood "safe blood". Blood-borne diseases are almost zero if the blood is from a healthy donor who is a volunteer.

Present day trauma, accidents, advanced surgery and treatment of blood related diseases such as hemophilia, blood cancer need almost care for safe blood.

WHO Day Theme 2001

Stop Exclusion—dare to care

The theme is devoted to mental health. Mental health and brain disorders are main cause of suffering and disability. We ignore the fact that mental patient needs assistance. Many mentally sick are not getting the help they need.

It is estimated that 400 million suffer from mental and neurological disorders or from psychosocial problems related to alcohol and drug.
- They are excluded
- They are not getting adequate care.

We need
- Community mental health service
- Fair insurance schemes
- Nondiscriminatory hiring practice.

Especially, we should note that for the first time WHO has devoted WHO day to mental health.

WHO Day Theme 2002

Move for Health

One of the major risk factor involved in CD and noncommunicable disease (NCD) of human race is getting to sedentary lifestyle in the attraction of civilization and urbanization. Absence of physical activity can lead to disease, disability or death. Improper diet can lead to either undernutrition or obesity. Habits such as eating, drinking, sleeping, working, playing, etc. matter much in determining happy life.

Physical activity is meant for burning calories or demolishing extra calorie which shall prevent or reduce disease, disability and death. In the century ahead of us has a few things such as unnecessary worry, unnecessary engagement, 24 hours watching TV, getting work done rather than doing by self-have-lead to sedentary lifestyle which is found greatly related to diseases such as cardiovascular diseases, coronary heart diseases, diabetes, cancer, osteoporosis, hypercholestremia, hypertension, obesity and the like. Developing and developed countries shows difference in communicable disease pattern and not in noncommunicable disease pattern.

The only solution left to man, for reducing disability and death, is to have regular physical activity and to move for his health. Move for health can include the following:
- Walk, brisk walk, cycling, get moving for shorter space, get moving for little longer if time permits, preferring staircase to elevators
- Attending to household, office and social work where you do the job to your satisfaction rather than getting the job done to get disease
- Advisable 0.5–1 hour moderate activity daily, vigorous activity once in 2 days for 15–20 minutes and if you sport there you go.

If you have started moving for health vide above, you will observe that considerable reduction of the following in your society:
- Violence
- Tobacco lifestyle
- Unsafe sex
- Drug abuse
- Loneliness
- Isolation.

Your move to health can revert deaths of 2 million, can reduce 80% of coronary heart disease, can reduce 50% of hypertension, hypercholestremia, osteoporosis, depression and anxiety. *Work while you work, play while you play, that is the way; to be happy and gay.*

WHO Day Theme 2003
Shape the future of Life—healthy Environment for Children

The Theme emphasizes to protect our asset, children. Health and environment are linked with healthy children. The very places of children for good healthy life are homes, schools and community. Every year over 5 million children aged 0–14 age group die of environment related diseases. Diarrhea, ARI, vector-borne diseases and injury are common problems. Unsafe water, poor hygiene, poor sanitation, air pollution are threats to health of our children.

Thus, future development of our children depends on our action today.

WHO Day Theme 2004
Road Safety is no Accident

Motorized road transport has become boon to our life and to our enjoyment. However, we are paying for that benefit and payment is too high. Majority of annual deaths are due to road accident. Victims and survivors are often young, leaving families to cope with the loss of breadwinner.

These deaths, injuries and economic losses can be prevented. Interventions can bring down death and loss to a considerable extent.

WHO Day Theme 2005
Make Every Mother and Child Count

Key messages of the theme are mothers and children who suffer and die to a greater extent, both in developing and developed countries. Health of mother and child are wealth of society. Our present knowledge can save them.

United family, multicultural diversity and powerful color to identify children are seen in *Tangram Puzzle* of design by WHO on the eve of its celebration.

Mother survives if child survive; society will prosper if mother and child survive.

Future will be healthier and more productive for all societies, if we act now to make every mother and child count.

WHO Theme 2006
Working Together for Health

Theme of 2006 gives us opportunity to celebrate the remarkable contribution to human health and development made by health workers. Potential gains to be made in human health by health workers are incalculable. We are finding it difficult to train, to sustain and to retain our health workers. There is ever growing demand for health workers as populations' age and chronic conditions increase.

Without a strong health workforce, advances in healthcare cannot reach and benefit the people who need them. If we can assess, deliver and monitor our health workers, more justification can be done. They are required for our millennium development goals, for our threat of pandemic and for our calamities.

Poor distribution of resource and unused skills, migration of health workers are making the situation worse. We should build support that health workers will be working where they are needed, when they are needed, to provide attainable level of health for people everywhere. HIV crisis management is possible with the achievement of goal through the theme of the year.

WHO Day Theme 2007

International Health Security

World Health Day 2007 theme of international health security has given the message to "Invest in health, build a safer future."

This will focus on threats to our collective health security. These include emerging and rapidly spreading diseases, environmental change, the danger of bioterrorism, sudden and intense humanitarian emergencies caused by natural disasters, chemical spills or radioactive accidents, and the impact of HIV/AIDS, a disease that is threatening the stability of communities in some

International Health Security Issues

- Emerging diseases: Severe acute respiratory distress syndrome (SARS), and avian influenza.
- Economic stability: Public health dangers have economic as well as health consequences. Containing international threats is good for economic well-being.
- International crises and humanitarian emergencies: Events like natural disasters kill and maim individuals and severely stress the health systems.
- Chemical, radioactive and biological terror threats: Deliberate or accidental like Anthrax-tainted letters, release of sarin on subway.
- Environmental change: Environmental and climate changes due to climate-related natural disasters, mainly in developing countries..
- HIV/AIDS–a key health and security issue: Impact of a public health issue on security.
- Building health security: National compliance for international health security.
- Strengthening health systems: Like health workers force in developing countries.

WHO Day Theme 2008

Protecting Health from Climate Change

The health impacts of climate change are already evident in different ways. These impacts will be disproportionately greater in vulnerable populations, which include the very young, elderly, medically infirm, poor and isolated populations.

We need to put public health at the heart of the climate change agenda, this includes mobilizing governments and stakeholders to collaborate on strengthening surveillance and control of infectious diseases, safer use of diminishing water supplies, and health action in emergencies.

Communities and organizations around the world will host activities to establish greater awareness and understanding of health consequences of climate change and to show the impact of the growing interdependency between these two areas on national and international decisions and policies.

WHO Day Theme 2009

Save Lives. Make Hospitals Safe in Emergencies

World Health Day 2009 focuses on the resilience and safety of health facilities and the health workers who treat those affected by emergencies. Events around the world will highlight successes, advocate for safe facility design and construction, and build momentum for widespread emergency preparedness.

The goal of raising awareness in this issue is to effect changes that will ensure that health facilities and services are able to function in the aftermath of emergencies and disasters,

protect the lives of patients, serve the affected population and keep health workers safe. This means:
- Ensuring the structural resilience of health structures with existing technologies
- Keeping the equipment and supplies of these health facilities intact should an emergency happen
- Improving the preparedness and risk reduction capacity of health workers
- Involving communities in this effort.

This World Health Day theme is intended to generate more momentum that will help sustain and mainstream disaster risk reduction into health sector initiatives. WHO together with its global partners will continue to work with governments, international and regional organizations, nongovernmental organizations and individuals will build and sustain efforts that ensure that health facilities can function during and in the aftermath of disasters.

WHO Day Theme 2010

World Health Day 2010 will Focus on Urbanization and Health

World Health Day 2010 will focus on urbanization and health. With the campaign "1,000 cities –1,000 lives", events will be organized worldwide calling on cities to open up streets for health activities. Stories of urban health champions will be gathered to illustrate what people are doing to improve health in their cities.

With the campaign 1,000 cities, 1,000 lives, events will be organized worldwide during the week of 7–11 April 2010.

The global goals of the campaign are 1,000 cities: To open up public spaces to health, whether it be activities in parks, town hall meetings, clean-up campaigns, or closing off portions of streets to motorized vehicles.

WHO Day Theme 2011

Antimicrobial Resistance:
No Action Today-No Cure Tomorrow

Antimicrobial resistance was the theme for this year's World Health Day. The world is on the brink of losing its miracle cures. The world has failed to handle these fragile medicines with appropriate care. **Irrational and inappropriate uses of antimicrobials are by far the biggest drivers of drug resistance.**

At a time of multiple calamities in the world, we cannot allow the loss of essential medicines, essential cures for many millions of people, to become the next global crisis.

This achievement has been made possible by dedicated country teams, committed health officials in endemic countries, generous donations from industry, and support from international partners.

Preventing the main killers of young children also calls for better use of the kind of basic interventions promoted by primary health care, such as safe water and sanitation.

It also calls for more aggressive and strategic implementation of cost-effective interventions, like oral rehydration therapy, antibiotics that can be administered in homes, micronutrient supplements, exclusive breastfeeding, and even something so simple as good hand hygiene.

This will have to change, especially if we want to reverse the growing burden of non-communicable diseases. In attempting to influence policies made in other sectors, it is good to have support from the recommendations of the Commission on Social Determinants of Health.

WHO Day Theme 2012

Good Health adds Life to Years

Aging and health, to which each and every one of us can relate is the theme of this year's World Health Day. Using the slogan "Good health adds life to years", campaign activities and materials focus on how good health throughout life can help older men and women lead full and productive lives and be a resource for their families and communities.

WHO Day Theme 2013

Control Your Blood Pressure

About high blood pressure

High blood pressure–also known as raised blood pressure or hypertension–increases the risk of heart attacks, strokes and kidney failure. If left uncontrolled, high blood pressure can also cause blindness, irregularities of the heartbeat and heart failure. The risk of developing these complications is higher in the presence of other cardiovascular risk factors such as diabetes. More than one in three adults worldwide has high blood pressure. The proportion increases with age, from 1 in 10 people in their 20s and 30s to 5 in 10 people in their 50s. However, high blood pressure is both preventable and treatable. In some developed countries, prevention and treatment of the condition, together with other cardiovascular risk factors, has brought about a reduction in deaths from heart disease. The risk of developing high blood pressure can be reduced by:

- Reducing salt intake
- Eating a balanced diet
- Avoiding harmful use of alcohol
- Taking regular physical activity
- Maintaining a healthy body weight, and
- Avoiding tobacco use.

Greater awareness, healthy behaviors, improved detection, and enabling environments always help to prevent risk of hypertension.

The ultimate goal of World Health Day 2013 is to reduce heart attacks and strokes. Specific objectives of the campaign are:

- To raise awareness of the causes and consequences of high blood pressure
- To provide information on how to prevent high blood pressure and related complications
- To encourage adults to check their blood pressure and to follow the advice of healthcare professionals
- To encourage self-care to prevent high blood pressure
- To make blood pressure measurement affordable to all, and
- To incite national and local authorities to create enabling environments for healthy behaviors.

WHO Day Theme 2014

Small Bite Big Threat

Vector-borne diseases are illnesses caused by these pathogens and parasites in human populations. They are most commonly found in tropical areas and places where access to safe drinking-water and sanitation systems is problematic.

The most deadly vector-borne disease, malaria, dengue, trade and travel and environmental challenges such as climate change and urbanization are having an impact on transmission of vector-borne diseases, and causing their appearance in countries where they were previously unknown.

World Health Day 2014 will spotlight some of the most commonly known vectors–such as mosquitoes, sandflies, bugs, ticks and snails–responsible for transmitting a wide range of parasites and pathogens that attack humans or animals. Mosquitoes, for example, not only transmit malaria and dengue, but also lymphatic filariasis, chikungunya, Japanese encephalitis, and yellow fever.

Better protection from vector-borne diseases

More broadly, through the campaign, we are aiming for the following:

Families living in areas where diseases are transmitted by vectors know how to protect themselves

Travelers know how to protect themselves from vectors and vector-borne diseases when traveling to countries where these pose a health threat.

In countries, where vector-borne diseases are a public health problem, ministries of health put in place measures to improve the protection of their populations, and

In countries, where vector-borne diseases are an emerging threat, health authorities work with environmental and relevant authorities locally and in neighboring countries to improve integrated surveillance of vectors and to take measures to prevent their proliferation.

WHO Day Theme 2015

How Safe is Your Food?

World Health Day will be celebrated on 7th April, with WHO highlighting the challenges and opportunities associated with food safety under the slogan "From farm to plate, make food safe."

Multiple new opportunities for food to become contaminated with harmful bacteria, viruses, parasites, or chemicals are becoming more.

Unsafe food can contain harmful bacteria, viruses, parasites or chemical substances, and cause more than 200 diseases—ranging from diarrhea to cancers.

There were an estimated 582 million cases of 22 different food-borne enteric diseases and 351,000 associated deaths.

The enteric disease agents responsible for most deaths were *Salmonella typhi* (52,000 deaths), enteropathogenic *Escherichia (E). coli* (37,000) and norovirus (35,000).

Over 40% people suffering from enteric diseases caused by contaminated food were children aged under 5 years.

Food safety is a cross-cutting issue and shared responsibility that requires participation of nonpublic health sectors (i.e., agriculture, trade and commerce, environment, tourism) and support of major international and regional agencies and organizations active in the fields of food, emergency aid, and education.

WHO Day Theme 2016

Beat Diabetes

In 2008, an estimated 347 million people in the world had diabetes and the prevalence is growing, particularly in low- and middle-income countries. In 2012, the disease was the direct cause of some 1.5 million deaths, with more than 80% of those occurring in low- and middle-income countries. WHO projects that diabetes will be the 7th leading cause of death by 2030.

There are 2 main forms of the diabetes. People with type 1 diabetes typically make none of their own insulin and therefore require insulin injections to survive. People with type 2 diabetes, the form that comprises some 90% of cases, usually produce their own insulin, but not enough or they are unable to use it properly. People with type 2 diabetes are typically overweight and sedentary, two conditions that raise a person's insulin needs.

Over time, high blood sugar can seriously compromise every major organ system in the body, causing heart attacks, strokes, nerve damage, kidney failure, blindness, impotence and infections that can lead to amputations.

WHO is focusing the next World Health Day, on 7th April 2016, on diabetes because:
1. The diabetes epidemic is rapidly increasing in many countries, with the documented increase most dramatic in low- and middle-income countries.
2. A large proportion of diabetes cases are preventable. Simple lifestyle measures have been shown to be effective in preventing or delaying the onset of type 2 diabetes. Maintaining normal body weight, engaging in regular physical activity, and eating a healthy diet can reduce the risk of type 2 diabetes.
3. Efforts to prevent and treat diabetes will be important to achieve the global sustainable development goal 3 target of reducing premature mortality from diabetes by one-third by 2030.

The main goals are:
1. Increase awareness
2. Set specific, effective, and affordable actions.

WHO Day Theme 2017

Depression–Let's Talk

The theme of 2017 World Health Day campaign is depression.

Depression affects people of all ages, from all walks of life, in all countries. It causes mental anguish and impacts on people's ability to carry out even the simplest everyday tasks, with sometimes devastating consequences for relationships with family and friends and the ability to earn a living. At worst, depression can lead to suicide, now the second leading cause of death among 15–29-year olds.

Yet, depression can be prevented and treated. A better understanding of what depression is, and how it can be prevented and treated, will help reduce the stigma associated with the condition, and lead to more people seeking help.

WHO Day Theme 2018

Universal Health Coverage: Everyone, Everywhere

The World Health Organization was founded on the principle that all people should be able to realize their right to the highest possible level of health. "Health for all" has therefore been our guiding vision for more than seven decades. It's also the impetus behind the current organization-wide drive to support countries in moving toward Universal Health Coverage.

Universal Health Coverage has emerged as a key strategy to make progress toward other health-related and broader development goals. Access to essential quality care and financial protection not only enhances people's health and life expectancy, it also protects countries from epidemics, reduces poverty and the risk of hunger, creates jobs, drives economic growth and enhances gender equality.

Throughout 2018, we aim to **inspire**, **motivate** and **guide** for the cause.

WHO Day Theme 2019

Health For All: Everyone, Everywhere

Although, we have made enormous progress in recent years against some of the world's leading causes of death and disease, we still have a lot of work to do to realize that vision.

Today, half the world's population cannot access essential health services. Millions of women give birth without help from a skilled attendant; millions of children miss out on vaccinations against killer diseases, and millions suffer and die because they cannot get treatment for HIV, TB, and malaria. In 2019, this is simply unacceptable. The good news is that there is a growing movement to address these inequalities.

Although, there will always be outbreaks and other disasters with health consequences, investing in stronger health systems can help to prevent or mitigate them.

In the sustainable development goals, all countries have committed to achieving universal health coverage by 2030. To meet that target, we need to see 1 billion people benefitting in the next 5 years.

Health for all is possible even with health systems that are less than perfect—countries at many different income levels are making progress with the resources they have.

WOMEN'S HYGIENE KIT (WHK)

Adolescent girls constitute a large segment of population which is of social significance for RCH status of the population at large, more so because they will shortly join the reproductive age group. The special needs of this group are not addressed in the past.

Health program for adolescent girls have special significance because it affects the health and nutrition of adolescent girls and their long-term intergenerational effect by reducing the risk of LBW and child mortality.

The population cover under women's hygiene comprises following two major groups;
1. Adolescent girls in age group of 10–14 years (10% of population).
2. Women of reproductive age group of 15–45 years (16% of population).

Women's hygiene kit is a necessary intervention under RCH program which can prevent RTI and RTI-induced gynecological problems. Women's hygiene kit is a suggested hygienic practice during menstrual cycle by adolescents and women in reproductive period.

A pilot study was undertaken up by the Government of Karnataka to implement WHK through the public distribution system, and through Anganwadi. To make the scheme a success following important additional components are undertaken.
a. IEC activities
b. Training
c. Research and evaluation.

ZIKA VIRAL INFECTION

- It was first noticed in Uganda in 1947. Microcephaly was found associated with this disease. It is transmitted by *Aedes aegypti*.
- Zika virus belongs to Flavivirus. Fever, Rashes, conjuntivitis, joint and muscular paid, headache which last for 1 week.
- Diagnostic test is polymerase chain reaction (PCR).
- No specific treatment is available.
- No vaccine is available.
- NIV Pune, NCDC Delhi provide diagnostic procedures.
- Preventive measures that can be suggested are:
  - Control of breeding places
  - Mosquito control
  - Mosquito repellent usage
  - Health education.

SUMMARY

Sixty-one areas of Recent Interest are described which are relevant in present day Public Health Practice.

VIVA VOCE

1. What is AAFP surveillance?
2. What is the theme of world AIDS day 2019?
3. Define baby friendly hospital initiative.
4. What is community psychiatry?
5. Define desmotology.
6. Define emporiatrics.
7. List common essential drugs.
8. List common method of hospital waste management.
9. Define IPPI.
10. National urban health programme.
11. Define ROME
12. Define PC PNDT.
13. Who day theme april 2020-09-03 women hygiene kit.
14. Impact of Corona Pandemic.
15. What are the basic preventive steps in the eradication of Corona Pandemic?

Appendix

PERFORMING CLINICO-SOCIOCULTURAL AND DEMOGRAPHIC ASSESSMENT OF INDIVIDUAL, FAMILY, AND COMMUNITY

MEDICOSOCIAL CASES

Is case of clinic-social case presentation in community medicine, students should attempt to elicit/correlate social and behavioral aspect of condition/illness/disease in the patient/case with the background of his/her family and his/her society. This can be in the hospital wards; can be in a family allotted to them. Most common conditions of public health importance are:

- Antenatal case (ANC)
- Gastroenteritis case
- Tuberculosis case
- Study of a family

Medicosocial Case-1

Antenatal Case (ANC)

- It is a physiological condition should be remembered in presentation. Do not use the word patient
- Present with identification data including socioeconomic status of the family.
- Elicit and present data
- Size, type and composition of family are relevant and present it.
- On examination—inspection, palpation and auscultation == to describe height of uterus corresponding to the period of amenorrhea, fetal movement and position, position like right occipito anterior or otherwise, etc.
- Provisional diagnosis shall be in terms of pregnancy (Normal or otherwise) mention if para-gravida
- Effect of pregnancy on her health which influence nutrition, personal hygiene, etc., should be mentioned.
- Attitude toward pregnancy in the family to be named, impact on financial condition, working condition, etc. should be borne in mind.
- Prepare from theory knowledge the following:
- Regarding levels of prevention
- Health education (HE), family planning (FP), ANC an Indian Nursing Council (INC)—check out and spell out.
- Management—check for completeness of AN care if incomplete, how to complete Normal delivery possible or not. Specify domiciliary care or institutional care.
- Mention HE material for her at AN care, at her family and at community—jot down measures.

Prepare and keep your answer for the following:

- Pregnancy changes
- Breast change is reliable sign in primi why?
- Reason for changes in cervix, vagina, vulva (extra venous blood in 2nd month onward)
- Period when abdominal change is evident (18th week)
- Weight gain in pregnancy (12.5 kg)
  - What is quickening
  - When pregnancy test is +ve (on or after 40 days of conception)
- Enumerate high risk—elderly primi, short stature primi, malpresentation, antepartum

hemorrhage (APH), threatened abortion, pre-eclampsia toxemia (PET), toxemia, anemia, twins, hydramnios, previous bad obstetrics and gynecology (OBG) history, pregnancy with systemic disorders
- Additional calorie in pregnancy (293)
- Specific health protection in pregnancy—correct anemia, iron-folic acid (IFA) detail, prevention of toxemia, tetanus toxoid (TT), diagnosis of reproductive tract infection/sexually transmitted infection (RTI/STD), attention for German measles, rhesus (Rh) incompatibility, prevention of human immunodeficiency virus (HIV) transmission, mental preparation, FP advice, and tackle child component
- Five clean practices
- DDK content (disposable delivery kit)
- When referral at domiciliary care—high temperature, heavy bleeding, collapse, placenta not separated within 30 minutes, cord collapse, prolonged labor.
- What is APGAR score?
- Hypothermia prevention in the new born
- Detail rooming in
- Comment ON exclusive breast feeding

Medicosocial Case-2

Gastroenteritis

- Present with identification data including socioeconomic status of the family.
- Elicit and present data for a child if patient is pediatric age group.
- Size, type, and composition of family are relevant and present it.
- On examination—general condition, dehydration, pallor, eye changes, skin changes
- Provisional diagnosis shall be in terms of bacterial/viral/chemical diarrhea.
- Effect of gastroenteritis (GE) on the health which influence nutrition, personal hygiene, etc. should be mentioned.
- Attitude toward loose motion, traditional home remedies if any to be mentioned, impact on financial condition, working condition, etc. should be borne in mind.

Prepare Theoretical Information
- Regarding levels of prevention
- HE, FP, personal hygiene, environmental (Env) hygiene—check out and spell out.
- Management—patient treatment, fluid replacement oral/intravenous (IV), etc.
- Mother's education, or patient education if adult, about ORS and home fluids
- Mention HE material at case level, at the family and at community—jot down measures.

Prepare and keep your answer for the following:
- **Difference between diarrhea and dysentery**
- **Differential diagnosis (DD) for the case depending upon positive findings**
- **Mortality rate and morbidity rate in India**
  - Coverage of protected water and good sanitation facility
  - IV fluid preparations
  - Detail about home fluid, ORS and action of each of them in ORS
  - About rota virus diarrhea
  - Why it is not cholera- substantiate
  - Human reservoir in transmission
  - Child feeding practices and diarrhea
  - Malnutrition and diarrhea
  - Illustration for water borne
  - Illustration for fecal borne
  - Composition of ORS and assessment of dehydration
  - ORS guidelines
  - Role of breast feeding in diarrhea in children
  - Comment on patient's malnutrition
  - Mention sanitation lacking, how will you improve that.
  - You are to give HE. Mention topic of importance.
  - Rotavirus vaccine is in use. Comment its efficacy.
  - Which are failed items under first level of prevention in this case?
  - What is digestive disorder center (DDC)? Explain.

Medicosocial Case-3

Tuberculosis

- Present with identification data including socioeconomic status of the family.
- History of past illness and family history is important.
- Elicit and present data for a child, if patient is pediatric age group.
- Size, type and composition of family are relevant and present it.
- On examination----general condition, weight loss, pallor, dyspnea, skin changes, body temperature, any symptoms of nonpulmonary tuberculosis, clinical examination such as inspection, palpation, percussion, and auscultation of chest
- Provisional diagnosis is made.
- Effect of chronic bacterial infection which is a social disease on the health which influence nutrition, personal hygiene, etc. should be mentioned.
- Attitude toward social stigma, marriage, occupation, if any to be mentioned, impact on financial condition, working condition, etc. should be borne in mind.

Keep a note on Theory Aspect of Following

- Regarding levels of prevention
- HE, FP, personal hygiene, Environmental hygiene—check out and spell out.
- No. 8 management—patient treatment, nutrition, etc.
- Mother's education, or patient education, if adult about drug reactions and hospital management

  Mention HE material at case level, at the family and at community—jot down measures.

Prepare and keep your answer for the following:

- Incidence/prevalence of tuberculosis (TB)
- Directly observed therapies (DOTs) as public health approach
- Epidemiological indices such as prevalence of infection, incidence of infection
- Prevalence of disease, incidence of new cases, mortality rate
- Definitions of case, new case
- What could be source of infection in this case?
- Social factors in the family responsible for the disease
- Mantoux test
- Bactericidal and bacteriostatic drugs
- Domiciliary treatment
- Importance of childhood tuberculosis
- Recent view on bacille calmette-guérin (BCG) vaccination
- DOTs plus
- Revised strategy of Revised National TB Control Program (RNTCP)
- Stop TB strategy of World Health Organization (WHO)
- Epidemiological impact on TB by HIV/acquired immunodeficiency syndrome (AIDS)

Medicosocial Case-4

Study of a Family

- **Importance of family case study** in community medicine
- It is a major case for the university examination.
- Practical training to view health problems in the background of family and society apart from at individual level
- Helps to study social and environmental condition which precipitates deviation from normal
- It is an insight for solving health problem at family level
- Learn interaction between health and different agencies
- Learn health education, counseling and prevention
- Learn rehabilitation in public health problems
- Basically, get geographical and demographic data of the field practice area from where the case is allotted.

When Allotted

- First get/elicit/find out:
  - General information
  - Child immunization status

- Check pregnant/lactating/child/disabled/chronic case/malnourished case/anemia case
- Vital events of family extracted (for the last 1 year)
- Tick relevant
  - Housing/sanitation
  - Culture, attitude
- Obtain data on diet survey
❖ Second get/elicit/find out
  - Tick individual health record
  - Child health record, if child +
  - ANC/postnatal care (PNC), if any

Third make note of special about family problem

HAVE THESE IN YOUR MIND

❖ TB patient in the family
❖ Leprosy patient in the family
❖ Mentally retarded in the family
❖ Any ANC–risk? With jaundice
❖ PNC in the family
❖ Requirement for family planning
❖ Any chronic case in the family
❖ Any physically handicapped in the family
❖ Any advanced illness in the family (incurable disease)

Index

Page numbers followed by *b* refer to box, *f* refer to figure, and *t* refer to table.

A

Abacavir 179
ABC analysis 315
Abdomen, pain in lower 389
Accident 215, 260
    determining factors in 216*f*
    prevention of 216, 262
    research 216
Accidentology 216
Accredited social health activist 433
Acid-fast bacilli 152, 185
Acquired immunodeficiency syndrome 114, 174, 175, 177, 178, 295, 329, 357, 384
    clinical diagnosis of 178
    complex 178
    education 71
    epidemiological triad in 177*f*
    natural history of 176
    red ribbon of 384
    surveillance 389
Actinomycosis 260
Activity therapy 276
Acupuncture 361
Acute flaccid paralysis 382
    surveillance 382
Acute respiratory infection 114, 145, 146*f*, 147*f*, 235-237, 297
    anatomical sites of 145*f*
    classification of 146
    concepts 145
    control 145, 234, 298
        program 147, 300
    prevention and control of 147
    risk factors in 145
Adolescent reproductive sexual health clinics 394
Advanced life directives 355
Adverse event following immunization 122, 382, 383
Adverse medical cascade 375
Aedes
    aegypti 54, 170, 198, 400
    albopictus 54, 400
    vittatus 54
Aerosol 391
Aflatoxin 84
Africanus 394
Aga Khan Foundation 344
Age sex pyramid 222, 222*f*
Agent-host-environment 7, 8
Agents, norwalk like 138
Agrochemicals 260
Air
    accidents 289
    composition of 34
    conditioning 36
    movement 39
    quality of 35
Air pollution 350
    control 35, 35*f*
    effects of 34
    indicators of 34
    inversion in 34
    source of 34
Aircraft disinfection 198
Albendazole 141
Alcohol 8, 276
    consumption 8
Alkaptonuria 270
Allopathic
    medicine 361
    practitioner 361
Alphavirus 395
Amantadine 159
Amebiasis 139
Amebic dysentery 139
Amino acids, essential 74
Amoxicillin 390, 391
Ampicillin 146
Amprenavir 180

Anatomical Gift Act 353
Ancylostoma 139
Anemia 82, 235, 446
    prevention of 297
Anesthesia, general 373
Anganwadi worker 248, 326
Angina pectoris 208
Animal plague 195
Anopheles 49, 52, 53, 161
    adult female 50, 50*f*
    adult male 50, 50*f*
    annularis 52
    culicifacies 52
    eggs 50*f*
    fluviatilis 52
    larva 50, 50*f*
    minimus 53
    mosquito 52*f*
    philippinensis 53
    stephensi 53
    subpictus 54
    sundaicus 54
    umbrosus 54
    varuna 54
Anorexia 258
    nervosa 276
ANOVA 106
Antenatal advice 235
Antenatal care 235, 297
Antenatal case 445
Anthracosis 259
Anthrax 199, 260, 390
    confirmation of 391
    epidemiological triad in 199*f*
    prevention and control of 200
Anthropology 13
Anthropometric examination 76
Anthroposophical medicine 373
Antibiotics 137
Anticipatory governance 289
Antigen 393

Antigenic drift 158
Antigenic shift 158
Antimicrobial resistance 440
Antiretroviral combination therapy 180
Anti-rodent measures 63
Antisera 121
Antitetanus serum 122
Antituberculosis treatment 152
Apoplexy 213
Appropriate technology 325
Aqua privy 44, 44*f*
Arachnida 49, 59
Arboviral infections 171
Armed force 22
Arsenic 259
Artemether 423
Artemisinin 423
Arthralgia 400
Arthritis 266, 276
Asbestosis 259
Ascaris
  lumbricoides 141
  pneumonia 141
Asexual blood stage 166
Aspergillus 85
  flavus 84
Asthma 273
Atmospheric pollution, ill-effects of 25
Atreya anushasana 356
Audio-video aid 68
Auditory aid 68
Autism 276
Autonomous ethic 352
Autosomal aberrations 271
Auxiliary nurse midwife 297, 395
Avian flu 289, 391
Avian influenza 391
Ayurveda 361
Ayushman Bharat Program 394

B

Baby care, support binders for 411*f*
Baby friendly hospital 244, 395
Bacillary dysentery 139
Bacillus
  anthracis 200, 390
  Calmette-Guérin 121, 233, 383, 431
  cereus 138

Back pain 262
Bacteria 83
Bacterial vaginosis 390
Bacteriological analysis 29, 33
Bacteriological index 185, 186
Bad genes 223
Bagassosis 259
Bajaj committee 312
Balanced diet 77, 79
  adult man 77
  adult woman 78
  children 78
  construction, guideline for 77
  elderly 80
  geriatric age 266
  special group 79
Bar diagram, multiple 102*f*
Basal metabolism 74
Basic Minimum Service Programme 307
Behavior
  criteria of abnormal 275
  health-seeking 16
  science 13
Benzene hexachloride 62
Benzylpenicillin 146
Beta-propiolactone 192
Bharat Sevak Samaj 341
Bias 97, 113
Bimodal distribution 125, 126*f*
Biohazard waste symbol, display 290*f*
Biological agents 260
Bioterrorism 390
  counter measure for 391
Biotin 74
Birds flu 391
Birth spacing, promoting 238
Black death 194
Bleaching powder 30
Blindness 211
  epidemiological triad in 212*f*
Blood 353
  borne 120
  loss, chronic 140
  saves lives 437
Blood films
  making 161
  staining of 162
Blood pressure
  control 440
  high 440

Blood transfusion 298
  services 320
Body building 73
Body louse 58
Body mass indexes 214
Boiled egg 76
Bone marrow 353
Bordetella pertussis 156
Bore-hole latrine 44, 45*f*
Brain fever 193
Break bone fever 170, 401
Breast milk 244
Breastfeeding 395
  exclusive 244, 395
Breathing, fast 145, 237
Breathlessness 258, 413
Broken family 14
Bronchial asthma 34
Bronchitis
  acute 34
  chronic 34, 413
Brucella 199
Brucellosis 198, 260
  epidemiological triad in 198*f*
Brudzinski's sign 159
Brugia malayi 168
Bubonic plague 194
Byssinosis 259

C

Calcium 74, 75, 244
Calorie 76
Cancer 114, 205, 207, 356, 438
  breast 205, 207
  causes of 206*f*
  cervix 205, 207
  colon 207
  common 206
  control approach 206
  education 71
  epidemiology 111
  occupational 261*f*
  prostate 207
  registry 207
  stomach 205, 207
  treatment for 206, 272
  warning signs of 207
Candidiasis 175, 390
Cane bagasse 259
Capsulitis 258
Carbohydrate 74, 76, 77
Carbon monoxide 34

Index

Carcinoembryonic antigen 208
Carcinoma 205
Cardiac failure 208
Cardiovascular disease 209, 438
Cardiovascular system 259
Caries 397
Carpal tunnel syndrome 258, 262
Case and control
   difference between 115
   study 95
Cat flea 58
Cataract 211, 398
Cell culture vaccine schedule 192
Census and sample, difference between 101
Central nervous system 259, 265
Central Social Welfare Board 340
Cerebral hemorrhage 213
Cerebral malaria 422
Cerebral thrombosis 213
Cerebrospinal fever 159
Certificate of death 124*f*
Cervical spondylosis 258
Chadah committee 311
Chancroid 174
Chandler index 140
Character disorders 275
Charaka Samhita 356
Chemical
   agents 119, 259, 262
   analysis 32
   closet 45, 45*f*
   oxygen demand 43
   toxin 138
   waste 288
Chemoprophylaxis 166, 188
Chemotherapy 150, 190
Chest pain 413
Chickenpox 157
Chikungunya 172, 395, 396
   fever 396
      epidemic 395
Child guidance clinic 242
Child survival 236
   and safe motherhood 232
   rate 241
Childhood blindness 211
Childhood disorders 276
Children, programs for 247

Child-to-Child Programme 70
Chlamydia 390
   trachomatis 189
Chloramine 181
Chloramphenicol 146, 159, 373
Chlorination, breakpoint 32, 32*f*
Chlorine tablet 30
Chloroquine 163-165, 369, 404, 423
   resistant cases 166
Chlorpromazine 369, 404
Cholera 120, 135, 348
   control of 137
   epidemiological triad in 136*f*
   organism, types of 135*f*
   vaccine 137
Chorioallantoin membrane 411
Chromium 75, 259
Chromosomal aberrations 271
Chromosome 269
Ciguatoxin 138
Ciprofloxacin 373, 390
Civil services 22
Claviceps 85
Claviceps fusiformis 85
Clean delivery 297
Cleft lip 273
Cleft palate 273
Clinical audit 404
Clinical genetic examination 270
Cloning 272, 354
Clostridium
   botulinum 138
   perfringens 29, 83, 138
Cobalt 75
Cognizable offense 427
Cohort 113
Cohort study 95
   design for 116*f*
Cold
   box 299
   chain equipment 122
   shock 258
Commercial product 424
Common foods, nutritive value of 76, 77
Common research design, use of 97
Communicability, period of 200
Communicable disease 112, 293, 329, 340, 403, 418
   epidemiology of 128

Communicable
   keratoconjunctivitis 189
Communication 10, 70
   barriers 11, 70
   behavioral change 14
   effective 10
   media 10, 70
   types 11, 70
Community dentistry 397
Community development 327, 341
   program 327
Community diagnosis 6, 7
   tool 214
Community health 6
   activities 339
   associations of 342
   center 151, 296, 325
   guide 326
   services 357
Community healthcare 324
Community Level Stroke
   Control Program 213
Community medicine 6, 381
Community ophthalmology 397
Community participation 325
Community psychiatry 277, 398, 399*f*
Community treatment 7
Compliance 374
Component bar diagram 102*f*
Condom 227
Conduct disorders 276
Congenital malformations 241
Conjunctivitis 189
Consumer Protection Act 399
Contagious disease 112
Contamination 27
Conversion 274
Cooked items, calorific value of 90
Cooked preparations, calorific value of 90
Copper 75
   T 227
Cornea 353
Corneal blindness 211
Corneal congestion 258
Corneal opacities 398
Corneal ulcer 398
Coronary artery disease 213
Coronary heart disease 207, 211, 438

community index of 208
prevention of 209
Coronavirus disease-2019 (COVID-19) 401
Corynebacterium diphtheriae 155
Cosmopolitan community 20
Cost inflation 18*t*
Cost-benefit analysis 316
Cost-effective analysis 316
Cough 141, 374, 413
Council of Medical Research 393
Counterfeit medicine 399
Cow's milk 244
Crab louse 58
Crab yaw 175
Critical health
  problems 93
  supplies 281
Critical path method 317
Critical velocity 27
Cross-sectional and longitudinal study, difference between 115
Crotalaria 85
Crustacea 49
Cryptococcal meningitis 179
Cryptosporidiosis 175
Culex 53, 395
  eggs 51, 53*f*
  fatigans 54
  female 51, 53*f*
  larva 51, 53*f*
  male 51, 53*f*
  mosquito 52*f*
  pupa 51, 53*f*
Cumulative health record 251
Cyclodevelopment 120
Cyclone 289
  aftermath of 286
Cyclonic storm, management of 286
Cyclops 49, 61
  female 61
  morphology of 61*f*
Cycloserine 150
Cystic fibrosis 272
Cytomegalovirus 206, 241
Cytotoxic drugs, common 206

D

Danger signs 237
Dangerous industries 350
Data
  analysis 100
  collection 101
    tool for 99
  compilation of 301
  presentation 101
  types of 102
  uses of 101
Death
  and dying 356
  certificate 124
Declining sex ratio, causes of 222
Deep springs 27
Deep trench latrine 46, 46*f*
Defense mechanisms, common 274
Deformity, grades of 186
Defunct National Health Programs 294
Delivery complications 249
Demographic cycle 224
Demographic data, sources of 224
Demographic values, estimates of 11, 223
Dengue 120, 400
  control 170
  hemorrhagic fever 171
  syndrome 170, 401
    history of 170
    natural history of 171*f*
  transmission dynamics 400
  vaccine 400
  virus 400
Dengvaxia® 400
Dental association 341
Dental caries 251
Deoxyribonucleic acid 130, 132, 177, 354
Depression 262, 374, 442
Depressive disorders 398
Dermacentor andersoni 60
Descriptive study, characteristics in 114
Desert Development Programme 20
Desk, type of 253*f*

Desmotology 118, 402
  priorities in 402*f*
Diabetes 210, 276, 438
  beat 442
  complications of 211
  development of 375
  epidemiological triad in 210*f*
  mellitus 210*t*
Diabetic diet 86
Diagnostic test 125
Diaphragm 227
Diarrhea 28, 134, 235, 237, 251, 446
  acute 134
  chronic 179
  epidemiological triad in 135*f*
  etiology of 134
  management 236, 237
  pathogenesis, algorithm in 134*f*
Diarrheal disease 295
  Control Programme 300
Dibothriocephalus latus 88
Dichlorodiphenyltrichlorethane 62
Didanosine 179, 180
Diet 73
  liquid 85
  low calorie 86
  low cholesterol 86
  low cost 79
  prudent 79
  social 14
  survey 77
  therapeutic 85
Dietetics 73
Diethylcarbamazine 169
Digestive diseases 266
Digestive problems 262
Digitalis 373
Digoxin 369, 404
Diphtheria 155, 233
  epidemiological triad in 155*f*
  pertussis and tetanus 233, 431
  tetanus, and acellular pertussis vaccine 431
Directly observed therapy agent 303
Directly observed treatment
  short course 302
  chemotherapy 152

Index

Disability 9
  indicators 11
  limitation 9
  prevention 9
Disablement benefit 264
Disabling conditions, chronic 204
Disaster 281, 284
  accidents 215
  areas 282
  chemical 289
  classification of 282
  conflict-related 282
  cyclone 286
  dynamics of 289
  effect of common 285*t*
  emergency preparedness in 283
  industrial 289
  man-made 282
  mine 289
  mitigation 281
  natural 282
  phases 283
  phases of 283, 286
  technological 282
  victim response phases 284
Disaster management 281
  action plan 285
  challenges in 282
  vulnerability reduction in 282
Disastrous situation 89
Disease
  causes of 5, 6*f*
  determinants of 113
  distribution of 113
  frequency of 113
  in man, prevention and control of 123, 123*f*
  natural history of 7, 8, 8*f*, 133*f*
  notification of 378
  spectrum 7
  transmission, dynamics of 120
  web of causation of 7
Disease Control Programs 294
Disease Eradication Programs 294
Disinfection 118
  and antiseptic, difference between 118
  procedures 183
Disposable delivery kit 236, 297
Disposable syringes 394
District Cancer Control Program 207
District Tuberculosis Center 302
  structure and function of 302
Doctor compliance 374
Doctor-patient relationship 11
Dog flea 58
Dog vaccine 192
Domiciliary care 236
Doxycycline 199, 390, 391
Dracunculus medinensis 140, 405
Drinking water
  quality, surveillance of 33
  standard for 33
Drought 285
  Prone Areas Programme 20
Drug 150
  abuse 425
  Act 364
  and equipment kits 233
  antimalarial 423
  complementary 373
  distribution center 305
  economics 376
  essential 403
  irrational use of 375
  kit 298
  modern 373
  oral 390
  proper store of 315
  pushing for cheaper 359
  recreational 400
  traditional 373
  treatment 390
  use of 372, 375
Duchenne muscular dystrophy 270, 271*f*
Dug hole latrine 45, 45*f*
Dysentery 446
Dyspnea 141

E

Early childhood development 403

Earthquake 284, 285, 289
  action plans on 285
Ecological barrier 189*f*
Economic cause 222
Economic problem 348
Economic rehabilitation 10
Ectoparasite 58
Ectopic ascariasis 141
Eczema 276
Edentulism 397
  mechanism of 397*f*
Education, types of 68
Efavirenz 180
Egg hygiene 88
Elderly citizen facility concept 267
Eligible couple 224*t*
Embryo, transfer of 354
Emergency care 234
Emergency management cycle 283*f*
Emergency nutritional rehabilitation 89
Emergency obstetric care 232, 234
Emphasis 203
Employees State Insurance Scheme 263
Employment Assurance Scheme 20
Emporiatrics 118, 403
Encephalitis 260
Endemic ascites 85
Endemic familial arthritis 407
Endemic index 140
Endemic typhus 172
Endogenous genetic factors 269*f*
Energy 244
  and protein supplement 80
  malnutrition 80
  yielding 73
Entamoeba histolytica 139
Enteric disease agents 442
Enteric fever 142
Enterovirus 130
Environmental health
  problems 25
  services 25
Environmental law 366
Environmental sanitation 25, 293
Epicondylitis 258

Epidemic dropsy 84
Epidemic hemorrhagic fever 172
Epidemic polyarthritis and rash 395
Epidemic typhus 172
Epidemiological triad 112
Epidemiology 111
- aims of 113
- analytic 114
- approach in 113
- changing concepts in 114, 115
- concept of 113
- descriptive 114
- future hold of 126
- milestones in 111
- terms used in 112
- types of 114
- use of 118

Epidemiometric analysis 123
Epilepsy 398
Epstein-Barr virus 206
Equipment 314
Eradication, epidemiology relevant to 129
Ergonomics 257, 262
Ergotism 85
Erythema marginatum 214
Erythrocyte sedimentation rate 214
Escherichia coli 29, 33, 85, 442
Essential Drug Program 372
Ethambutol 150, 153
Ethical interest, areas of 358
Ethical issue 358
Ethionamide 150
Euthanasia 356, 359
- active 356
- nonvoluntary 356
- passive 356
- types 356
- voluntary 356

Excreta disposal
- policy 350
- sociological aspect of 48

Exotoxin canned bottle 83
Expectoration 413
Experimental epidemiology 117
Extended sickness benefit 263
Eye
- care, primary 212
- health care 212
- infection 398
- redness 251
- strain 262

F

Face masks 394
Factory Act 363
Family
- crisis 405
- loss of 9
- medicine 404
- problem 14, 17
- situation 89
- type of 19

Family planning 224, 225*f*, 226, 227, 229, 295, 329, 330
- administration 229*f*
- association 341
- disincentive in 225, 225*t*
- evaluation 229
- incentive in 225, 225*t*
- measures 226, 228
- methods of 225-228
- present concept of 224, 227
- voluntary organizations in 227

Family welfare 229
- planning 224, 341
Farmer's lung 259
Fasciola hepatica 87
Fat 74, 76
- invisible 74
Fatigue 258
Fatty acids, unsaturated 74
Favism 85
Fecal-borne diseases 44
- barriers in 44*f*
Fernandez 185
Fertility 222
- rates 222
- regulation 231
Fetal brain tissue 353
Fetal growth retardation 235
Fever 141
- and chills 251
- high 400, 423
- prolonged 179
- treatment depots 305
- undulant 198
Field and Health Centers 382
Filaria 49, 168
- control 169
- indicators of 169
- epidemiological triad in 168*f*
- survey 169
Filariometric values 169
Financial management 315, 316
Fire 289
First five-year plan to tenth plan 311
First referral unit 325
Fish hygiene 88
Five clean practices, application of 236
Five-year plan outlay 311
Fixed virus 191
Flea 49, 54, 57
Float ridges 49
Floods 285, 289
Fluorine 75
Fluorosis 82
Flushed face 251
Folic acid 75, 76, 77
Folk media 69
Food 73
- Act 364
- additives 88
- and agricultural organization 337
- fortification 88
- free 86
- hygiene 87
- myths 89
- poisoning 83, 138
- sanitation 83
- standards 88
- surveillance 87
- toxins 83
- unsafe 442
Food adulteration 88
- Act, prevention of 88
Food-borne diseases 85
Foodstuff, nutritional profile of 75
Footpad culture 185
Force field analysis 317
Ford foundation 344
Formaldehyde 181
Fowl plague 391
Freedom, degree of 92
Fruit 76
- and vegetable hygiene 88
- portion 86
Functional index test 76

Funeral benefit 264
Fungal infection 260
Fungal toxins 85
Fusarium toxin 85

G

Galactosemia 270
Gamete
  micromanipulation of 354
  transfer of 354
Gamma-glutamyl transferase 131
Gammexane 62
Gangosa 175
Garbage recycling policy 350
Gastroenteritis 114, 134, 138, 446
  effect of 446
  investigation of 139
Gastrointestinal tract 208
Gender issues 406
Gene 269
  behavior of 223
  cloning 405
  therapy 272, 355
Genetic basis 270
Genetic disorders 270
  autosomal dominant 270
  autosomal recessive 270
  lifetime frequency of 269
  prevention of 271
Genetic engineering 405
Genetic epidemiology 111
Genetic inheritance 243
Genetic liability 273f
Genetic origin 206f
Genetic predisposition 271, 273f
Genetics and health 269
Genital molluscum 174
Genital ulcer 174, 389
Genital warts 174
Genitourinary system malfunctions 266
Genome 269
Genotype 269
Gentamicin 146
Geographic pathology 21
Geriatric
  and health 265
  economic aspect of 266
  health problems 266
  psychological problems of 266
  social problems of 266
Germ theory 7
German measles 157
  infection 157
Giemsa stain 162
Glaucoma 398
Global warming 350, 405
Globe thermometer 39f
Glucose tolerance 210
Gonorrhea 173, 174
Good health 440
  habits 267
  information system, qualities of 377
  planning, characteristics of 310
Good housing, indicators of 40
Gram panchayat 327
Granuloma inguinale 174
Green leaves 76
Greenhouse
  effect 350
  gases 405
Groundnut 76
Group behavior 15
Group discussion 69f
Group disorders 275
Growth 242
  and development 243
  chart 242, 243f
  monitoring 87
  normal 243
Guinea worm
  eradication 405
  impact of 406
  free of 406
  infection 140
Gulick's posdcorb 313

H

H5N1 influenza 393
Habitual diet, supplement to 79
Haemaphysalis spinigera 60
Hand pain 262
Handicap 9
  children 242
Handigodu syndrome 407
Hansen's disease 184
Hard ticks 59, 60f
Hardness, degree of 27
Harpenden skin caliper method 215
Hazard 281, 288
  description scales 286
Head
  and chest circumference 244
  loss of 31, 31f
Headache 251, 258, 262, 276, 400
Health 3, 5, 225f, 314
  activities 91
  administration 313
  and development 5
  and service 5
  appraisal 251
  assistant 330
  centers 330
  committee reports 311
  concepts 4, 328
  demand 309
  determinants of 5
  dimension 4
  ecology of 5
  equality in 5
  ethics 362
  examinations 5
  hazards 41
  holistic approach of 4
  indicators 11
  information 67, 377
  infrastructure 311
  insurance 330
  law 362, 363
  model 316
  move for 437
  need 309
  policy 318
  problem 10, 250, 261, 266, 329
  professionals, occupational risks of 261, 262
  programs 329
  propaganda 69
  protection measures 262
  relation to 25
  resources 309, 329
  sciences, development of 339
  sector planning 311
  situation 316
  spectrum of 5
  statistics 377

status, influencing factors in 5t
survey and planning 311
system 4, 320, 321
team 4
worker 330
working together for 438
Health and disease
concept of 3
sociocultural factors in 16
Health and family welfare 233
training centers 296
Health education 68, 69, 202, 251
administration 71
approach 69
in health programs, role of 11, 70
management of 71
methods of 68
principles of 68
Health for all 4, 328, 443
basic principles of 328
targets of 328
Health information system 377
components of 377
sources of 378
uses of 378
Health management 313
basic activity of 316
Health planning 309, 310
elements of 310
Health promotion 9, 81, 271
and education, principles of 67
Health service 307
evaluation of 322
utilization 377
Healthcare
basic 324
component of 324
comprehensive 324
concepts of 324
delivery systems 330
essential 327
facilities 321
indicators 11
levels of 330
Healthy carriers 120
Healthy school environment 253
Hearing
defect 251

loss 258, 262
Heart 353
disease, congenital 273
Heat
cramps 39
exhaustion 38
hyperpyrexia 39
stress 38, 39
effect 38
stroke 39
syncope 39
Heavy metals, wastes of 288
Hemagglutinin protein 391
Hemoglobinuria 423
Hemophilia 270
Hemorrhage 170
antepartum 235, 445
manifestations 400
postpartum 235
Hepatitis 28, 402, 431
A 120, 130, 403
epidemiological triad in 131f
immunization 433
vaccine, live attenuated 431
virus 28, 130
B 121, 131-133, 174
core antigen 131, 132
epidemiological triad in 132f
surface antigen 131, 132
vaccination 207
viral infection 133f
virus 28, 130
B antigen 131, 132
serum level of 132f
C 133
virus 28
D virus 28
delta 133
E 133
antigen 131, 132
virus 28
G 134
virus 28
infections 131
vaccines 134
Herbal medicine 361
Herd immunity 121
Hereditary disease 242
Heritability 273t
Herpes simplex 174

Heteronomous ethic 352
Heterozygote 269
High temperature
causes 258
heat stroke 39
Hill's criteria 99
Hind Kusht Nivaran Sangh 340
Hippocratic oath 356
Histogram and frequency polygon 102f
Histoid leproma 184
Homemade fluids 135
Homeopathy 361, 373
Homozygote 269
Hookworm
infection 139
infestation, epidemiology of 140f
Horizontal Health Program 295, 295t
Horrock's test 30
Hospital
acquired infections 202
and health centers 7
cross infection 202
disinfection 119
sociology 21
Hospital waste 407
disposal, treatment option for 287t, 408
management 287, 288, 290, 407
system 287
treatment option for 288
House type 19
Housefly 54, 55
adult 55, 55f
eggs 55f
larva 55, 55f
Household food security 319
Housing activity promotion organization 40
Housing and town planning 39
Housing standards 40f
Human behavior 68, 400
Human chorionic gonadotropin 208
Human control 199
Human dead body disposal 48
Human development index 3
Human engineering 257
Human experimentation 357
Human flea 58

Index

Human genome project 272
  steps in 273f
Human immunodeficiency
    virus 120, 174-178, 301,
    353, 357, 446
  distribution of 176
  epidemiological triad in 177f
  natural history of 176
  prevention 388
  vaccine 180
Human life, ethics of 354
Human Organ Transplant Act 354
Human papillomavirus
  vaccination 432, 433
Human rights 3
  universal declaration of 433
Human values, teaching of 351
Human voluntary research 357
Human-fibroblast cell 192
Humanitarian assistance, effects
  of inappropriate 282
Humanitarian supplies 281
Humidity 39, 258
Hunger, freedom from 344
Hydatid cyst 260
Hydramnios 446
Hydrogen peroxide 181
Hydrophobia 191
Hygiene 4, 5
Hymenolepis diminuta 58
Hyperargininemia 270
Hypercholestremia 438
Hyperparasitemia 423
Hypertension 9, 126f, 209, 209t, 273, 438
  eye in 398
  prevention of 209
Hypnosis 276
Hypoglycemia 422
Hypothermia 407, 408
Hysteria 274

I

Iatrogenic disease 113
Iatrogenic disorders 375
Ice-lined refrigerator 299
Illegal drug 400
Immersion hypothermia 258
Immune deficiency 385
Immunity 121
Immunization 251, 397
  active 183
  coverage, high level 238
  hazards 122
  passive 183
  schedule 122
Immunizing agents 121
Immunoglobulin 121, 157, 244
  common 121
Incinerate human anatomical
  waste 290f
Indian Factory Act 263
Indian Red Cross Society 341, 359
Indinavir 180
Industrial hygiene 257
Industrial workers 23
Infant feeding practices 244
Infant mortality rate
  causes of 240
  factors influencing 235t
Infection 112, 201, 235, 239
  emerging 200
  re-emerging 200
  reservoir of 193
  source of 178f
  surface 173
  types of 202
Infectious disease 112
Influence, zone of 27, 27f
Influenza 158, 378
  virus 145, 158
Information
  conventional 67
  education and
    communication 68f, 297, 409, 419
  prepare theoretical 446
  progressive 67
  system 202
Injury 275, 398
  unintentional 215
Inorganic dust 259
Input-output analysis 316
Insecticides 62, 63, 407
  classification of 62f
Insects 49
Insomnia 258, 262
Institutional surveillance 382
Insulin 442
Integrated child development
  services 90, 247
Integrated Rural Development
  Program 20

Integrated vector control 64, 166
Intensive pulse polio
  immunization 408
Intentional injuries 216
International health,
  development of 335
Interviewing technique 21
  types 21
Intestinal amebiasis, specific
  treatment of 139
Intestinal immunity 129
Intramuscular schedule 192
Intranatal care 235
Intraocular lenses 212
Intraperitoneal sperm transfer 354
Intrauterine
  device 297, 326, 330
  insemination 354
Invasive pneumococcal disease 237
Inventory management 314
Iodine 30, 75
Iodine deficiency disorder 6, 82, 295
  analysis of 83f
  ill effects of 83f
Ionizing radiation 37
Iron 74, 75, 77, 244, 259
Irrational drug
  risks to 375
  use, types of 373
Irritable bowel syndrome 276
Ischemic heart disease 272, 273
Itch mite, morphology of 61f

J

Janam gutti 245
Janani Suraksha Yojana 410
Japanese B encephalitis 193
Japanese encephalitis 120, 171
  epidemiological triad in 193f
  mode of transmission of 193f
Jaundice 28, 423
Jawahar Rojgar Yojana 20
Job-fitting
  code 257, 257t
  examination 258
Jungalwalla committee 312
Juvenile delinquency 242

K

Kala-azar 169
   control 170
   epidemiological triad in 170f
   laboratory tests in 171f
Kanamycin 150
Kangaroo mother care 410
   basis of 410
Kangaroo position 410
Kaposi sarcoma 175, 179
Karnataka Private Nursing Home (Regulation) Act 364
Kartar Singh committee 312
Karunakaran committee 312
Kasturba Memorial Fund 340
Kata thermometer 39f
Kernig's sign 159
Kesari dal 76
Kidney 353
Killed vaccine 121, 122, 159
Kirlian photography 373
Koplik's spot 154
Krishnan committee 312, 350
Kuppuswamy classification 18t
Kyasanur forest disease 121, 171, 196
   epidemiological triad in 196f

L

Labor Act 263
Lactalbumin 244
Lactate dehydrogenase 208
Lactose 244
Lamivudine 179, 180
Lathyrism 83
   preventive measures in 84
Lathyrus sativus 84
Lead 259
Leishman stain 162
Lepra reaction 186
Lepromin test 185
Leprosy 184, 189f, 245
   control unit 190
   elimination campaign 187
     modified 186, 304
   elimination of 187
   epidemiological triad in 185f
   prominent history in 184
   types of 185f
   work 187
Leptospira 411f
Leptospirosis 199, 410

Liberating information 67
Lice 49, 58
Lids, drooping of 398
Life
   after death, organ donation for 354
   index, physical quality of 3
   prolongation of 355
   quality of 3
Lime 29
Lipoprotein
   low-density 204
   very-low-density 213
Lippes loop 227
Liquid waste 42
   composition of 43
Live and let live 385
Live viral vaccine, modified 193
Liver 353
Living, standard of 3, 16
Locomotor system impairment 266
Lopinavir 180
Low altitude 258
Low birth weight 246
Lower respiratory infection, acute 237
Lung
   cancer 205, 206
   carcinoma 34
Lymphadenopathy 179
   persistent generalized 178
Lymphogranuloma venereum 174, 390
Lymphoma 205
Lysozyme 244

M

Macronutrient 73
Magnesium 75
Magnetotherapy 361
Mala
   D 225, 228, 373
   N 225, 228
Malaria 49, 120, 160, 378, 418
   Action Program 305
   border 161
   chronic 160
   containment of severe 305
   control 163
   drug resistance 166
   effective control 304

   epidemiological triad in 165f
   history of 160
   management of severe 423
   project area 161
   severe 422, 423
   statistics 163
   transmission, elements of 161
   uncomplicated severe 422
Malaria parasite 162, 164f, 422
   algorithm for 167
   identification of 163
   smear 161
Malariol 63
Malariometric values 163
Male and female health
   assistants, duties of 330
   workers, duties of 331
Malnutrition 235, 348
   classification of 80
   ecology of 80
   grades of 80
   mild 81
   moderate 81
Malta fever 198
Manganese 259
Manpower training 233
Mansonia 63, 395
   annularis 54
   eggs 51, 54f
   Indiana 54
   longipalpis 54
   uniformis 54
Manure pit 42
Marfan syndrome 270
Marriages 222
Mask use 290f
Mass media 69
Massage 361
Maternal and child health 231, 395
   indicators 238
   problem 234
Maternal and neonatal sepsis, prevention of 236
Maternal death, cause of 419
Maternal mortality rate 239, 302
Maternity
   benefit 263
   improvident 224
Measles 122, 153, 431
   elimination strategy 154
   epidemiological triad in 154f

Index

mumps, and rubella vaccination 431
Meat hygiene 87
Mebendazole 141, 369, 404
Medical association 341
Medical audit 322
Medical benefits 263
Medical care 293
Medical economics 21
Medical education, re-orientation of 421
Medical entomology 49
Medical ethics 351, 352
   demerits of 351b
   merits of 351b
   perspectives of 352
Medical examination 251
Medical informatics 377, 412
   activities of 412
Medical profession, confidentiality in 353
Medical rehabilitation 9
Medical sociology 13
Medical statistics 92
Medical supplies 314
Medical termination of pregnancy 226, 228, 233, 296, 297, 326
   Act 365
   person to perform 365
   place to perform 365
Medicine
   alternative 361
   deletion of 370
   essential 369
   list of essential 369
   preventive 6
   systems of 330
   uses of essential 370
Medicosocial cases 16, 445
Medina worm 140
Mediterranean fever 198
Mefloquine 423
Meiosis 269
Memory impairment 258
Meningococcal meningitis 159
   acute infection of 159
Mental health 274, 275
Mental illness 275, 348
   prevention of 276
Mental retardation 276, 398
Mentally ill 275
Mercury 259

Meta-analysis 413
Metabolic diseases 266
Metabolic status 265
Metabolism, inborn errors of 270, 270t
Meta-ethics 351
Meteorology 38
Methane 405
Metronidazole 369, 404
Micronutrient 73
Mid-day school meal 252
Migratory birds 392
Milk hygiene 87
Milk-borne diseases 87
Millennium development goals 413
Miner's nystagmus 258
Minerals
   effects and requirements of 75
   requirements of 75
   springs 27
Mission wells scheme 20
Mites 49, 60
   morphology of 60f
Mitosis 269
Modern medicine 356, 361, 363
Modern sewage treatment 46, 47
   plant 47f
Modern therapy 276
Molecular genetics 270
Molybdenum 75
Monkey fever 196
Monkeypox 201
Monovalent rotavirus vaccine 431
Morbidity 113
   indicators 11
   rate 124
Morphological index 186
Mortality 113, 222
   indicators 11
Mortality rate 124
   infant 240
   neonatal 240
Mosquito 49, 193f, 397
   control 198
   measures 54f
   repellents, use of 396
   species of 52
Mother yaw 175
Mouse brain vaccine 193

Mudhok committee 312
Mukherjee committee 311
Multibacillary treatment, blister pack for 188f
Multifactorial cause 7
Multipurpose worker 115, 233
Mumps 158
   attenuated 158
Municipal Act 48, 365
Municipality Act 353
Musca domestica 55
Musculoskeletal system 258
Mutation 269
Myalgia 400
Mycobacterium tuberculosis 148
Myeloma 205
Myocardial infarction 114, 208, 211

N

Nalgonda technique 84f
Nasopharyngeal swab 393
Nasopharyngeal wash 393
National Acquired Immunodeficiency Syndrome Control Programme 301
National Acute Respiratory Infections Control Programme 294
National Aids Control Organization 417
National Aids Control Program 181
National Anti-Malaria Program 167, 304
National Blood Policy 320
National Cancer Control Program 206, 207
National Cholera Control Program 137, 294
National Days 413
National Diabetic Control Program 211, 306
National Disaster Response Fund 289
National Drug Policy 375
National Education Policy 318, 319
National Family Planning Program 293, 294, 300

National Family Welfare
    Program 229, 300
National Filaria Control
    Programme 303
National Goiter Control
    Programme 293
National Guinea Worm
    Eradication Program 406
National Health Goals 415
National Health Policy 312, 318,
    418
    components of 318
    goals 318
    report 312
National Health Problems 293
National Health Programs 294,
    296, 329
National Health Protection
    Scheme 394
National Housing Policy 320
National Immunization Days
    409
National Immunization
    Schedule 122
National Institute for
    Communicable Diseases
    143
National Institution for
    Transforming India 418
National Leprosy Control
    Programme 293
National Leprosy Eradication
    Program 303
    strategies of 186
National Level Control
    Programs 166
National List of Essential
    Medicines 370
National Malaria Control
    Programme 294
National Malaria Eradication
    Programme 304, 305
National Malaria Surveillance
    167
National Mental Health
    Programme 277, 306
National Nutrition Policy 318,
    319
National Nutritional Programs
    294
National Polio Surveillance
    Project 130

National Population Policy 229,
    230, 298, 318, 319
    report 312
National Registry of Diseases
    378
National Rural Health Mission
    415, 416
    strategies under 416
National Sexually Transmitted
    Disease 294
    Control Programme 300
National Social Assistance
    Program 20
National Sociodemographic
    Goals 417
National Surveillance Program
    for Communicable
    Diseases 306
National TB Control Program
    293, 302
    revised 151, 302
National Trachoma Control
    Programme 294
National Urban Health Mission
    417
National Water Supply and
    Sanitation Program 34,
    294, 329
Natural agents 119
Natural disasters
    common 284
    management of 286
Naturopathy 361
Nausea 258
Neck
    pain 262
    rigidity 251
Needle prick injury 180
Neisseria meningitidis 159
Nelfinavir 180
Neonatal causes 240
Network analysis 316, 317*f*
Neuraminidase protein 391
Neuritic manifestation 122
Neuroepidemiology 111
Neurofibromatosis 270
Neurolathyrism 83
Neuroparalysis, less 192
Neuropsychiatric illness 402
Neurosis 275
Nevirapine 180
Newborn care, essential 234,
    237, 297, 327

Niacin 74, 75, 76
Nickel 259
Nicotine 259
Nicotinic acid 77
Night soil
    disposal of 43
    methods of disposal of 44
Nipah viral infection 418
Nitrous oxide 405
No action today-no cure
    tomorrow 440
Noise 36, 258
    pollution, effect and control
    of 37*f*
Nonbailable offense 427
Noncommunicable disease
    112, 204, 205, 329, 340
    epidemiology of 204
    prevention of 205
Noncompoundable offense 427
Nonexperimental design 98
Nongovernmental health
    organizations 343
Nongovernmental organization
    234, 297
Nonhuman viral 121
Nonmedical supplies 314
Nonnucleoside reverse
    transcriptase inhibitors
    180
Nonsteroidal anti-inflammatory
    drugs 396
Norethisterone 369, 404
Normative ethics 351
Nose and throat, irritation of
    413
Nosocomial infection 113, 202
Nosopsyllus fasciatus 58
Nuclear incidents 289
Nucleoside analogs 179
Null hypothesis 91
Nutrient 73, 75, 76, 267
Nutrition
    adequate 243
    and health 73
    education 71, 89
    rehabilitation 89
    source of 73
    status 265
    supplementation 7
Nutritional advice, indirect 267
Nutritional anemia 82
Nutritional assessment 76

Nutritional diseases 79
Nutritional health problems 293
Nutritional indicators 11
Nutritional program 88
Nutritional requirement 266
Nutritional service 252
Nutritional status 88
Nutritional surveillance 87

O

Obesity 214, 276, 438
   community assessment of 215
   consequences 215
   determinants of 215f
Obstetric care, essential 234, 297, 327
Obstetric fistulae 419
Occupational cancer 260, 261t
Occupational dermatitis 260
Occupational diseases, prevention of 262
Occupational environment 257
Occupational hazards 258-260
   agriculture 260
   industry 260
Occupational health 257
   research institutes of 264
Ointment 190
Oncology, screening test in 207, 207t
One's own law 352
Operation theater disinfection 119
Oral cancer 206, 397
Oral contraceptive 213, 238, 330
Oral pills 225
Oral polio vaccine 130, 431
Oral rehydration 137
   solution 137
   therapy 296, 297
Oral typhoid 121
Oral vaccine 142, 193
Organ donation 353
   requirements in 353
Organ replacement 353
Organic dust 259
Organic lead 259
Ornithodoros moubata 60
Oropharyngeal swab 393
Oseltamivir 393
Osteoarthritic changes 407
Osteoarthritis 266
Osteolathyrism 84
Osteoporosis 438
Oxidation
   ditches 47
   pond 47
Oxygen 369, 404
Ozone 29
   depletion 350

P

Pain management 396
Panchayat Raj 20
   system 327
Panchayat Samiti at block level 327
Pantothenic acid 74, 75
Para-aminosalicylic acid 150
Paracetamol 396
Paralysis 258
   infantile 128
Paralytic polio 129
Paramyxovirus 153
Paratyphoid 142
Pareek method 19
Parenteral nutrition, indications for 87
Paris green 63
Parkinson's disease 355
Partogram 419
Patient's compliance 374
Paucibacillary treatment, blister pack for 189f
Pediculus humanus
   female 58
   male 58, 59f
Pelvic inflammatory disease 174, 390
Penicillin 159
   G 390
Penicillium 85
Peptic ulcer 273
Perinatal mortality rate 239
Periodontal disease 397
Peritonitis, mortality from 105
Perpetual inventory method 315
Personal health service 250
Personal prophylaxis 174
Personal protection 216
Personality disorders 275
Personnel protective equipment 393
Pertussis 431
   immunization 432, 433
Phenobarbitone 369, 404
Phenotype 269
Phenylketonuria 126f, 270
Phlebotomus sandfly 56
Phosphorus 74, 75, 244, 259
Phthirus pubis 58
Physical activity 437
Physical agents 119, 258, 261
Physical analysis 32
Physical environment, components of 25
Physical examination 29
Physical stressors 258
Physical therapy 276
Pitch 36
Placebo 374
Plague 49, 120, 121, 194
   control cell 195
   domestic 194
   epidemiological triad in 194f
   prevention and control 195f
Planning cycle 310, 310f
Planning programming budgeting system 317
Plant toxin 138
Plasma cholesterol, total 213
Plasmodium 160, 163, 165
   falciparum 166
   infection 422
   treatment in 165
Play therapy 276
Plumbism 259
Pneumoconiosis 260
Pneumocystis carinii
   pneumonia 175
Pneumonia 237
Pneumonic plague 194
Poison 64
   control information 418
Polio 120, 378
   epidemiological triad in 129f
   vaccine, inactivated 130, 431
   virus isolation 410
Poliomyelitis 128
Pollutants, measurement of 43
Pollution 27
Polyethylene glycol 355
Polymerase chain reaction 391
Polyposis coli 270

Polysacharide vaccine 432
Polyvidone iodine 181
Population
　control 227
　dynamics 221
　education 71, 221, 227, 229, 251
　estimation 224
　explosion 293
　　malthusian theory of 224
　genetics 272
　law 365
　medicine 7
　nutrient 90
　statistics 92
Porcelain 30
Porcine circovirus 431
Postdelivery complications 249
Postnatal care 236
Postneonatal causes 240
Postneonatal mortality rate 240
Postpartum
　center 296
　program 419
Potassium 75
Poverty line 14
Prabhakara classification 20t
Pradhan Mantri Jan Arogya Yojna 394
Prasad classification 17t
Preconception prenatal diagnostic techniques 427
Predisaster phase 286
Pre-eclampsia toxemia 446
Pregnancy, specific protection during 235
Pregnant and lactating woman, habitual diet of 79
Prenatal diagnostic techniques 426
Pressor amines 85
Prestroke warning 213
Preterm baby 247
Preventive and social medicine 6
Primaquine 165
Primary health center 151, 190, 295-297, 325, 326, 382
Primary healthcare 4, 229, 233, 324, 325, 328
　principles of 325
Primary immune response 121
Professional activities 341

Professional ethics 356
Property, loss of 9
Prophylactic therapy 373
Prophylaxis 61, 392, 397
　postexposure 388
Prostate specific antigen 208
Protein 74, 76
　basic etiology of 80
Protein-energy malnutrition 6, 79
　community action in 81
　manifestations 80
　prevention of 80
Psittacosis 260
Psychiatry 13
Psychogenic pain 276
Psychological phases 284
Psychological rehabilitation 10
Psychological status 265
Psychology 13
Psychoneurosis 275
Psychopharmacology 276
Psychophysiological disorders 275
Psychosis 275
　acute 398
　chronic 398
Psychosocial agents 262
Psychosomatic disorders 275
Pthirus pubis 59f
Pubic distribution system 307
Pubic louse 58, 59f
Public health 6
　Act 364
　importance 27, 40, 43, 60, 74, 119
　informatics 377
　interventions 282
　law 362
　legal aspect in 362
　measure 33, 166, 193
　milestones in 322
　problem, emerging 410
　relevance 173
Puerperal sepsis 235
Pulmonary function impairment 266
Pulmonary tuberculosis 149f
Pulse immunization 129
Pulse polio immunization 128, 408, 409
Purine free foods 86
Pyrazinamide 153

Pyrethrum extract 63
Pyrexia, mild 411
Pyridoxine 74, 77
Pyrimethamine 423

Q

Qualitative method 317
Quantitative methods 316
Quarantinable diseases 118
Quarantine 118
　ship disinfection for 119
Quetelet's index 214
Quinine 373, 423

R

Rabies 122, 191, 192, 378
　epidemiological triad in 191f
　immunization 433
　prophylaxis for 432
Radiation 8, 37
　by rays 258t
　hazards, prevention of 38f
Radio frequency 400
Rail accidents 289
Rain forest area 407
Rain water 26
　harvesting 421
Ramalingaswami committee 312
Ramp method tipping 42f
Rapid sand filter 31, 32f
Rat flea 57, 57f, 58
Rational drug management 372, 372f
　process of 376f
Rational treatment, rationale of 372
Rats and rat flea, control of 58
Rattus
　norvegicus 63f, 64
　rattus 63f, 64
Rauvolfia serpentina 373
Rays, penetrating ability of 37
Reaction formation 274
Recent immunization, trends in 428
Record system 251
Red cross day 420
Refractive error 398
Rehabilitation 9, 81
Rehydration 137
Relapsing fever 378

Index

Repression 274
Reproduction, uncontrolled 235
Reproductive and child health 231-233, 297, 329, 330, 340
   activity, initiatives of 234
   administration 233f
   basic elements of 232
   differential approach 232
   indicators in 248
   interventions 232, 297
   programme 296
Reproductive health, concept of 296
Reproductive maternal and child health 231
Reproductive tract infection 230, 296, 297, 417
   control of 233
   prevention of 296
Research
   design 97
   ethics 357
   hypothesis 97
   methods 94
   process 96
   types of blinding in 95
Reserpine 373
Reservoirs, impounding 26
Respiratory allergy 34
Respiratory changes 265
Respiratory infection 143
   chronic 348
Respiratory symptoms 251
Retinoblastoma 270
Retinol 77
Retro-orbital pain 400
Rhabdovirus 191
Rheumatic fever 214
   prevention chart of 214
Rheumatic heart disease 213
   epidemiological triad in 214f
Riboflavin 73, 75, 76, 77
Ribonucleic acid 144, 154, 157, 177, 191, 355, 385
Rickettsia 121
Rickettsial infections 172
Rickettsial pox 172
Rifampicin 153
Rights of persons with disability bill 420
Rimantadine therapy 159
Ring immunization 129

Ritonavir 180
Rockefeller foundation 343
Rocky mountain spotted fever 172
Rodents 63
Romanowsky stain 162
Rotavirus vaccine 431
Round worm 141
   epidemiology of 141f
Rubella 157
   congenital 157
   epidemiological triad in 157f
Rule of half 209f
Rural community 20
Rural development 322
   scheme of 322f
Rural family welfare center 296
Rural health 341
   scheme 312
   services 327
Rural malaria 161
Rural medical practitioners 426
Rural water supply 307
   Programme 306
Rural youth for self employment, training of 20

S

Safe and wholesome water 26
Safe blood starts 437
Safe drinking water 350
Safe motherhood 235
   Program 232, 236
Safety 314
   education 216, 251
Salmonella
   paratyphi 142
   poisoning 138
   typhi 142, 442
   typhimurium 138
Salmonellosis 378
Sample registration system 378
Sampling, types of 99
Sand flea 58
Sandfly 56
   egg 56f
   female 57f
   fever 172
   larva 56, 56f
   male 56, 56f
Sanitary landfill, controlled 41
Sanitary latrines 44

Sanitary well, criteria for 27
Sanitation 6
   control 55
Saquinavir 180
Sarcoma 205
Sarcoptes scabiei 60
Sarpagandha 373
Saturated fatty acids 74
Save children fund 344
Save lives 439
Schick results 155
Schick test 155
Schizophrenia 273-275
School education 251
School health 250
   administration 253, 253f
School immunization 251
Screening test 124, 125
   and diagnostic test, difference between 125, 125t
Scrub typhus 172
Security cause 223
Selenium 75
Self-medication 374
Sensitivity, precision of 97
Sentinel surveillance 7
Septic tank 45, 45f
Septicemic plague 194
Serological epidemiology 111
Serum glutamic
   oxaloacetic transaminase 131
   pyruvic transaminase 131
Severe acute respiratory syndrome 143-145
   epidemiology of 144f
Sewage farming 47
Sex attitude, learning of 252
Sex chromosomes 270
Sex education 251
Sex emotion 252
Sex ratio, declining 223
Sex-linked disorders 270
Sex-linked genetic expressions 271f
Sexually transmitted disease 173, 174, 177, 245, 295, 297, 300
   causative agents of 174
   control of 233
   epidemiological triad in 173f

Sexually transmitted infections 230
Shallow springs 27
Shallow trench latrine 46, 46f
Shivaraman committee 312
Shoulder pain 262
Sickness
　absenteeism 261
　benefit 263
Siddha 361
Silicosis 259
Simple bar diagram 102f
Single vaccines preferred 156
Skin
　diseases 245
　infection 235, 250
　rash 251
　to skin contact 408
Sleeplessness 374
Sling psychrometer 39
Slow sand filter 31, 31f
Small bite big threat 441
Small-for-date babies 247
Smoking 8
Social
　agencies 21
　agents 260
　anatomy 15
　and behavioral to health and disease, relationship of 13
　assistance 23
　causes 222
　classification 17, 17t
　defense 14, 23
　disease 14
　factors 16, 243
　insurance 14, 23
　mobility 221
　obstetrics 15
　participation 19
　pathology 15
　pediatrics 15
　physiology 15
　problems 15
　product 424
　reforms, role in 340
　rehabilitation 10
　science 13
　therapy 15
Social marketing 424
　advantages of 425
　process of 424
Social medicine 6

special terms in 14
Social security 14, 23
　and health care 22
　comprehensive 23
　legislative support for 23
Social welfare
　measures 267
　schemes 247
Socioeconomic
　indicators 11
　programs 20
Sociometric analysis 425
Sodium 75
Soft ticks 59, 60, 60f
Sound pressure level 258
Soybean 76
Special group
　balanced diet allowance 79
　requirement of 79
Special sense impairment 266
Species 60
Specific protection 9
Sperm
　intrafallopian transfer 354
　intraovarian transfer 354
Spondylitis 266
Springs 27
Sputum
　negative 148
　positive 148
Squint 398
Staff development 314
Standard urban area 20
Staphylococcal food poisoning 138
State Public Health Act 364
Statistics
　scope of 101
　sources of 101
Stavudine 179, 180
Stenosis 213
Stillbirth rate 240
Strain injury, repetitive 262
Street virus 191
Stroke 213
　types of 213
Student's T test 106
Subcenter drug kits 298
Subcutaneous nodule 214
Substance abuse 425
　causes of 425
Substance dependence 276
Sudden death 208

Sudden infant death syndrome 383
Sulabh Shauchalaya 425
Sulfadoxine 423
Sunstroke 39
Supervision and leadership quality 317
Surface water 26
Surrogate motherhood 354
Surveillance 113
　flowchart 382f
　function 33
Survey education training unit 190
Sushruta Samhita 356
Swimming pool sanitation 33
Swollen face 251
Syndrome approach 301, 389
Syphilis 173, 174
Systems analysis 316

T

Taenia
　saginata 87
　solium 87
Tapeworm 88
Target couple 224t
Technological cause 222
Teeth
　care of 397
　loss of 397
Temperature 258
　causes, low 258
Temporary hardness 27
Tendinitis 258
Tenosynovitis 258
Tension neck syndrome 258
Terminal care 356
Tertian fever 422
Testicular feminization 270
Tetanus 122, 182, 233, 260, 431
　epidemiological triad in 183f
　neonatal 182, 183
　postinjury 183
　toxoid 233, 297, 417, 446
Thalassemia 355
Thalidomide 241
Thermal springs 27
Thiacetazone 150
Thiamine 75, 77
Thoracic outlet syndrome 258
Threatened abortion 446

Three-tier health system 320
Ticks 49, 59
Tiny liposome 355
Tissue cultured measles vaccine 154
Tobacco chewing and oral cancer 106
Tobacosis 259
Toga virus family 157
Tolerable daily intake 29
Toxemia 235, 446
Toxicokinetics 259
Toxin 85
   source of 138
   type 83
Toxoid 121
Toxoplasmosis 175, 241
Trachoma 189, 398
   epidemiological triad in 190f
Traditional birth attendance 229, 408
Trained nurses association 341
Transgenesis 269
Transient ischemic attack 211, 213
Transovarian transmission 193f
Trap 44f
Trauma, occupational 258
Trench fever 173
Trench method tipping 42f
Triage 281
Tribal health 433
Trichinella spiralis 87
Trichomonas vaginalis 174
Trimethoprim 369, 404
Trombicula
   akamushi 60
   deliensis 60
Tropical eosinophilia 97
Tsetse fly 57
Tube well 27
Tuberculin test 148, 149
Tuberculoid 184
Tuberculosis 114, 147, 149, 151, 175, 178, 238, 245, 329, 390, 418, 447
   association 340
   concepts in 148
   control of 148
   epidemiological triad in 148f
   strategies 420
Tumor markers 208
Twins 446

Typhoid 142
   conjugate vaccine 431, 432
   epidemiological triad in 143f
   immunization 432
   transmission, dynamics of 142f
   vaccine 432
Typhus 172

U

Ulcerative colitis 276
Ultrasound machine, sale of 428
Ultraviolet rays 29
Unani 361
Uncinariasis 139
Under-five clinics, functions of 242f
Under-five mortality rate 241
Unhygienic practice 398
Unimodal distribution 125, 126f
United Nations Development Programme 337
United Nations Fund for Population Activities 337
United Nations International Children's Emergency Fund 336
Universal access and human rights 386, 387
Universal Health Coverage 443
Universal Immunization Program 230, 233, 295, 299, 329, 330
Upper respiratory tract infection 114
Urban agglomeration 20
Urban community 20
Urban health 347, 350
   history of 348
   problems 348
   process of 348
Urban life, process of 348, 349f
Urban malaria 161
   control scheme 305
Urban population, growth of 347
Urban revamping scheme 350
Urban water supply programme 306
Urethral discharge 174, 389
Urinary infection 262

V

Vaccination, catch-up 154
Vaccine 121, 142, 159, 160, 166, 188, 192, 197, 198, 393
   attenuated 121, 122
   carrier 300
   development cycle 402
   newer 159
   pentavalent 432
   reaction 383
   treatment 391
   ventures 402
   vial monitor 238f
Vaginal discharge 174, 389
Vaginal sponge 227
Vancomycin 150
Vancouver style 100
Variability, measures of 104
Varicella 157
Varicella-zoster immune globulin 157
Vector bionomics 161
Vector transmission 120
Vector-borne
   diseases 49, 441
   infections 160
Vegetable milk 76
Vehicular accidents 215
Velvet mites 60
Ventilation 35, 262
   cross 35
   mechanical 35
   natural 35
   standards of 35f
Vertical Health Program 295, 295t
Vibration 258
Vibrio
   cholera 135
   infection 88
Village health guide 229
Village panchayat 327
Viral hepatitis 130
Virological examination 29
Virus 129
   coat protein 396
Vision 423
   defect 251
   impairment 258
Visual aid 68
Vital statistics 77, 92
   sources of 101

Vitamin 75, 76
  A 73, 75, 76, 236
    prophylaxis 234, 238, 298, 398
  A deficiency 81, 81*f*, 238
    treatment schedule 81
  B 73
  B12 75, 76, 77
  B6 75
  C 73, 75-77, 244
  D 73, 75, 244
  E 73, 75
  effect 75
    and requirements of 75
  K 73, 75, 76
  requirements of 75
Vocational rehabilitation 10
Voluntary health
  agencies 330
  association 341
Voluntary health organization 339
  functions of 340
  role of 339
Vomiting 258
von Gierke's disease 270
Vulnerability reduction
  horizontal integration of 283*f*
  vertical integration of 283*f*

W

Waste
  disposal 41
  disposal container code 288
  general 290*f*
  genotoxic 288
  hazardous 287
  infected sharp 407
  infectious 288
  liquid 42
  noninfective 407
  pathological 288
  pharmaceutical 288
  radioactive 288
  solid 41

Water
  and other components 25
  carriage system 43*f*
  current access of 34
  disease 28
  for domestic purposes, purification of 29
  hardness of 27
  source of 26*f*
  underground 26
Water pollution 27
  chemical indicators of 29
  law 34
Water sampling 32, 33
  time limit of 33
Water seal latrine 45
  direct type 46*f*
  indirect type 44*f*
Waterborne diseases 28
  etiology of 28
Wealth, loss of 9
Weaning and supplementation 246
  age-related guidelines for 246
Weaning foods, desirable qualities of 246
Weil's disease 28
Weil-Felix reaction 172
Well
  deep 26
  disinfection 30
  mentally 275
  shallow 26
  types of 26
West Nile fever 171, 172
Wheezing 413
White plague 204
  source of 204*t*
Whooping cough 156
  epidemiological triad in 156*f*
Widow marriage 10
Wild plague 194
Women and children in rural areas, development of 20
Women empowerment 406

Women's hygiene kit 443
Woolsorter's disease 199
Work and mental health 261
World Bank 337
World Disaster Reduction Day 282
World Health Assembly Proclamation 354
World Health Organization 231, 335, 436
Wound
  classification 192
  treatment strategy 183
Wrist pain 262
Wuchereria bancrofti 168

X

Xenodiagnosis 169
Xenopsylla
  astia 58
  brasiliensis 58
  cheopis 58
Xerophthalmia 398
XYY chromosomes 242

Y

Yate's correction 106
Yaws 175
  epidemiological triad in 175*f*
Yellow fever 197, 198
  epidemiological triad in 197*f*
Yoga 361

Z

Zalcitabine 179, 180
Zidovudine 179, 180
Zika viral infection 173, 444
Zinc 75
Zoonoses 64, 112
Zoonotic disease 112
Zoonotic infections 191